Equine Clinical Pharmacology

For Saunders:

Commissioning Editor: **Joyce Rodenhuis**
Senior Development Editor: **Zoë A Youd**
Project Manager: **Samantha Ross**
Designer: **Andrew Chapman**

Equine Clinical Pharmacology

Edited by

Joseph J. Bertone DVM MS Diplomate ACVIM
Professor of Equine Medicine, Western University of Health Sciences, Pomona, USA

Linda J. I. Horspool BVMS PhD Diplomate ECVPT MRCVS
Technical Manager Companion Animals, Intervet International, Boxmeer, The Netherlands

SAUNDERS

EDINBURGH   LONDON   NEW YORK   OXFORD   PHILADELPHIA   ST LOUIS   SYDNEY   TORONTO   2004

SAUNDERS
An imprint of Elsevier Limited

First published 2004

ISBN 0 7020 2484 8

British Library Cataloguing in Publication Data
A catalogue record for this book is available from the British Library

Library of Congress Cataloguing in Publication Data
A catalogue record for this book is available from the Library of Congress

Note
Medical knowledge is constantly changing. Standard safety precautions
must be followed, but as new research and clinical experience broaden our
knowledge, changes in treatment and drug therapy may become necessary
or appropriate. Readers are advised to check the most current product
information provided by the manufacturer of each drug to be administered
to verify the recommended dose, the method and duration of administration,
and contraindications. It is the responsibility of the practitioner, relying on
experience and knowledge of the patient, to determine dosages and the
best treatment for each individual patient. Neither the Publisher nor the
editors assume any liability for any injury and/or damage to persons or
property arising from this publication.

The Publisher

ELSEVIER   your source for books,
            journals and multimedia
            in the health sciences
www.elsevierhealth.com

Working together to grow
libraries in developing countries

www.elsevier.com | www.bookaid.org | www.sabre.org

ELSEVIER   BOOK AID   Sabre Foundation
            International

Transferred to digital print 2008
Printed and bound by CPI Antony Rowe, Eastbourne

The
Publisher's
policy is to use
**paper manufactured
from sustainable forests**

Contents

List of contributors vi
Preface vii
Acknowledgements viii

1 **Basic principles of veterinary pharmacology for equine practitioners 1**
Joseph J. Bertone

2 **Antimicrobial therapy 13**
Patricia M. Dowling

3 **Antiprotozoal drugs 49**
Clara K. Fenger

4 **Parasiticides 63**
Sandy Love and Robert M. Christley

5 **Drugs acting on the endocrine system 75**
Janice E. Sojka, Michel Levy and Laurent Couetil

6 **Drugs acting on the gastrointestinal system 85**
Michael J. Murray

7 **Intraarticular medication 121**
Tom Yarbrough

8 **Drugs affecting skeletal muscle 135**
Jennifer M. MacLeay

9 **Drugs acting on the neurological system and behavior modification 145**
Patricia M. Dowling

10 **Drugs acting on the urinary system 155**
Harold C. Schott II

11 **Drugs acting on the reproductive system 177**
Sally Vivrette

12 **Drugs acting on the cardiovascular system 193**
I. Mark Bowen, Celia M. Marr and Jonathan Elliott

13 **Ophthalmic therapeutics 217**
Andrew Matthews

14 **Non-steroidal anti-inflammatory drugs 247**
Cynthia Kollias-Baker and Karina Cox

15 **Anesthetics, tranquillizers and opioid analgesics 267**
Diane E. Mason

16 **Inhalation therapy for the respiratory system 311**
Bonnie R. Rush

17 **Fluid therapy 327**
Kevin T. T. Corley

Appendix Drugs and dosages for use in equines **365**

Index 381

Contributors

Joseph J. Bertone DVM MS Diplomate ACVIM
Professor of Equine Medicine, Western University of Health Sciences, Pomona, CA, USA

I. Mark Bowen BvetMed Cert VA Cert EM (IntMed) MRCVS
Royal Veterinary College, University of London, UK

Robert M. Christley BVSc PhD Dipl VCS MVCS Diplomate ECVPH MRVCS
Department of Veterinary Clinical Science,
University of Liverpool, Neston, South Wirral, UK

Kevin T. T. Corley BSc BVM&S MS PhD Diplomate ACVIM & ACVECC MRCVS
Royal Veterinary College, University of London, UK

Laurent Couetil DVM Diplomate ACVIM
Purdue University, School of Veterinary Medicine,
West Lafayette, IN, USA

Karina Cox BS
KL Maddy Equine Analytical Chemistry Laboratory,
School of Veterinary Medicine, University of California,
Davis, USA

Patricia M. Dowling DVM MS Diplomate ACVIM & ACVCP
Department of Veterinary Biomedical Sciences
Western College of Veterinary Medicine,
Saskatoon, Canada

Jonathan Elliott MA VetMB PhD Cert SAC Diplomate ECVPT MRCVS
Royal Veterinary College, University of London, UK

Clara K. Fenger DVM PhD Diplomate ACVIM
Equine Internal Medicine Consulting, Georgetown, KY, USA

Linda J. I. Horspool BVMS PhD DipECVPT MRCVS
Intervet International, Boxmeer, Netherlands

Cynthia Kollias-Baker DVM PhD Diplomate ACVCP
Racing Laboratory, College of Veterinary Medicine,
University of Florida, Gainesville, USA

Michel Levy DVM Diplomate ACVIM
Purdue University, School of Veterinary Medicine,
West Lafayette, IN, USA

Sandy Love BVMS PhD MRCVS
Department of Veterinary Clinical Studies,
University of Glasgow, UK

Jennifer M. MacLeay DVM PhD Diplomate ACVIM
Department of Clinical Sciences, Colorado State University,
Fort Collins, CO, USA

Celia M. Marr BVMS MVM PhD DEIM Diplomate ECEIM MRCVS
Beaufort Cottage, Equine Hospital, Newmarket, UK

Diane E. Mason DVM MS PhD Diplomate ACVA
Department of Clinical Sciences, Kansas State University,
Manhattan, USA

Andrew Matthews BVM&S PhD FRCVS
McKenzie, Bryson and Marshall, Kilmarnock, UK

Michael J. Murray DVM MS Diplomate ACVIM
Merial Ltd, Duluth, GA, USA

Bonnie R. Rush DVM MS Diplomate ACVIM
Department of Clinical Science, Kansas State University,
Manhattan, USA

Harold C. Schott II DVM PhD Diplomate ACVIM
Department of Large Animal Clinical Sciences,
Veterinary Medical Center, Michigan State University,
East Lansing, USA

Janice E. Sojka VMD MS Diplomate ACVIM
Purdue University, School of Veterinary Medicine,
West Lafayette, IN, USA

Sally Vivrette DVM PhD Diplomate ACVIM
Triangle Equine Mobile Veterinary Services, Cary, NC, USA

Tom Yarbrough DVM Diplomate ACVS
School of Veterinary Medicine, University of
California, Davis, USA

Preface

Equine clinical pharmacology is by definition 'the study of drugs in equine clinical cases'. Rational drug therapy, founded on pharmacological principles, requires a medical diagnosis. In fact, without this diagnosis and an understanding of the relevant pathophysiology, knowledge of pharmacologic principles and specific therapeutic objectives, one cannot rationally prescribe drug therapy.

This first edition of *Equine Clinical Pharmacology* brings together many of the topics pertinent to daily practice for equine veterinarians. This book has a number of goals. It aims to provide both veterinarians and veterinary students with a source of current information about the rational use of drugs, including best practice principles, in the treatment of specific diseases in the horse. Secondly, it aims to provide an incentive for adopting a rational approach to drug therapy in clinical cases and in addition to stimulating sustained interest in the conducting of controlled studies of the safety and efficacy of drugs in diseased horses.

This book has been organized mainly around bodily systems, since many clinical problems in horses are related to disorders of one or more of these systems. The editors have made an effort to include information on pathophysiology and the dosage, best practice guidelines, precautions and potential adverse effects of the drugs discussed. It is hoped that this information will help the reader in making risk/benefit assessments and in determining the therapeutic objectives for each equine treated.

The contributors to this volume, recognized experts in their specialties, were selected on the basis of their particular research and/or clinical specialization and expertise. Their recommendations for drug therapy are based on studies reported in veterinary medical literature, where possible, and on their own personal experience. The medications described do not necessarily have specific approval from the European Medicines Evaluation Agency, Food and Drugs Administration or other similar agencies, for the treatment of the diseases for which they are recommended. Whilst every effort has been made to include the most up-to-date recommendations, information about drug dose rates and dosage forms is constantly changing. The dose rates given should generally be considered as averages or starting points and thus require individualization. Similarly, new drugs that were not approved at the time of publication may appear on the market and other drugs or dosage forms may no longer be available.

This book could not be all-inclusive. It is hoped, however, that it will stimulate the continuation of interest and studies in equine clinical pharmacology and help better arm the equine veterinarian for the therapeutic decisions they make on a daily basis.

Joseph J. Bertone
Linda J.I. Horspool

Acknowledgements

This 1st Edition of *Equine Clinical Pharmacology* would not have been possible without the generous support and contributions of many people. The contributors, selected because each is recognized as among the most accomplished in their respective disciplines, provided up-to-date chapters discussing both modern trends and best practice principles and managed to adhere to sometimes apparently impossible deadlines. This work would of course not exist without the excellent and well focused contributions of: Mark Bowen, Rob Christley, Kevin Corley, Laurent Couetil, Karina Cox, Patricia Dowling, Jonathan Elliott, Clara Fenger, Cindy Kollias-Baker, Michael Levy, Sandy Love, Diane Mason, Andy Matthews, Celia Marr, Michael Murray, Jen MacLeay, Bonnie Rush, Harold Schott II, Janice Sojka, Sally Vivrette and Tom Yarbrough. A special thank you also to Michele Doucet and Jill Price for critiquing chapters of the manuscript for technical content and for providing many beneficial suggestions. The manuscript was greatly enhanced by their thoughtful attentions. Thanks also to Joyce Rodenhuis, Samantha Ross and Zoë Youd at Elsevier Limited for their guidance and support particularly during the final stages of preparation of the manuscript and for their encouragement in getting this project back on track.

Joseph J Bertone would like to dedicate this work to Mel and the children, Tina and Carmine, and to his parents Tina and John.

Linda Horspool would like to express her heartfelt thanks to her parents Bill and Una Horspool for their continued encouragement and support and to Marco Franken and his family, Wily, Patricia and Frank Franken, Kim Konings, and Francis and Lola Kuenen, for their patience and understanding. She dedicates this work to the memory of Tonny Franken-Franssen.

CHAPTER CONTENTS

Introduction 1

Physicochemical factors in drug
transfer across membranes 2

Absorption 2
  Drug administration 3

Distribution 4

Biotransformation 5

Elimination 6
  Urinary excretion 6
  Gastrointestinal excretion 6
  Excretion in milk 6

Pharmacokinetics 7
  Clearance 7
  Half-life 7
  Mean residence time 8
  Volumes of distribution 8
  Bioavailability 10

Other clinically relevant concepts 10
  The loading dose 10
  Maximum plasma concentration 10

References 10

Suggested reading 11

1

Basic principles of veterinary pharmacology for equine practitioners

Joseph J. Bertone

INTRODUCTION

Unfortunately, drugs do not distribute in living organisms as though injected into balloons filled with fluid. The study of how drugs react in living tissues and organisms is pharmacology. The science of pharmacology includes many different fields. The relationship between the dose of a drug given to an animal and the use of that drug in treating diseases is pharmacokinetics; what the body does to a drug and what a drug does in the body is pharmacodynamics, and whether it is desirable or undesirable is toxicology.

Pharmacokinetics is the study of absorption, distribution, biotransformation (metabolism) and excretion of drugs. The end result is determined by the physical, chemical and biochemical principles that govern the transfer and distribution of drugs across biological membranes. These factors and the dosage (route, dose and frequency) determine the drug concentration at the site of action and the intensity of a drug's effects as a function of time. Pharmacodynamics is the study of the mechanisms of action of drugs and their biochemical and physiological effects. Toxicology is the field of pharmacology that deals with the adverse effects of drugs used in therapy and of other non-drug chemicals.

A drug's usefulness as a therapeutic agent is critically dependent on its ability to produce desirable effects and a tolerable level of undesirable effects. Therefore, the selectivity of a drug's effects is one of its most important characteristics. Drug therapy is based on the correlation of the effects of drugs with the physiological, biochemical,

1

microbiological and/or immunological aspects of the disease in question. Disease may modify the pharmacokinetic properties of drugs by altering absorption into the systemic circulation and drug disposition (distribution, metabolism and elimination). In addition, sufficient concentrations of a drug must be present at its sites of action in order to produce its characteristic effects. Clearly this depends on the concentrations produced in the milieu around the cells in question, which is a function of dosage, the extent and rates of absorption, distribution, biotransformation and excretion, and the rate of transfer of the drug across biological membranes.

PHYSICOCHEMICAL FACTORS IN DRUG TRANSFER ACROSS MEMBRANES

Drugs are transported in the aqueous phase of blood plasma. To have an effect, drugs must enter cells or reach cell membrane receptors. All aspects of the absorption, distribution, biotransformation and elimination of drugs involve transfer across cell membranes. Other barriers, including multiple layers of cells (e.g. the intestinal epithelium or epidermis), also exist.

Biological membranes are essentially lipid; consequently, the rate at which drug molecules cross these barriers is dictated primarily by their lipid solubility. Molecular size and shape and the solubility at the site of absorption also directly affect the absorption of drugs. The other important factor that determines the ability of a drug to cross these biological barriers is the degree of ionization.

Most drugs are weak acids or bases and are present in solution as both the ionized and unionized forms. Ionized molecules are usually unable to penetrate lipid cell membranes because they are hydrophilic and poorly lipid soluble. Unionized molecules are usually lipid soluble and can diffuse across cell membranes. "Like is unionized in like", meaning that a weak acid will be most unionized in a fluid with an acidic pH and a weak base will be most unionized in a fluid with a basic pH. Under most circumstances, the

transmembrane distribution of a weak acid or base is determined by its acidic dissociation constant (pK_a) and by the pH gradient across the membrane. The proportions of drug in each state are calculated using the Henderson–Hasselbach equation. For a weak acid:

$$pH = pK_a + \log(A^-/HA)$$

where A^- is the ionized drug and HA the unionized drug. For a weak base:

$$pH = pK_a + \log(B/HB^+)$$

where B is the unionized drug and HB^+ is the ionized drug. Therefore, when the local pH is equal to the pK_a of a drug, the drug will be 50% ionized and 50% unionized ($\log 1 = 0$). There is further information on this area in the suggested reading.

Passive diffusion across cell membranes dominates the absorption and distribution of most drugs. Drugs enter cells down concentration gradients. This transfer is directly proportional to the magnitude of the concentration gradient across the membrane and to the oil to water partition coefficient of the drug (lipid solubility). Therefore, diffusion is fastest when there is a large partition coefficient and large concentration gradient across the membrane. For ionized compounds, the equilibrium concentrations are dependent on the differences in pH across the membrane and the pK_a of the drug. For unionized compounds, once the equilibrium is reached, the concentration of free drug is the same on both sides of the membrane.

Active, selective mechanisms play an important role in the absorption of some drugs. Energy is used to move drugs across membranes, often against the concentration gradient. There is active transport of some drugs in the kidneys (tubular cells), liver and nervous system. Facilitated diffusion is a carrier-mediated transport process that requires no input of energy and that does not occur against an electrochemical gradient.

ABSORPTION

Absorption is the rate and extent to which a drug leaves its site of administration. Many variables affect the transport of drugs across membranes and hence influence the absorption of drugs. Absorption is dependent on drug solubility. Drugs given in aqueous solution are absorbed more rapidly than those given in lipid solutions because they mix more readily with the aqueous phase at the absorption site. Drugs in solid form must first dissolve, and this may be the limiting factor in absorption.

Bioavailability indicates the extent to which a drug enters the systemic circulation. Factors that modify the absorption of a drug can change its bioavailability. A drug that is absorbed from the gastrointestinal tract enters the portal circulation and must first pass through the liver before it reaches the systemic circulation. Drugs that are not absorbed from the gastrointestinal tract, or are metabolized extensively in the liver and/or excreted in bile, will be inactivated or diverted before reaching the general circulation. If the metabolic or excretory capacity of the liver for a drug is excessive, the bioavailability of the drug will be substantially decreased (i.e. the first-pass effect). Reduced bioavailability not only is a function of the anatomical site of absorption but also is affected by many physiological and pathological factors. The choice of the route of drug administration is based on understanding these conditions. Table 1.1 lists common routes of drug administration.

DRUG ADMINISTRATION

Intravenous administration

Problems with absorption can be circumvented using intravenous (i.v.) administration of an aqueous solution of a drug. The desired concentration of a drug in blood is obtained with great accuracy and immediacy. The dosage can be titrated to effect, such as in the induction of anesthesia, where the drug dose is not predetermined but adjusted to the animal's response. In addition, irritant solutions can be given in this manner, since blood vessel walls are relatively insensitive to drug forms that are highly irritant when given by other routes. The major liability of intravenous administration is that adverse reactions are more likely to occur since high concentrations of drug are reached rapidly both in plasma and tissues. Repeated intravenous injections require an intact vein or, often, catheter placement.

Table 1.1 Common routes of drug administration and their characteristics

Route	Absorption	Use	Precautions
Intravenous	None (directly into the circulation); potentially immediate effects	Emergency use or large volumes; Absorption is bypassed	Increased risk of adverse effects; inject solutions slowly Not suitable for most lipid solutions or insoluble substances
Subcutaneous	Rapid if an aqueous solution; less rapid if depot formulations	Some less-soluble suspensions and implantation of solid pellets or depot forms	Not suitable for large volumes; irritant substances cause pain and/or necrosis
Intramuscular	Rapid if an aqueous solution; less rapid if depot forms	Moderate volumes; lipid vehicles; irritant drugs	Inadvertent intravenous injection; pain or necrosis at injection site
Oral	Rate and extent are highly variable and dependent on many factors	Maximize compliance (convenient); economical; usually safe	Absorption (bioavailability) may be erratic and incomplete
Pulmonary	Rapid; local application for pulmonary disease	Usually for the treatment of pulmonary disease	Irritant substances must be avoided; rapid absorption may induce high plasma concentrations and adverse effects

Intramuscular administration

Drugs in aqueous solution are absorbed rapidly following intramuscular (i.m.) injection, although this varies depending on factors such as the blood flow to the injection site. In humans, absorption from the deltoid or vastus lateralis muscles is faster than from the gluteus maximus. Absorption from this site is slower in females than in males. This has been attributed to sex differences in the distribution of subcutaneous fat, since fat is a relatively poorly perfused tissue.

Subcutaneous administration

Non-irritant drugs can be administered by subcutaneous (s.c.) injection. The rate of absorption may be sufficiently constant and slow to provide a sustained effect.

Oral administration

Absorption from the gastrointestinal tract is governed by a number of factors, such as the physical state of the drug, the surface area for absorption, blood flow to the absorption site and the drug concentration at the absorption site. Most drug absorption is by passive diffusion; consequently, absorption from the gastrointestinal tract is favored when a drug is in its unionized, more lipophilic form. In general, the absorption of weak acids is optimal from the acidic environment of the stomach whereas the relatively alkaline environment of the small intestine facilitates the absorption of weak bases. This is, of course, an oversimplification.

Pulmonary administration

Drugs may be administered directly into the respiratory tract for activity on, or through, the pulmonary epithelium and mucous membranes. Access to the systemic circulation is relatively enhanced and rapid following administration by this route because the pulmonary surface area is large. A drug solution can be administered as an aerosol that is inhaled. The advantage of this route of administration is the almost instantaneous absorption of drugs into the bloodstream, avoidance of the hepatic first-pass effect and local (topical) application of the drug in the case of pulmonary disease.

Topical application

Drugs are applied topically primarily for local effects; however, this route can be used to administer drugs for systemic action. Few drugs readily penetrate intact skin. The absorption of drugs that do penetrate the skin is proportional to the surface area over which they are applied and to their lipid solubility. Increased cutaneous blood flow also enhances absorption. Systemic toxicity can become evident when highly lipid-soluble substances (e.g. lipid-soluble insecticides) are absorbed through the skin. Controlled-release patches are now commonly used in human medicine for transcutaneous drug administration.

Other routes of administration

Intraarticular administration, local infiltration and ocular administration are useful in equine medicine and are covered in Chapters 7, 15, and 13, respectively.

The intraarterial, intrathecal and intraperitoneal routes are used only rarely in equine medicine.

DISTRIBUTION

Once a drug is absorbed, it distributes to many tissues, including its sites of action. The pattern of drug distribution reflects the physiological and physicochemical properties of the drug. The initial phase of distribution often reflects cardiac output and regional blood flow. The drug is delivered to the heart, liver, kidney, brain and other well-perfused organs during the first few minutes after absorption. The second much slower phase of drug distribution involves delivery of the drug to skeletal muscle, other viscera, skin and fat. These tissues may require several minutes to several hours before steady-state concentrations are reached.

Distribution can be limited by binding of drugs to plasma proteins, particularly albumin, for acidic drugs and α_1-acid glycoprotein for basic drugs. Protein-bound drug is too large to pass through biological membranes; drug that is extensively protein bound will have limited access to intracellular sites of action (Martinez 1998a). Bound and free drug are in equilibrium on either side of membranes and free (unionized) drug is in equilibrium across cell membranes. The ability of a bound drug to contribute to these equilibriums is determined by the strength of its adherence to the protein moiety.

Protein-bound drugs may be metabolized and eliminated more slowly than expected. They may also accumulate in tissues in greater concentrations than would be expected from their physicochemical properties because of intracellular binding, partitioning into lipid and ion trapping (pH partitioning). This may provide a reservoir that prolongs drug action. Protein binding also limits the glomerular filtration of a drug. However, it does not generally limit renal tubular secretion or biotransformation, since these processes lower the free drug concentration in plasma, which rapidly causes dissociation of the drug–protein complex and increases the total unbound fraction.

The degree of protein binding is only clinically significant for those drugs that are more than 90% protein bound. For these drugs, conditions that decrease plasma protein concentrations, such as liver and kidney disease, will cause significant increases in the amount of free drug available for pharmacological actions. Protein binding may also be involved in drug interactions. If a highly protein-bound drug is coadministered with a drug that uses the same protein-binding site, it can displace the first drug from the plasma protein and thus increase the amount of the first drug available for pharmacological action. The classical example of this is the interaction between phenylbutazone and warfarin, where phenylbutazone displaces warfarin from the protein-binding site. Reducing the amount of protein-bound warfarin from 99% to 98% effectively doubles the plasma concentrations of free warfarin (which has anticoagulant activity) and can lead to bleeding problems.

Central nervous system

Entry of drugs into the cerebrospinal fluid (CSF) and extracellular space of the central nervous system (CNS) is relatively restricted. The endothelial cells of the CNS have tight junctions and do not have intercellular pores and pinocytotic vesicles.

Bone

Divalent metal ion chelating agents (e.g. tetracyclines) and heavy metals accumulate in bone by adsorption onto the bone-crystal surface and eventual incorporation into the crystal lattice.

Placental transfer

If drugs are transferred across the placenta, they may be potentially hazardous to the fetus. Drugs primarily cross the placenta by passive diffusion. Lipid-soluble, unionized drugs can enter the fetal bloodstream. The fetal bloodstream is protected from drugs that are relatively lipid insoluble and/or highly ionized in plasma. However, the fetus is, at least to some extent, exposed to essentially all drugs administered to the pregnant mare.

Transcellular compartments

Drugs may accumulate in the transcellular fluids. The major transcellular fluid compartment is in the gastrointestinal tract. Weak bases can enter the stomach from the circulation and concentrate. Drugs may also be secreted in bile either in an active form or as a conjugate that can be hydrolyzed in the intestines. Thus, the gastrointestinal tract can serve as a drug reservoir. Under normal circumstances, the CSF, aqueous humor, and joint fluids generally do not accumulate significant total quantities of drugs.

BIOTRANSFORMATION

Biotransformation detoxifies and/or removes foreign chemicals from the body and thus promotes survival. The main metabolic enzyme systems are located in the hepatic smooth endoplasmic reticulum. Some enzyme systems are also located in the kidneys, lungs and gastrointestinal epithelium. The first-pass effect (presystemic metabolism) can thus be a combination of gastrointestinal and hepatic enzyme systems. Biotransformation can also improve therapeutic activity by activating an inactive prodrug or by converting a drug to a more active metabolite (e.g. metabolic activation of ceftiofur to desfuroylceftiofur).

The chemical peculiarities of drug molecules that allow for their rapid passage across cellular membranes during absorption and distribution also delay elimination. The enzymatic biotransformation of drugs into more polar, less lipid-soluble (more water-soluble) metabolites promotes elimination. Conjugation of drugs further increases their water solubility and hence elimination. Horses tend to conjugate drugs to glucuronide (Dirikolu et al 2000, Harkins et al 2000).

ELIMINATION

Drugs are eliminated from the body either unchanged or after biotransformation (metabolites). The excretory organs tend to eliminate polar, less lipid-soluble compounds more efficiently than compounds with high lipid solubility.

The kidney is the most important organ for elimination of drugs and metabolites. Some substances are excreted via the gastrointestinal tract, for the most part drugs that were unabsorbed or metabolites excreted in the bile and not reabsorbed. Pulmonary excretion is important mainly for the elimination of anesthetic gases. The efficacy of some drugs may be partially dependent on excretion in the pulmonary secretions. Drugs are also excreted into milk, skin, sweat, saliva and tears but these routes are usually of minor importance. In lactating mares, excretion of drugs in milk may be significant and affect suckling foals. Elimination by the latter routes is via diffusion of the unionized lipid-soluble moiety through the gland epithelial cells and is pH dependent.

URINARY EXCRETION

Elimination of drugs and metabolites by the kidneys is by three mechanisms: glomerular filtration, active tubular secretion and passive tubular reabsorption. The amount of drug filtered through the glomeruli is dependent on the degree of plasma protein binding and the glomerular filtration rate. Organic anions and cations are added to the glomerular filtrate by active tubular secretion in the proximal tubule. Most organic acids (e.g. penicillin) and glucuronide metabolites are transported by the same system that is used for excretion of natural metabolites, such as uric acid. Organic bases are transported by a separate system that is designed to excrete bases such as choline and histamine. Both of these systems are relatively non-selective and may be bidirectional, with some drugs being both eliminated and reabsorbed. However, the main direction of transport is into the renal tubules for excretion. Clearly, the rate of passage into the renal tubules is dependent on the pK_a of the drug and its metabolites and on urine pH. As an example, increasing urine pH can produce a dramatic increase in excretion of acidic compounds such as salicylate.

GASTROINTESTINAL EXCRETION

Many metabolites produced by hepatic metabolism are eliminated into the intestinal tract via the bile. These metabolites may be excreted in feces but are often reabsorbed. Organic anions (i.e. glucuronides) and cations are actively transported into bile by carrier systems that are similar to those in the renal tubules. Similarly, charged ions can compete for transport by these systems because both are non-selective. Steroidal and related substances are transported by a third carrier mechanism. Glucuronide-conjugated metabolites undergo extensive enterohepatic recirculation— a cycle of absorption from the gastrointestinal tract, metabolism in the liver and excretion in bile—and this cycle delays elimination when the final step in elimination from the body is via the kidneys.

EXCRETION IN MILK

Suckling foals may potentially receive high doses of drug via milk. Normal milk is more acidic than plasma. Weak bases are highly unionized in plasma and the unionized drug fraction crosses readily into the mammary gland and then becomes "ion trapped" in the more acidic milk. Weak acids are highly ionized in plasma and, therefore, do not penetrate the mammary glands very well. These factors are used in the systemic treatment of mastitis but should be borne in mind when treating lactating mares with any therapeutic agent.

PHARMACOKINETICS

Clinical pharmacokinetics assumes that there is a relationship between the serum concentration versus time profile and the response to a drug. Drug concentration versus time data can be described using compartmental (model-dependent) or non-compartmental (model-independent) pharmacokinetics. The majority of publications use compartmental pharmacokinetics, where the models used to describe the drug concentration versus time data assume that drug in the central compartment (blood and rapidly equilibrating tissues) is distributed to one or more peripheral or tissue compartments and that drug is eliminated only from the central compartment. A graph of the plasma drug concentration (on a logarithmic scale) versus time (on a linear scale) following intravenous administration can be divided into a series of linear segments and can be described using mono-, bi- or triexponential equations, which reflect the number of compartments in the model. One-, two- and three-compartment models have been used to describe drug disposition in the horse. Some authors use the non-compartmental approach, which is based on statistical moment theory.

The three most important indices in pharmacokinetics are clearance (related to the rate of elimination), apparent volume of distribution (V_d: the volume into which a drug distributes in the body) and bioavailability (the fraction of a drug absorbed into the systemic circulation).

CLEARANCE

Clearance can be used to design an appropriate dosage regimen for long-term drug administration.

The total systemic clearance is the sum of clearance by all mechanisms (e.g. renal, hepatic, etc.). Clearance is defined as the volume of plasma that is completely depleted of drug per unit time to account for the rate of elimination. It is usually constant for a drug, within the desired clinical concentrations, but does not indicate how much drug is being removed.

$$\text{Clearance} = k_{el}/C_p$$

where k_{el} is the rate of elimination and C_p is the concentration in plasma. Excretion systems have a high ceiling and so are rarely saturated under clinical circumstances. The elimination rate is essentially a linear function of the drug concentration in plasma; elimination follows first-order kinetics. This means that there is a constant fraction of drug eliminated per unit time. This is why doubling the dose (e.g. of intravenous penicillin) does not reduce the need for frequent dosing. If elimination mechanisms become saturated, the kinetics follow a zero-order pattern and a constant quantity of drug is eliminated per unit of time. In this situation, clearance varies with time.

HALF-LIFE

The elimination or terminal half-life is the time needed for the drug concentration in plasma to decrease by 50%. For most drugs, the half-life remains constant for the duration of the drug dose in the body. The elimination half-life can be calculated following intravenous drug administration whereas the terminal half-life is calculated following drug administration via other routes (non-intravenous).

$$\text{Half-life} = 0.693/k_{el}$$

where 0.693 is the natural logarithm of 2. Terminal half-life is calculated using λ_n, the terminal slope of the concentration versus time profile for the nth compartment, in place of k_{el}.

Clinically, the half-life determines the inter-dosing interval, how long a pharmacological or toxic effect will persist and drug withdrawal times in food-producing animals and performance horses (Martinez 1998b). The plasma concentration of drug remaining at any given time ($C_p(t)$) can be calculated as:

$$C_p(t = 0)e^{-(0.693/t^{1/2})(t)}$$

where $C_p(t = 0)$ equals the plasma concentration of drug at time zero and t is the time interval. Table 1.2 shows the relationship between half-life and the amount of drug in the body. With each half-life, the amount of drug remaining reduces by 50%. Note it takes 10 half-lives to eliminate 99.9% of a drug from the body. Also recognize that doubling the dose of a drug (so that the table would start at 200%) does not double the withdrawal time but merely adds one additional half-life to reach the same concentration endpoint (Baggot 1992). Steady-state concentrations are reached after three to five half-lives have elapsed.

MEAN RESIDENCE TIME

The mean residence time is the equivalent of half-life and is the parameter calculated when non-compartmental methods are used to determine pharmacokinetic values. Some pharmacokinetic studies report mean residence time instead of half-life. The mean residence time is actually the time taken for the plasma drug concentration to decrease by 63.2% and should thus be somewhat greater than half-life.

Table 1.2 Relationship of the elimination half-life to the amount of drug in the body

Number of half-lives	Fraction of drug remaining (%)
0	100
1	50
2	25
3	12.5
4	6.25
5	3.125
6	1.56
7	0.78
8	0.39
9	0.195
10	0.0975

VOLUMES OF DISTRIBUTION

The V_d is used as an indication of a drug's ability to escape the vascular compartment. It is a mathematical term that describe the apparent volume in the body into which a drug is dissolved with units in milliliters or liters per kilogram (ml/kg or l/kg) (Riviere 1999). The apparent V_d values vary with the physical characteristics of the drug molecules, including ionization (pK_a), lipid solubility, molecular size and protein binding, that determine their ability to cross membranes (Martinez 1998a).

To understand the concept of V_d, think of the body as a beaker filled with fluid (Fig. 1.1), where the fluid represents the plasma and the other extracellular fluid (ECF). If the drug does not readily cross lipid membranes, it will be confined mainly to the ECF. If this drug is administered intravenously, it will distribute rapidly in the ECF, as represented by the stars in the beaker on the left. A sample taken from this beaker will have a high drug concentration. The higher the measured concentration in relation to the original dose, the lower the numerical value of V_d. Some drugs readily cross lipid membranes and distribute into tissues. This is represented by the beaker on the right, where the stars at the bottom of the beaker represent drug molecules that have

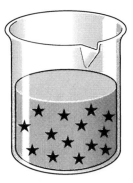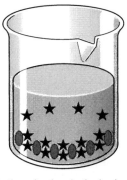

Figure 1.1 The volume of distribution of a drug in the body can be compared with the stars in the beakers. For a drug that stays confined to the vascular system (the fluid) in the beaker on the left, taking a sample will yield a high drug concentration. For a drug that leaves the vascular system and binds to tissues, as in the stars bound to the ovals in the beaker on the right, then sampling the fluid will yield a lower concentration.

been taken up by tissues. A sample taken from the fluid in this beaker will have a low drug concentration in proportion to the original dose and will have a high numerical value for V_d.

The three most important volume terms used in compartmental analysis are the volume of the central compartment (V_c), the volume of distribution based on elimination (V_d, or $V_d\beta$ or $V_d$area) and the volume of distribution at steady state ($V_d$ss). The numerical values of these terms differ slightly, but they all give an indication of a drug's ability to cross membranes. Although similar in magnitude, V_d is usually greater than $V_d$ss because the latter describes the volume that the drug occupies after equilibration has taken place, which is usually greater than V_c. The value of $V_d$ss and hence clearance and dose rate can also be calculated using non-compartmental methods.

The term V_c is the proportionality constant that relates the drug dose to the amount of drug measured in a blood/plasma sample (C_p).

For a one-compartment model, the distribution phase occurs rapidly compared with elimination:

$$V_c = \text{Dose}/C_p(t = 0)$$

In this model, the drug concentration in the blood or plasma is proportional to both the concentration in other tissues (e.g. muscle) and to the total amount of drug in the body. When the equilibration of a drug between the central and peripheral compartments occurs less rapidly, relative to elimination, then the disposition kinetics of the drug can be described by assuming that there are two (or sometimes more) distribution compartments. The apparent V_d varies with time after drug administration in these models because of the time required for equilibration between the compartments. Thus, for a two-compartment model, V_c is dose/(A + B), where A and B are the y intercepts (plasma concentrations at time 0) associated with the distribution and elimination phases, respectively.

$$V_d = \text{Dose}/(\beta.\text{AUC})$$

where β is the slope of the terminal phase and AUC is the area under the plasma concentration versus time curve from time 0 to infinity. The $V_d$ss is

quoted in most reference texts and is the value when the rate of drug entry from the bloodstream into the tissues is equal to its exit rate from the tissues back into the circulation. It is directly proportional to the tissue-binding affinity and the fraction of drug remaining unbound in the blood.

Adult animals are considered to be approximately 60% water; the total body water has a volume of 0.6 l/kg. The ECF compartment is approximately 30% of body weight and has a volume of 0.3 l/kg. Neonates are considered to have total body water closer to 80% and the additional 20% is found primarily in the ECF compartment. Geriatric animals tend to have reduced total body water primarily because of a reduction in ECF volume.

Compounds may be distributed and confined to the vascular space or may be distribute into intracellular and extracellular compartments. In the latter, $V_d$ss approximates the volume associated with total body water. Weakly lipid-soluble compounds (e.g. cephalosporins, aminoglycosides, penicillins) generally penetrate poorly into cells. Their natural distribution space tends to be extracellular and the value of $V_d$ss approximates extracellular fluid volume, about 30% of an animal's body weight (Baggot 1990). The value for gentamicin approximates 0.254 l/kg (Pedersoli et al 1980), which implies an ECF distribution, while that for metronidazole is 0.69 l/kg (Specht et al 1992). Highly lipophilic compounds are associated with large $V_d$ss values (e.g. propranolol is 3.9 l/kg). Therefore, a drug with V_d of 0.3 l/kg will be distributed primarily into the ECF, while a drug with a V_d of 3.4 l/kg will be distributed beyond the body water compartments and will achieve high concentrations in tissues yet relatively low concentrations in plasma. Some of these drugs (e.g. macrolides, fluoroquinolones) are sequestered within cells or have extensive tissue binding, reflected by estimates of $V_d$ss that exceed the volume of total body water (Atkinson et al 1996). If the value of V_d is greater than 1 l/kg, the drug concentration will be greater in tissues than in plasma (Evans 1992). While a large value for $V_d$ss suggests excellent extravascular distribution, it does not guarantee adequate active drug concentrations at the sites of action.

Drug doses are usually determined in normal, healthy adult animals and the V_d value is constant for any drug and only changes if there are physiological or pathological changes that alter drug distribution. Any condition that changes ECF volume will dramatically affect the plasma concentrations of drugs with low V_d values. Drugs with high V_d values normally distribute throughout the fluid and tissue compartments and so are not significantly affected by changes in body water status. ECF volume contraction and dehydration occur in conditions such as shock, colic and enteritis. Parasitism, heart failure and vasculitis can all cause edema and an increase in the ECF volume. Local changes in acid–base status can alter the ionization of drugs and affect their movement across membrane barriers. Conditions that alter the amount or affinity of plasma proteins will change the V_d value of highly protein-bound drugs.

BIOAVAILABILITY

Bioavailability is a measure of the extent of absorption. It is an indication of the amount of drug that is absorbed from the administration site. Drugs administered intravenously essentially have a bioavailability of 100%. Drugs administered orally will have variable bioavailability. The rate of absorption is clearly important because if the rate is very slow, the drug may not reach active concentrations before it is eliminated and if it is very rapid, unsafe plasma concentrations may be reached.

AUC is a frequency distribution of the number of molecules within the body versus time. When measured out to infinity (∞), the AUC value ($AUC_{0-\infty}$) represents the total drug exposure. Its value is unaffected by the rate of absorption (assuming linear kinetics) but is affected by dose, clearance and bioavailability. Bioavailability is calculated by comparing the total amount of drug in the body (AUC) following administration by a non-i.v. route with that obtained following i.v. administration (100%), corrected for dose.

$$\text{Bioavailability} = \frac{AUC_{\text{non-i.v.}} \times Dose_{\text{i.v.}}}{AUC_{\text{i.v.}} \times Dose_{\text{non-i.v.}}}$$

OTHER CLINICALLY RELEVANT CONCEPTS

THE LOADING DOSE

A loading dose is an initial dose of drug that is administered at a dose rate higher than that normally used. A loading dose is used when the time needed to reach steady-state concentrations (i.e. about three to five half-lives) is long relative to the need for treatment. It rapidly increases plasma concentrations so that steady-state concentrations are approached more rapidly.

MAXIMUM PLASMA CONCENTRATION

The maximum plasma concentration reflects the extent of drug bioavailability. It can be used in relation to minimum inhibitory concentration (MIC) to predict the efficacy of concentration-dependent antimicrobial agents (e.g. fluoroquinolones, aminoglycosides). Both the maximum (peak) and minimum (trough) plasma concentrations are used during therapeutic drug monitoring to maximize efficacy and minimize the occurrence of undesirable effects.

REFERENCES

Atkinson A J, Ruo T, Frederiksen M C 1996 Physiological basis of multicompartmental models of drug distribution. Trends in Pharmacological Sciences 12:96–101

Baggot J D 1990 Pharmacokinetic-pharmcodynamic relationship. Annals de Recherches Veterinaires 21(suppl):29–40

Baggot J D 1992 Bioavailability and bioequivalence of veterinary drug dosage forms, with particular reference to horses: an overview. Journal of Veterinary Pharmacology and Therapeutics 15:160–173

Dirikolu L, Lehner A F, Karpiesiuk W et al 2000 Identification of lidocaine and its metabolites in post-administration equine urine by ELISA and MS/MS. Journal of Veterinary Pharmacology and Therapeutics 23:215–222

Evans W E 1992 General principles of applied pharmacokinetics. In: Evans W E, Schentag J J, Jusko W J et al (eds) Applied pharmacokinetics, principles of therapeutic drug monitoring, 3rd edn. Applied Therapeutics Inc, Vancouver, pp. 1–8

Harkins J D, Karpiesiuk W, Tobin T et al 2000 Identification of hydroxyropivacaine glucuronide in equine urine by ESI+/MS/MS. Canadian Journal of Veterinary Research 64:178–183

Martinez M N 1998a Physicochemical properties of pharmaceuticals. Journal of the American Veterinary Medical Association 213:1274–1277

Martinez M N 1998b Volume, clearance and half-life. Journal of the American Veterinary Medical Association 213:1122–1127

Pedersoli W M, Belmonte A, Purohit R C et al 1980 Pharmacokinetics of gentamicin in the horse. American Journal of Veterinary Research 41:351–354

Riviere J E 1999 Comparative pharmacokinetics: principles, techniques and applications. Iowa State University Press, Ames, IA, pp. 47–61

Specht T E, Brown M P, Gronwall R R et al 1992 Pharmacokinetics of metronidazole and its concentration in body fluids and endometrial tissues of mares. American Journal of Veterinary Research 53:1807–1812

SUGGESTED READING

Gilman A G, Rall T W, Nies A S et al (eds) 1990 The pharmacological basis of therapeutics, 8th edn. Pergamon Press, New York

Rowland P E, Towser T N (eds) 1995 Clinical pharmacokinetics: concepts and applications. Lea and Febiger, Philadelphia, PA

CHAPTER CONTENTS

Rational use of antimicrobial agents   13

Documenting an infection   17

Dosage regimen design   18
  Inhibitory drug dosage   18
  Bacteriostatic versus bactericidal agents   19
  Antimicrobial drug concentration   20
  Calculating the drug dosage regimen   20
  Site of the infection   21
  Combination antimicrobial therapy   21
  Prophylactic use of antimicrobial drugs   22

Beta-lactam antibiotics   22
  Penicillin G (benzylpenicillin)   23
  Aminopenicillins: amoxicillin and ampicillin   24
  Extended-spectrum penicillins   25
  Cephalosporins   25
  Imipenem   28

Aminoglycoside antibiotics   28
  Streptomycin/dihydrostreptomycin   32
  Neomycin   32
  Gentamicin   32
  Amikacin   33
  Tobramycin   33

Chloramphenicol and florfenicol   33

Potentiated sulfonamides   35

Tetracyclines   38

Fluoroquinolones   40

Macrolides   43

Rifampin   44

Metronidazole   45

Vancomycin   45

References   46

2

Antimicrobial therapy

Patricia M. Dowling

RATIONAL USE OF ANTIMICROBIAL AGENTS

In recent years, there have been important changes in antimicrobial therapy. New antimicrobial agents have become available and there is a greater database of species-specific pharmacokinetic and pharmacodynamic information on the agents used in veterinary medicine. Concerns over drug residues in food-producing and performance animals and the continued development of bacterial resistance to antimicrobial agents have heightened the awareness of the rational use of these agents. By definition, antibiotics are natural products of microorganisms. The term antimicrobial agent is more encompassing as it includes synthetic drugs, such as the fluoroquinolones, and organic compounds, such as the sulfonamides.

The equine practitioner must consider several questions when developing an antimicrobial treatment regimen

- does the diagnosis warrant antimicrobial therapy?
- which organisms are likely to be involved?
- what is the *in-vitro* antimicrobial susceptibility of the pathogen?
- where is the infection located and is it accessible to the drug?
- will the agent be effective in the environment at the site?
- what formulation and treatment regimen will maintain the appropriate antimicrobial concentrations for sufficient time?

- what adverse reactions or toxicities might occur?
- is there a product suitable for horses?

Does the diagnosis warrant antimicrobial therapy?

Much of the use of antimicrobial agents is irrational. Antimicrobial therapy for superficial wounds and single doses of penicillin administered after the elective castration of normal horses has no real therapeutic benefit and encourages antimicrobial resistance.

Which organisms are likely to be involved?

For many equine infections, it is possible to predict which microorganisms will be involved. Traumatic wounds are usually contaminated with skin and fecal flora. Respiratory tract infections routinely involve *Streptococcus* (*Strep.*) species (spp.). Septic neonates routinely have positive blood cultures for *Escherichia coli* and other Gram-negative enteric bacteria.

What is the *in-vitro* antimicrobial susceptibility of the pathogen?

The antimicrobial susceptibility of many pathogens is very predictable (Prescott & Holgate 1993). For example, *Streptococcus* spp. and most anaerobes are usually susceptible to penicillin. However, pathogens such as Gram-negative enteric bacteria are very efficient at transmitting and acquiring resistance genes and, therefore, have unpredictable susceptibility patterns: susceptibility testing should always be carried out in order to choose effective therapy.

Where is the infection located and will the agent reach the site of infection?

Practitioners must consider the effects of physiology and pathology on the distribution of drugs in order to adjust dosages to achieve effective therapy. Many infections occur in sequestered areas of the body. For example, an abscess may be

walled off by a thick fibrous capsule. It is difficult for many drugs to reach therapeutic concentrations in the central nervous system (CNS), mammary glands and accessory sex glands because of specialized blood and tissue barriers.

Chapter 1 discussed the principles of drug pharmacokinetics; here the importance of volumes of distribution (V_d), drug ionization and protein binding are outlined for antimicrobial drugs.

Volumes of distribution

The V_d is a pharmacokinetic parameter that indicates the apparent distribution of a drug within the body (Riviere 1999). The relative value of V_d indicates how well a drug is going to distribute to the tissues. Antimicrobial agents can be categorized as having V_d values that are low (<0.3 l/kg, similar to the volume of the extracellular fluid (ECF)), medium (0.3–1 l/kg) and high (>1 l/kg, greater than the total body water volume) (Table 2.1 and the Appendix to this chapter).

Physiological or pathological changes in the V_d are very important in determining the dose rate of drugs that are predominantly confined to the ECF compartment. Foals have a total body water of 80%, whereas adult horses are 60% water. For a given dose of any drug with a low V_d, such as gentamicin, foals will have a lower plasma concentration than adult horses. Therefore, a higher dose must be given to foals to achieve the same *effective* plasma drug concentrations (Fig. 2.1). This is not intuitive; it is commonly thought that neonates should be given a lower dose than adult horses because of concerns about gentamicin

Table 2.1   Categories of antimicrobial agents based on their volume of distribution (V_d)

Volume of distribution (l/kg)		
Low (<0.3)	Medium (0.3–1)	High (>1)
Penicillins	Sulfonamides	Fluoroquinolones
Cephalosporins	Florfenicol	Trimethoprim
Aminoglycosides		Tetracyclines
		Macrolides
		Chloramphenicol
		Metronidazole
		Rifampin

nephrotoxicity. This can unfortunately lead to under-dosing and ineffective therapy.

Drug ionization

Changes in acid–base balance are very common in disease states. Antimicrobial drugs are weak acids or weak bases (Table 2.2, Appendix). Their lipid solubility depends greatly on their degree of ionization (charged state) (Martinez 1998a). An ionized drug is hydrophilic and poorly lipid soluble. A drug that is nonionized is lipophilic and can cross biological membranes. The degree of ionization of a weak acid or base depends on both the acidic dissociation constant (pK_a) of the drug and the pH of the surrounding fluid.

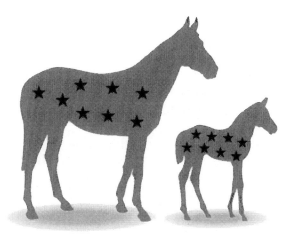

Figure 2.1 For a drug with a low volume of distribution, when the same dose is given to an adult horse and a foal, the increased extracellular fluid volume of the foal dilutes the drug, resulting in lower plasma concentrations. To achieve the same plasma concentrations, the foal must be given a higher dose than the adult horse.

Table 2.2 Classification of antimicrobial agents according to their dissociation constant (pK_a)

Acidic drugs	Basic drugs	Amphoteric drugs
Penicillins	Aminoglycosides	Fluoroquinolones
Cephalosporins	Macrolides	Tetracyclines
Sulfonamides	Chloramphenicol/ florfenicol	
	Trimethoprim	

Clinically, it is sufficient to remember that only nonionized drug crosses membranes readily and that "like is nonionized in like". This concept dictates the distribution of antimicrobial agents into sequestered infections. For example, mastitis is treated parenterally with antimicrobial agents that are weak bases (Fig. 2.2) because milk is more acidic than plasma. Weak bases are highly unionized (UI) in plasma and thus can cross readily into the mammary gland, where they become "ion trapped" in the more acidic environment of the mammary gland (milk). A new equilibrium is established between the ionized and unionized drug. Although smaller than the fraction in plasma, the unionized fraction in the milk can enter pathogenic bacteria and produce the desired antimicrobial action. By comparison, weak acids are highly ionized in plasma and, therefore, do not penetrate into the mammary gland very well. Successful therapy of mastitis using agents that are weak acids requires local (intramammary) infusion, as is routinely done in cattle, where the high local drug concentrations overcome any effects of drug ionization. Other sequestered infections such as abscesses, metritis and meningitis are also typically acidic compared with plasma; consequently,

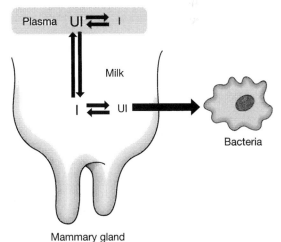

Figure 2.2 A weak base is not highly ionized in plasma and this fraction is available to cross the blood–mammary gland barrier and enter the milk. A new equilibrium is established between unionized (UI) and ionized (I) drug in the more acidic milk. The unionized fraction in milk is available to cross the cell wall of pathogenic bacteria to produce desired antimicrobial action.

parenteral therapy is most effective using basic antimicrobial agents.

Acidic antimicrobial agents are also drugs with low V_d values and most weak bases have high V_d values (Table 2.2). The exception to this rule is the aminoglycosides. The aminoglycosides are weak bases but are very large, hydrophilic molecules that are highly ionized at physiological pH and do not readily cross lipid membranes. Therefore, aminoglycosides that are administered parenterally do not achieve therapeutic concentrations in milk, abscesses or cerebrospinal fluid (CSF). Amphoteric drugs, such as the fluoroquinolones and tetracyclines, have both acidic and basic groups as part of their chemical structures. These drugs have a range of pH where they are maximally UI. For example, fluoroquinolones are most lipid soluble in the pH range 6–8 and so are lipid soluble in most situations. These drugs are significantly ionized in acidic urine, which reduces their antibacterial activity. However, the fluoroquinolones are primarily eliminated in urine, so any reduction in activity caused by low environmental pH is offset by the extremely high urine concentrations of these agents and is thus of no clinical importance. The fluoroquinolones and tetracyclines are highly UI at most physiological pH, so are similar to weak bases in that they have high V_d values.

Protein binding

Many drugs are bound to plasma proteins (mainly albumin) in the circulation, bound drug is too large to pass through biological membranes, so only a free drug is available for delivery to the tissues and to produce the desired pharmacological actions (Martinez 1998a). However, just like the relationship between ionized and UI drugs, free and bound drugs are in equilibrium.

The degree of protein binding is only clinically significant for those drugs that are more than 90% protein bound. The only antimicrobial agent that is significantly protein bound is ceftiofur. The efficacy of ceftiofur is attributed to its binding to acute-phase proteins, such as α_1-antitrypsin, which acts as a reservoir of the active drug and carries the bound drug to sites of inflammation,

where a new equilibrium is established between the free and bound drug. Because of its high degree of protein binding, ceftiofur does not readily cross into milk when administered parenterally, hence the "zero" milk withdrawal time in lactating dairy cattle. There is no interaction with other highly protein-bound drugs, such as phenylbutazone, since ceftiofur and phenylbutazone do not compete for the same protein-binding site.

Will the antimicrobial be effective in the infection site environment?

Even when the pharmacokinetic parameters of a drug are such to suggest that it will reach the site of the infection, local factors can influence its antimicrobial activity. Aminoglycosides are ineffective in hyperosmolar, anaerobic acidic environments, such as the purulent environment of abscesses. Sulfonamides act by replacing para-aminobenzoic acid (PABA) in the folic acid synthetic pathway of bacteria and are ineffective in purulent material and necrotic tissue, which provide alternative sources of PABA.

What drug formulation and treatment regimen will maintain appropriate antimicrobial concentrations for sufficient time?

The formulation of a drug influences its availability to the systemic circulation (Baggot 1992). Administration intravenously (i.v.) achieves the most rapid onset of drug action. With intramuscular (i.m.) or subcutaneous (s.c.) injections, absorption can be delayed as drug moves from the injection site into the vascular system. The absorption rate can also vary depending on the site of injection (e.g. absorption is usually more rapid from the neck muscles than from the muscles of the hindquarters). Some formulations are designed to have a slow release profile from the injection site making the antimicrobial agent "long acting".

Preparations for oral (p.o.) administration may have reduced or erratic systemic availability in herbivores because of adsorption onto feedstuffs and incomplete absorption. The liver may inactivate some drugs that are easily absorbed as they pass via the portal circulation (first-pass effect). Drugs with large molecular weights may not be well absorbed, unless attached to a "carrier" that allows absorption through the lymphatic system.

Elimination half-life

Infectious diseases are typically treated using multiple doses of an antimicrobial agent. The timing of these repeated doses is determined by the elimination half-life of the drug (Martinez 1998b). The elimination half-life is the time required for the drug concentration to decrease by one-half. For most drugs, half-life remains constant for the duration of the drug dose in the body. Clinically, the half-life determines (a) the inter-dosing interval; (b) how long a pharmacological or toxic effect will persist; and (c) drug withdrawal times for food-producing animals and performance horses.

What adverse drug reactions or toxicity might be expected?

Most drugs have some potential adverse/toxic effects and the practitioner must decide if the risks of therapy outweigh the benefits. Antimicrobial drugs frequently cause adverse reactions in horses. Because of their digestive physiology, horses are prone to developing antimicrobial-associated colitis that can be fatal (Freeman 1999). Antimicrobial agents with activity against anaerobic bacteria, combinations of broad-spectrum agents and those agents that undergo extensive enterohepatic recirculation are often incriminated in disturbing the normal gastrointestinal flora and allowing the proliferation of *Clostridium* spp. and pathogens such as *Salmonella* spp. Anaphylactic reactions and immune-mediated hemolytic anemia are associated with penicillin administration. Fatal cardiac arrhythmias are associated with the concurrent i.v. administration of potentiated sulfonamides and the α_2-adrenergic agonist detomidine.

The use of antimicrobial agents for relatively trivial infections encourages the selection of resistant organisms. Consequently, in the absence of evidence of a susceptible pathogen, antimicrobial use is irrational and may expose treated horses to unnecessary risks.

Is there a suitable product approved for use in horses?

In addition to finding a suitable product, the practitioner must also determine an appropriate withdrawal time for an antimicrobial agent used in a horse intended for human consumption or performance.

Whenever possible, veterinarians should use approved products. If there is no suitable approved product, then agents approved for use in other species may be used in horses as long as there is a valid veterinarian–client–animal relationship. The veterinarian must be available in the case of treatment failure or adverse reactions and must be able to provide information on the withdrawal time prior to slaughter or competition. For information on withdrawal periods, veterinarians should consult a database such as the Food Animal Residue Avoidance Databank (FARAD) in the USA (Riviere et al 1998). FARAD centers are being established worldwide. Drug withdrawal times for performance horses will vary between sports and countries. The governing body of a particular discipline should be consulted for the appropriate current guidelines.

DOCUMENTING AN INFECTION

A diagnosis must be established before any therapy can be administered. It is not always necessary to isolate bacteria from all horses with microbial infections in order to identify the organisms involved. The diagnosis can be based on clinical experience. The signs of some particular infections are so obvious that the need for microbiological confirmation is minimal; however, for those diseases of unknown cause or attributable to organisms with unpredictable antimicrobial susceptibility, there is no substitute for bacterial culture and identification of the causative agent. For these organisms, initial therapy, while waiting for the culture results, should include an antimicrobial agent with a broad spectrum of activity, although these agents are usually more toxic and more expensive.

Representative samples of infected material should be taken from clinical cases. Beware of sampling grossly contaminated sites, such as wounds and purulent nasal discharges. Correct samples may improve the odds of isolating the relevant pathogen: septic arthritis is best diagnosed using synovial fluid samples rather than a synovial membrane biopsy, salmonellosis from rectal biopsy and septicemias from blood culture. A Gram stain can be performed immediately on a direct smear and will direct initial therapy until the laboratory results are obtained. Samples should be submitted for appropriate culture and identification and the type of culture required should be specified: aerobic, anaerobic, mycoplasma. In some cases, the pathogen may be identified using serology to demonstrate antibodies (e.g. leptospirosis, brucellosis, ehrlichiosis).

DOSAGE REGIMEN DESIGN

Successful antimicrobial therapy relies on administering sufficient doses to suppress or kill pathogens effectively at the site of infection so that they can be eliminated by the host's defenses. The relationship between the host, the organism and the drug can be very complex. High plasma antimicrobial concentrations are *assumed* to be advantageous in that a large amount of drug will diffuse into various tissues and body fluids. The drug concentration at the infection site is assumed to be of major importance in determining drug efficacy. Remember, the ability of a drug to diffuse out of the plasma into the extravascular tissues depends on its molecular size, lipid solubility, pK_a, and the degree of protein binding, as well as local pH and specific cellular transport mechanisms.

INHIBITORY DRUG DOSAGE

In the laboratory, the relationship between an antimicrobial drug and a pathogen is described by the minimum inhibitory concentration (MIC) and the minimum bactericidal concentration (MBC). The MIC is the lowest drug concentration that inhibits bacterial growth. The MBC is the lowest drug concentration that kills 99.9% of the bacteria.

MIC values are used to determine a drug dose, that should achieve blood and tissue concentrations that exceed the *in vitro* MIC of the pathogen. Antimicrobial susceptibility is described as the following:

- susceptible ("S") pathogen is when MIC < local drug concentration: successful therapy
- intermediate ("I") pathogen is when MIC = local drug concentration: doubtful therapeutic effect
- resistant ("R") pathogen is when MIC > local drug concentration: drug will have no effect.

The "S", "I", "R" designations are assigned by laboratories based on safely achievable plasma concentrations. A culture and susceptibility report should contain the name of the organism and a list of common antimicrobial agents designated as susceptible, intermediate or resistant. This information is intended to guide antimicrobial selection; however, these reports must be interpreted carefully. There are a number of important factors that are not taken into account in these data (Verbist 1993).

Host defenses

The interaction between an antimicrobial and a pathogen in the laboratory does not take normal host defense systems into account. Humoral and cell-mediated immune systems play a major role in pathogen eradication; their contribution is underestimated in susceptibility reports. Antimicrobial agents act in concert with endogenous microbial inhibitors such as immunoglobulins, T lymphocytes, phagocytes, complement components, lactoferrin, lactoperoxidase and lysozymes.

Drug distribution in the body

Susceptibility designations are based on achievable plasma concentrations and do not take preferential drug accumulation at specific sites into account: most antimicrobial agents are eliminated by the kidneys, achieving concentrations in urine that are hundreds of times higher than those in plasma; tetracyclines accumulate in pneumonic lung tissue, resulting in successful therapy, which would not be predicted by *in vitro* susceptibility testing. Direct application of an antimicrobial drug, such as a topical or an ophthalmic formulation, produces such high concentrations that the susceptibility report may be inapplicable.

Growth rates and the size of inoculum at the infection site

MIC is measured using standardized methods and a standardized inoculum size. In clinical cases, there may be sites of infection with only a few bacteria and other sites with many. Some bacteria grow and multiply very slowly at infection sites, while the laboratory incubator and optimal conditions encourage rapid growth and multiplication. Rapidly multiplying bacteria under optimal test conditions are very sensitive to antimicrobial treatment.

Mixed infections

In the laboratory, cultured organisms are separated prior to susceptibility testing. This prevents the observation of any synergism between pathogens. For example, *Pasteurella* spp. and anaerobes demonstrate synergistic pathogenicity *in vivo* that cannot be seen when they are cultured separately *in vitro*.

Infection environment

Laboratory culture plates provide an ideal environment for the drug–organism interactions. In clinical cases, the local environment at the infection site has a large effect on antimicrobial action. In diseases characterized by abscess formation, treatment failure may occur when the chosen antimicrobial agent is ineffective in acidic, anaerobic and hyperosmolar environments. The action of many antimicrobial drugs is decreased in milk.

Route of administration

Unless specifically requested, topically administered antimicrobial agents are not tested. Systemically toxic antimicrobial agents, such as polymixin B, bacitracin and mupirocin, are often not included

Table 2.3 Classification of antimicrobial agents as bactericidal or bacteriostatic

Bactericidal	Bacteriostatic
Fluoroquinolones	Chloramphenicol
Aminoglycosides	Florfenicol
Penicillins	Macrolides
Cephalosporins	Tetracyclines
Trimethoprim/sulfonamides	Sulfonamides

in susceptibility profiles, yet they have great value in veterinary medicine. In addition, agents not listed in susceptibility reports are often not considered for therapy, even when they may be both suitable and effective.

The use of *in vitro* MIC values to predict the results of antimicrobial therapy *in vivo* is questionable. Yet, by convention, drug dosage regimens target a plasma drug concentration that is based on some multiple (usually 2–10) of the MIC. Proposed treatment regimens are then evaluated in clinical cases and modified, as required, to maximize efficacy.

BACTERIOSTATIC VERSUS BACTERICIDAL AGENTS

It is common to classify antimicrobial agents as either bactericidal or bacteriostatic (Table 2.3). If the ratio of the MBC to the MIC is small (<4–6), the agent is considered to be bactericidal and it is possible to obtain drug concentrations that will kill 99.9% of the organisms exposed. If the ratio of the MBC to the MIC is large, it may not be possible to administer safely dosages of the drug to kill 99.9% of the bacteria and the agent is considered to be bacteriostatic. For many drugs, the distinction between bactericidal and bacteriostatic is not exact and depends on the pathogen involved and the drug concentration attained in the target tissues. For example, florfenicol is considered bactericidal in very susceptible pathogens of the bovine respiratory tract but bacteriostatic in enteric pathogens. A bactericidal drug may be preferred over a bacteriostatic drug in specific situations including immunosuppressed patients (e.g. septic neonates), life-threatening conditions (e.g. bacterial endocarditis and meningitis) and for surgical prophylaxis.

Table 2.4 Postantibiotic effect (PAE) of various antimicrobial agents

	Postantibiotic effect (h)		
	Long (>3)	Intermediate (1–3)	Short (<1)
Gram-positives	Fluoroquinolones Macrolides Chloramphenicol Tetracyclines	Aminoglycosides Penicillins Cephalosporins	
Gram-negatives	Fluoroquinolones Aminoglycosides		Penicillins Cephalosporins Trimethoprim/sulphonamides
Anaerobes	Metronidazole		

For some bacteria–drug interactions, bacterial growth remains suppressed for a period after the drug concentration has decreased below the MIC. This period when antimicrobial concentrations have fallen below MIC but the damaged bacteria are more susceptible to host defenses is called the postantibiotic effect (PAE). PAE may explain why dosage regimens that allow antimicrobial concentrations to fall below the MIC for a significant portion of the interdosing interval are still efficacious. The PAE depends on both the antimicrobial agent and the specific bacterial pathogen (Table 2.4).

ANTIMICROBIAL DRUG CONCENTRATION

Bacterial killing curve studies show that antimicrobial agents exhibit either concentration-dependent or time-dependent bacterial killing (Table 2.5) (Martinez 1998c). For concentration-dependent killers, such as the aminoglycosides, a high maximum plasma concentration (C_{max}) relative to the MIC is the major determinant of clinical efficacy. These drugs also have prolonged PAE values, thereby allowing long interdosing intervals that maximize clinical efficacy and minimize side-effects. For time-dependent agents, such as the penicillins and cephalosporins, the time that the antimicrobial concentration exceeds the MIC determines the clinical efficacy. Once the MIC of the bacteria has been exceeded, further increases in the plasma concentrations do not increase the bactericidal activity of these agents.

Table 2.5 Concentration-dependent versus time-dependent antimicrobial agents

Concentration dependent	Time dependent
Aminoglycosides	Penicillins
Fluoroquinolones (in Gram-negative aerobes)	Cephalosporins
Metronidazole	Other "bacteriostatic" antimicrobial agents

CALCULATING THE DRUG DOSAGE REGIMEN

Antimicrobial dosage regimens are designed in one of two ways: either to maximize the plasma concentration or to provide a plasma concentration above the MIC for most of the interdosing interval (Vogelman et al 1988).

For concentration-dependent killers with a prolonged PAE, it is suggested that the peak plasma drug concentration be 8- to 10-fold higher than the MIC of the pathogen. If the V_d of the antimicrobial is known, a precise drug dosage regimen for the pathogen can be calculated using the following equation:

Dose rate = V_d [desired plasma concentration]

For example, a foal with *Klebsiella* spp. pneumonia is to be treated with gentamicin. The MIC of gentamicin for *Klebsiella* spp. is 2 μg/ml. The desired plasma concentration would be 10 times the MIC, which is 20 μg/ml. The V_d of gentamicin in the foal is 0.3 l/kg. The dose rate calculated is:

Dose rate = (300 ml/kg)(0.02 mg/ml) = 6 mg/kg

Given once daily, this dosage would provide effective concentration-dependent bacterial killing, while limiting the renal accumulation of gentamicin and any associated nephrotoxicity.

For time-dependent killers, the objective is to keep the average plasma drug concentration above the MIC of the pathogen for the entire duration of the interdosing interval. Again, utilizing V_d and half-life, you can calculate a dosing regimen.

Therapeutic index

The therapeutic index assesses a drug in terms of the ratio between the average minimum effective dose and the average maximum tolerated dose in normal subjects. This does not take into account variation between individuals and it is now usually defined as the median lethal dose (LD_{50}) divided by the median effective dose (ED_{50}). It is intended to indicate the margin of safety of a drug, a high therapeutic index implying a better safety margin.

SITE OF THE INFECTION

The pathophysiology of an infection influences the distribution and activity of antimicrobial agents. Abscess formation poses a significant therapeutic problem: the walls of an abscess limit the penetration of non-lipid-soluble drugs; the acidic environment encourages weak bases to accumulate; the low pH and the presence of cellular debris interfere with the activity of some antimicrobial agents. Penicillins and cephalosporins do not penetrate abscesses well. Aminoglycosides do not penetrate abscesses well and are inactivated in acidic, anaerobic, hyperosmolar environments. Potentiated sulfonamides achieve adequate concentrations, but the competitive mechanism of action of the sulfonamides is overwhelmed by the abundance of free PABA from lysed phagocytes. The fluoroquinolones and macrolides achieve high concentrations, but the acidic environment lessens their activity. Rifampin (rifampicin), chloramphenicol, florfenicol, the tetracyclines and metronidazole all achieve high concentrations in abscesses and retain their antimicrobial efficacy in purulent environments.

COMBINATION ANTIMICROBIAL THERAPY

Combination antimicrobial therapy is commonplace in equine practice. However, combination therapy has never been demonstrated to be superior to single drug therapy in controlled clinical trials. The use of multiple antimicrobial agents should be limited to certain situations.

1. Combinations with known synergism against specific organisms. Synergism occurs when the antimicrobial effect of a combination of drugs is greater than the sum of their independent effects. For example, penicillins and cephalosporins are synergistic with aminoglycosides. Disruption of the bacterial cell wall by the beta-lactam antibiotic allows for greater uptake of the aminoglycoside and results in a synergistic killing effect.
2. To prevent the rapid development of bacterial resistance. Erythromycin and rifampin are used in combination in the treatment of foals with *Rhodococcus* (*R.*) *equi* infections. Each drug has a completely different mechanism of antimicrobial action; their combination reduces the chance of chromosomal mutations conferring bacterial resistance.
3. To extend the spectrum of activity for the initial antimicrobial therapy of life-threatening infections. In emergency situations, such as septicemia or meningitis, where the causative organism is unknown, combination therapy may be initiated to provide antimicrobial activity against Gram-positive, Gram-negative and anaerobic bacteria.
4. To treat mixed bacterial infections. For example, it is rational to combine gentamicin plus a beta-lactam plus metronidazole for cases of equine pleuropneumonia, which predictably involve mixed infections of *Strep. zooepidemicus*, Gram-negative enteric bacteria and anaerobes.
5. Non-synergistic or antagonistic combinations should be avoided. Classically, penicillins are not administered concurrently with tetracyclines. The penicillins require actively dividing bacterial cells to be effective as they act against bacterial cell wall formation,

while the tetracyclines' bacteriostatic action inhibits bacterial replication. The combination of procaine benzylpenicillin (procaine penicillin) and a potentiated sulfonamide has minimally additive effects against pathogens but does have additive effects against the commensal microflora; so this combination therapy increases the risk of colitis.

PROPHYLACTIC USE OF ANTIMICROBIAL DRUGS

The principles upon which drugs are used prophylactically to prevent surgical infections are based on human studies; there are few veterinary studies that evaluate these recommendations.

1. **The relative risk of infection must warrant the use of prophylactic antimicrobial agents**. Typically, they are used in surgical procedures associated with an infection rate that exceeds 5%. The risks of the prophylactic antimicrobial therapy must be less than the risk and consequences of infection.
2. **The organisms that are likely to cause the infection and their antimicrobial susceptibility should be known or predicted accurately**. Routine monitoring in surgical hospitals provides information on the normal equine flora and nosocomial pathogens that are involved commonly in hospital-acquired infections.
3. **The drug must be administered and distribute to the potential infection site before the onset of the infection**. To achieve high concentrations rapidly, antimicrobial agents are administered i.v. to provide prophylaxis.
4. **Drugs used prophylactically should not be those that are used routinely for therapy, to avoid bacterial resistance caused by previous exposure to that antimicrobial agent.**
5. **The duration of antimicrobial prophylaxis should be as short as possible**. Most studies demonstrate that prolonging treatment for longer than 24 hours after the procedure has no additional benefits.
6. **The selected agent should be bactericidal rather than bacteriostatic**. It is assumed that

surgical patients are immunocompromised to some degree.
7. **The selected protocol should be cost effective**.

BETA-LACTAM ANTIBIOTICS

The beta-lactam antibiotics are commonly used because of their safety, efficacy, relatively low cost and the variety of dosage forms available. Both *penicillins* and *cephalosporins* have a four-membered beta-lactam ring that is responsible for the instability of these compounds. The penicillins are also relatively insoluble; they are prepared as various salts by the substitution of the hydroxyl group or the hydrogen of the carboxyl group with sodium, potassium, benzathine or procaine.

Mechanism of action

Beta-lactam antibiotics act on enzymes called penicillin-binding proteins (PBP) near the bacterial cell wall. When beta-lactam antibiotics bind covalently and irreversibly to the PBP, they interfere with the production of cell-wall peptidoglycans, causing cell lysis in hypoosmotic environments. Differences in the spectrum of activity and actions of beta-lactam antibiotics result from their relative affinity for different PBP.

Resistance mechanisms

Resistance to the beta-lactams develops via a number of mechanisms.

1. Failure of the antibiotic to penetrate the outer layers of bacterial cells. In order to bind to the PBP, the beta-lactam antibiotic must first diffuse through the bacterial cell wall. Gram-negative organisms have an additional lipopolysaccharide layer that decreases antibiotic penetration. Therefore, Gram-positive bacteria are usually more susceptible to the action of beta-lactams than Gram-negative bacteria.
2. Genetic alteration of PBP decreases the affinity of the PBP for the antibiotic. This is the

mechanism of resistance in methicillin-resistant staphylococci (MRSA).

3.   Production of beta-lactamase enzymes. There may be as many as 50 beta-lactamase enzymes (penicillinases, cephalosporinases) produced by bacteria. These enzymes hydrolyze the cyclic amide bond of the beta-lactam ring and inactivate these antibiotics. Staphylococcal beta-lactamase is produced by coagulase-positive staphylococci. This is the most clinically relevant beta-lactamase. The genes controlling the synthesis of these enzymes are encoded on plasmids and the enzymes are exocellular. These enzymes typically do not inactivate cephalosporins and antistaphylococcal penicillins (e.g. cloxacillin, oxacillin). The beta-lactamase enzymes produced by Gram-negative bacteria form a diverse group that can be encoded on the chromosome and/or a plasmid. Chromosome-mediated beta-lactamases hydrolyze both penicillins and cephalosporins. *E. coli* beta-lactamase genes are transferred by plasmids and also hydrolyze both groups of drug. Inhibitors such as clavulanic acid and sulbactam can inactivate most beta-lactamases.

PENICILLIN G (BENZYLPENICILLIN)

Indications

Penicillin G (benzylpenicillin) remains the agent of first choice for the treatment of streptococcal infections in horses and is, therefore, indicated for the treatment of strangles, pneumonia and pleuropneumonia. Its efficacy may be limited by poor drug penetration into abscesses, as is seen in strangles. Penicillin G is also indicated in the treatment of most anaerobic infections; however, *Bacteroides* (*B.*) *fragilis* is often resistant. Penicillin G is usually combined with other drugs to achieve a broad spectrum of activity. Its activity may be synergistic with the aminoglycosides and additive with the fluoroquinolones.

Pharmacokinetics

The sodium and potassium salts of penicillin G are the only formulations suitable for i.v. administration. They are also the most rapidly absorbed from i.m. and s.c. injection sites. Procaine benzylpenicillin (procaine penicillin) is more slowly absorbed from i.m. sites than the sodium or potassium salts, so it produces lower but more sustained plasma concentrations. Procaine benzylpenicillin (procaine penicillin) is more rapidly absorbed and reaches higher plasma concentrations when injected into the muscles of the neck muscles than those of the hindquarters and when injected i.m. rather than by s.c. injection. Benzathine benzylpenicillin (benzathine penicillin) produces the longest duration of penicillin concentrations, but concentrations remain below the MIC of most pathogens; consequently, it is of no therapeutic value and should not be used in equine practice. The absorption of penicillin in horses following p.o. administration is too poor to be of practical use.

Being weak acids with a pK_a of 2.7, penicillins have low V_d values (typically 0.2–0.31/kg). After absorption, penicillins distribute mainly into the ECF. CSF concentrations are 10% of plasma concentrations unless the meninges are inflamed. Penicillins distribute into milk but reach only subtherapeutic concentrations for most bacteria. Penicillins cross the placenta but are not associated with producing adverse effects in the fetus. Protein binding is considered to be moderate (52–54%).

Elimination of the penicillins is primarily via the kidneys, by glomerular filtration and active tubular secretion. The half-life is approximately 1 h after i.v. injection. Because of slow absorption from the injection site, the half-life of procaine benzylpenicillin (procaine penicillin) is approximately 7 h.

Drug interactions and adverse effects

Concurrent administration with phenylbutazone increases plasma concentrations, but lowers tissue concentrations, of penicillin G. Bacteriostatic antimicrobial agents, such as chloramphenicol and the tetracyclines, antagonize the antibacterial activity of penicillin G.

Immune-mediated reactions to penicillin G include anaphylaxis (a type I hypersensitivity reaction), hemolytic anemia and thrombocytopenia (type II hypersensitivity reactions). Anaphylactic reactions can be fatal, so epinephrine (adrenaline) should be kept near at hand when administering penicillins.

Adverse CNS effects occur when the procaine portion of the procaine benzylpenicillin (procaine penicillin) formulation is given intravascularly. The signs of toxicity include hyperexcitability, muscle tremors, ataxia, apnea and cardiac arrest. There is no specific treatment for procaine toxicity; one can only attempt to prevent the horse from injuring itself and others until the effects of the procaine wear off. The CNS reaction can be prevented by pretreatment with diazepam. The solubility of the procaine fraction of procaine benzylpenicillin (procaine penicillin) formulations increases with increasing ambient temperature, so these products should be stored in a cool place to reduce the risk of reactions. Procaine is a common cause of positive drug tests in racehorses and other performance horses. Procaine benzylpenicillin (procaine penicillin) should be avoided in these animals.

The sodium or potassium content of i.v. formulations can contribute to electrolyte imbalances associated with congestive heart failure and renal function impairment. Care should be taken when using these formulations in neonates.

Formulations

Penicillin G is available in injectable formulations. The sodium and potassium salts (crystalline penicillin) are water-soluble formulations and may be injected i.v., i.m. or s.c. They rapidly produce high plasma concentrations but have very short half-lives, so must be administered frequently. The potassium salt must be administered more carefully than the sodium salt, as rapid i.v. administration can cause cardiac arrhythmias. These formulations are frequently used for their Gram-positive activity in life-threatening diseases and conditions such as surgical colic, neonatal septicemia and clostridial myositis.

Procaine benzylpenicillin (procaine penicillin) is a poorly soluble salt that is absorbed slowly following i.m. or s.c. injection. It is the most commonly used formulation of penicillin in horses. Injections s.c. cause severe local inflammation and hemorrhage, as well as leaving deposits of

penicillin that can lead to residues in food-producing animals.

Benzathine benzylpenicillin is a very insoluble salt. It is administered i.m. in "long-acting" formulations that contain one-half procaine benzylpenicillin (procaine penicillin) and one-half benzathine benzylpenicillin. Any clinical effect is from the procaine benzylpenicillin (procaine penicillin) portion of these formulations since the benzathine penicillin provides persistent but subtherapeutic plasma concentrations.

AMINOPENICILLINS: AMOXICILLIN AND AMPICILLIN

Indications

The aminopenicillins are able to penetrate the outer layer of Gram-negative bacteria better than penicillin G; they have activity against Gram-positive bacteria and many Gram-negative bacteria (*E. coli* and *Salmonella* and *Pasteurella* spp.). Amoxicillin is superior to ampicillin in its ability to penetrate Gram-negative bacteria. Resistance to the aminopenicillins is easily acquired by some Gram-positive and Gram-negative bacteria via plasmids; therefore, these agents are not usually effective against *Staph. aureus* and *Klebsiella*, *Proteus* and *Pseudomonas* (*Ps.*) spp. Most anaerobes, except beta-lactamase-producing strains of *Bacteroides* spp., are susceptible to the aminopenicillins.

Pharmacokinetics

In horses, amoxicillin or ampicillin sodium are well absorbed following i.m. or s.c. administration. Amoxicillin or ampicillin trihydrate are poorly soluble salts that are given i.m. and produce lower plasma concentrations that extend over a longer period of time. Amoxicillin and ampicillin are too poorly absorbed following p.o. administration to be clinically useful in horses. The ampicillin esters, pivampicillin and bacampicillin, show promise for p.o. use but are currently not available for use in horses.

The aminopenicillins are distributed rapidly and widely into most tissues, except the eye and the accessory sex glands. They distribute poorly into the CSF unless the meninges are inflamed. Their penetration into synovial fluid is high. The V_d of amoxicillin is 0.192 l/kg in adult horses and 0.265 l/kg in foals. The V_d of ampicillin is 0.18 l/kg in adult horses. Amoxicillin is moderately protein bound (38%), while ampicillin is minimally protein bound (6.8–8%). Following an i.m. dose of ampicillin sodium at 10 mg/kg, peak serum concentrations of 6.2–9.7 μg/ml are reached in 16 min.

Amoxicillin and ampicillin are excreted primarily unchanged in the urine. The half-life of amoxicillin is 0.5–1.5 h in adults and 0.75 h in 1-week-old foals. The half-life of ampicillin is 0.5–1.5 h.

Drug interactions and adverse effects

The drug interactions and adverse effects of the aminopenicillins are the same as for penicillin G. Ampicillin trihydrate may cause i.m. injection site reactions in horses: mild to moderate heat, pain and/or swelling.

Formulations

Sodium ampicillin is approved for i.v. or i.m. administration to humans and horses. These formulations have a very short shelf-life after reconstitution. The human approved formulation come in a variety of presentations that are more convenient for use in different sizes of horses. The trihydrate salts of amoxicillin and ampicillin are available for i.m. administration to cattle.

EXTENDED-SPECTRUM PENICILLINS

Indications

The extended-spectrum penicillins include carbenicillin and ticarcillin. Ticarcillin has been shown to be the most efficacious antimicrobial drug tested versus Gram-positive bacteria, with 93% being susceptible in vitro. This group of penicillins can penetrate the outer cell wall of *Pseudomonas* spp. and other Gram-negative bacteria. They are active against anaerobes and are synergistic when

administered with the aminoglycosides. They are susceptible to beta-lactamase enzyme degradation. Extended-spectrum penicillins are of limited use in horses because of the expense of therapy. Ticarcillin is primarily used by intrauterine administration for the treatment of streptococcal and pseudomonad metritis (see Ch. 11) in mares. Both ticarcillin and carbenicillin are used for the treatment of infectious keratitis.

Pharmacokinetics

Although there is limited pharmacokinetic information available in horses, these agents appear to be similar to other penicillins. Following i.v. injection of ticarcillin to horses, at a dose rate of 44 mg/kg, the serum concentration at 30 min was 104.3 μg/l and the mean peak peritoneal fluid concentration (61.4 μg/l) was reached 2 h after injection. The half-life of ticarcillin was 0.94 h. Following i.m. injection (44 mg/kg), the peak serum (28.3 μg/l) and peritoneal fluid (19.2 μg/l) concentrations were reached after 2 h. The bioavailability of ticarcillin was 64.9%.

Drug interactions and adverse effects

Drug interactions and adverse effects of the extended-spectrum agents are the same as for penicillin G.

Formulations

These drugs are available as sodium salts. In general, they are expensive and their use in equine practice is limited. A veterinary approved formulation of ticarcillin is available in the USA for intrauterine administration to mares.

CEPHALOSPORINS

Indications

The widespread emergence of penicillin-resistant staphylococci in the 1950s led to the development of the cephalosporins. The cephalosporins have the same mechanism of action as the penicillins but are more resistant to bacterial defenses. The cephalosporins are usually grouped into three "generations" based primarily on their antibacterial activity. However, some of the newer cephalosporins do not fit easily into this scheme. Cephalosporins are used widely for prophylaxis in cardiovascular, orthopedic, biliary and abdominal surgery.

First-generation cephalosporins are effective against most Gram-positive cocci, including beta-lactamase-producing staphylococci, by virtue of their higher affinity for PBP. They are very active against staphylococci and streptococci, with the exception of MRSA and enterococci. Although most corynebacteria are susceptible, *R.* (formerly *Corynebacterium*) *equi* is usually resistant. They also have greater activity against Enterobacteriaceae than other beta-lactam antibiotics, but may be degraded by Gram-negative beta-lactamases, making them ineffective against some Gram-negative bacteria. Among the commonly encountered Gram-negative bacteria, *E. coli* and *Klebsiella, Haemophilus, Proteus, Actinobacillus, Pasteurella* and *Salmonella* spp. are usually susceptible to the first-generation cephalosporins. Indole-positive *Proteus, Enterobacter, Serratia* and *Pseudomonas* spp. are resistant. Most anaerobic bacteria are susceptible, with the exception of beta-lactamase-producing *Bacteroides* spp. and *Clostridium difficile*.

First-generation cephalosporins are an effective alternative to penicillins. Only 3–7% of humans allergic to penicillin are allergic to cephalosporins; therefore, they may usually be used in penicillin-sensitive individuals. First-generation cephalosporins do not cross the blood–brain barrier. All of the first-generation cephalosporins have essentially the same spectrum of activity, so the choice of an individual drug is usually based on pharmacokinetic and economic considerations. The first-generation cephalosporins used most commonly in horses are cefalotin and cefazolin. Cefazolin is promoted as being better tolerated after i.m. injection than the other first-generation cephalosporins.

Second-generation cephalosporins are no more active against Gram-positive bacteria and may be less active against staphylococci than the first-generation drugs but have greater activity against Gram-negative bacteria that are resistant to first-generation agents (e.g. *E. coli* and *Klebsiella, Proteus* and *Enterobacter* spp.). Their increased spectrum of activity results from increased resistance to Gram-negative beta-lactamases. Second-generation cephalosporins are usually active against anaerobes, and cefoxitin is effective against *B. fragilis*. The cost of these agents is roughly twice that of the first-generation cephalosporins; therefore, their use is limited to situations where the infection is resistant to a first-generation drug, susceptible to a second-generation drug and the only other therapeutic options produce unacceptable side-effects.

Third-generation cephalosporins have increased activity against Gram-negative bacteria because of their resistance to beta-lactamases. In the past, they were considered to have unreliable and erratic effects against Gram-positive organisms. However, good activity against Gram-positive organisms, except for enterococci and *Listeria* spp., has been demonstrated recently. Some of the third-generation products (ceftazidime and cefoperazone) have good activity against *Pseudomonas* spp. The use of the third-generation cephalosporins is usually restricted to bacterial infections caused by multiple drug-resistant strains. These drugs are most likely to be useful in equines with neonatal septicemia, nosocomial pneumonia, postoperative wound infections and urinary tract infections related to catheterization. Cefotaxime has been investigated in the treatment of meningitis and septicemia in neonatal foals. All of the third-generation cephalosporins are extremely expensive and are, therefore, rarely used in veterinary medicine.

Ceftiofur is marketed as a "new" generation cephalosporin as it does not clearly fall into the previous classification scheme. It is currently approved for the treatment of streptococcal infections in horses. It has broader Gram-positive spectrum of activity than the third-generation cephalosporins and has activity against anaerobes. Ceftiofur has no activity against *Pseudomonas* spp. and does not penetrate into the CNS. It is metabolized very rapidly *in vivo* to its active metabolite desfuroylceftiofur. Desfuroylceftiofur is very highly protein bound because of a sulfhydryl group in its chemical structure. The efficacy of ceftiofur is attributed to desfuroylceftiofur binding to acute phase proteins, such as α_1-antitrypsin, that act as a reservoir of active drug and carry it to sites of inflammation. Because of the high degree of protein binding, ceftiofur does not readily cross into the milk when administered parenterally. Desfuroylceftiofur does not have the same activity as ceftiofur against certain pathogens, so the results of susceptibility tests using ceftiofur disks may be misleading: *Staph. aureus* is four to eight times less sensitive to desfuroylceftiofur than to ceftiofur; *Proteus mirabilis* has widely variable susceptibility to desfuroylceftiofur.

Pharmacokinetics

The absorption of the cephalosporins is rapid following i.m. or s.c. administration. The extent of absorption depends on the drug used and the species treated. The absorption of cephalosporins is erratic following p.o. administration to horses.

Cephalosporins distribute into most body fluids and tissues, including pleural fluid, synovial fluid, pericardial fluid and urine. Cephalosporins distribute into milk, but therapeutic concentrations are not reached following systemic administration at accepted dose rates. Cephalosporins cross the placenta but do not appear to cause adverse effects in the fetus. Their penetration into cortical and cancellous bone is usually adequate. Most cephalosporins penetrate poorly into the aqueous humor, accessory sex glands and CSF. Cephalosporins have typically low V_d values in horses: 0.19 l/kg for cefazolin, 0.15 l/kg for cefalotin, 0.17 l/kg for cefapirin, 0.4 l/kg for cefradine and 0.12 l/kg for cefoxitin.

Ceftiofur and its active metabolite desfuroylceftiofur distribute differently to the other cephalosporins because of their high degree of protein binding. Reversible covalent bonding with plasma and tissue proteins produces lower than expected free concentrations of ceftiofur and desfuroylceftiofur following the administration of clinically effective doses. Tissue chamber studies have shown that concentrations of parent drug and active metabolite are higher in infected than in normal tissues.

Most cephalosporins are excreted unchanged in the urine. Renal elimination of the cephalosporins occurs through a combination of glomerular filtration and active tubular secretion. The dosage regimen for most cephalosporins must be modified in renal failure. Cefalotin, cefapirin, cefotaxime and ceftiofur are deacetylated by the liver. Their metabolites have significant antibacterial activity. For the cephalosporins that undergo hepatic metabolism, hepatic insufficiency may result in decreased metabolism and increased drug accumulation. Most cephalosporins are eliminated rapidly after systemic administration; with halflives of 0.25–1 h. Ceftiofur has a relatively long half-life (3–5 h).

Drug interactions and adverse effects

In general, the cephalosporins have a high therapeutic index. Most of the adverse effects produced are the same as those reported for the penicillins. In humans, there is a low incidence of crosssensitivity with the penicillins for type I and type II hypersensitivity reactions. Bleeding disorders, caused by vitamin K antagonism, are associated with some of the cephalosporins used in humans but have not been reported in animals. Anemia and thrombocytopenia develop in dogs administered high doses of ceftiofur for an extended period. Horses may develop diarrhea after treatment with ceftiofur. The currently available cephalosporins are considered to be potentially nephrotoxic, either via the deposition of immune complexes in the glomerular basement membrane or as a direct effect that leads to acute tubular necrosis. However, animal studies have shown that the cephalosporins protect against nephrotoxicity. In human medicine, it is recommended that cephalosporins not be used in conjunction with aminoglycosides.

Formulations

Cefazolin, cefotaxime, cefoxitin, cefalotin, cefapirin and ceftiofur are all available as sodium salts for injection. Ceftiofur is the only approved veterinary formulation.

IMIPENEM

The carbapenem antibiotics such as imipenem were developed to deal with the beta-lactamase-producing Gram-negative organisms resistant to the penicillins.

Indications

Imipenem is a carbapenem antibiotic. It has the broadest spectrum of activity of all antibiotics. It is the most potent of the newer agents against Gram-positive cocci and anaerobes and more than 90% of Gram-negative organisms including those resistant to other beta-lactam antibiotics and the aminoglycosides, are susceptible. Imipenem is highly resistant to most beta-lactamases. Resistance to imipenem develops rapidly in *Pseudomonas aeruginosa* through changes in its outer membrane proteins that reduce permeability. Imipenem is rarely used in veterinary medicine because of the expense of therapy.

Pharmacokinetics

Pharmacokinetic studies have not been performed in horses; however, i.v. doses of 0.7–1.1 mg/kg three times a day have been suggested as being suitable for use in small animals. Imipenem has to be administered i.v. because it is not absorbed following p.o. administration. Imipenem has been shown to penetrate inflamed meninges. It is metabolized extensively by the renal tubules to a potentially toxic compound. Therefore, it is usually combined with cilastatin, a drug that inhibits the renal tubular enzymes. The combined product produces high urine concentrations of active antibiotic and avoids renal toxicity. In the presence of cilastatin, 70% of a dose of imipenem is excreted unchanged in the urine. The half-life of imipenem in the dog is 30–45 min.

AMINOGLYCOSIDE ANTIBIOTICS

The aminoglycoside antibiotics include streptomycin, neomycin, gentamicin, amikacin, tobramycin and kanamycin. They have a chemical structure of amino sugars joined by a glycoside linkage. Streptomycin was originally developed for the treatment of tuberculosis in humans (its discoverer was awarded a Nobel Prize), but the newer aminoglycosides such as gentamicin and tobramycin have been targeted to treat *Pseudomonas* spp. infections. In veterinary medicine, these agents are important in the treatment of Gram-negative infections caused by enteric pathogens such as *E. coli*.

Mechanism of action

Aminoglycosides must penetrate bacteria to assert their effects. Susceptible, aerobic Gram-negative bacteria actively pump aminoglycoside into their cells. This is initiated by an oxygen-dependent interaction of the antibiotic cations and the negatively charged ions of the bacterial membrane lipopolysaccharides. This interaction affects membrane permeability by displacing divalent cations (calcium, magnesium). Once inside the bacterial cell, aminoglycosides bind to the 30S ribosomal subunit and cause misreading of the genetic code, thus interrupting normal bacterial protein synthesis. This leads to changes in cell membrane permeability, resulting in additional antibiotic uptake, further cell disruption and ultimately cell death.

Aminoglycosides are bactericidal and produce dose- (concentration-) dependent effects. For example, gentamicin concentrations of 0.5–5.0 µg/ml are bactericidal in Gram-positive and some Gram-negative bacteria. Gentamicin concentrations of 10–15 µg/ml are effective against more resistant bacteria such as *Pseudomonas*, *Klebsiella* and *Proteus* spp. The clinical implication is that high initial doses of aminoglycosides increase ionic bonding, which enhances the initial, rapid, concentration-dependent phase of antibiotic internalization and leads to greater immediate bactericidal activity. Clinical studies in humans have demonstrated that proper initial therapeutic doses of aminoglycosides are critical in reducing the mortality from Gram-negative septicemia.

The aminoglycosides are effective against most Gram-negative bacteria, including *Pseudomonas* spp. They are usually effective against staphylococci, although resistance can occur. They are often effective against enterococci, but their action against streptococci is more effective when combined with a beta-lactam antibiotic. *Salmonella* and *Brucella* spp. are intracellular pathogens that are often resistant because of poor intracellular drug penetration. Aminoglycosides are ineffective against anaerobic bacteria because bacterial penetration is oxygen dependent. The aminoglycosides induce significant PAEs. The duration of these PAEs tends to increase as the initial drug concentration increases.

The antimicrobial activity of aminoglycosides is enhanced in an alkaline environment (pH 6–8). They also bind to and are inactivated by the nucleic acid material released by decaying white blood cells. They are, therefore, usually ineffective in the acidic, hyperosmolar, anaerobic environment of abscesses.

Resistance mechanisms

Bacteria have a number of mechanisms that confer resistance to the aminoglycosides. Penetration of the bacterial cell wall is essential for antimicrobial activity. Strict anaerobes respire without a functioning electron-transport system and are unable to drive the energy-requiring phases of aminoglycoside uptake. Exposure to the aminoglycosides results in the development of bacterial mutants with altered cell membrane structure that prevents such penetration. Bacterial enzymes have been identified that attack different parts of the aminoglycoside molecule. The members of the aminoglycoside group vary in their susceptibility to these enzymes and thus cross-resistance is not uniform. Production of these enzymes by bacteria is plasmid encoded and so is transferable both within and between bacterial strains. Amikacin is the least susceptible to enzymatic inactivation.

Aminoglycoside antibiotics also have a unique method of bacterial resistance known as first-exposure adaptive resistance. Both inhibitory and subinhibitory concentrations of aminoglycosides can result in resistant bacterial cells, which survive the initial ionic bonding. This adaptive resistance results from decreased transport of aminoglycosides into the bacteria. Exposure to one dose of an aminoglycoside is sufficient to produce resistant

variants with altered metabolism and impaired aminoglycoside uptake. This resistance develops within 2 h of exposure to the aminoglycoside but it reverses if the drug is absent for a period (usually hours). If the aminoglycoside concentration remains constant, such as during a constant i.v. infusion, adaptive resistance persists and increases. Therefore, intermittent dosing regimens are most effective for aminoglycoside therapy.

Pharmacokinetics

The aminoglycosides are well absorbed following i.m. and s.c. administration because of large pores in the capillary walls of the subcutaneous tissues and muscle and the bioavailability approaches 100%. Aminoglycosides are absorbed poorly after p.o. administration but enough may be absorbed in animals with enteritis to result in drug residues in food-producing animals.

The aminoglycosides are large polar drug molecules that remain primarily in the ECF space; they are highly ionized at physiological pH. The V_d of aminoglycosides is higher in neonates, because of their increased ECF volume, than in adult horses. Therefore, to achieve the same plasma concentrations, a foal must be given a higher dose than an adult horse. Following parenteral administration, effective concentrations are obtained in synovial, perilymph, pleural, peritoneal and pericardial fluids. Therapeutic concentrations are not achieved in bile, milk, CSF, respiratory secretions, accessory sex glands and ocular fluids. Aminoglycosides readily cross the placenta and may be hazardous to fetal kidneys. The protein binding of the aminoglycosides is low.

Aminoglycosides are almost exclusively eliminated by glomerular filtration. Elimination is dependent on cardiovascular and renal function, age, fever, other physiological factors and the V_d. The half-lives are usually 1–2 h in normal adult horses but are increased in horses with renal dysfunction and in neonates. Increased dosage intervals must be used in these patients to prevent nephrotoxicity. The renal elimination of the aminoglycosides increases with age. The half-life of gentamicin is approximately 50% longer in 1-day-old than in 30-day-old foals.

Drug interactions and adverse effects

Aminoglycosides are inactivated when combined *in vitro* with many other drugs because of pH incompatibilities. Aminoglycosides exhibit synergism with beta-lactam antibiotics against streptococci, enterococci, *Pseudomonas* spp. and other Gram-negative bacteria. Ticarcillin binds aminoglycoside molecules *in vivo* and may decrease aminoglycoside toxicity after an accidental overdose. Supplemental iron increases the risk of nephrotoxicity and ototoxicity. Halothane anesthesia reduces the V_d and increases the half-life of gentamicin. Concurrent administration of gentamicin and phenylbutazone reduces the V_d of gentamicin by 26% and the half-life by 23%. These alterations are thought to be caused by increased entry of gentamicin into tissues; concurrent phenylbutazone therapy may improve the efficacy of gentamicin in treating Gram-negative tissue infections. Fluid administration i.v. does not change the pharmacokinetics of concurrently administered aminoglycosides. Coadministration of aminoglycosides and other nephrotoxic drugs should be avoided.

The nephrotoxicity caused by aminoglycosides (acute tubular necrosis) is of great concern and limits the practical use of these agents. The aminoglycosides enter the renal tubule after filtration through the glomerulus. A small amount of drug binds to phospholipid receptors on the luminal surface of the proximal tubular cells via a charge-mediated process. The phospholipid receptor is a common anionic binding site that is competed for with amino acids, cationic polypeptides and electrolytes. The aminoglycoside is taken into the cells via carrier-mediated pinocytosis. The drug is translocated into cytoplasmic vacuoles, which fuse with lysosomes. The aminoglycoside is sequestered unchanged in the lysosomes. With continued pinocytosis, the drug continues to accumulate within the lysosomes. The accumulated aminoglycoside interferes with normal lysosomal function and eventually overloaded lysosomes swell and rupture. Lysosomal enzymes, phospholipid and the aminoglycoside are released into the cytosol of the proximal tubular cells, disrupting other organelles and causing cell death.

Approximately 10–26% of human patients reportedly develop nephrotoxicosis associated with aminoglycoside therapy. Individual cases of aminoglycoside nephrotoxicity have been reported in horses but the incidence is not known.

There are several risk factors for aminoglycoside nephrotoxicity.

1. **Prolonged therapy**. Nephrotoxicity is associated with prolonged therapy (longer than 7–10 days), which allows substantial amounts of drug to accumulate within the renal tubular cells. Overdosing within the first 1–2 days of aminoglycoside therapy does not lead to nephrotoxicity provided that renal function is within normal limits.
2. **Metabolic acidosis and electrolyte disturbances**. Acidic environments increase the ionization of aminoglycosides and positive cations compete with the aminoglycosides for binding sites. Consequently, metabolic acidosis and electrolyte imbalances such as hypokalemia and hyponatremia increase the binding of aminoglycosides to the phospholipid receptors on the renal tubular cells, increasing intracellular accumulation.
3. **Volume depletion**. Dehydration, sodium depletion, shock, endotoxemia and diuretic drugs decrease the ECF volume, thereby increasing aminoglycoside concentration and necessitating changes in drug dose.
4. **Concurrent nephrotoxic drug therapy**. Concurrent therapy with other nephrotoxic drugs, such as non-steroidal anti-inflammatory drugs (NSAIDs) and amphotericin B, potentiates the nephrotoxicity of the aminoglycosides.
5. **Pre-existing renal disease**. Aminoglycosides are eliminated by renal excretion and a decrease in renal function prolongs the persistence of these nephrotoxic drugs. The glomerular filtration rate decreases with age, as a result of progressive vascular changes in the glomeruli; therefore, renal excretion may be reduced in aged horses.
6. **Elevated trough plasma concentrations**. The uptake of the aminoglycosides by the renal tubular cells is a saturable process. Sustained

high trough plasma concentrations result in greater drug accumulation and nephrotoxicosis. Dosage regimens that result in high peak concentrations and low to undetectable trough concentrations reduce the risk of nephrotoxicity.

High-protein diets protect against the development of aminoglycoside nephrotoxicity. Increased dietary protein increases the glomerular filtration rate and renal blood flow, promoting aminoglycoside excretion. Dietary proteins also compete with the aminoglycosides for the phospholipid receptors on the renal tubular cells. Increased dietary protein also increases the V_d of the aminoglycosides, increasing tissue concentrations while decreasing plasma concentrations. Horses fed an alfalfa diet have a significantly lower degree of gentamicin-induced nephrotoxicity than horses fed an oat grain diet. Calcium supplementation (20 mg/kg calcium gluconate i.v. three times a day) also decreases aminoglycoside nephrotoxicity through cation competition for the renal binding sites.

Clinically, aminoglycoside nephrotoxicity most commonly manifests as an asymptomatic rise in serum creatinine concentrations 7–10 days after the initiation of treatment. Acute renal failure is generally not oliguric; oliguria is a poor prognostic sign. Significant tubular dysfunction actually precedes the decline in the glomerular filtration rate. Increased urinary excretion of lysosomal enzymes and β_2-microglobulin, decreased reabsorption of potassium and magnesium ions and tubular resistance to vasopressin (antidiuretic hormone), resulting in polyuria and partial nephrogenic diabetes insipidus, can also be seen. Nephrotoxicity is usually reversible on discontinuing the drug treatment; however, renal dysfunction may persist for some time as a result of renal cortical drug accumulation. Nephrotoxicity increases the half-lives of the aminoglycosides to 24–45 h in horses. Peritoneal dialysis is useful for lowering creatinine and blood urea nitrogen concentrations, but it does not effectively increase the clearance of the accumulated aminoglycoside. If there is enough healthy renal tissue remaining, regeneration and hypertrophy of nephrons will restore normal renal function.

Therapeutic drug monitoring, to optimize peak and trough drug concentrations and monitor changes in the drug elimination rate, can be used to prevent aminoglycoside nephrotoxicity. If this is not available, then once daily, high-dose therapy is recommended. The development of nephrotoxicity can initially be identified by increases in urine gamma-glutamyltransferase (GGT) and β-N-acetylglucosaminidase (AGS) enzymes and increases in the urine GGT:creatinine and urine AGS:creatinine ratios. Urinary GGT and AGS activity increases within 5 days of aminoglycoside administration and provides an earlier indication of renal tubular disease than any other indices in clinical pathology. Elevations of blood urea nitrogen and serum creatinine concentrations are not typically seen for at least 6 days after starting aminoglycoside therapy. Proteinuria, urine casts and a decrease in urine specific gravity all occur after approximately 1 week of aminoglycoside therapy.

Aminoglycosides should be used cautiously in horses with endotoxemia. Even a low serum endotoxin concentration may increase toxicity by increasing kidney aminoglycoside concentrations. The bactericidal action of the aminoglycosides against Gram-negative bacteria may transiently increase endotoxin concentrations. Bacterial toxins may have local synergism with the aminoglycosides in damaging the renal tubular cells. Administration of a NSAID prior to aminoglycoside administration may prevent the deleterious effects of endotoxin.

Aminoglycoside ototoxicity is a significant problem in human medicine but has not been investigated in horses. Aminoglycosides accumulate in the tissues of the inner ear by binding to a phospholipid receptor. Streptomycin, tobramycin and gentamicin damage the cochlear division of the 8th cranial nerve, resulting in vertigo. Dihydrostreptomycin, amikacin, kanamycin and neomycin damage the auditory division of the 8th cranial nerve, resulting in deafness.

Neuromuscular blockade is a rare side-effect of the aminoglycosides, related to blockade of acetylcholine at the nicotinic cholinergic receptor. This is most often seen as respiratory depression and apnea when anesthetic agents are administered concurrently with aminoglycosides. Postsynaptic blockade can be reversed using a cholinesterase inhibitor such as neostigmine. Presynaptic blockade can be antagonized by calcium ions, administered i.v.

Amikacin, as a 2 g intrauterine dose, was not found to impair fertility when administered to mares 8 h prior to breeding. Mares should not be bred within 8 h of intrauterine treatment with amikacin and gentamicin should not be administered to these mares on the day of breeding.

STREPTOMYCIN/ DIHYDROSTREPTOMYCIN

Dihydrostreptomycin was developed as a non-ototoxic alternative to streptomycin, however it was just as ototoxic. Clinically, dihydrostreptomycin used to be given in combination with penicillin G, but most of these injectable products are no longer available.

NEOMYCIN

Neomycin is not usually administered parenterally to animals because of nephrotoxicity and ototoxicity. Only 3% of a dose of neomycin is absorbed following p.o. administration; it is, therefore, used in the therapy of coliform enteritis in small and large animals. It is available as tablets, boluses and water additives, in many different combinations with antibiotics, corticosteroids and anticholinergic agents. It can also be used to decrease nitrogenous waste production by the normal gastrointestinal flora in animals with hepatic encephalopathy. Neomycin is not absorbed through the skin, so it is frequently utilized as the antibacterial constituent in ophthalmic formulations (especially in combination with bacitracin and polymyxin B) and in preparations for the treatment of otitis externa in small animals.

GENTAMICIN

Indications

Gentamicin is more active against a wide range of bacteria, particularly against *Pseudomonas* spp. than the earlier aminoglycosides. It is also very effective against *Proteus* and *Klebsiella* spp., *E. coli* and staphylococci. It has only moderate activity against streptococci and poor activity against anaerobes. Transmissible resistance by Gram-negative bacteria occurs in proportion to gentamicin use. Bacteria that are resistant to gentamicin are also resistant to neomycin, streptomycin and kanamycin. The reverse is not true, as many strains resistant to the other aminoglycosides will remain susceptible to gentamicin. Gentamicin is approved only for intrauterine administration to horses. However, it is often used parenterally in the therapy of Gram-negative septicemia and infectious arthritis and prophylactically before abdominal surgery.

Pharmacokinetics

In adult horses, the V_d of gentamicin ranges from 0.12 l/kg to 0.24 l/kg. In foals, it is approximately 0.3 l/kg and this decreases to adult values by 6 months of age. The predominant site of drug accumulation is the renal cortex. When repeated doses of gentamicin are given, tissue concentrations (from highest to lowest) are found in the renal cortex, renal medulla, liver/lung/spleen and skeletal muscle. Gentamicin is distributed rapidly into synovial fluid in normal horses and 2 h after an i.v. dose, at a dose rate of 4.4 mg/kg, reaches a peak concentration of 6.4 µg/ml. Local inflammation and repeated dosing may further increase synovial fluid concentrations. After intraarticular administration of gentamicin (150 mg), peak synovial concentrations of approximately 2 mg/ml are reached within 15 min. Gentamicin (2.5 g) administered once daily for 5 days by the intrauterine route produced concentrations of 42 µg/ml in endometrial tissue 24 h after the last dose. The protein binding of gentamicin is <30%.

In horses, 75–100% of a gentamicin dose is excreted unchanged in the urine in the first 8–24 h after administration. The half-life is 1–2 h and is longer in neonatal foals than in older foals and adult horses. Any gentamicin that accumulates in the renal cortical tissue is eliminated slowly; however, these levels are often below the limits of quantification of the assays used and are, therefore, not demonstrated in pharmacokinetic studies.

Therapeutic drug monitoring

The gentamicin dosage regimen should be determined using therapeutic drug monitoring so as to maximize efficacy and minimize toxicity. Plasma concentrations of gentamicin differ widely between individual horses treated with the same dosage regimen. This variability in the relationship between the dose and plasma drug concentrations, combined with the narrow therapeutic range of the aminoglycosides, makes the monitoring of plasma concentrations in clinical cases very desirable. The desired peak plasma concentration is eight to ten times the MIC of the suspected pathogen. With once daily dosing, peak concentrations can be measured in plasma 1–2 h after dosing. The desired trough concentration is $<2 \mu g/ml$ and it is thought that the longer the period in the dosing interval that plasma concentrations are $<2 \mu g/ml$, the lower the risk of nephrotoxicity.

Formulations

Gentamicin sulfate is approved for intrauterine use in mares. Other unapproved routes of administration (i.v., i.m., s.c. and intraarticular routes) are used frequently. An ophthalmic solution of gentamicin is also approved for veterinary use.

AMIKACIN

Indications

Amikacin is derived from kanamycin and has the broadest spectrum of activity of the aminoglycosides. It is less susceptible to bacterial enzyme inactivation than the other aminoglycosides, so it is usually reserved for therapy of gentamicin-resistant bacterial infections.

Pharmacokinetics

The V_d of amikacin is 0.14–0.22 l/kg in adult horses and 0.4–0.6 l/kg in foals. The distribution into tissues is similar to that for gentamicin. One hour after i.v. administration of gentamicin (6.6 mg/kg) peak concentrations were 14 μg/ml in peritoneal fluid and 17 μg/ml in synovial fluid. Concentrations of greater than 40 μg/g endometrial tissue

were reached within 1 h of intrauterine administration of 2 g amikacin. Regional i.v. perfusion of amikacin (125 mg) produced sufficiently high concentrations to be effective in the treatment of most equine pathogens in the joint fluid, bone and serum of the treated limb.

The elimination of amikacin is similar to gentamicin. The half-life of amikacin ranges from 1 to 3 h in adult horses but may be as long as 5 h in neonatal foals.

Therapeutic drug monitoring

The amikacin dosing regimen is best determined using therapeutic drug monitoring. The suggested peak concentration of amikacin (1 h after administration) is 25 μg/ml and the trough concentration should be $<5 \mu g$/ml.

Formulations

Amikacin sulfate is approved for i.m. or s.c. injection in horses (50 or 250 mg/ml solution) and for intrauterine infusion (250 mg/ml solution). Other routes of administration that are not within the label indications (i.v. and intraarticular) are used frequently.

TOBRAMYCIN

Tobramycin is structurally related to kanamycin and has four times the activity of gentamicin against *Pseudomonas* spp. It is an extremely expensive drug. Its use in animals is usually limited to the topical treatment of melting corneal ulcers caused by gentamicin-resistant *Pseudomonas* spp. using the ophthalmic solution approved for use in humans.

CHLORAMPHENICOL AND FLORFENICOL

Indications

Chloramphenicol was isolated in 1947 from a soil actinomycete from Venezuela. Florfenicol is a fluorinated derivative of chloramphenicol. These antibiotics have a very broad spectrum of activity, being active against streptococci, staphylococci, *Haemophilus*, *Salmonella*, *Pasteurella* and *Brucella* spp., anaerobes and *Mycoplasma* spp. Florfenicol has activity against chloramphenicol-resistant strains of *Staph. aureus*, *E. coli* and *Klebsiella*, *Proteus* and *Salmonella* spp. These agents are also active against *Rickettsia*, *Chlamydia* and *Hemobartonella* spp. The use of chloramphenicol in food-producing animals is prohibited because of its association with idiosyncratic aplastic anemia in humans. It is used in horses to treat a variety of bacterial infections, especially where penetration into the CNS or sequestered infections is desired.

Mechanism of action

Chloramphenicol and florfenicol act by binding to the 50S ribosomal subunit and blocking transfer RNA, inhibiting bacterial protein synthesis. They are considered bacteriostatic, but the MBCs of florfenicol for some respiratory pathogens are low enough to consider it bactericidal.

Resistance mechanisms

Bacterial resistance to chloramphenicol occurs from plasmid-mediated bacterial production of acetylase enzymes. Acetylation of hydroxyl groups prevents the drug binding to the 50S ribosomal subunit. There is less bacterial resistance to florfenicol because of the substitution of a fluorine molecule for one of the hydroxyl groups.

Pharmacokinetics

Chloramphenicol is not administered i.v. to horses because of its short half-life, which precludes achieving therapeutic plasma concentrations. Injections of chloramphenicol i.m. are associated with severe pain in horses and are not recommended. Chloramphenicol and florfenicol are absorbed rapidly and extensively after p.o. administration to horses. The bioavailability was 83% after p.o. administration of chloramphenicol to neonatal foals and of florfenicol in an organic solvent.

Chloramphenicol and florfenicol distribute widely throughout the body. The highest drug levels are attained in the liver and kidneys, but therapeutic drug concentrations are attained in most tissues and fluids, including the ocular humors and synovial fluid. Chloramphenicol may achieve CSF concentrations of up to 50% of plasma concentrations, when the meninges are normal, or higher, when inflammation is present. Florfenicol does not penetrate the blood–brain barrier as readily as chloramphenicol but may reach therapeutic concentrations for some sensitive pathogens in the CSF. The V_d of chloramphenicol is 1.41 l/kg in adult horses and 1.6 l/kg in neonatal foals. The V_d of florfenicol is 0.72 l/kg in adult horses. After a single i.m. administration of a long-acting florfenicol preparation to horses at a dose rate of 20 mg/kg, peak plasma concentrations of 1–2 µg/ml were reached after 3 h and plasma concentrations were still >0.25 µg/ml after 72 h.

Chloramphenicol and florfenicol undergo hepatic metabolism (glucuronide conjugation) followed by active renal tubular secretion. Only 5–15% of the dose is excreted unchanged (glomerular filtration) in urine. The half-life of chloramphenicol and florfenicol are <1 h and 1.8 h, respectively, following i.v. administration to horses.

Drug interactions and adverse effects

Chloramphenicol is a hepatic microsomal enzyme inhibitor. It decreases the clearance of other drugs that are metabolized by the same enzymes (e.g. phenytoin, phenobarbital, pentobarbital and cyclophosphamide). It is not known if florfenicol has this effect. Chloramphenicol also profoundly prolongs the duration of barbiturate anesthesia. Therapeutic drug monitoring should be carried out when any of these drugs are used concurrently with chloramphenicol. Chloramphenicol may suppress antibody production if given prior to an antigenic stimulus and may affect the response to vaccination. Chloramphenicol and florfenicol should not be administered concurrently with the penicillins and aminoglycosides (they may antagonize the activity of the penicillins and aminoglycosides), fluoroquinolones (they inhibit protein synthesis and thus interfere with the production of autolysins responsible for cell lysis after the fluoroquinolones interfere with DNA supercoiling) or macrolides (they act at the same site as the macrolides).

Idiosyncratic aplastic anemia occurs only in humans exposed to chloramphenicol. The reaction is rare (1 in 30 000) and not dose related. The toxic effects are related to the presence of the para-nitro group on the chloramphenicol molecule. Florfenicol lacks this group and is not associated with aplastic anemia in any species. Long-term chloramphenicol therapy (>14 days) is associated with dose-related anemia and pancytopenia through a decrease in protein synthesis in the bone marrow, especially in cats. Florfenicol may cause similar reversible suppression of the myeloid series in bone marrow, but this does not appear to be clinically significant during short-term treatment regimens.

Florfenicol is associated with producing transient diarrhea in calves and has been associated anecdotally with severe colitis in horses. In one pharmacokinetic study, all of the horses and ponies developed mild diarrhea following i.v., i.m. or p.o. administration of florfenicol. In a recent study where the commercial florfenicol formulation was administered i.m. to horses at 20 mg/kg every 48 h, all of the horses remained clinically normal but showed significant changes in commensal fecal flora. High numbers of *Clostridium perfringens* and *Salmonella* spp. were isolated from some of the treated horses. Florfenicol should be used with caution in horses because of its potential to induce antimicrobial-associated colitis.

Formulations

A water-soluble formulation of chloramphenicol sodium succinate is available for i.v. use. Chloramphenicol succinate is hydrolyzed to chloramphenicol in the liver. Chloramphenicol palmitate is an insoluble ester suitable for p.o. administration. Chloramphenicol palmitate is hydrolyzed to chloramphenicol in the gastrointestinal tract. Chloramphenicol (generic and veterinary labeled) is also available in a variety of tablet and capsule strengths. A long-acting formulation of florfenicol is approved for i.m. and s.c. administration to cattle. This formulation contains three carriers (propylene glycol, polyethylene glycol and 2-pyrrolidone) that make it unsuitable for i.v. administration. This product causes minor pain and swelling following administration into the neck muscles in horses.

POTENTIATED SULFONAMIDES

Indications

The sulfonamides are a group of organic compounds with chemotherapeutic activity; they are antimicrobial agents and not antibiotics. They have a common chemical nucleus that is closely related to PABA, an essential component in the folic acid pathway of nucleic acid synthesis. The sulfonamides are synergistic with the diaminopyrimidines, which inhibit an essential step further along the folate pathway. The combination of a sulfonamide and a diaminopyrimidine is advantageous because it is relatively non-toxic to mammalian cells (less sulfonamide is administered) and is less likely to select for resistant bacteria. Only these so-called potentiated sulfonamides are used in equine medicine. These drugs are formulated in a ratio of one part diaminopyrimidine to five parts sulfonamide, but the optimal antimicrobial ratio at the tissue level is 1:20, which is achieved because the diaminopyrimidines are excreted more rapidly than the sulfonamides.

Potentiated sulfonamides are usually active against streptococci, staphylococci, *C. perfringens* and some *Fusobacterium* and *Bacteroides* spp., *Nocardia* spp. and some Gram-negative bacteria, including strains of *E. coli* and *Shigella, Salmonella, Klebsiella, Pasteurella* and *Proteus* spp. They are considered ineffective against most obligate anaerobes and should not be used to treat serious anaerobic infections. Trimethoprim and pyrimethamine are diaminopyrimidines that are used most commonly in combination with the sulfonamides and the MIC of pathogens is generally lowered in such a combination.

Pyrimethamine is an aminopyrimidine agent that is structurally related to trimethoprim but is more active against protozoa than bacteria. It is most effective against protozoa when administered in conjunction with a sulfonamide. In humans, pyrimethamine is used in the treatment of toxoplasmosis and malaria. In horses, it is used in combination with a sulfonamide drug in the treatment of equine protozoal myeloencephalitis (EPM) caused by *Sarcocystis neurona* (see Chs 3 and 9).

Mechanism of action

In the folic acid pathway, the sulfonamides inhibit the bacterial enzyme dihydropteroate synthetase (DPS), thereby blocking bacterial nucleic acid synthesis. Sulfonamides substitute for PABA, preventing its conversion into dihydrofolic acid. This action is considered bacteriostatic. Since the antimicrobial activity is by competitive substitution, tissue concentrations of sulfonamides must be high enough to prevent bacterial access to PABA. Sulfonamides are ineffective in pus and necrotic tissue where there are additional sources of PABA. They are safe to mammalian cells because mammalian cells do not require PABA and synthesize dihydrofolic acid from dietary folate. Trimethoprim and pyrimethamine inhibit bacterial folic-acid synthesis at the step subsequent to that affected by sulfonamides. They inhibit the conversion of dihydrofolic acid to tetrahydrofolic acid by inhibiting dihydrofolate reductase (DHFR). Bacterial and protozoal DHFR are significantly more tightly bound by the diaminopyrimidines than mammalian DHFR. When a diaminopyrimidine is combined with a sulfonamide, the action is synergistic and the combination is bactericidal.

Mechanisms of resistance

Resistance to the sulfonamides occurs via chromosomal mutation or is plasmid mediated. Chromosomal mutation results in hyperproduction of PABA in bacteria, which overcomes the competitive substitution of the sulfonamides. These mutations are of minor clinical significance. The most common form of bacterial resistance to sulfonamides is via the plasmid-encoded production of altered forms of DPS. More than 50 years of widespread use of the sulfonamides in animal health has resulted in widespread resistance.

Resistance to the diaminopyrimidines usually occurs by plasmid-encoded production of diaminopyrimidine-resistant DHFR. Excessive bacterial production of DHFR and a reduction in the ability of the drug to penetrate the bacterial cell wall also results in resistance. There is less resistance to the potentiated sulfonamides than to the individual agents.

Pharmacokinetics

In general, the sulfonamides are readily absorbed from the gastrointestinal tract of non-ruminants. Absorption may be delayed when the potentiated sulfonamides are administered with feed. Initial serum concentrations are lower in a fed horse than a fasted horse but the food effect is greatly reduced by the third treatment day. The bioavailability of one formulation of pyrimethamine is 56% following p.o. administration.

Sulfonamides are weak acids. They distribute well but relatively slowly (compared with trimethoprim), and tissue concentrations are lower than plasma concentrations. Some sulfonamides reach significant concentrations in the CSF. The highest drug concentrations are in the liver, kidneys and lungs; lower levels are achieved in muscle and bone. Sulfonamides cross the placenta and some may achieve therapeutic concentrations in milk. Some are highly protein bound; protein binding varies with both the species and the drug. The V_d values in horses for sulfamethazine, sulfadoxine and sulfadiazine are 0.63, 0.39 and 0.58 l/kg, respectively.

Diaminopyrimidines are weak bases. Peak plasma concentrations are reached early and diaminopyrimidines are soon found in high concentrations in tissues. In fact, the tissue concentrations are often higher than the concentrations in serum. When inflammation is present, trimethoprim levels in the CSF may reach 50% of the plasma concentrations. CSF concentrations of pyrimethamine are 25–50% of the plasma concentrations. The V_d for trimethoprim and pyrimethamine is 1.5 l/kg in horses. The protein binding of trimethoprim is moderate (50%). There is no protein-binding interaction between the sulfonamides and the diaminopyrimidines.

Sulfonamides are metabolized in the liver, usually by acetylation, glucuronidation and aromatic hydroxylation. The type of metabolite formed and the amount of each varies depending on the sulfonamide administered and the species, age, diet and environment of the animal treated. The metabolites have little antimicrobial effect but may compete with the parent drug in folic acid synthesis. The kidneys eliminate parent drug and metabolites by glomerular filtration and active tubular secretion. Reabsorption, by passive diffusion, occurs in the distal tubules. Most sulfonamides are weak acids; therefore, they are predominantly ionized and excreted in alkaline urine. In acidic urine they are unionized and reabsorbed. In horses, only 43% of a dose of sulfamethazine is excreted in the urine and only 7.8% of this is in the form of the unchanged parent drug. Relatively small amounts of the sulfonamides are distributed into milk, saliva and the gastrointestinal tract. The half-lives in horses of sulfamethazine, sulfadoxine, sulfadiazine and sulfamethoxazole are 5.4–11, 10–14, 3–4 and 3.5–5 h, respectively.

Trimethoprim is metabolized in the liver to oxide and hydroxyl metabolites. It is eliminated by glomerular filtration and active tubular secretion in the kidneys. In horses, a large percentage of trimethoprim is metabolized before excretion in urine (46%) and feces (52%). The clearance of trimethoprim is affected by urine pH, plasma concentrations and the degree of hydration. In horses, the half-life of trimethoprim is 2–3 h and for pyrimethamine it is 12 h.

There is considerable controversy regarding dosage regimens of the potentiated sulfonamides, which are very difficult to determine based on pharmacokinetic principles since each drug has a different absorption, distribution and elimination. Different pathogens have different MICs and the optimal ratio of diaminopyrimidine to sulfonamide varies depending on the pathogen. Clinically, the most important component of the formulation appears to be the diaminopyrimidine; the choice of sulfonamide seems not to be nearly as important. Registered veterinary potentiated sulfonamide products are indicated for once daily administration based on the pharmacokinetics of the sulfonamides; however, twice daily dosing is required to attain therapeutic plasma concentrations of the diaminopyrimidines.

Drug interactions and adverse effects

Sulfonamides should not be administered with coumarin anticoagulants (e.g. warfarin) as their antimicrobial activity against vitamin K-synthesizing bacteria in the gastrointestinal tract can increase the toxicity of the anticoagulant. Concurrent use of bone marrow depressants may increase the leukopenic and thrombocytopenic effects of folate antagonism of the sulfonamides or diaminopyrimidines. It is assumed that animals have the same tendency as humans to develop signs of folate deficiency during long-term administration or with high doses of folic acid antagonists. Signs of folate deficiency include agranulocytosis, megaloblastic anemia and thrombocytopenia. Complete blood and platelet counts should be performed on a regular basis, especially during long-term or high-dose treatment.

Sulfonamides cross the placenta and are teratogenic at very high doses. Potentiated sulfonamides have been associated with abortion in pregnant mares treated for equine protozoal myeloencephalitis (EPM; see Ch. 3) in the absence of folate supplementation. However, folate administration did not prevent fetal defects (renal and bone marrow hypoplasia) in foals born to one group of treated pregnant mares. Despite folate supplementation, both mares and foals had lower than normal serum folate levels. Folate and the diaminopyrimidines use the same intestinal carrier for absorption, so if used concurrently they should be administered at least 2 h apart. The risk of congenital defects should be considered when treating pregnant mares with potentiated sulfonamides. When trimethoprim/sulfamethoxazole was given at recommended doses to pony stallions, no changes in spermatogenesis were noted. However, these stallions developed neurological signs that could be mistaken for clinical signs of EPM.

Phenylbutazone may displace the sulfonamides from plasma protein-binding sites, increasing plasma sulfonamide concentrations. Procaine (in procaine benzylpenicillin (procaine penicillin)) is a PABA analog and may reduce the antimicrobial activity of the sulfonamides. Crystallization of the sulfonamides may occur in the kidneys or in urine in dehydrated animals or following the administration of high doses. The solubility of the sulfonamides in urine is dependent on urine pH, urine drug concentration and the animal's hydration status. The risk of crystalluria can be minimized by maintaining a high urine flow and by alkalizing the urine. Hepatic insufficiency may reduce sulfonamide metabolism and renal function impairment may reduce elimination, thereby increasing the risk of adverse effects. Rifampin increases the elimination rate of trimethoprim and these agents should not be used concurrently.

The potentiated sulfonamides have been associated with producing diarrhea in horses. In one study, changes in coliforms and clostridia were not seen following p.o. administration of tri-methoprim/sulfadiazine. However, in a study of hospitalized horses, the risk of diarrhea was significantly increased when horses had been given a potentiated sulfonamide and procaine benzyl-penicillin (procaine penicillin) concurrently.

The injectable formulations of potentiated sulfonamides are suspensions; consequently, rapid i.v. administration causes hypotension and collapse. Fatal dysrhythmias are associated with the potentiated sulfonamides administered i.v. concurrently with the α_2-adrenergic agonist deto-midine. It is suspected that the potentiated sulfonamide formulation potentiates the cardiac changes produced by detomidine. This adverse reaction has not been reported for the other α_2-adrenergic agonists xylazine and romifidine.

Formulations

Oral paste and powder formulations of trimetho-prim/sulfadiazine are approved for use in horses. An injectable suspension of trimetho-prim/sulfadiazine (48%) is available for i.v. or i.m. administration to horses. Injections must be administered slowly i.v. to avoid collapse and i.m.

injections are painful. An injectable suspension of trimethoprim/sulfadoxine that is approved for administration to cattle is often used in horses (extra label). An injectable solution and oral tablets and suspension containing trimethoprim/sulfamethoxazole are approved for use in humans and are used frequently in horses. Pyrimethamine is available as 25 mg tablets for p.o. administration. Veterinary compounding pharmacies commonly concoct a pyrimethamine/sulfadiazine powder, which can easily be added to a horse's feed, for the treatment of EPM.

TETRACYCLINES

Indications

Tetracycline was discovered after a team of workers examined 100 000 soil samples from around the world. Tetracycline derivatives include chlor-tetracycline, oxytetracycline, doxycycline and minocycline. The tetracyclines have a broad spectrum of activity; they are effective against Gram-positive and Gram-negative bacteria, some anaerobes, *Chlamydia*, *Mycoplasma*, *Ehrlichia* and *Rickettsia* spp. and some protozoa. Their activity against staphylococci is usually limited and they are not active against enterococci. *E. coli*, *Klebsiella*, *Proteus* and *Pseudomonas* spp. are usually resistant. Doxycycline and minocycline are usually more active in vitro than the other tetra-cyclines. Differences in the clinical efficacy of the tetracyclines can be attributed to differences in the absorption, distribution and excretion of the individual drugs rather than to differences in bacterial susceptibility.

Oxytetracycline and doxycycline are used in horses. Oxytetracycline is the drug of choice for Potomac horse fever, caused by *Ehrlichia risticii*, and equine ehrlichiosis, caused by *Ehrlichia equi*. It is also used to treat contracted flexor tendons in foals, where the effects may be caused by calcium chelation at the myotendinous junction resulting in the relaxation of the flexor tendons. Some clinicians use parenteral oxytetracycline or p.o. doxycycline to treat horses with EPM.

Mechanism of action

Tetracyclines bind to the 30S ribosomal subunit and interfere with bacterial protein synthesis. They are bacteriostatic at normal therapeutic concentrations, but bactericidal at high concentrations. They enter bacteria by passive diffusion and an active carrier-mediated process. Mammalian cells do not possess the tetracycline transport mechanism. The tetracyclines are most active at acidic pH, which is of benefit in the treatment of abscesses.

Mechanisms of resistance

Acquired bacterial resistance to the tetracyclines has become widespread in animal populations and has severely reduced the usefulness of these drugs. Resistance to the tetracyclines results from plasmid-mediated mechanisms that prevent the active transport of the drug into the bacterial cell or increase the efflux of drug from the bacterial cell.

Pharmacokinetics

The tetracyclines are amphoteric compounds with high lipid solubility. The absorption and bioavailability of oxytetracycline following parenteral administration varies depending on the formulation and the injection site. Oxytetracycline formulated in polyethylene glycol (PEG) has a bioavailability of 83% following i.m. administration to horses. Long-acting formulations, approved for use in cattle, have a rapid absorption phase that is followed by a slow absorption phase to produce the "long-acting" effect. Absorption from the neck muscles is typically more rapid and complete than from the hindquarters. Tetracyclines are often administered p.o. but their absorption can be erratic and unpredictable and may be decreased by food. The bioavailability following p.o. administration is lowest for chlortetracycline (30%), intermediate for tetracycline and oxytetracycline (60–80%) and highest for doxycycline (95%).

The tetracyclines are distributed into most tissues, except the CNS (therapeutic levels may be achieved when the meninges are inflamed). Doxycycline is the most lipid-soluble tetracycline and has the greatest degree of tissue penetration. The tetracyclines diffuse readily into milk. The V_d of oxytetracycline is 0.34–0.95 l/kg in adult horses and 2.17 l/kg in foals. The pharmacokinetics of doxycycline in horses has not been published. Oxytetracycline is moderately protein bound in horses (50%). Doxycycline is highly protein bound in other species (90%).

Tetracycline, chlortetracycline and oxytetracycline are excreted unchanged in urine, primarily by glomerular filtration. Parent drug is also eliminated unchanged into the gastrointestinal tract in bile. Doxycycline is excreted primarily in an inactive form in the feces via non-biliary routes. Doxycycline does not accumulate in subjects with renal insufficiency. After i.v. administration to horses of oxytetracycline-PEG the half-life of drug is 6 h. Following i.m. administration, it has a "long-acting effect" and a half-life of 22 h.

Drug interactions and adverse effects

In horses, oxytetracycline administration has been associated with proliferation of *Clostridium* and *Salmonella* spp., resulting in potentially fatal colitis. However, the cases reported typically involved stress, surgery, transportation and the concurrent use of multiple antimicrobial agents. Recent studies have demonstrated minimal changes in the fecal flora and no other adverse effects in horses given multiple i.m. doses of oxytetracycline-PEG.

Rapid i.v. administration of tetracyclines can result in hypotension and collapse. This has been attributed to intravascular chelation of calcium and/or a decrease in blood pressure owing to the drug vehicle. The i.v. administration of doxycycline to horses causes tachycardia, systemic arterial hypertension, collapse and death. This reaction may be caused by the highly lipid-soluble doxycycline chelating intracellular calcium, resulting in cardiac neuromuscular blockade.

Renal tubular necrosis following oxytetracycline administration is associated with high doses, expired parenteral products and concurrent endotoxemia, dehydration and/or pigment nephropathy.

Tetracyclines bind to teeth and bone. This may result in discoloration of the teeth and inhibition of bone growth in fetuses exposed *in utero*. Tooth discoloration may occur in young animals when tetracyclines are administered during permanent tooth development.

Formulations

Many formulations containing oxytetracycline (50 or 100 mg/ml) in propylene glycol (approved for i.v. or i.m. administration to food-producing animals) are used extra label in horses. Long-acting formulations of oxytetracycline (200 mg/ml) formulated in PEG, 2-pyrrolidone, glycerol formal or *N,N*-dimethylacetamide are approved for use in cattle. Only the oxytetracycline in PEG formulation can be administered i.m. to horses; the other formulations are irritant. Oxytetracycline in PEG or 2-pyrrolidone may be administered i.v. but as such will not be long acting.

FLUOROQUINOLONES

Indications

The quinolones are a group of synthetic antimicrobial agents. The first, nalidixic acid, was introduced in 1964. Nalidixic acid had good activity against Gram-negative bacteria, but had a low V_d and produced serious side-effects, so its use was limited to treatment of urinary tract infections. Further chemical manipulation resulted in the development of the fluorinated quinolones, agents with an extended spectrum of activity and improved safety. This group includes ciprofloxacin, enrofloxacin, danofloxacin, difloxacin, sarafloxacin, norfloxacin, orbifloxacin, marbofloxacin, ofloxacin and ibafloxacin. New fluoroquinolones are being developed for use in human and veterinary medicine.

The fluoroquinolones have a broad spectrum of activity including most aerobic Gram-negative bacteria, some aerobic Gram-positive bacteria and *Mycoplasma*, *Chlamydia* and *Rickettsia* spp. They are particularly effective against the enteric Gram-negative pathogens, including some strains resistant to the cephalosporins and the aminoglycosides. The MICs reported for the fluoroquinolones are very low and the MBCs are one to two times the MIC for most pathogens. These are the only p.o. antimicrobial agents available that have efficacy against *Pseudomonas* spp. They are usually active against staphylococci, including MRSA. They have variable activity against streptococci and enterococci and are ineffective against anaerobic bacteria. This may confer a therapeutic advantage in the treatment of enteric infections in large animals, where anaerobes rarely cause disease and usually protect the gastrointestinal tract by competitively inhibiting the colonization by pathogenic aerobic organisms.

Mechanism of action

The fluoroquinolones have a unique mechanism of action. They act directly on the bacterial cell nucleus by inhibiting bacterial DNA gyrase (topoisomerase). Bacteria have a single chromosome that consists of double-stranded DNA. Within the bacterial cell, the chromosome is folded around a RNA core and each DNA fold is supercoiled by DNA gyrase. DNA gyrase has four subunits: two A monomers and two B monomers. The enzyme forms a heart-shaped molecule, with the A monomers forming the "atria" and the B monomers the "ventricles". Bacterial DNA binds to the topoisomerase in the cleft between the A and B subunits. The enzyme nicks the double-stranded DNA, introduces negative supercoils and reseals the DNA. The fluoroquinolones bind to the DNA–DNA gyrase complex and inhibit this resealing, resulting in an abnormal spatial configuration of the DNA, which leads to its degradation by bacterial autolysins.

Fluoroquinolone activity is concentration dependent. All of the fluoroquinolones are bactericidal; however, these drugs have an optimal bactericidal concentration: higher or lower drug concentrations result in reduced bactericidal activity. It is thought that the DNA–DNA gyrase complex has two binding sites for fluoroquinolones. At low drug concentrations, only one binding site is occupied, resulting in single-stranded nicks remaining in the DNA. Reduced killing at high concentrations is thought to be a consequence of the dose-dependent inhibition of RNA or protein synthesis. RNA and protein synthesis are required for the production of the bacterial autolysins that are responsible for quinolone-induced cell lysis. This explains the antagonism between fluoroquinolones and antimicrobial agents that inhibit RNA and protein synthesis such as chloramphenicol and rifampin.

The fluoroquinolones are concentrated within phagocytic cells by simple diffusion. Intracellular concentrations may be several times greater than plasma concentrations. Intracellular drug is microbiologically active; *in vitro* studies indicate that ciprofloxacin reduces the survival of intracellular pathogens such as *Brucella*, *Mycoplasma* and *Mycobacterium* spp. Exposure of Gram-negative bacteria to fluoroquinolones at concentrations several times the MIC for 1–2 h results in a PAE of 1–6 h. This suggests that fluoroquinolone dosage regimens can include extended periods where plasma concentrations are below the MIC of a pathogen.

Resistance mechanisms

Microbial resistance to the fluoroquinolones results from chromosomal mutations that alter bacterial DNA gyrase, decrease cell wall permeability or increase fluoroquinolone efflux from bacterial cells. The most common mechanism of resistance is an alteration in the bacterial DNA gyrase that results in decreased fluoroquinolone binding to the DNA–DNA gyrase complex. This occurs as a result of point mutations in the gene coding for the A subunit of the enzyme. Most mutations identified involve substitution of the serine at position 83 by leucine or tryptophan. The substitution of the hydroxyl group of the serine residue with the bulkier hydrophilic groups of leucine and tryptophan results in physical obstruction of the binding of the fluoroquinolone to the DNA–DNA gyrase complex. The quinolone-sensitive A subunit (A_s) is dominant over the quinolone-resistant A subunit (A_r): DNA gyrase composed of both A_s and A_r subunits is as sensitive as gyrase composed of A_s subunits alone. Gyrase mutations confer a high level of cross-resistance to all fluoroquinolones

but are not associated with resistance to other unrelated antimicrobial agents.

Fluoroquinolones must penetrate bacteria to reach their target, DNA gyrase. The second mechanism of fluoroquinolone resistance is decreased cell wall permeability. The fluoroquinolones diffuse through porin channels in the outer membrane of Gram-negative bacteria. Mutation results in a decrease in porin channel proteins, resulting in decreased uptake of the fluoroquinolones into bacterial cells. Alterations in a wide range of outer membrane proteins in *Pseudomonas* spp. result in resistance. From these mutations, the increase in MIC of the fluoroquinolones is relatively low (2- to 32-fold). However, there is cross-resistance with unrelated antibiotics, most frequently cefoxitin, chloramphenicol, trimethoprim and tetracycline.

The third mechanism of resistance is increased fluoroquinolone efflux, an energy-dependent process in the inner bacterial membrane that exports drug into the periplasm or out of the cell. This type of resistance has only been identified in *Staph. aureus* and is associated with the presence of a resistance gene, *norA*. This appears to be a single point mutation, where alanine is substituted for asparagine. The degree of resistance conferred by this mechanism is less than that caused by *gyrA* mutation, but the increases in the MICs are sufficient to produce resistant mutants during fluoroquinolone therapy. In addition, this mechanism of resistance has the potential to become plasmid mediated.

The fluoroquinolones have been used intensively in human medicine in the 1990s, resulting in a high level of resistance in some pathogens. In resistant strains, more than one mechanism is responsible for resistance; usually two or three mechanisms operating in conjunction. In resistant *Staph. aureus*, increased efflux is often coupled with *gyrA* mutation. In resistant *E. coli*, *gyrA* mutation is usually associated with changes in the outer membrane proteins.

Pharmacokinetics

Injections of enrofloxacin i.v. are well tolerated by horses. Enrofloxacin is well absorbed after i.m. administration but is irritant. The fluoroquinolones are rapidly and well absorbed from the gastrointestinal tract of monogastric animals and preruminant calves. The bioavailability of enrofloxacin is 50–60% after p.o. administration to horses, but for ciprofloxacin in ponies it is only 6%.

The fluoroquinolones are extremely lipid soluble and distribute well. The V_d of enrofloxacin is 2–51/kg in most species. Tissue concentrations greatly exceed plasma concentrations during therapy. Extremely high concentrations are achieved in the kidneys, urine, liver and bile. After multiple p.o. doses, urine, endometrial tissue and synovial fluid concentrations in horses are higher than serum concentrations. Therapeutic concentrations may be achieved in the CSF. High concentrations occur in milk. The protein binding is low (22%).

The fluoroquinolones are predominantly excreted unchanged in urine following glomerular filtration and active tubular secretion. Enrofloxacin is partially metabolized (de-ethylated) to ciprofloxacin and other active metabolites. Ciprofloxacin concentrations reach 20–35% of enrofloxacin concentrations in serum. For some pathogens, the MICs for ciprofloxacin are lower than for enrofloxacin; therefore, ciprofloxacin contributes to the efficacy of enrofloxacin. The half-life of enrofloxacin in horses is 6–7h, while for ciprofloxacin in ponies it is 2.5h.

Drug interactions and adverse effects

The fluoroquinolones have been used in combination with other antimicrobial agents to expand their therapeutic spectrum, to suppress the emergence of drug-resistant bacterial populations or to exploit inhibitory or bactericidal synergism (a four-fold or greater decrease in MIC or MBC for each antimicrobial) against drug-resistant populations. There is minimal synergy between the fluoroquinolones and the beta-lactams or aminoglycosides against Gram-negative enteric bacteria. This may be because of the already high susceptibility of these organisms to the fluoroquinolones. Combination with the beta-lactams, aminoglycosides or vancomycin is additive or indifferent against staphylococci. The fluoroquinolones are antagonistic to chloramphenicol or rifampin owing to the inhibition of bacterial autolysin synthesis following the concurrent administration of bacterial protein synthesis inhibitors. The fluoroquinolones interfere with the metabolism of methylxanthines such as theophylline. Serum concentrations of theophylline or aminophylline may double and so must be monitored during concurrent therapy.

Chronic administration of high doses of the fluoroquinolones causes articular cartilage lesions in young puppies. Transient arthropathy occurs when ciprofloxacin is used in the therapy of *Pseudomonas* spp. pneumonia in children with cystic fibrosis. Arthropathy has not been reported in calves, swine, or poultry. Arthropathy has been documented in 2-week-old foals given enrofloxacin p.o. at a dose rate of 10mg/kg but was not seen in adult horses given enrofloxacin i.v. at up to 25mg/kg for 3 weeks. Despite the risk of arthropathy, the fluoroquinolones have been used with clinical success in septic foals when the treatment options were limited. Joint lesions are most severe in weight-bearing, diarthrodial joints, so if fluoroquinolones are administered to foals exercise should be severely limited.

In general, the fluoroquinolones are not recommended for use during pregnancy. However, the fluoroquinolones available currently are not teratogenic in laboratory animals. Moreover, women treated with ciprofloxacin and pregnant mares treated with enrofloxacin did not have an increase in abortions or birth defects.

Hallucinations, photosensitivity reactions and Achilles tendon rupture have been associated with fluoroquinolone use in humans but have not been reported in animals.

Formulations

Ciprofloxacin (40mg/ml) is approved for i.v. administration to humans. This formulation must be diluted and administered slowly and is extremely expensive. Enrofloxacin is available as an injectable solution (50mg/ml) and tablets for p.o. administration to small animals and as a solution (100mg/ml) for s.c. administration to cattle. Both of these injectable solutions may be administered safely by i.v. injection (extra label) to horses and the tablets for small animal may be ground up and administered p.o. to horses.

MACROLIDES

Indications

The macrolide antibiotics include erythromycin, clarithromycin, azithromycin, tylosin, tilmicosin and tiamulin. Clindamycin and lincomycin are related lincosamides. Susceptible bacteria include staphylococci, streptococci, *Campylobacter jejunii*, *Clostridium* spp., *R. equi*, *Mycoplasma pneumoniae* and *Chlamydia* spp. Drugs in this group are only effective against a few Gram-negative bacteria in cattle, namely some strains of *Pasteurella* and *Haemophilus* spp. Macrolides and lincosamides are associated with causing colitis in horses, so their use is usually restricted to p.o. erythromycin for the treatment of *R. equi* infections in foals. Subantimicrobial doses of erythromycin are administered i.v. to horses for gastrointestinal prokinetic action.

Mechanism of action

Macrolides bind to the 50S ribosomal subunit, in a manner similar to chloramphenicol and florfenicol, and interfere with bacterial protein synthesis. They are usually considered bacteriostatic but may be bactericidal at high concentrations. The antimicrobial activity of erythromycin is pH dependent. Optimum activity occurs at a pH of 8.8; activity is reduced in acidic environments such as abscesses.

Mechanisms of resistance

The routine use of the macrolides is limited because bacterial resistance develops quickly following repeated exposure. There can be cross-resistance between the drugs in this class. The mechanisms of resistance include decreased drug entry into bacteria, inability to bind to the 50S ribosomal subunit and the plasmid-mediated production of macrolide-destroying esterase.

Pharmacokinetics

Erythromycin formulations are highly irritant if administered by i.m. injection and are not used in horses. Many p.o. preparations of erythromycin are enteric coated to allow passage into the small intestine, where absorption is higher because of the higher pH. In horses, erythromycin stearate and erythromycin phosphate produce peak plasma concentrations faster than the ester formulations following p.o. administration.

The macrolides distribute well and tissue concentrations may be higher than serum concentrations. Erythromycin concentrates and is active in leukocytes because of its high lipid solubility and ion trapping. The V_d of erythromycin is 3.7–7.21/kg in adult horses and foals. The protein binding is low. The hepatic clearance of the macrolides may be slower in animals of up to 1 month of age than in adult animals.

Erythromycin is extensively metabolized, with much of the unchanged parent drug and active metabolite eliminated in bile, resulting in a short half-life (1–3 h). Erythromycin undergoes enterohepatic recirculation, which may contribute to the adverse gastrointestinal effects seen in adult horses.

Drug interactions and adverse effects

Macrolides are metabolized in the liver via the microsomal (cytochrome P450) enzyme system. The alkylxanthines (e.g. theophylline, aminophylline) utilize the same enzyme system, so concurrent administration with macrolides leads to a doubling of the alkylxanthine concentration and toxicity. Because of similar mechanisms of action, concurrent administration of other macrolides, lincosamides, chloramphenicol or florfenicol is not recommended.

Agents in this group, especially clindamycin and lincomycin, are associated with bacterial overgrowth in the colon. Serious and potentially fatal diarrhea may occur in humans, rabbits, ruminants and horses. Foals appear to be less susceptible to erythromycin-induced diarrhea than adult horses and the ethylsuccinate formulation seems to be the least likely to induce diarrhea.

Fatal colitis has been reported in mares with foals that were being treated with p.o. erythromycin. Erythromycin may also induce diarrhea because of its prokinetic action. It mimics the effects of the hormone motilin on the enteric nervous system, and subantimicrobial doses stimulate small intestinal, cecal and colonic motility.

Administration of erythromycin i.m. is very painful and this route is not used in horses. The i.m. formulation cannot be safely administered i.v.

Erythromycin may reduce the normal thermoregulatory response to hyperthermia. Erythromycin has been associated with hyperthermia in foals. Treated foals that are turned out on hot, sunny, humid days develop fever, tachypnea and distress, which may result in fatal heat stroke.

Formulations

Erythromycin glucceptate and erythromycin lactobionate are approved for i.v. use in humans. Several delayed-release p.o. formulations are available because erythromycin is unstable in gastric acid: enteric-coated erythromycin tablets and erythromycin stearate, ethylsuccinate and estolate.

RIFAMPIN

Indications

Rifampin is effective against *Staph. aureus*, *Haemophilus* spp., *R. equi* and a variety of mycobacteria. At very high concentrations, it has activity against poxviruses and adenoviruses. Rifampin also has antifungal activity when combined with other antifungal agents. Resistance develops rapidly; therefore, it is usually administered concurrently with another antimicrobial agent. In equine practice, is most commonly used in combination with erythromycin for the treatment of *R. equi* infections in foals. It may also be used in the treatment of refractory osteomyelitis and endocarditis caused by *Staph. aureus*.

Mechanism of action

Rifampin suppresses RNA synthesis by selectively inhibiting DNA-dependent RNA polymerase in susceptible organisms. It has no effect on the mammalian enzyme. Its action is bacteriostatic or bactericidal depending on the susceptibility of the organism and the concentration of the drug.

Mechanisms of resistance

Chromosomal mutation develops readily in most bacteria exposed to rifampin and leads to a high level of resistance. These mutants show stable changes in RNA polymerase that prevent binding. Resistance to rifampin is not transferable and there is no cross-resistance with other antibiotics.

Pharmacokinetics

The bioavailability of rifampin following p.o. administration to horses is 40–70%. The bioavailability is reduced if given with feed, but the current dosage regimens compensate for this.

Rifampin is very lipophilic and penetrates most tissues including mammary glands (milk), bone, abscesses and the CNS. It is concentrated in neutrophils and macrophages and is effective against intracellular pathogens. It is most active at acid pH, making it a rational choice for the treatment of septic foci and granulomatous infections. In horses, the V_d of rifampin is 0.9 l/kg. Rifampin is highly protein bound.

Rifampin is metabolized in the liver to a deacetylated metabolite that also has antibacterial activity. Unchanged drug and the active metabolite are eliminated primarily in bile, but up to 30% may be excreted in urine. The parent drug undergoes extensive enterohepatic recirculation, but the metabolite does not. The half-life of rifampin is 6–8 h in adult horses and 17 h in foals. Repeated dosing results in a decrease in the half-life of rifampin through induction of hepatic enzymes; this may also affect the metabolism of concurrently administered drugs.

Drug interactions and adverse effects

Microsomal enzyme induction may shorten the half-life of rifampin and decrease drug concentrations of concurrently administered chloramphenicol, corticosteroids, itraconazole, ketoconazole, warfarin and barbiturates. Rifampin stains everything it contacts red and treated horses will also produce red urine, feces, tears, sweat and saliva. This has no harmful consequences!

Formulations

Capsules for p.o. administration are approved for use in humans.

METRONIDAZOLE

Indications

Metronidazole is a unique antimicrobial agent that has very little effect on most aerobic Gram-positive and Gram-negative bacteria but is highly effective against anaerobic bacteria, including *B. fragilis* (penicillin-resistant) and *Fusobacterium* and *Clostridium* spp. It also has good activity against protozoa (e.g. *Giardia and Trichomonas* spp.). In horses, it is used to treat sequestered anaerobic infections or infections caused by bacteria resistant to the beta-lactam antibiotics.

Mechanism of action

Bacteria rapidly take up metronidazole and reduce it to cytotoxic short-lived free radicals. These compounds damage DNA and other critical intracellular macromolecules. Aerobic bacteria lack the reductive pathway necessary to produce these free radicals.

Mechanisms of resistance

Resistance involves reduced intracellular drug activation and is rare among usually susceptible bacteria. There is one report of metronidazole-resistant isolates of *B. fragilis* from a horse with pleuropneumonia.

Pharmacokinetics

Metronidazole is rapidly and well absorbed after p.o. administration to horses, with a bioavailability of 58–91%. Therapeutic concentrations are attained after administration of metronidazole per rectum to horses with gastrointestinal stasis.

Metronidazole is lipophilic and distributes widely. Peritoneal fluid and milk concentrations approach plasma concentrations. It reaches therapeutic concentrations in bone, abscesses and the CNS. It readily crosses the placenta and enters the fetal circulation. In most species, the V_d is 1–2 l/kg.

Metronidazole is metabolized primarily in the liver. Both unchanged drug and metabolites are eliminated in urine and feces. The half-life of metronidazole in horses is 3–4 h.

Drug interactions and adverse effects

Metronidazole is mutagenic (in bacteria) and carcinogenic (following prolonged treatment of laboratory mice); therefore, its use is prohibited in food-producing animals. It has also been implicated as being teratogenic in laboratory animals and so should be avoided in pregnant animals.

Neurotoxicity may occur with metronidazole at recommended doses during prolonged use or at high doses. The signs of this include ataxia, lethargy, anorexia, nystagmus and seizures. Affected animals may recover with supportive therapy.

Formulations

Metronidazole is available as tablets and capsules for human use.

VANCOMYCIN

Indications

Vancomycin is a glycopeptide antibiotic that is very important in human medicine because of its activity against multidrug-resistant organisms such as MRSA and enterococci. Vancomycin is only active against Gram-positive bacteria. In recent years, nosocomial infections of vancomycin-resistant enterococci (VRE) have become a major problem in human hospitals. Recently, a MRSA resistant to vancomycin was isolated from human clinical patients, causing a great deal of concern in human medicine because of the lack of treatment options. Vancomycin inhibits synthesis of bacterial cell wall phospholipids and polymerization of peptidoglycan. Vancomycin resistance results from plasmid-mediated changes in cell wall permeability and decreased binding of vancomycin to receptor molecules. Vancomycin is expensive, must be given parenterally and causes serious adverse effects. There are only a few reports of the use of vancomycin in veterinary medicine.

REFERENCES

Baggot J D 1992 Bioavailability and bioequivalence of veterinary drug dosage forms, with particular reference to horses: an overview. Journal of Veterinary Pharmacology and Therapeutics 15:160–173

Freeman D E 1999 Gastrointestinal pharmacology. Veterinary Clinics of North America Equine Practice 15:535–559

Martinez M N 1998a Physicochemical properties of pharmaceuticals. Journal of the American Veterinary Medical Association 213:1274–1277

Martinez M N 1998b Volume, clearance and half-life. Journal of the American Veterinary Medical Association 213:1122–1127

Martinez M N 1998c Clinical application of pharmacokinetics. Journal of the American Veterinary Medical Association 213:1418–1420

Prescott J F, Holgate S T 1993 Antimicrobial susceptibility and drug dosage prediction. In: Prescott J F, Baggot J D (eds) Antimicrobial therapy in veterinary medicine, 2nd edn. Iowa State University Press, Ames, IA, pp. 11–20

Riviere J E 1999 Comparative pharmacokinetics: principles, techniques and applications. Iowa State University Press, Ames, IA, pp. 47–61

Riviere J E, Webb A I, Craigmill A L 1998 Primer on estimating withdrawal times after extra label drug use. Journal of the American Veterinary Medical Association 213:966–968

Verbist L 1993 Relevance of antibiotic susceptibility testing for clinical practice. European Journal of Clinical Microbiology and Infectious Diseases 12(suppl 1):2–5

Vogelman B, Gudmundsson S, Leggett J et al 1988 Correlation of antimicrobial pharmacokinetic parameters with therapeutic efficacy in an animal model. Journal of Infectious Diseases 158:831–847

Appendix: Overview of the pharmacokinetics, indications and dose rates of antimicrobial agents used in the horse

Antimicrobial agent	Volume of distribution (l/kg)	Half-life (h)	Acid–base status	Protein binding (%)	Elimination	Indications	Dose
Potassium penicillin, sodium penicillin	0.2–0.3	1	Acid	52–54	RE	Streptococcal infections; anaerobic infections	20 000 IU/kg, q.i.d.
Procaine benzylpenicillin (procaine penicillin)		7	Acid		RE	Streptococcal infections; anaerobic infections	25 000 IU/kg, b.i.d.
Ampicillin	0.18	0.5–1.5	Acid	6.8–8	RE	Gram-positive, some Gram-negative and anaerobic infections	10–20 mg/kg i.v. or i.m., t.i.d. to q.i.d.
Cefazolin	0.19	0.6–0.8	Acid	8	HM, RE	Gram-positive, some Gram-negative and anaerobic infections	15 mg/kg i.v., b.i.d. to t.i.d.
Cefalotin	0.15	0.25	Acid	18	HM, RE	Gram-positive, some Gram-negative and anaerobic infections	20–40 mg/kg i.v. or i.m., t.i.d. to q.i.d.
Cefapirin	0.17	0.9	Acid		RE	Gram-positive, some Gram-negative and anaerobic infections	30 mg/kg i.v. or i.m. every 4–6 h
Cefoxitin	0.12	0.8	Acid		RE	Gram-positive, some Gram-negative and anaerobic infections	20 mg/kg i.v. every 4–6 h

(continued)

(continued)

Antimicrobial agent	Volume of distribution (l/kg)	Half-life (h)	Acid–base status	Protein binding (%)	Elimination	Indications	Dose
Ceftiofur		3–5	Acid	99	HM, RE	Gram-positive, some Gram-negative and anaerobic infections	2.2 mg/kg i.m. once daily
Gentamicin	0.12–0.24 (adult), 0.3 (foal)	1–2 (adult)	Base	<30	RE	Staphylococcal and Gram-negative infections	5–7 mg/kg i.v., i.m., s.c. once daily
Amikacin	0.14–0.22 (adult), 0.4–0.6 (foal)	1–3 (adult), 5 (foal)	Base		RE	Infections with bacteria resistant to gentamicin	6 mg/kg i.v., i.m., s.c. once daily; 20 mg/kg i.v. once daily in neonatal foals
Chloramphenicol	1.4 (adult), 1.6 (foal)	<1	Base	Low	HM, RE	Gram-positive, some Gram-negative and anaerobic infections	45–60 mg/kg i.v., i.m., s.c. or p.o., t.i.d. to q.i.d.
Florfenicol	0.72	1.8	Base	Low	HM, RE	Cautious use with infections from resistant bacteria	20 mg/kg i.m. every 4–8 h
Sulfonamides	0.3–0.6	Variable	Acid	Varies	HM, RE	Gram-positive, some Gram-negative and protozoal infections	25 mg p.o. b.i.d.
Trimethoprim	1.5	2–3	Base	50	HM, RE	Gram-positive, some Gram-negative and anaerobic infections	5 mg p.o. b.i.d.
Pyrimethamine	1.5	12	Base	70–80	HM, RE	Protozoal infections	1 mg/kg p.o. once daily
Oxytetracycline	0.34–0.95 (adult), 2.2–4 (foal)	6 (i.v.), 22 (i.m., long acting)	Amphoteric	50	HM, RE	Gram-positive, some Gram-negative and anaerobic infections	7–10 mg/kg i.v. once daily; 20 mg/kg i.m. every 72 h (long acting)
Enrofloxacin	2–5	6–7	Amphoteric	22	HM, RE	Staphylococcal and Gram-negative infections	5–10 mg/kg i.v. or p.o. once daily
Erythromycin	3.7–7.2	1–3	Base	Low	HM, RE	*R. equi* infections	25 mg/kg p.o. once daily
Rifampin	0.9	6–8 (adults), 17 (foals)	Amphoteric	89	HM, RE	*R. equi* infections	5–10 mg/kg p.o. once daily
Metronidazole	1–2	3–4	Base		HM, RE	Anaerobic infections	15–25 mg/kg q.i.d

HM, hepatic metabolism; RE, renal elimination; IU, international units; q.i.d., four times daily; b.i.d., twice daily; i.v., intravenous; i.m., intramuscular; t.i.d., three times daily; s.c., subcutaneous

CHAPTER CONTENTS

Introduction 49

Piroplasmosis/babesiosis 49
Parasite biology 49
Pathogenesis, clinical signs and diagnosis 50
Treatment 51

Trypanosomiasis 53
Parasite biology 53
Pathogenesis, clinical signs and diagnosis 53
Treatment 55

Giardiasis 57
Parasite biology 57
Treatment 57

Coccidiosis (globidiosis) 57
Parasite biology 57
Pathogenesis, clinical signs and diagnosis 57
Treatment 57

Sarcocystis infections: equine protozoal
myeloencephalitis 58
Parasite biology 58
Pathogenesis, clinical signs and diagnosis 58
Treatment 59

Other Sarcocystis infections 61
Parasite biology 61
Pathogenesis, clinical signs and diagnosis 62
Treatment 62

References 62

3

Antiprotozoal drugs

Clara K. Fenger

INTRODUCTION

Horses act as the natural and aberrant hosts for a number of protozoan species spanning a wide range of phyla. This wide diversity means that the drug classes used for the treatment of these different protozoa may be effective against one species and not others. Thus, this chapter is organized by pathogen rather than by drug class.

PIROPLASMOSIS/BABESIOSIS

Protista Apicomplexa Pyroplasma Pyroplasmida Babesiidae *Babesia*.

PARASITE BIOLOGY

Species of the genus *Babesia* are intracellular erythrocyte pathogens transmitted by ticks, with mechanical transmission possible by biting flies such as *Tabanus* spp. Equine piroplasmosis is caused by *B. caballi* and *B. equi*, both of which utilize horses, mules and donkeys as hosts. *B. caballi* is distributed throughout temperate Eurasia (transmitted by *Dermacenter reticulatus* and *D. marginatus*), the Mediterranean basin and central-western Asia (transmitted by *Hyalomma m. marginatum*), North Africa (transmitted by *Hyalomma* spp.) and tropicoequatorial America (transmitted by *Dermacenter nitens*). The known natural tick vectors for *B. equi* are the tropical horse tick, *D. nitens* in the western hemisphere, *Rhipicephalus bursa* in the Mediterranean basin and *Rhipicephalus evertsi* in tropicoequatorial Africa. *Dermacenter* and *Hyalomma* spp. may be implicated in other regions of Africa and *Boophilus microplus* has been shown to be capable of supporting complete development of *B. equi* experimentally.

The *B. caballi* vectors are ticks with two and three hosts and only the adult ticks feed on horses and transmit this protozoan. The adult female tick ingests the *B. caballi* merozoite-infected erythrocyte during its final blood meal before egg laying. The merozoites develop into macrogametocytes, which may continue development as a macrogametocyte (female) or develop into microgametocytes (male) by exflagellation. After fertilization, the zygote goes on to develop into a sporoblast in the cells of the digestive epithelium of the tick. The blasto-zoites develop within these cells, elongate and then escape into the hemocoel of the tick. These blastokinetes (motile protozoa) penetrate multiple tissues of the tick including the ovaries, resulting in transovarial transmission. During the embryo-genesis of the tick, the protozoans multiply, going through several stages of blastozoite, sporoblast and then blastokinete. The terminal blastozoites in the salivary glands of the juvenile tick develop into trophoblasts, which develop into terminal sporocysts; these produce the infective form of the parasite, the metacyclic sporozoites.

The vector ticks of *B. equi* are infected at the nymph stage by feeding on an infected equine host and the protozoan is passed transstadially, through the development stages of the tick to the adult tick, where the infection can be transmitted to another susceptible equine host. *B. equi* differs from *B. caballi* and other *Babesia* spp. in terms of biological behavior, molecular phylogenetics and chemosensitivity, suggesting that it may belong to a different genus. Some authors have, in fact, reclassified this organism as *Theileria equi* (Melhorn & Schein 1998). However, it will be con-sidered here in the section on piroplasmosis and the differences in chemosensitivity discussed.

PATHOGENESIS, CLINICAL SIGNS AND DIAGNOSIS

Infective metacyclic sporozoites in tick saliva are passed directly into the host, where they immedi-ately enter erythrocytes and begin to undergo

asexual reproduction or schizogony. The mero-zoites of *B. equi* have a developmental stage in lymphocytes prior to entry into erythrocytes. As the protozoa reproduce, the erythrocytes are destroyed releasing the piroplasms into the blood-stream and clinical signs of hemolytic anemia occur. The severity of these clinical signs is corre-lated to the degree of parasitemia in both forms of piroplasmosis.

B. caballi produces a great variety of clinical signs and variable disease progression: it may be acute or chronic and mild or severe. The incubation period is 7–19 days; the level of parasitemia is high (50–100%) and there is 10–20% mortality. Anemia and icterus without hemoglobinuria are typical. Locomotor disorders and pelvic limb paralysis, related to cortical congestion, are seen in the acute forms of this disease. Lymphadenitis, peritonitis and pericarditis are usually evident. Horses with chronic disease may have poor gen-eral condition, colic, lethargy and inappetance. Although the mortality rate may be as high as 20% in naive populations of horses, it is much lower in endemic regions. If untreated, horses that recover remain persistently infected. In general, horses that have recovered have a subclinical infection and act as a reservoir of infection for other horses. The disease is considered exotic in the USA, Canada, Australia, New Zealand and Japan, where control measures are in place to prevent its intro-duction. These controls limit the movement of equines and have a profound effect on the equine industry in endemic regions.

B. equi usually causes subacute or acute dis-ease after an incubation period of 10–21 days. Moderate (10–30%) and transient (3–5 days) parasitemia occur and there is 20–50% mortality. If the disease is peracute, death may occur within 2 days of the onset of infection. In acute cases, the process lasts for 8–10 days, after which the ani-mal recovers and becomes a carrier. The first clin-ical sign, around 10 days after a tick bite, is typically high fever (up to 41°C/105.8°F) accom-panied by anemia, hemoglobinuria, icterus and a rapid respiratory rate. Lethargy, depression, anorexia and edema of the head, ventral abdomen and limbs ensue as the disease progresses. Ascites and petechial hemorrhages may be evident.

Equine piroplasmosis is usually diagnosed by examining (peripheral) blood smears for the parasites. This is most sensitive during the acute phase of the infection because the parasites are not usually visible during the latent phase. In the latent phase and in subclinical disease, serology is the most effective method of disease detection. There are complement fixation tests specific for *B. caballi* and *B. equi*, respectively, although there may be some cross-reactivity between the two tests. Both false-positive and false-negative test results can occur, confounding any attempt to view the results of these tests as absolute.

TREATMENT

B. caballi can be treated effectively but there is not a comparable chemotherapeutic approach to the treatment of *B. equi*, where drugs may control the clinical signs of infection but horses often remain life-long carriers. In regions where piroplasmosis is endemic, elimination of the infection may not be desirable because these horses will then be susceptible to reinfection. In these areas, premunition is used: the horses are infected or allowed to become infected and are then treated with sufficient chemotherapy to control the clinical signs but not to eliminate the infection. Horses that have been premunised are thus infected but not affected. This technique permits the development of the carrier state and as a result some resistance (immunity) to reinfection.

Aromatic diamidines

The mechanism of action of this group of compounds is not known but is related to their guanyl group $NH=(NH_2)$. Ultrastructural studies show that these compounds cause dilatation of membrane-bound organelles, dissolution of the cytoplasm and destruction of the nucleus in *Babesia* spp. Compounds with two guanyl groups separated by a hydrocarbon chain have a high level of babesicidal activity, which increases with the length of the hydrocarbon chain. There are three compounds in this class that are used in the treatment of piroplasmosis in horses: diminazene aceturate, phenamidine isoethionate and pentamidine.

Diminazene aceturate

Diminazene aceturate is an odorless, yellow powder that is soluble in water up to a concentration of 7%. It is active, stable, has low toxicity and has bactericidal, babesicidal and trypanocidal properties; it appears to bind directly to parasites. It is effective in the treatment of babesiosis in cattle, sheep and dogs: intramuscular (i.m.) administration of diminazene aceturate at 3.5 mg/kg is followed by the disappearance of the clinical signs of babesiosis within 24 h. In horses, the recommended regimen is two doses administered intramuscularly 24 h apart at 5 mg/kg for the treatment of *B. caballi* and at 6–12 mg/kg for *B. equi*. At these dose rates, the drug effectively clears *B. caballi* infection and eliminates the clinical signs but does not clear *B. equi* infection. It is effective at similar dose rates against *Trypanosoma congolense* and *T. vivax* infections but less active against *T. brucei*, which requires a dose of 7 mg/kg. In persistent trypanosome infections, dose rates of up to 8 mg/kg should be given, divided into two doses administered 4 h apart and split between two or three different injection sites.

In horses, diminazene aceturate should be administered by deep i.m. injection divided between several injection sites. The injection sites should be massaged in order to promote drug absorption. At the dose rates suggested here, signs of toxicity are uncommon but local reactions, caused by muscle necrosis, may be severe. Diminazene aceturate should be avoided in horses unless other drugs are either ineffective or unavailable. Toxic doses result in respiratory distress, depression, cardiac signs, hypersalivation and diarrhea. Toxic doses may be treated with calcium salts.

Phenamidine isoethionate

Phenamidine isoethionate is a bitter, white, odorless, water-soluble compound. In horses, it is used at 8–13 mg/kg i.m. or subcutaneous (s.c.); it is limited to the treatment of *B. caballi* infections because it is ineffective in the treatment of *B. equi* infections and trypanosomiasis.

Pentamidine

Pentamidine is rarely used in horses but may be effective against *B. caballi, T. brucei* and *T. evansi*. It must be administered by slow intravenous (i.v.) injection or i.m. injection using multiple small injection sites and the treatment repeated after 48 h.

Complex urea compounds

The complex urea compounds are related to the aromatic diamidines. Their mechanism of action is unknown.

Quinuronium sulfate

Quinuronium sulfate is a bitter, white to yellow, crystalline powder that is usually available as a stable 5% aqueous solution. This compound is effective in the treatment of *B. caballi* infections but is associated with relapses, making it more effective for premunition than for the elimination of infection. One treatment consists of two doses of a 5% solution of quinuronium sulfate, administered s.c. at 0.3 mg/kg, 6 h apart. Quinuronium sulfate has a narrow margin of safety and overdosing produces parasympathomimetic effects including tremors, salivation, urination and defecation. These signs usually respond to treatment with atropine, epinephrine (adrenaline) and calcium gluconate. The interval between treatments should not be shorter than 2 weeks and should preferably be 3 months because sensitization occurs, which results in shock, with a profound drop in blood pressure, and death.

Amicarbalide

Low doses of amicarbalide can be used for premunition; however, relapses are frequent. Two doses administered i.m. at 8.8 mg/kg 24 h apart are effective in eliminating *B. caballi* infections. However, 22 mg/kg administered i.m. once daily for 7 days is only 50% effective in eliminating *B. equi* infections. At therapeutic doses, there is swelling, inflammation and necrosis at the i.m. injection site, resulting in increased serum concentrations of muscle enzymes and mild hepatic peripheral lobular necrosis (Taylor et al 1972). Amicarbalide is toxic at very high doses and the toxicity includes hepatic and renal tubular necrosis.

Imidocarb dipropionate

Imidocarb is an off-white, water-soluble powder. This compound distributes well and can be found in tissues up to 4 weeks after a single i.m. injection. Imidocarb is mainly eliminated unchanged in urine; about 10% is excreted in feces. A single i.m. injection of imidocarb diprorionate 2.2 mg/kg can be used to ameliorate the clinical signs of *B. caballi*, with two doses administered 24 h apart required to clear this infection. However, four doses at 4 mg/kg administered 72 h apart are not consistently effective in eliminating *B. equi* infection. Imidocarb dipropionate is well tolerated at i.m. injection sites. Horses may exhibit marked transient side-effects, including extreme restlessness, sweating, colic and persistent anorexia following imidocarb diprorionate administration. These side-effects can be ameliorated or avoided by pretreatment with atropine sulfate (1% solution 1 ml/100 kg) and by dividing the imidocarb dose into two injections given 3 h apart.

Tetracyclines (oxytetracycline)

The tetracyclines are amphoteric antimicrobial agents that can form salts with bases or acids (see Chs 1 and 2). Oxytetracycline is a bitter, yellow, odorless crystalline powder. The base is slightly water soluble and the hydrochloride is readily water soluble and is typically administered to horses by slow i.v. injection. It is effective at 5.5 mg/kg once daily for 2 days or more in the treatment of *B. equi* but is unlikely to completely clear this infection. It is, therefore, used for premunition. Rapid i.v. injection may cause a precipitous drop in blood pressure and collapse owing to the effects of calcium chelation on the myocardium. Intramuscular injection causes objectionable local reactions in horses and should be avoided. Oral administration may be more likely to be associated with colitis in horses than i.v. administration, although colitis may occur following administration by any route.

Other compounds

Trypan blue (Trypan red)

The Trypan dyes are bisazo compounds distantly related to the sulfonamides. Trypan blue, a bluish-gray, water-soluble powder, was one of the first drugs to be used for the treatment of piroplasmosis and trypanosomiasis. Trypan blue is effective against *B. caballi* but not *B. equi*. In horses, a freshly prepared 1–2% solution of Trypan blue can be administered by slow i.v. injection at 2–3 mg/kg for premunition. Rapid i.v. administration of Trypan blue may result in shock. Subcutaneous administration of Trypan blue should be avoided because it causes skin sloughing. Trypan blue stains the mucous membranes and other tissues blue and is, therefore, not used commonly.

Efluvane

Efluvane is a derivative of acridine, a non-specific bacteriostatic compound. It is an orange–red crystalline powder that is slightly soluble in saline. It is thought to intercalate with, and, therefore, interfere with, the normal coiling of parasite DNA. For premunition (this compound does not eliminate *Babesia* spp.), a 5% solution of efluvane is administered i.v. at 4–8 ml/100 kg up to a maximum dose of 20 ml.

Buparvaquone/parvaquone

The similarity of *B. equi* to *Theileria* spp. has led many investigators to look at the efficacy of some theilericidal drugs in the treatment of *B. equi* infections. Preliminary studies suggest that these drugs may be effective in eliminating *B. equi* when used in combination with imidocarb.

TRYPANOSOMIASIS

Protista Sarcomastigophora Zoomastigophorea Kinetoplastida Trypanosomatidae *Trypanosoma*.

PARASITE BIOLOGY

Trypanosomes are flagellate hemoprotozoans that live extracellularly in the blood. Most *Trypanosoma* spp. are transmitted by tsetse flies (*Glossina* spp.) in endemic regions of tropicoequatorial Africa but they may also be transmitted by mechanical vectors, including horse flies (*Tabanus* spp.), or by the venereal route, in the case of *T. equiperdum* (dourine). Mechanical transmission is the primary source of infection in non-tsetse regions including parts of Africa, Central and South America, West India and Mauritania.

Trypanosomes are ingested by the tsetse fly during a blood meal and enter the midgut, where they transform into procyclic trypomastigotes that are capable of multiplication. These migrate to the fly's salivary glands and go through the epimastigote stage followed by the metacyclic (infective) stage where division ceases. These metatrypanosomes are injected into the animal host during a blood meal and become the bloodstream form of the organism. Trypanosomes do not have a sexual stage of reproduction.

Horses are susceptible to several *Trypanosoma* spp. with various transmission vectors:

- tsetse fly: *T. brucei, T. congolense, T. vivax*;
- mechanical: *T. evansi* (surra), *T. vivax*;
- venereal: *T. equiperdum* (dourine).

PATHOGENESIS, CLINICAL SIGNS AND DIAGNOSIS

In tsetse fly transmitted trypanosomiasis, metatrypanosomes are injected into the skin of the animal by the tsetse fly during a blood meal and cause localized swelling. The trypanosomes migrate to the lymph nodes and then into the bloodstream, where they undergo rapid asexual multiplication. The clinical signs, incubation period and mortality rate vary with the *Trypanosoma* spp. involved.

Equids are highly susceptible to *T. brucei* infection, with a very high mortality rate within 14–90 days in untreated horses. The prepatent period, the period from infection to parasitemia, is approximately 6–10 days. Locomotor ataxia is the earliest clinical sign. Remittent high fever (41.7°C/107°F) occurs between intervening periods when the rectal temperature is normal. Anemia and icterus are evident in the early stages of the disease. Depression, unthriftiness, lymphadenopathy, penile prolapse, urticarial plaques, edema and keratitis are also seen.

Disease caused by *T. congolense* is rare in horses. The prepatent period is 17 days and the parasitemia is unimpressive. Edematous plaques become evident after about 10 days, and may recur during the infection. Generalized edema becomes evident from about 14 days postinfection. Keratitis may develop. *T. congolense* infection is relatively mild in horses: normal appetite despite a moderate anemia and clinical signs that resolve spontaneously in about 6 weeks.

Equine disease caused by *T. vivax* is usually, but not always, relatively innocuous. The prepatent period is about 16 days. Parasitemia is cyclic and is accompanied by fever. Between these febrile episodes, urticarial plaques may become evident in the skin and dependent edema develops. In more severe cases, ataxia may develop in the first few days after infection, with muscle tremors occurring around 2 weeks after infection. The ataxia and anorexia are progressive. Keratitis with associated corneal opacity may develop.

Surra or murrina (*T. evansi* also known as *T. equinum*) is transmitted mechanically. The most significant effect of this mode of transmission is that the disease is not limited to the geographical range of the tsetse fly. This disease can be found in North Africa, the Middle East, Asia and Central and South America. The genera of bloodsucking flies that may act as mechanical vectors, by transferring blood on their mouthparts from an infected animal to a new host, include *Tabanus*, *Stomoxys*, *Atylotus* and *Leperosia* spp., although *Tabanus* spp. is the most commonly implicated. The vampire bat (*Desmodus rotundus*) is also responsible for transmission in South America. The pathogenesis, clinical signs and treatment of *T. evansi* are similar to those of the tsetse-transmitted trypanosomiases. The prepatent/latent period is highly variable but is probably approximately 4–7 days. There is a reaction at the site of the infective bite. Parasitemia is accompanied by fever, which is sometimes extremely high, ataxia and occasionally excessive thirst.

Chronic wasting occurs in the face of a normal appetite and progressive anemia is evident. Urticaria is irregular and can be localized or generalized. Lymphadenopathy, icterus and edema are also seen. The mortality rate is high and occurs in days to months. The course of disease is more chronic in donkeys and mules. Ataxia, from cortical involvement, occurs late in this disease.

Dourine (*T. equiperdum*) is a venereal disease of horses that is limited in geographical distribution to Africa, the Middle East, southern and eastern Europe, Russia and Central and South America. This trypanosome passes through intact mucous membranes. The incubation period is from 2 weeks to 3 months or more. The infection is chronic and persists for years with a mortality rate of about 50% within 2 years. The clinical signs of dourine develop over a period of weeks to months and are more variable than in the other forms of trypanosomiasis. The signs may be more evident in some locations than others: for example, the most evident sign may be in the genitalia or the central nervous system (CNS) without significant clinical signs elsewhere. Most commonly fever, swelling and edema, anemia, wasting, ocular lesions, ataxia and facial paralysis are seen, with the appetite remaining normal. The earliest signs are edema of the external genitalia and mucopurulent discharge from the urethra of affected stallions or the vagina of affected mares. Fever is intermittent and is more common in the early stages of this disease. As the disease progresses, a skin rash consisting of large plaques (2–10 cm in diameter) develops. In the late stages of dourine, progressive paralysis occurs, starting with the face and neck and progressing to the pelvic limbs. Abortion is also observed. The mortality rate is high in untreated horses, while donkeys and mules may be infected without developing obvious clinical signs. Treatment is not recommended unless the infected equine is not going to be used for breeding since these horses may remain a source of infection for other horses.

The diagnosis of trypanosomiasis is based on the direct demonstration of the parasite or on serology. Direct detection includes the examination of blood smears, anion-exchange chromatography or mouse inoculation. The latter method is not effective in the diagnosis of *T. equiperdum* because it rarely produces hemoparasitism. However, direct smears of fluid from the edematous genitalia of affected animals may reveal these trypanosomes. Alternatively, a centrifuged sample of blood may reveal parasites. Indirect serological tests including latex agglutination tests, enzyme-linked immunosorbant assays (ELISAs) and complement fixation tests are available. The last is of particular benefit in the diagnosis of *T. equiperdum*.

TREATMENT

The treatment of trypanosomiasis in horses is taken directly from the treatment regimens used in other species. The choice of drug and the administration route depend upon the management and chemosensitivity of the trypanosome strain in question. The recent development of in vitro assays to determine trypanosome chemosensitivity mean that the choice of drug can be based on local drug resistance patterns.

Aromatic diminazenes

The use of this class of drugs for the treatment of trypanosomiasis is included in the section on piroplasmosis.

Quinapyramine salts

The mode of action of this class of drugs is related to the inhibition of cell growth and division.

Quinapyramine

Quinapyramine sulfate and chloride are bitter, odorless, white to pale yellow crystalline powders. The sulfate salt is readily soluble in water and the chloride salt is soluble in boiling water up to a concentration of 2%. The sulfate salt has a rapid onset of action but a short duration effect, whereas the chloride salt has a long-acting effect and is used for prophylaxis.

Quinapyramine sulfate is the most effective treatment for trypanosomiasis in horses but is often poorly tolerated and there is widespread

resistance as a result of extensive drug use. It is less effective against *T. brucei* but is used for the treatment of *T. congolense*, *T. vivax*, *T. evansi* and *T. equiperdum*. For the treatment of *T. brucei*, *T. evansi* and *T. equiperdum* infections, a 5% solution of quinapyramine sulfate is administered to horses at 3–5 mg/kg at 6 h intervals, by s.c. or deep i.m. injection, split between three injection sites. There may be edema and skin sloughing at the injection site after s.c. injection and these reactions are often marked and resolve very slowly (many months). Systemic signs of toxicity include intense hypersalivation, dyspnea, hyperhidrosis, colic and sometimes collapse. The systemic reactions are most common is young animals and may occur within a few minutes of drug administration.

Quinapyramine prosalt is a solution containing 10% (three parts) sulfate and 6.67% (two parts) chloride that is administered s.c. at 0.025 ml/kg. The chloride salt is not very soluble and produces a s.c. deposit of the drug that is then absorbed slowly from the injection site, providing a prophylactic effect that lasts for up to 3 months. The addition of suramin markedly enhances the prophylactic effect of the quinapyramine. In endemic areas, a combination of quinapyramine prosalt and suramin is administered to stallions every 90 days during the breeding season and to mares at least 18 days before breeding to protect against dourine (*T. equiperdum*) infection.

Suramin

Suramin is a synthetic complex aromatic organic compound. The sodium salt is a white or pinkish crystalline powder with some solubility in water. It is useful in the treatment of *T. brucei*, *T. evansi* and *T. equiperdum*. Suramin markedly enhances the prophylactic effect of quinapyramine and the phenanthridinium compounds, although it has no prophylactic effects when used alone. It is most effective when given in the early stages of the disease because it attacks the *Trypanosoma* spp. as they concentrate in the lymph nodes and circulate in the bloodstream. This drug is less effective during the later stages of the disease when the trypanosomes invade the CNS.

A 10% solution of suramin sodium is administered i.v. to horses at 7–10 mg/kg and the treatment repeated up to three times at weekly intervals. This drug is generally well tolerated but systemic reactions may occur after i.v. administration. Edema, urticaria and laminitis are among the systemic reactions observed and prolonged use may result in chronic nephritis with albuminuria. Local reactions occur after i.m. administration. The widespread existence of stable suramin resistance among trypanosomes has rendered this compound of little use.

Phenanthridinium compounds

Homidium bromide

Homidium bromide is available as purple tablets (250 mg) that dissolve in boiling water. The drug is prepared as a 1–2.5% solution that is administered s.c. or i.m. at 1 mg/kg to horses. This dose is both prophylactic (for at least 1 month) and curative in susceptible trypanosome infections. Ethidium bromide can produce severe local reactions, which are less pronounced following deep i.m. injection. This compound is most effective against *T. vivax*, has lower efficacy against *T. brucei* and *T. congolense* and no activity against *T. evansi*. There is widespread resistance to this compound in tsetse regions.

Pyrithidium bromide

Pyrithidium bromide (prothidium) is available as red tablets (500 mg) that are dissolved in boiling water to make a 2.5% solution (1 tablet per 10 ml water). It is administered to horses by deep i.m. injection at 2–2.5 mg/kg and confers protection for 4 months. Systemic reactions are rare but severe local reactions may occur. This drug rapidly induces trypanosomal resistance, which includes cross-resistance to quinapyramine and ethidium.

Isometamidium chloride

Isometamidium chloride hydrochlorate is a red powder that is readily soluble in water. A 1–2% solution is administered by deep i.m. injection at 0.25–1 mg/kg bwt. It is effective against *T. vivax* at 0.5 mg/kg i.m. and *T. brucei* and *T. congolense* at 0.5–1 mg/kg i.m. It has prophylactic activity for up to 6 months but is commonly administered as frequently as every 2 months. This drug causes severe local reactions and should be given by deep i.m. injection divided between several injection sites. Other transient toxic effects included nasal discharge, flatulence, hypersalivation and prostration. The side-effects observed in horses are substantial and warrant careful deliberation when considering using this drug. Drug resistance occurs in regions where this compound is used widely for prophylaxis.

Aromatic diamidines

Diminazene aceturate is used for the treatment of *T. brucei* infections in horses and minimal resistance is reported (see Piroplasmosis, p. 51). However, it should only be used in horses when no other treatment is available because it produces severe local reactions (muscle necrosis). If diminazene aceturate is used, the dose should be divided into two or three portions administered 4 h apart.

Treatment recommendations

Isometamidium 0.5 mg/kg administered by deep i.m. injection divided between three injection sites is used for the treatment of *T. congolense* and *T. vivax* in horses. A 5% solution of quinapyramine 3–5 mg/kg administered by s.c. or deep i.m. injection divided between three injection sites and administered as divided doses (three doses given at 6 h intervals) is used for the treatment of *T. brucei* and *T. evansi* in horses.

Prophylaxis recommendations

Isometamidium 0.5–1 mg/kg administered by deep i.m. injection into the neck muscles and withers, divided between several injection sites, protects horses for 2–4 months against *T. congolense* and *T. vivax*. Prothidium bromide administered by deep i.m. injection 2 mg/kg protects horses for at least 3 months against *T. congolense* and

T. vivax. Quinapyramine prosalt 7.4 mg/kg provides 3 to 4 months protection against *T. congolense, T. vivax* and *T. equiperdum* but causes severe local reactions. Suramin–quinapyramine complex administered s.c. at a dose rate of 10 mg/kg provides protection for at least 6 months against *T. evansi.*

GIARDIASIS

PARASITE BIOLOGY

Giardia spp. are intestinal parasites that are found in horses of all ages but rarely produce clinical signs. Infection is found commonly in foals of 2–22 weeks of age (17–35%) and less commonly in older horses. On rare occasions, chronic diarrhea has been associated with giardial infection. A diagnosis of giardiasis requires the identification of *Giardia* spp. cysts in feces, usually using the zinc sulfate centrifugal flotation method. The shedding of cysts is inconsistent and, therefore, fresh fecal samples should be tested daily for 5 days. Other causes of diarrhea should be ruled out before *Giardia* infection is diagnosed since *Giardia* spp. is shed commonly in equine feces in the absence of clinical signs.

TREATMENT

The nitroimidazole metronidazole 5 mg/kg orally three times a day for 10 days is effective in the treatment of equine giardiasis. The benzimidazole anthelmintic fenbendazole is used in the treatment of giardiasis in dogs and cats.

COCCIDIOSIS (GLOBIDIOSIS)

PARASITE BIOLOGY

Eimeria leukarti is the intestinal coccidian of horses. Infection with *E. leukarti* follows the ingestion of sporulated oocysts in contaminated food or water. After exposure to bile in the small intestine, the oocysts excyst and individual protozoa, the sporozoites, emerge. The sporozoites penetrate the intestinal epithelium and differentiate

into trophozoites, which increase in size to form schizonts; these divide into many daughter cells called merozoites. The merozoites are released from the infected intestinal cells and infect adjoining cells to continue the asexual reproductive cycle (schizogony). After one or more cycles of schizogony, the merozoites differentiate into the sexual forms, the micro- and macrogametocytes, for sexual reproduction or gametogony. The final product of the sexual reproductive cycle is the oocyst or egg, which is then shed in feces and is infective to new hosts. The prepatent period, the time from the ingestion of sporulated oocysts to the production of infective oocysts, is 16–35 days.

PATHOGENESIS, CLINICAL SIGNS AND DIAGNOSIS

Coccidia are found in the small intestine of young horses and donkeys around the world. They are found commonly in the feces of normal foals aged 30–125 days, suggesting that this organism does not usually cause diarrhea or other clinical signs in foals. However, severe diarrheic episodes have been attributed to massive coccidial infection in foals. A diagnosis of coccidiosis is made by examining fecal sediment for oocysts or by flotation of oocysts using saturated sucrose solution. Before a diagnosis of intestinal coccidiosis is made, other causes of diarrhea must be excluded because coccidia are rarely pathogenic in horses.

TREATMENT

The treatment of choice for coccidiosis is the sulfonamide antimicrobial agents (see Ch. 2). The sulfonamides disrupt folic acid and nicotinamide metabolism and coenzymes I and II by competing with para-aminobenzoic acid (PABA). Coccidia must manufacture their own folic acid and, therefore, this step is mandatory in the pyrimidine pathway of these parasites. Sulfamethazine (sulfadimidine) at 220 mg/kg i.v. or orally, or sulfadimethoxine (55 mg/kg) orally or sulfathiazole (66 mg/kg) orally, all once daily for 5–7 days, are used commonly for the treatment of equine coccidiosis. The signs of toxicity of the sulfonamides are covered extensively in Chapter 2. Crystalluria, a sign of toxicity in other species, is uncommonly observed in horses.

SARCOCYSTIS INFECTIONS: EQUINE PROTOZOAL MYELOENCEPHALITIS

PARASITE BIOLOGY

Equine protozoal myeloencephalitis (EPM) is caused by *Sarcocystis neurona* (the most recognized cause) or by *Neospora hughesi* (possibly transplacentally). *Sarcocystis* spp. has a heteroxenous (two host species) life cycle with gametogony (sexual reproduction) taking place in the definitive host (usually a predator or scavenger species) and schizogony or merogony (asexual reproduction) in the intermediate host (usually a prey species). Sexual division begins in the intestinal tract of the definitive host within 18 h of the ingestion of cysts in the muscle of the intermediate host. However, the time required for the development of the sexual stages (gametogony) is not known. Ingested bradyzoites rapidly penetrate enterocytes and develop into the sexual stages of the organism, the micro- and macrogametes. Motile male microgametes penetrate the macrogamete to cause fertilization. Sporulation occurs within the oocyst in the enterocytes of the definitive host. Two sporocysts, each of which contains four infective sporozoites, form within the oocyst. Oocysts are passed in the feces of the definitive host and ingested by the intermediate host. Upon exposure to bile in the duodenum of the intermediate host, or in the case of *S. neurona* the aberrant intermediate host the horse, the sporozoites excyst from the protective sporocysts. The sporozoites then enter the intestinal epithelial cells and undergo the first of many stages of asexual reproduction (schizogony or merogony) to produce tachyzoites (merozoites). The merozoites undergo several cycles of replication in this manner.

PATHOGENESIS, CLINICAL SIGNS AND DIAGNOSIS

Horses are presumed to become infected with *S. neurona* by the ingestion of infective sporocysts in feed, hay or pasture that is contaminated with feces of the definitive host; the route of infection of the natural intermediate host. The sporocysts are ingested, excyst, penetrate enterocytes and ultimately enter the circulation, but they apparently never encyst in the tissues of the horse. Instead, in some horses, they migrate to the CNS and continue to undergo schizogony intracellularly in neurons and microglial cells without forming tissue cysts. The merozoites are found free in the cytoplasm of cells in the CNS, suggesting that the merozoites of *S. neurona* never mature beyond what would normally be the second generation of division. Horses cannot transmit *S. neurona* to other animals, including other horses.

The time from exposure to *S. neurona* to the development of marked clinical signs of EPM is highly variable. The disease has been identified in a 2-month-old foal and there is no evidence that transplacental transmission occurs, suggesting that 2 months may be around the minimum time required for the development of this disease in horses. An older horse with acute onset spinal ataxia was seronegative (antibody) for *S. neurona* in both serum and cerebrospinal fluid (CSF) when the clinical signs of EPM developed, but became seropositive in both fluids within 3.5 weeks of the onset of these signs. This suggests that the merozoites of *S. neurona* migrated into the CNS of this horse before antibodies could be detected in the bloodstream, which takes around 10–14 days after the exposure to merozoites. Therefore, it appears that horses may develop clinical signs of EPM within only a few weeks of infection. However, the development of clinical signs of EPM may require as long as 2 years, since it has been seen in horses that have been exported. In fact, EPM has only been reported outside North America in exported horses, although there have been no comprehensive studies to determine whether exposure to *S. neurona* occurs in other countries.

The clinical signs of EPM are the result of both direct damage to neurons, by protozoal proliferation within the neuronal cell bodies, and indirect damage to neural elements, produced by edema and inflammation in response to the merozoites and meronts in the CNS. Deposition of the parasite within the CNS is presumed to occur by hematogenous spread, because of the parasite's predilection for endothelial cells. Although the spinal cord seems to be the most commonly affected region, the protozoa may begin to proliferate and cause dysfunction at any site in the CNS. The disease is often insidious in onset, misdiagnosed until late in its course and may culminate in death if untreated.

The classic presentation for EPM is progressive asymmetric ataxia and focal muscle atrophy. Although the most common presenting sign of EPM is ataxia (incoordination), any neurological dysfunction or even lameness can occur. In fact, the neurological signs that occur are referable to the site or sites of infection. Both white and gray matter damage, resulting in upper and lower motor neuron signs, respectively, produce locomotor deficits. Upper motor neuron damage results in ataxia and spasticity while lower motor neuron damage results in dragging of one or more toes and weakness. There is no consistent pattern of gait deficits found in horses with EPM and quadriplegia may be present in severe cases.

Signs of cranial nerve dysfunction are seen in at least 10% of cases of EPM. Any cranial nerve nucleus (collection of nerve cell bodies demarcated within the CNS) may be affected if the infection is in the brainstem. Airway abnormalities, such as laryngeal hemiplegia (vagus nerve) or dorsal displacement of the soft palate (glossopharyngeal nerve), may result from infection of the nuclei of the respective cranial nerves. Most horses with airway abnormalities do not have EPM; therefore, a diagnosis of EPM may be overlooked. Atrophy of the temporalis or masseter muscles (trigeminal nerve) may be observed. This can be accompanied by dysphagia, which may also be caused by abnormalities of the glossopharyngeal, hypoglossal or vagus nerves. Difficulty in the prehension, mastication and deglutition of food may be difficult to assess unless the horse is observed eating. Evidence of quidding (dropping chewed feed) or aspiration or reflux of chewed material into the nostrils may occur as a result of cranial nerve dysfunction. Abnormalities of the facial and vestibulocochlear nerves are often observed together because of the proximity of these nuclei to each other in the brainstem. Facial nerve paralysis is associated with muzzle deviation away from the affected side, ptosis and ear droop. Vestibular signs, including nystagmus, and head tilt and a wide-based stance can occur.

Infection of the cerebrum, basal ganglia and cerebellum are observed less commonly. Depression is associated with other cerebral abnormalities but is uncommon in EPM. Protozoal infections in the cerebrum may be focal and associated with seizure activity and electroencephalographic abnormalities. Alternatively, asymmetric amaurosis (central blindness) and facial hypalgesia may be observed. Infection of the cerebellum results in cerebellar ataxia that is usually not associated with weakness or proprioceptive deficits. Involvement of the reticular activating system is also uncommon but may produce a narcolepsy-like syndrome in the absence of any other neurological signs. Occasionally, lameness that cannot be eliminated with nerve and joint local anesthesia may be the only evidence of a neurological deficit.

Low numbers of protozoa in the CNS produce this disease, rendering direct methods of parasite detection of little use in the diagnosis of EPM. Therefore, it is diagnosed indirectly using serology (immunoblot). Both serum and CSF is tested, with a positive serum antibody titer indicating exposure to the parasite and a positive CSF titer indicating either blood contamination of the CSF during sampling or intrathecal antibody production.

TREATMENT

Potentiated sulfonamides (pyrimethamine plus sulfadiazine)

The recommendations for the treatment of EPM using pyrimethamine, trimethoprim and sulfadiazine were originally based on the use of these drugs for the treatment of malaria and toxoplasmosis in humans. Either pyrimethamine or trimethoprim in combination with sulfadiazine or sulfamethoxazole have been used with some success and have gained widespread acceptance as the treatment of choice for EPM. Pyrimethamine and trimethoprim are diaminopyrimidine antimicrobial agents that inhibit dihydrofolate reductase (DHFR; see Ch. 2). These agents interfere with the production of the enzyme cofactor tetrahydro-folate from dihydrofolate. Diaminopyrimidines interfere with both the de novo production of tetrahydrofolate and the recycling of this cofactor, interfering with bacterial and protozoal DNA synthesis. The antimicrobial effect of the diaminopyrimidines is potentiated by the addition of a sulfonamide agent.

The sulfonamides are analogs of PABA that compete in the production of dihydrofolate by the enzyme dihydropteroate synthase (see Ch. 2). Sulfadiazine is the sulfonamide of choice for the treatment of EPM because it penetrates the CNS better than other sulfonamides, producing concentrations of 10–60% of serum concentrations (Boger 1959, Shoaf et al 1989). In general, most protozoa are resistant to the sulfonamides but the effects of these drugs are greatly enhanced by the presence of pyrimethamine. Horses should remain on both drugs for the duration of treatment. Apicomplexan protozoa that are ordinarily susceptible to pyrimeth-amine, including *Plasmodium* spp. (malaria), have been shown to become rapidly resistant to pyrimethamine in the absence of the sulfonamides (Watkins & Mosobo 1993).

Based upon pharmacokinetic information and minimal inhibitory concentrations (MIC) for pyrimethamine, an oral daily dose of 1 mg/kg in combination with 22 mg/kg sulfadiazine is recommended in horses. The duration of treatment is controversial and the recommendations range from a minimum of 3 months (least conservative) to the point at which the CSF is seronegative (most conservative). It is clear that the latter course of treatment is least likely to result in relapse of the clinical signs (Fenger 1997), but it is likely that this exceeds what is absolutely necessary in most cases.

Trimethoprim should not be used in combination with pyrimethamine since both drugs are DHFR inhibitors, although pyrimethamine is more selective for the protozoal enzyme and trimethoprim for the bacterial enzyme. When used together, trimethoprim competitively inhibits pyrimethamine, thus decreasing the efficacy of this more effective compound. In addition, pyrimethamine and trimethoprim have at least additive effects on mammalian DHFR (Burchall 1973). The most commonly observed sign of toxicity of pyrimethamine and sulfadiazine combinations is bone marrow suppression (see Ch. 2). This effect causes a gradual increase in red blood cell size during treatment, anemia and neutropenia, which can be profound (Fenger 1997). Rarely, the chronic administration of pyrimethamine and sulfadiazine, particularly at higher than the recommended dose rates, also causes a neurological syndrome. This syndrome includes symmetric ataxia, dysphagia and bilateral facial nerve paralysis in addition to anemia and neutropenia (Polk, unpublished data, 2003). Incoordination has also been reported in a study where healthy ponies were given pyrimethamine with trimethoprim and sulfamethoxazole (Bedford & McDonnell 1999); however, this effect has not been observed in clinical cases. This side-effect may confuse the assessment of the neurological signs of EPM. However, this neurological syndrome is always accompanied by bone marrow suppression and, therefore, a complete blood count may help to confirm or exclude pyrimethamine toxicity as the cause of the ataxia.

Benzeneacetonitriles (diclazuril)

The benzeneacetonitrile diclazuril has been used in the treatment of EPM in horses. Its mode of action is not completely understood but it is believed to have efficacy against a plastid-like organelle in protozoa. Oral administration of diclazuril to horses at 5.5 mg/kg for 21 days provides CSF concentrations of 100–250 ng/ml, which exceed the concentrations required to inhibit 95% of the proliferation of *S. neurona* in tissue culture (Dirikolu et al 1999). This compound is currently undergoing safety and efficacy trials in the USA for the treatment of EPM in horses.

Symmetrical triazinones

Toltrazuril and ponazuril (toltrazuril sulfone) are water-soluble, coccidicidal agents that are effective against the schizogony stage of most coccidia. Oral toltrazuril at 5 mg/kg once daily for

60–90 days or, more frequently, 10 mg/kg for 28 days is recommended and appears to produce few side-effects in horses. There are some veterinarians that use large doses administered by nasogastric tube 10 days apart. Unfortunately, there is a high rate of relapses associated with this practice and the properties of this drug, such as drug half-life in the body, do not support this practice. The dosage of ponazuril is 5 mg/kg orally once daily for 28 days. Large doses of ponazuril produce few side-effects apart from uterine edema, suggesting that the uterus may be one of the target organs for toxicity. Ponazuril has recently been approved in the USA for the treatment of EPM in horses.

Nitrothiazoles (nitazoxanide)

Nitazoxanide is a nitrothiazolyl–salicylamide compound that has a wide range of activity against bacteria, intestinal parasites and protozoa. Its mechanism of action is not known but the compound is structurally related to the antimicrobial agent metronidazole. This compound is unusual in that it is effective against gastrointestinal protozoan and helminth parasites, *Trichomonas vaginalis*, and some Gram-positive and Gram-negative bacteria. It has also been reported to be effective in treating metronidazole-resistant giardiasis. It is highly lipophilic and, therefore, has greater bioavailability when administered with oil or oil-containing feeds, such as typical equine grain rations. Nitazoxanide is marketed throughout most of Latin America for use in treating intestinal parasitism in humans. It is currently under registration in other parts of the world and is available ("orphan drug" status) in the USA for the treatment of cryptosporidiosis inpatients with acquired immunodeficiency syndrome (AIDS). Preliminary studies indicate that 77% of horses treated with nitazoxanide paste, either at 25 mg/kg for 5 days followed by 50 mg/kg for an additional 23 days or at 50 mg/kg for 28 days, improved with treatment. Side-effects occur in less than 15% of horses and include fever, diarrhea, colic, limb edema and laminitis. Pregnant mares have been treated without any pregnancy-related problems or the production of abnormal foals. Nitazoxanide is currently undergoing safety and efficacy trials in the USA for the treatment of EPM in horses.

OTHER *SARCOCYSTIS* INFECTIONS

PARASITE BIOLOGY

Sarcocystis bertrami, S. equicanis and *S. fayeri* use horses as their natural intermediate host. *S. bertrami* was first described in horses in 1901. Subsequently, muscle cysts have been identified in horses in Germany, Austria, Morocco, the UK and the USA; in donkeys in Sardinia, Egypt and Morocco; and in a zebra in South Africa, perhaps representing two or three separate *Sarcocystis* spp. *S. bertrami* and *S. equicanis* can be distinguished based on their unique cyst wall morphology. Cysts of both species are macroscopic, ranging in length from 9–15 mm for *S. bertrami* to 1–9 mm for *S. equicanis*. *S. fayeri* is clearly a distinct species: sarcocysts from this species are microscopic and exhibit unique cyst wall morphology, smaller sporocysts and a longer prepatent period than *S. bertrami*. Dogs serve as the definitive hosts for *S. equicanis* and *S. fayeri*.

S. fayeri infection has been estimated to occur in as many as 88% of horses in Chile and as few as 30% of horses in the USA. This parasite encysts in microscopic cysts that may be up to 990 µm long and 136 µm wide. Sporocysts are ingested and two generations of schizogony take place in the endothelial cells of the arteries or capillaries in the heart, brain and kidney 10–25 days post-infection. After several cycles of replication in the horse, the merozoites enter the myocytes of the esophagus, tongue and skeletal muscles and form sarcocysts. By the 77th day postinfection, the sarcocysts are infectious to the definitive host, the dog. Once a dog ingests horse muscle containing sarcocysts, infective sporocysts are shed after a prepatent period of 12–15 days. Transplacental infection of *S. fayeri* also occurs.

All three *Sarcocystis* spp. identified so far are minimally pathogenic in horses. Natural infections are often found incidentally during postmortem examination. Feeding studies suggest that there are both dose- and strain-specific factors that determine sporocyst pathogenicity. For example, a pony fed 1 million sporocysts of *S. fayeri* developed mild transient anemia and fever, while a horse fed 10 million sporocysts of *S. fayeri* developed a stiff gait. Another pony fed 2 million sporocysts from a different source developed lethargy, depression and unthriftiness 150 days after infection. A German isolate of *S. fayeri* was even more pathogenic; causing similar clinical signs in five ponies fed only 200 000 sporocysts each. Myositis has been associated with the presence of sarcocysts in equine muscle; however, inflammation is rarely found in association with the muscle cysts. Nonetheless, in some cases, inflammation and increased serum concentrations of creatine phosphokinase and aspartate aminotranferase are found in association with the tissue cysts.

PATHOGENESIS, CLINICAL SIGNS AND DIAGNOSIS

Natural disease caused by *Sarcocystis* spp. is uncommon in horses, so diagnosis is rarely necessary. However, histopathological evidence of inflammation associated with cysts in muscle biopsy samples would be highly suggestive of sarcocystis-related myositis.

TREATMENT

Oxytetracycline or pyrimethamine plus sulfadiazine may be effective in eliminating *Sarcocystis* spp. cysts.

REFERENCES

Bedford S J, McDonnell S M 1999 Measurements of reproductive function in stallions treated with trimethoprim-sulfamethoxazole and pyrimethamine. Journal of the American Veterinary Medical Association 215:1317–1319

Boger W P 1959 The diffusion of sulfonamides into the cerebrospinal fluid: a comparative study. Antibiotic Medicine and Clinical Therapy 6:32–40

Burchall J J 1973 Mechanism of action of trimethoprim-sulfamethoxazole. Journal of Infectious Diseases 128(suppl):437–441

Dirikolu L, Lehner F, Nattrass C et al 1999 Diclazuril in the horse: its identification and detection and preliminary pharmacokinetics. Journal of Veterinary Pharmacology and Therapeutics 22:374–379

Fenger C K 1997 Equine protozoal myeloencephalitis. Compendium on Continuing Education for the Practicing Veterinarian 19:513

Melhorn H, Schein E 1998 Redescription of *Babesia equi* Laveran, 1901 as *Theileria equi*. Parasitology Research 84:467–475

Shoaf S E, Schwark W S, Guard C L 1989 Pharmacokinetics of sulfadiazine/trimethoprim in neonatal male calves: effect of age and penetration into cerebrospinal fluid. American Journal of Veterinary Research 50:396–402

Taylor W M, Simpson C F, Martin F G 1972 Certain aspects of toxicity of an amicarbalide formulation to ponies. American Journal of Veterinary Research 33:533–541

Watkins W M, Mosobo M 1993 Treatment of *Plasmodium falciparium* malaria with pyrimethamine and sulphadoxine: a selective pressure for resistance is a function of long elimination half-life. Transactions of the Royal Society of Tropical Medicine and Hygiene 87:75–79

CHAPTER CONTENTS

Introduction 63

Endoparasiticides 64
Drugs 64
Control programs for internal parasites 67

Ectoparasiticides 71
Drugs 71
Control programs for ectoparasites 72

Miscellaneous parasiticides 72

References 73

4

Parasiticides

Sandy Love   Robert M. Christley

INTRODUCTION

Since 1917, only 11 new endoparasiticides have been developed for use in the horse. Many of the early compounds had very narrow spectra of activity and/or high potential for toxicity such that they have become obsolete. Febantel, levamisole, trichlorfon, dichlorvos, phenothiazine and carbon disulfide are no longer used routinely in the horse (Lyons et al 1999).

Following the landmark studies of Drudge & Lyons (1966), the concept of interval anthelmintic dosing has been the mainstay of equine parasite control programs. Since the initial efficacy reports for drugs against equine parasites—benzimidazoles (Drudge et al 1963), pyrantel (Cornwell & Jones 1968), ivermectin (DiPietro et al 1982) and moxidectin (Lyons et al 1992)—intensive, interval dosing with these potent, broad-spectrum anthelmintics has been practiced widely, which has resulted in major changes in clinical parasitism. Cyathostomes have superseded *Strongylus vulgaris* as the major equine parasitic pathogens (Love et al 1999) and the results of quantitative epidemiological studies have provided evidence that tapeworms, previously considered a minor pathogen, are important in the etiopathogenesis of certain forms of colic (Proudman et al 1998). In essence, this reflects the excellent efficacy of modern anthelmintics against *S. vulgaris*, which now rarely infects well-managed horses (Drudge & Lyons 1986) and highlights the generally poor efficacy of the same compounds against early mucosal stages of cyathostomes.

Concurrent with widespread application of intensive interval anthelmintic dosing, there has been worldwide documentation of benzimidazole resistance in cyathostome populations and, on a more limited scale, resistance has also been reported to piperazine and pyrantel (Lyons et al 1999). To date, the only class of equine anthelmintics that cyathostomes have not developed resistance to are the macrocyclic lactones (ivermectin and moxidectin) but Sangster (1999) forecasted that this would occur by 2004. Importantly, there is no evidence of reversion to susceptibility after protracted period of withdrawal of benzimidazoles from parasite control programs (Uhlinger & Johnstone 1984).

With regard to ectoparasiticides, public health and environmental concerns have led to the withdrawal of the organochlorines and organophosphates in many countries. Since Elliot (1973) reported the first photostable synthetic pyrethroid, these compounds have both replaced the naturally occurring pyrethrins (extracted from chrysanthemum flowers) and progressively become the mainstay of external parasite control programs.

Overall, much more is known about the pharmacology of endoparasiticides than is known about the biology of the target parasites. With development and marketing of new anthelmintics with novel modes of action extremely unlikely in the foreseeable future (Hennessy 1997), and against the background of the eventual possibility of resistance to ivermectin and/or moxidectin (Sangster 1999), education in the clinical pharmacology and responsible use of equine anthelmintics in parasite control programs are major issues in veterinary medicine. With regard to equine ectoparasites, there is huge regional and international variation in their importance both as primary causes of disease and also as vectors of other microbial pathogens. Equine protozoal myeloencephalitis (EPM), a major disease of the horse, has created many issues for clinicians with regard to achieving successful therapeutic protocols; these are addressed in Chapters 3 and 9.

ENDOPARASITICIDES

Three principal chemical classes of anthelmintic with a broad spectrum of activity are in common usage in equids, namely the macrocyclic lactones, benzimidazoles and pyrimidines (Table 4.1). In addition, two compounds with a narrow spectrum of activity, piperazine and praziquantel, are used in combination preparations, with the benzimidazoles and ivermectin, respectively. Each class of anthelmintic has a discrete mode of action, which dictates the spectra of parasites on which the anthelmintics will have toxic effects (Martin 1997). Anthelmintic efficacy depends on both the presence of specific drug receptors within the parasite and on achieving sustained high concentrations of anthelmintic at the location of the parasite within the host tissues (Lanusse & Prichard 1993). The absorption, distribution and elimination of anthelmintic compounds can be affected by dosage formulation, route of administration and animal species (Baggot & McKellar 1994).

DRUGS
Macrocyclic lactones

There are five macrocyclic lactones utilized in veterinary practice of which ivermectin (an avermectin) and moxidectin (a milbemycin) are approved for use in the horse. Ivermectin and moxidectin selectively paralyze parasites by increasing muscle chloride permeability through interaction with glutamate-gated chloride ion channels (McKellar & Benchaoui 1996). There is evidence that ivermectin and moxidectin may have several sites of action within the parasite and the effects of these compounds may also differ between the nematode species (McKellar & Benchaoui 1996, Martin 1997).

Macrocyclic lactones are highly lipophilic and are distributed widely to and eliminated slowly from the body compartments such that they have persistent anthelmintic activity. There are physicochemical differences between ivermectin and moxidectin that confers different lipid solubility on each drug: moxidectin has a much longer half-life in body fat (Afzal et al 1997). This constitutes at least a partial explanation for the longer period of suppression of equine fecal worm egg output achieved following dosing with moxidectin compared with ivermectin (Jacob et al 1995,

Table 4.1 Pharmacological and therapeutic features of equine anthelmintics

Class	Anthelmintic	Administration route	Dose (mg/kg)[a]	Mode of action	Duration of action (weeks)[b]	Lethal to major parasites						
						LS	MLS	SS	SSML	T	A	B
Macrocyclic lactones	Ivermectin	p.o.	0.2	Affect glutamate-gated chloride ion channels	6–8	✓	✓	✓	–	–	✓	✓
	Moxidectin	p.o.	0.4		13	✓	✓[e]	✓	✓[c]	–	✓	✓[d]
Benzimidazoles	Fenbendazole	p.o.	5–10[e]	Beta-tubulin binding and inhibition of microtubule formation	4–6	✓	✓[e]	✓[e,i]	✓	–	✓[e]	–
	Mebendazole	p.o.	8.8		4–6	✓	–	✓	–	–	–	–
	Oxibendazole	p.o.	10–15		4–6	✓	–	✓	–	–	–	–
	Oxfendazole	p.o.	10		4–6	✓	✓[g]	✓	–	–	–	–
	Tiabendazole	p.o.	44		4–6	✓	✓[h]	✓	–	–	✓[h]	–
Pyrimidines	Pyrantel pamoate	p.o.	6.6 (13.2)	Cholinergic effect on parasite ganglia	4	✓	–	✓	–	✓	–	–
	Pyrantel embonate	p.o.	19 (32)		4							
	Pyrantel tartrate	p.o.	2.6[f]		Continuous	✓[f]	✓[c]	✓[f]	–	✓	–	–
Heterocyclics	Piperazine	p.o.	88	Neuromuscular Hyperpolarization	4–6	✓[f]	.	✓	–	–	✓[k]	–
Pyrazinoisoquinolines	Praziquantel	p.o.	1.5	Increased Ca^{2+} permeability	Unknown	–	–	–	–	–	✓[l]	–

p.o., oral; s.c., subcutaneous; LS, adult large strongyles; MLS, migrating large strongyle larvae; SS, adult small strongyles (cyathostomes); SSML, inhibited mucosal larval small strongyles; T, tapeworm; A, ascarids; B, bots

[a] Regional differences exist in recommended dose rates and label claims

[b] Duration of action is the time from dosing until worm eggs appear in feces, i.e. the so-called egg reappearance period (ERP)

[c] 30–40% efficacy

[d] 90% efficacy

[e] Standard dose rate in USA is 5mg/kg; standard dose rate in Europe is 7.5mg/kg, ascarid dose is 10mg/kg. MLS dose is either 10mg/kg (7.5mg/kg, in Europe) on 5 consecutive days or 50mg/kg on 3 consecutive days or single dose 60mg/kg. SSML dose is 10mg/kg on 5 consecutive days

[f] Anthelmintic resistance may affect efficacy

[g] 60–75% efficacy

[h] 50% efficacy

[i] MLS dose is 440mg/kg on 2 consecutive days; ascarid dose is 88mg/kg

[j] Standard dose rate in USA is 6mg/kg pyrantel pamoate; standard dose in Europe is 19mg/kg pyrantel embonate; pyrantel tartrate dose is 2.6mg/kg daily in feed; tapeworm dose is twice standard dose

[k] The mode of action results in rapid death of parasites such that they may cause intestinal obstruction/rupture if given to animals with high burdens of Parascaris equorum

[l] Combination product with ivermectin

Taylor & Kenny 1995, DiPietro et al 1997, Demeulenaere et al 1997). However, while there are significant differences in the pharmacokinetic profile (longer plasma residence time and higher peak plasma concentrations) following oral dosing with commercial preparations of moxidectin and ivermectin, this may also reflect differences in the product formulation (oral gel versus oral paste) and manufacturer's recommended dose rates (0.4 mg/kg versus 0.2 mg/kg) as well as the different lipophilicity of the two compounds (Perez et al 1999).

There are diverse formulations and delivery systems for macrocyclic lactones in ruminants, including injectable, oral, sustained-release bolus and transdermal ("pour on") products. In Europe, it is popular clinical practice to administer injectable solutions of ivermectin intravenously (i.v.) to horses. This constitutes extra-label (unlicensed) use and there are no objective data to support the perceived improved efficacy following administration by this route. Specifically, in relation to hypobiotic cyathostome larvae, Klei et al (1993) reported no increase in efficacy when horses were administered 10 µg/kg, which is five times the recommended dose rate.

Ivermectin and moxidectin have a broad spectrum of activity and high efficacy against the adult stages of the major parasites of the horse with the notable exception of the tapeworm (Costa et al 1998). However, ivermectin has only limited activity against fourth-stage cyathostome larvae. Although moxidectin has in the region of 60% activity against late third-stage and fourth-stage cyathostomes, neither ivermectin nor moxidectin are consistently effective against hypobiotic third-stage cyathostome larvae, with reported efficacies ranging from 10 to 90% (Eysker et al 1992, Klei et al 1993, Xiao et al 1994, Monahan et al 1995, Bairden et al 2001). Ivermectin has variable activity against fourth-stage ascarids (Campbell et al 1989). There are marked differences in the activity against bots (*Gasterophilus* spp. larvae), with ivermectin 95% effective (Britt & Preston 1985) and moxidectin only 20% effective (Xiao et al 1994). Ivermectin is also documented as being active against *Strongyloides westeri* (Ryan & Best 1985), *Dictyocaulus arnfeldi* (Britt & Preston 1985) and

the microfilariae of *Onchocerca cervicalis* (French et al 1988). In ruminants and dogs, macrocyclic lactones are marketed as 'endectocides,' reflecting their activity against both nematodes and arthropods. However, the formulations indicated for use in the horse have no label claim for efficacy against equine lice, mites or ticks.

Generally, the exceptional antiparasitic potency of macrocyclic lactones (in the microgram per kilogram body weight range) renders them extremely safe in mammals; toxic doses are normally in the tens of milligrams per kilogram ranges (McKellar & Benchaoui 1996). However, the particularly high lipophilicity of moxidectin can predispose to toxicosis in young foals and in emaciated animals with insufficient adipose tissue. This results in adverse neurological reactions, including prolonged coma and, in some cases, death (Johnson et al 1999). Although the product label contains a specific contraindication to the use of moxidectin in foals less than 4 months of age, this may be because of a lack of specific data in foals of this age group rather than an observed toxicity.

The possibility of environmental effects of ivermectin has been a contentious issue since Wall & Strong (1987) reported differences in rate of degradation of fecal pats from treated compared with untreated ruminants. There are no published data on similar studies in Equidae following oral administration of either ivermectin or moxidectin.

Benzimidazoles

Currently, four benzimidazole compounds are in common use in equine practice: fenbendazole, oxibendazole, mebendazole and oxfendazole. The benzimidazoles selectively bind to the nematode β-tubulin and inhibit the formation of microtubules, which are intracellular organelles with a variety of functions including the movement of both energy metabolites and chromosomes during cell division and the provision of the skeletal structure of the cell (Martin 1997). The benzimidazoles essentially starve the nematodes via intestinal cell disruption and inhibit worm egg production. From a clinical standpoint, the most important aspect of the mode of action of the benzimidazoles is that, compared with anthelmintic compounds that disrupt parasite neurotransmission, the onset of the anthelmintic effect is slow. The individual benzimidazoles have different absorption, distribution and elimination characteristics such that there are differences in the dose rates required to achieve comparable antiparasitic efficacy. Furthermore, efficacy is achieved with the more-soluble benzimidazoles, which are eliminated rapidly, by exposing parasites to lethal plasma levels for longer by administering the drugs over a prolonged period (Prichard et al 1978, McKellar & Scott 1990). In the horse, this has led to the development of specific "5 day" dosing protocols with fenbendazole (Duncan et al 1980, 1998, Lyons et al 1986).

The benzimidazoles have a broad spectrum of activity against adult strongyles (assuming susceptible cyathostome populations) ascarids and lungworm but not tapeworm and bots. Multiple dosing strategies of fenbendazole are effective against migrating *S. vulgaris* larvae, mucosal hypobiotic third-stage cyathostome larvae, migrating ascarid larvae and lungworm (Clayton & Neave 1979, Duncan et al 1980, 1998, Lyons et al 1986, Vandermyde et al 1987).

Pyrimidines

Three pyrantel salts (pamoate, embonate and tartrate) are indicated for use in the horse. The pyrimidines are selective agonists at synaptic and extrasynaptic nicotinic acetylcholine receptors on nematode muscle cells, which produce spastic paralysis of the parasites.

Pyrantel salts are active against adult and luminal stages of strongyles and ascarids but have only limited efficacy against migrating larval parasites and no activity against bots in the stomach. At double dose rates, either 13.2 mg pamoate salt/kg (Lyons et al 1986) or 38 mg embonate salt/kg, pyrantel salts are effective in the treatment of tapeworm infections. Pyrantel tartrate, administered at a continuous low level of 2.6 mg/kg in feed, is effective against adult strongyles and ascarids, as well as being active against newly ingested infective third-stage larvae (Valdez et al 1995).

Piperazine

Piperazine is a gamma-aminobutyric acid (GABA) agonist that hyperpolarizes the muscle membrane potential and so increases membrane conductance, which produces spastic paralysis of the parasite. Piperazine on its own has a narrow spectrum of activity against adult stages of cyathostomes and ascarids but is also marketed in a variety of combinations with individual benzimidazoles. Such combination products have a broad spectrum of activity and may be effective against benzimidazole-resistant cyathostomes, but separate piperazine-resistant cyathostome populations have also been identified (Britt & Clarkson 1988, Drudge et al 1988, Pereira et al 1991).

Praziquantel

Praziquantel is indicated for use in the horse in several countries as a component of a combination ivermectin product (Mercier et al 2001). The mode of action of praziquantel has been studied extensively in trematodes (Harnett 1998) and the anticestodal effects of this compound are assumed to have a similar basis. Praziquantel increases the permeability of tegumental and muscle cells to calcium ions, which results in parasitic muscular contraction and paralysis. In the horse, praziquantel has a narrow spectrum of activity against tapeworm, with 89–100% efficacy at dose rates of 0.75–1 mg/kg (Lyons et al 1992).

CONTROL PROGRAMS FOR INTERNAL PARASITES

The fundamental concept of the control of equine internal parasites is to reduce the transmission of parasites between animals. Although it is possible to achieve this by exclusively non-chemical means, such as either frequent collection of pasture fecal pats (Herd 1986) or feeding grazing animals nematode-trapping fungi (Larsen 1996), typical control programs for internal parasites are based on anthelmintic dosing (Table 4.2). The program should be designed on the basis of epidemiological features of interest. Most commonly, these are strongyles (especially cyathostomes), tapeworms and ascarids (when young stock are present).

Table 4.2 Guidelines for internal parasite control programs

Program	Dosing regimen	Comments
Targeted dosing	Monthly FWEC all grazing animals	Appropriate on farms with: strictly controlled grazing management; mature horses only; minimal new intake animals; efficient and compliant owner/manager prepared to undertake frequent sampling
	Dose all FWEC positive (or arbitrary level, say > 200 epg) with principal anthelmintic at "standard" dose rate	Standard faecal tests have very poor sensitivity for tapeworm detection: modified test has been developed that is 61% sensitive and 98% specific (Proudman & Edwards 1992)
	Biannual tapeworm faecal analysis or tapeworm serology	Tapeworm quantitative serological test available in Europe
	Dose all tapeworm-positive animals with pyrantel pamoate 13.2 mg/kg p.o. (USA) or pyrantel embonate 38 mg/kg p.o. (Europe)	
Strategic dosing	Only spring/summer dosing	Regional variations in climate affect the total period for which suppression of faecal worm egg output is required
	All grazing animals dosed at same time points with principal anthelmintic	
	Dosing with principal anthelmintics repeated on one or two occasions at predetermined intervals (based on ERP associated with each drug class; see Table 4.1)	Appropriate on premises in areas which have discrete periods of weather detrimental to parasite survival on pasture
Interval dosing	Year round synchronized dosing all grazing animals	Intensive usage anthelmintics predisposes to development of resistance so requires vigilant post-treatment FWEC monitoring
	Dosing with principal anthelmintic at predetermined intervals (based on ERP associated with each drug class, see Table 4.1)	Appropriate for situations where: grazing group is casually managed (e.g. multiowner self-care livery premises); young animals grazing; frequent new intake animals
Continuous in-feed dosing	Daily administration in feed pyrantel 2.6 mg/kg (not licenced in Europe)	Most appropriate if grazing group are mature animals

FWEC, fecal worm egg count; ERP, egg reappearance period; epg, eggs per gram; p.o., oral dosing

Although stomach bots are non-pathogenic, it is common to incorporate boticidal dosing into the control programs. The programs designed to control the major species incidentally control other minor parasite species. The epidemiology of the major internal parasite species of the horse varies with the climate, geographical region, host demographics, grazing practices and grassland management. As a result, there is no single program for parasite control that is applicable to all equine premises (Proudman & Matthews 2000).

General points that apply to the use of anthelmintics in parasite control programs are:

• monitoring for anthelmintic resistance should be performed at least annually by either fecal egg count reduction tests or *in vitro* assays (Craven et al 1999);

• the class(es) of drug(s) to which anthelmintic resistance has developed should be indefinitely omitted as a principal anthelmintic from any premises where anthelmintic resistance occurs; and

• the efficacy of anthelmintics has been reported to be markedly less in young than in adult horses (Herd & Gabel 1990, Herd & Majewski 1994).

Guidelines for the options for chemical control of equine internal parasites are given in Table 4.3.

Although the consensus is that discrete drug classes should be used in a slow (annual) rotational basis in order to delay the selection for anthelmintic resistance (Herd & Coles 1995), this issue remains unresolved and contentious. In field situations where multiple parasite species

Table 4.3 Parasiticide regimens in clinical endoparasitic disease

Disease	Treatment regimen	Comments
Cyathostomosis	Intensive protocol combining ivermectin and benzimidazoles Ivermectin, 0.2 mg/kg p.o. on days 1, 16, 31, 61 and 91 Fenbendazole 10 mg/kg p.o. (7.5 mg/kg in Europe) on days 2–6, 17–21, 32–36, 62–66 and 92–96	Moxidectin has the potential for toxicity in thin, debilitated animals, such that it is probably inappropriate to use in the therapy of clinical cases with cyathostomosis. Grazing cohorts of animals with cyathostomosis are likely to harbour immature mucosal cyathostome burdens and the owner/manager should be warned that treatment per se has some risk of precipitating overt clinical disease. For the cohorts a slightly less-intensive protocol is advised. ivermectin 0.2 mg/kg p.o. or moxidectin 0.4 mg/kg p.o. on days 1, 31, 61 and 91 or fenbendazole 10 mg/kg (7.5 mg/kg in Europe) p.o. on day 2–6, 32–36, 62–66 and 92–96.
Large strongyloid infection	Protocol should be directed at both parasites within the intestinal lumen and also those migrating within the vasculature. Use ivermectin 0.2 mg/kg p.o., or moxidectin 0.4 mg/kg p.o., or fenbendazole 10 mg/kg (Europe 7.5 mg/kg) p.o. for 5 consecutive days, or fenbendazole 60 mg/kg p.o. as a single dose	Typically there will be concurrent luminal cyathostomes and immature cyathostome larval infection such that intensive repeated parasiticide therapeutic dosing at 10-day intervals may be indicated (see above). When colic is a clinical feature, administration of anthelmintics might exacerbate signs, and recent anthelmintic dosing is a known risk factor for the onset of overt cyathostomosis.
Ascarid infection	Use fenbendazole 10 mg/kg p.o. for 5 consecutive days, or levamisole 8.8 mg/kg p.o. (not licenced in Europe), or ivermectin 0.2 mg/kg, p.o., or moxidectin 0.4 mg/kg, p.o.	Recommended to repeat 3–4 weeks after first treatment and avoid further grazing of ascarid egg-contaminated paddocks for 12 months. The mode of action results in rapid death of parasites such that they may cause intestinal obstruction/rupture if given to animals with high burdens of *Parascaris equorum*.
Tapeworm infection	Only pyrantel salts have label claim for good efficacy (> 90%) for the removal of tapeworm infections. Use pyrantel pamoate 13.2 mg/kg p.o. (USA), or pyrantel embonate 38 mg/kg p.o. (Europe), or praziquantel 1 mg/kg p.o.	
Bot infection	Use ivermectin 0.2 mg/kg p.o., or organophosphates: trichlorfon 40 mg/kg p.o. or dichlorvos 35 mg/kg p.o.	Bots do not cause disease such that prescribing treatment for clinical purposes is likely, but annual inclusion of a boticidal anthelmintic is often part of a control program (mid-winter dosing)
Lungworm infection	ivermectin 0.2 mg/kg p.o.	
Strongyloides westeri infection	Use fenbendazole 50 mg/kg p.o., or oxibendazole 10 mg/kg p.o., or thiabendazole 44 mg/kg p.o., or ivermectin 0.2 mg/kg p.o., or moxidectin 0.4 mg/kg p.o.	
Pinworm infection	Any anthelmintics at 'standard' dose rates but efficacy of piperazine is <70%	

(continued)

Table 4.3 *(continued)*

Disease	Treatment regimen	Comments
Stomach worm infection	Ivermectin 0.2 mg/kg p.o.	Gastric lesions unlikely to be treated as entity; summer sores treated with ivermectin.
Eyeworm infection	Physical removal/ophthalmic irrigation; fenbendazole 10 mg/kg p.o. for 5 consecutive days partially effective	
Onchocerca spp. infection	Ivermectin 0.2 mg/kg p.o.	May get recurrences because this kills only cutaneous microfilaria and not adult stages.
Liver fluke infection	Triclabendazole (extra-label use) 15 mg/kg p.o.	

p.o., oral dosing

require to be controlled, it is necessary to use more than one drug class during 1 year (Proudman & Matthews 2000). In a recent study, it was found that 86% of horse owners/managers administered either two or three classes of anthelmintic drug per annum (Lloyd et al 2000).

Ultimately, the success of a parasite control program is best assessed by evidence of a reduced incidence or prevalence of parasite-associated disease. However, apart from the general observation of reduced prevalence of colic following *S. vulgaris* infection (Drudge & Lyons 1986), there is only a single report that provides evidence of the effectiveness of specific equine parasite control programs in reducing the incidence of disease (Uhlinger 1990).

Anthelmintic regimens for parasite-associated disease

The guidelines for anthelmintic regimens as a component of therapeutic protocols in disease states are summarized in Table 4.4. These recommendations are derived from anthelmintic efficacy studies in healthy animals and/or clinical observation, because there are no data from controlled clinical trials. In equine practice, it is not uncommon to make a generic diagnosis of 'intestinal parasitism,' in which concurrent treatment with several classes of anthelmintic drug with different spectra of activity may be justified (this contrasts with the general recommendations for ideal control programs). Also, in disease states, high dosage rates are often appropriate and these

may be repeated in a much shorter timeframe than recommended for control programs.

Anthelmintic resistance

Anthelmintic resistance is an inherited trait that develops in response to selection pressure favoring survival of those worms that have the inherent genetic ability to survive anthelmintic treatment. Typically, as the selection pressure is a result of prolonged and/or frequent usage of deworming doses in parasite control programs (Sangster 1999). Once resistance develops, it appears that reversion to susceptibility does not occur (Uhlinger & Johnstone 1984). To date in equine parasites, anthelmintic resistance has only been documented in cyathostomes. There is widespread and well-documented resistance to the benzimidazoles and there are also reports of resistance to pyrantel, piperazine and phenothiazine (Lyons et al 1999). It has been hypothesized that resistance to the macrocylic lactones will occur within around 5 years of the introduction of moxidectin as an equine parasiticide. This is likely because the persistent effect of moxidectin (compared with ivermectin) on cyathostomes means that there is a prolonged period of exposure at which drug concentrations in the host favor the survival of resistant worms (Sangster 1999). The same author has suggested that the first evidence of developing macrocyclic lactone resistance will be a reduction in the egg reappearance period (ERP) following ivermectin or moxidectin dosing and it is most likely to first occur in foals (Sangster 1999). With the

Table 4.4 Parasiticide regimens in clinical ectoparasitic disease

Disease	Treatment regimen	Notes
Lice infestation	Piperonyl butoxide: pyrethrum shampoo	Skin contact for 10 min then wash out, repeat after 10–14 days
	Permethrin citronella solution	Topical sponge or spray, repeat after 14 days
Chorioptic mange	Doramectin injection 0.3 mg/kg s.c.	Repeat after 30 days
	Fipronil spray applied to affected areas	Repeat three times at 5 day intervals
	Selenium sulfide shampoo	
	Ivermectin injectable applied topically to affected areas	Do not use ivermectin as a 'pour' on as it is irritant to equine skin; repeat after 14 days
		All listed treatments are extra-label use; topical treatments applied after clipping leg hair and general skin hygiene
Onchocerciasis	Ivermectin 0.2 mg/kg p.o.	Repeat after 14 days
	Moxidectin 0.4 mg/kg p.o.	
Sarcoptic and psoroptic mange	Ivermectin 0.3 mg/kg p.o.	Extra-label; should be effective
Demodectic mange		Extremely rare infection, suggestive of underlying immunosuppressive illness; do not treat with amitraz as it is highly toxic to horses
Tick infection	Fipronil, direct topical application	Extra-label

p.o., oral; s.c., subcutaneous

prevalence of anthelmintic resistance recently reported to be 90% and 30% for fenbendazole and pyrantel, respectively, in specific regions (Tarigo-Martinie et al 2001), the importance of vigilant monitoring for developing anthelmintic resistance cannot be understated. The options for this are fecal egg count reduction tests or in vitro assays (Ihler & Bjorn 1996, Craven et al 1999, Pook et al 2002, von Samson-Himmelstjerna et al 2002). Recommendations for slowing the spread of anthelmintic resistance necessitate much greater veterinary intervention in parasite control programs, with considerable horse owner/manager compliance and improved dissemination of accurate information on "best practice" parasite control strategies (Herd & Coles 1995, Reinemeyer 1999).

ECTOPARASITICIDES

DRUGS

Pyrethroids

Pyrethroids are contact poisons that enter insects through their cuticular (skin) surface and disrupt neural activity by action on the ion exchange associated with action potentials. There is rapid development of insect muscle contractions, convulsions, paralysis and death. As a class, the synthetic pyrethroids have very low mammalian toxicity as absorbed pyrethroids are oxidized rapidly and they are used widely as residual insecticides in the horse, formulated as solutions or emulsions and powders. Currently permethrin, cypermethrin, fenvalerate and deltamethrin are indicated for use in horses. These are often formulated as combination products containing the synergistic compound piperonyl butoxide; citronella; insect repellent molecules such as the natural pyrethrin, pyrethrum and stabilene (butoxypolypropylene glycols); or a combination of these. The duration of action of pyrethroid products varies from 4 to 14 days depending on the formulation.

Miscellaneous ectoparasiticides

Macrocyclic lactones

The macrocyclic lactones (p. 64) are less effective against ectoparasites in the horse than in ruminants, but extra-label use of the injectable solution of ivermectin for cattle applied topically to chorioptic mange lesions has, anecdotally, some therapeutic effect. Similarly, extra-label systemic administration of doramectin appears to have good efficacy in cases of chorioptic mange.

Selenium sulfide

Selenium sulfide (off label) has been reported to have efficacy for the treatment of lice in the horse (Paterson & Orrell 1995) and it has also been used in chorioptic mange (Curtis 1999).

Fipronil

Fipronil, a product indicated for the treatment of fleas in small animals, has anecdotal reports of efficacy against equine ticks (Littlewood 1999). The use of fipronil in an individual case of chorioptic mange has been reported (Littlewood 2000).

CONTROL PROGRAMS FOR ECTOPARASITES

Because of regional differences in the prevalence of external parasites, control programs should be tailored to suit local requirements. In addition to topical and systemic treatments, control should aim to minimize exposure to parasites.

Generally, the control of lice and mites involves the treatment of both affected individuals and contact animals. Preventative programs are rarely used. However, systemic use of ivermectin reduces the extent of egg laying by lice and mites. While ivermectin and moxidectin may have some effect against adult stages, alone they are unlikely to treat or prevent infestation effectively (Littlewood 2000).

Prevention of exposure of grazing animals to flies, mosquitoes and ticks is difficult. For control of flying insects (*Diptera* spp.), stabling and the provision of face masks, hoods and body rugs, particularly at times of increased parasite activity, can help to reduce exposure. In addition, the effect of stabling can be enhanced by using electric fans to induce air movement and by fitting screens, treated with insecticide, to windows. Limiting grazing to mowed pastures can reduce exposure to ticks.

The topical application of insecticides and/or repellents can reduce exposure. Suggested regimens include the application of 200 ml 0.5% fenvalerate along the line of the back. Alternatively 1 litre 0.1% fenvalerate may be applied as a body spray. This should be repeated every 7 days, or following exposure to rain. Permethrin insecticidal repellents are also effective and are used as a pour on preparation (30–40 ml 4% permethrin). However, adverse skin reactions have been reported following application. Cypermethrin and permethrin are also used in plastic tags or strips that can be attached to the head collar, mane and tail.

Repellents may be applied to the horse or to rugs and hoods. However, this usually has only limited efficacy.

Regimens for ectoparasitic disease

Guidelines for specific ectoparasite disease entities are listed in Table 4.4. These are largely based on clinical observations and include extra-label use of several products.

It is important to apply control measures to all horses in a group rather than only treating those that demonstrate clinical signs of fly, mosquito or tick problems.

MISCELLANEOUS PARASITICIDES

Sulfonamides and diaminopyrimidines

The treatment of EPM is covered extensively in Chapters 3 and 9. Further information on these antimicrobial agents is presented in Chapter 2.

Toltrazuril

The use of toltrazuril and other similar agents in horses is covered in Chapter 3.

Imidocarb diprionate

Imidocarb has a direct effect on the structure of *Babesia* spp. and is the drug of choice for equine piroplasmosis (see Ch. 3). Imidocarb has cholinergic effects and may cause adverse, potentially fatal effects (colic, ptyalism and diarrhea) in the donkey.

Trypanocidal drugs

There are significant problems with resistance to trypanocidal drugs (see Ch. 3). Several formulations cause significant necrosis at injection sites. In the horse, the most commonly used trypanocides are sumarin, quinapyramine sulfate and isometamidium, which have efficacy against *T. evansii* and *T. congolense*. Quinapyramine is also used to treat *T. brucei* and *T. vivax*.

REFERENCES

Afzal J, Burke A B, Balten P L et al 1997 Moxidectin: metabolic fate and blood pharmacokinetics of ^{14}C-labeled moxidectin in horses. Journal of Agricultural and Food Chemistry 45:3627–3633

Baggot J D, McKellar Q A 1994 The absorption distribution and elimination of anthelmintic drugs: the role of pharmacokinetics. Journal of Veterinary Pharmacology and Therapeutics 17:409–419

Bairden K, Brown S R, McGoldrick J et al 2001 Efficacy of moxidectin 2% gel against naturally acquired strongyle infections in horses, with particular reference to larval cyathostomes. Veterinary Record 148:138–141

Britt D P, Clarkson M J 1988 Experimental chemotherapy in horses infected with benzimidazole-resistant small strongyles. Veterinary Record 123:219–221

Britt D P, Preston J M 1985 Efficacy of ivermectin against *Dictyocaulus arnfieldi* in ponies. Veterinary Record 116:343–345

Campbell W C, Leaning W H D, Seward R L 1989 Use of ivermectin in horses. In Campbell WC (ed) Ivermectin and abamectin. Springer Verlag, New York, pp. 245–259

Clayton H, Neave R M 1979 Efficacy of mebendazole against *Dictyocaulus arnfeldi* in the donkey. Veterinary Record 104:571–572

Cornwell R L, Jones R M 1968 Field trials in horses with pyrantel tartrate. Veterinary Record 82:586–587

Costa A J, Barbosa O F, Moraes F R et al 1998 Comparative efficacy evaluation of moxidectin gel and ivermectin paste against internal parasites of equines in Brazil. Veterinary Parasitology 80:29–36

Craven J, Bjorn H, Barnes E H et al 1999 A comparison of in vitro tests and a faecal egg count reduction test in detecting anthelmintic resistance in horse strongyles. Veterinary Parasitology 85:49–59

Curtis C F 1999 Pilot study to investigate the efficiency of 1 per cent sulphide selenium shampoo in the treatment of equine chorioptic mange. Veterinary Record 144:674–675

Demeulenaere D, Vercruysse J, Dorny P et al 1997 Comparative studies of ivermectin and moxidectin in the control of naturally acquired cyathostome infections in horses. Veterinary Record 141:383–386

DiPietro J A, Todd K S, Lock T F et al 1982 Anthelmintic efficacy of ivermectin given intramuscularly in horses. American Journal of Veterinary Research 43:145–148

DiPietro J A, Hutchens D E, Lock T F et al 1997 Clinical trial of moxidectin oral gel in horses. Veterinary Parasitology 72(2):167–177

Drudge J H, Lyons E T 1966 Control of internal parasites of the horse. Journal of the American Veterinary Medical Association 148:378–383

Drudge J H, Lyons E T 1986 Large strongyles: recent advances. Veterinary Clinics of North America 2:263–280

Drudge J H, Szanto T, Wyant A M 1963 Critical tests of thiabendazole as an anthelmintic in the horse. American Journal of Veterinary Research 35:1409–1412

Drudge J H, Lyons E T, Tolliver S C et al 1988 Piperazine resistance in population *B. equine* strongyles: a study of selection in thoroughbreds in Kentucky from 1966 through 1983. American Journal of Veterinary Research 49:986–994

Duncan J L, McBeath D G, Preston N K 1980 Studies on the efficacy of fenbendazole used in a divided dosage regime against strongyle infection in ponies. Equine Veterinary Journal 12:78–80

Duncan J L, Bairden K, Abbott E M 1998 Elimination of mucosal cyathostome larvae by five daily treatments with fenbendazole. Veterinary Record 142:268–271

Elliot M 1973 A photostable pyrethroid. Nature 246: 169–170

Eysker M, Boersema J H, Kooyman F N 1992 The effect of ivermectin treatment against inhibited early third stage, late third stage and fourth stage larvae and adult stages of the cyathostomes in Shetland ponies and spontaneous expulsion of these helminths. Veterinary Parasitology 42:295–302

French D D, Klei T M, Foil C S et al 1988 Efficacy of ivermectin in paste and injectable formulations against microfilariae of *Onchocerca cervicalis* and resolution of associated dermatitis in horses. American Journal of Veterinary Research 49:1550–1554

Harnett W 1998 The anthelmintic action of praziquantel. Parasitology Today 4:144–146

Hennessy D 1997 Modifying the formulation or delivery mechanism to increase the activity of anthelmintic compounds. Veterinary Parasitology 72:367–390

Herd R P 1986 Epidemiology and control of equine strongylosis at Newmarket. Equine Veterinary Journal 18:447–452

Herd R P, Coles G C 1995 Slowing the spread of anthelmintic resistant nematodes of horses in United Kingdom. Veterinary Record 136:481–485

Herd R P, Gabel A A 1990 Reduced efficacy of anthelmintics in young compared with adult horses. Equine Veterinary Journal 2:164–169

Herd R P, Majewski G A 1994 Comparison of daily and monthly pyrantel treatment in yearling thoroughbreds and the protective effect of strategic medication of mares on their foals. Veterinary Parasitology 55: 93–104

Ihler C F, Bjorn H 1996 Use of two in-vitro methods for detection of benzimidazole resistance in equine small strongyles. Veterinary Parasitology 65:117–125

Jacob D E, Huchinson M J, Gibbons L M 1995 Equine cyathostome infection: suppression of faecal egg output with moxidectin. Veterinary Record 137:545

Johnson P J, Mrad D R, Shwartz A T et al 1999 Presumed moxidectin toxicosis in three foals. Journal of American Veterinary Association 214:678–680

Klei T R, Chapman M R, French D D et al 1993 Evalution of ivermectin at an evaluated dose against encysted equine cyathostome larvae. Veterinary Parasitology 47:99–106

Lanusse C, Prichard R 1993 Relationship between pharmacological properties and clinical efficacy of ruminant anthelmintics. Veterinary Parasitology 49:123–158

Larsen M, Nansen P, Grondahl C et al 1996 The capacity of the fungus *Duddingtonia flagrans* to prevent strongyle infections in foals on pasture. Parasitology 113:1–6

Littlewood J 1999 Control of ectoparasites in horses. In Practice 21:418–424

Littlewood J 2000 Chorioptic mange: successful treatment of a case with fipronil. Equine Veterinary Education 12:144–146

Lloyd S, Smith J, Connan R M et al 2000 Parasite control methods used by horse owners: factors predisposing to the development of anthelmintic resistance in nemotodes. Veterinary Record 146:487–492

Love S, Murphy D, Mellor D 1999 Pathogenicity of cyathostome infection. Veterinary Parasitology 85:113–122

Lyons E T, Drudge J H, Tolliver S C et al 1986 Pyrantel pamoate: evaluating its activity against equine tapeworms. Veterinary Medicine 81:280–285

Lyons E T, Tolliver S C, Drudge J H 1992 Activity of praziquantel against *Anoplocephala perfoliata* (cestode) in horses. Journal of the Helminthology Society of Washington 59:1–4

Lyons E T, Tolliver S C, Drudge J H 1999 Historical perspective of cyathostome: prevalence, treatment and control programs. Veterinary Parasitology 85:97–112

Martin R J 1997 Modes of action of anthelmintic drugs. Veterinary Journal 154:11–34

McKellar Q A, Benchaoui H A 1996 Avermectins and millbemycins. Journal of Veterinary Pharmacology and Therapeutics 19:331–351

McKellar Q A, Scott E W 1990 The benzimidazole anthelmintic agents: a review. Journal of Veterinary Pharmacology and Therapeutics 13:223–247

Mercier P, Chick B, Alves-Branco F et al 2001 Comparative efficacy, persistent effect, and treatment intervals of anthelmintic pastes in naturally infected horses. Veterinary Parasitology 99:29–39

Monahan C M, Chapman M R, French D D et al 1995 Efficacy of moxidectin oral gel against *Onchocerca cervicalis* microfilariae. Journal of Parasitology 81:117–118

Paterson S, Orrell S 1995 Treatment of biting lice (*Damalinia equi*) in 25 horses using 1% selenium sulphide. Equine Veterinary Education 7:304–306

Pereira M C, Kohek I Jr, Campos R et al 1991 A field evaluation of anthelmintics for control of cyathostomes of horses in Brazil. Veterinary Parasitology 38:121–129

Perez R, Cabezas I, Garcia M et al 1999 Comparison of the pharmacokinetics of moxidectin (Equest®) and ivermectin (Eqvalan®) in horses. Journal of Veterinary Pharmacology and Therapeutics 22:174–180

Pook J F, Power M L, Sangster N C et al 2002 Evaluation of tests for anthelmintic resistance in cyathostomes. Veterinary Parasitology 106:331–343

Prichard R K, Hennessy D R, Steel J W 1978 Prolonged administration: a new concept for increasing the spectrum of effectiveness of anthelmintics. Veterinary Parasitology 4:309–315

Proudman C J, Edwards G B 1992 Validation of a centrifugation/flotation technique for the diagnosis of equine cestodiasis. Veterinary Record 131:71–72

Proudman C J, Matthews J B 2000 Control of intestinal parasites in horses. In Practice 22:90–97

Proudman C J, French N P, Trees A J 1998 Tapeworm infection as a significant risk factor for spasmodic colic and ileal impaction colic in the horse. Equine Veterinary Journal 30:194–199

Reinemeyer C R 1999 Current concerns about control programs in temperate climates. Veterinary Parasitology 85:163–172

Ryan W G, Best P J 1985 Efficacy of ivermectin paste against *Strongyloides westeri* in foals. Veterinary Record 117:169–170

Sangster N C 1999 Pharmacology of anthelmintic resistance in cyathostomes: will it occur with the avermectin millbemycins. Veterinary Parasitology 85:189–204

Tarigo-Martinie J L, Wyatt A R, Kaplan R M 2001 Prevalence and clinical implications of anthelmintic resistance in cyathostomes in horses. Journal of the American Veterinary Medical Association 218:1957–1960

Taylor S M, Kenny J 1995 Comparison of moxidectin with ivermectin and pyrantel embonate for reduction of faecal egg count in horses. Veterinary Record 137:516–518

Uhlinger C 1990 Effects of three anthelmintic schedules on the incidence of colic in horses. Equine Veterinary Journal 22:251–254

Uhlinger C, Johnstone C 1984 Failure to re-establish benzimidazole susceptible populations of small strongyles after prolonged treatment with non-benzimidazole drugs. Equine Veterinary Science 4:7–9

Valdez R A, Dipietro J A, Paul A J et al 1995 Controlled efficacy study of the bioequivalence of Strongid C® and generic pyrantel tartrate in horses. Veterinary Parasitology 60:83–102

Vandermyde C R, DiPietro J A, Todd K S Jr et al 1987 Evaluation of fenbendazole for larvacidal effect in experimentally induced *Parascaris equorum* infections in pony foals. Journal of the American Veterinary Medical Association 190:1548–1549

von Samson-Himmelstjerna G, von Witzendorff C, Sievers G et al 2002 Comparative use of faecal egg count reduction test, egg hatch assay and beta-tubulin codon 200 genotyping in small strongyles (cyathostominae) before and after benzimidazole treatment. Veterinary Parasitology 108:227–235

Wall R, Strong L 1987 Environmental consequences of treating cattle with the antiparasitic drug ivermectin. Nature 327:418–421

Xiao L, Herd R P, Majewski G A 1994 Comparative efficacy of moxidectin and ivermectin against hypobiotic and encysted cyathostomes and other equine parasites. Veterinary Parasitology 53:83–90

CHAPTER CONTENTS

Introduction 75

Pituitary and adrenal glands 75
  Corticosteroids 75
  Equine Cushing's disease 76

Brain 80
  Endophyte infected fescue toxicosis 80

Thyroid gland 80

References 82

5

Drugs acting on the endocrine system

*Janice E. Sojka   Michel Levy
Laurent Couetil*

INTRODUCTION

The endocrine system consists of not one but multiple systems with distinct functions, some of which overlap. Most endocrine systems were originally believed to be simple feedback loops, but this is now viewed as an oversimplification and agents may up- or downregulate hormonal responses at numerous points in a cycle. This chapter will attempt to give an overview of the drugs that affect the various endocrine systems in the horse. The reader must bear in mind that most of what is known about these interactions has been elucidated in other species, primarily in humans. There is a danger in overgeneralizing or applying the findings too rigorously to the equine. Unfortunately, until more information is available in horses, the data that are available must be applied.

For the sake of clarity, this chapter will be subdivided into sections. The adrenal and pituitary glands will be described first, followed by the brain and then the thyroid glands. Reproductive endocrinology is a separate topic and as such has been given its own chapter in this book (see Ch. 11).

PITUITARY AND ADRENAL GLANDS

CORTICOSTEROIDS

The class of drug that undoubtedly has the most effect on the various endocrine systems is the corticosteroids (glucocorticoids).

Glucocorticoids enjoy a large range of applications including topical ocular therapy, intralesional, intraarticular and systemic therapy. The most common reason for systemic therapy is the treatment of chronic obstructive pulmonary disease (COPD). Other uses include the treatment of immune-mediated diseases, dermatological conditions and other chronic inflammatory diseases.

Corticosteroids exert their systemic effects on the pituitary–adrenal axis by binding to receptors on the corticotrophs in the pituitary gland and other cells throughout the body. They exert negative feedback in this way and suppress the secretion of adrenocorticotropic hormone (ACTH) from the pituitary gland and cortisol from the adrenal glands. The horse is extremely sensitive to these effects. A single injection of dexamethasone at 0.04 mg/kg is sufficient to inhibit endogenous cortisol secretion and keep it at extremely low levels for more than 24 h. It can take the pituitary–adrenal axis up to 72 h to recover from a single dose of corticosteroid. In addition, repeated topical application or intraarticular injections have been implicated in producing systemic corticosteroid effects in horses. The degree and duration of the suppression of the pituitary–adrenal axis that is produced by depot and longer-acting corticosteroid preparations have not been as well documented in horses; however, by and large, the potency of the corticosteroid correlates with the duration of its suppressive effects.

In an effort to minimize the systemic side-effects of the corticosteroids, short-acting, less-potent forms, including topical or local therapy, should be used whenever possible. Prednisone is short acting but is poorly absorbed from the gastrointestinal tract and for that reason is of questionable efficacy in the treatment of pulmonary and other disorders. It should not be considered when treating severe conditions such as *purpura hemorrhagica* and advanced COPD, when potent corticosteroid effects are required. Depot forms of the corticosteroids are potent but may lead to an increased incidence of side-effects; consequently, aqueous formulations, such as dexamethasone, are used most commonly. Some of the undesirable side-effects of the systemic corticosteroids include immunosuppression, iatrogenic Cushing's disease, adrenocortical suppression and laminitis (Lavoie 2003).

Excessive or prolonged administration of exogenous corticosteroids has been reported to produce adverse effects in horses turned out after a prolonged racing season. This effect is termed the "steroid wash-out" or "steroid let down" syndrome. These horses exhibit lack of thrift, depression, weight loss and a poor hair coat. The etiology of this syndrome is hypothesized to be adrenal atrophy secondary to prolonged corticosteroid use. However, it has been difficult to reproduce experimentally using the administration of exogenous corticosteroids.

Glucocorticoids also have weak mineralocorticoid effects as they have some affinity for mineralocorticoid receptors. The laminitis-producing effects of the glucocorticoids have recently been linked to their ability to stimulate mineralocorticoid receptors and produce changes in blood flow and electrolyte balance.

Corticosteroids are also inhibitors of thyroid gland secretion and low thyroid hormone levels may be demonstrable in horses at times when excessive (exogenous or endogenous) corticosteroid concentrations exist. Older horses with equine Cushing's disease (ECD) and decreased muscle mass frequently have low thyroid hormone concentrations. These animals have euthyroid sick syndrome and should not be confused with true hypothyroidism. In these horses, the thyroid gland is capable of producing adequate hormone concentrations and will respond normally when stimulated with either thyroid-stimulating hormone (TSH) or thyroid-releasing hormone (TRH). Thyroid supplementation should not be administered to these horses; rather their primary problem should be addressed.

EQUINE CUSHING'S DISEASE

ECD is nearly always associated with hypertrophy, adenomatous hyperplasia or, in the most advanced cases, a functional adenoma of the *pars intermedia* of the pituitary gland. This condition was first described in 1932; however the exact pathogenesis, diagnostic plan and appropriate treatment regimen are still under dispute. Although, all breeds of horses and both sexes may be affected, there is an increased incidence of ECD in ponies.

Functional adenomas of the *pars intermedia* of the pituitary gland usually occur in aged horses. The average age at diagnosis is 19–21 years. However, ECD is being recognized increasingly in younger horses. It is no longer unusual to diagnose ECD in horses aged 8–10 years, which exhibit subtle clinical signs of ECD.

The first sign observed is often abnormal fat distribution and the owner noticing that the horse or pony is an "easy keeper" that requires much less grain or feed than other animals. With time, other clinical signs also appear. The clinical signs most often associated with advanced ECD include hirsutism, an abnormal hair shedding pattern, hyperhidrosis, polyuria and polydipsia, weight loss and decreased muscle tone. Other clinical signs, including infertility, chronic laminitis, lethargy, blindness, seizures, delayed wound healing, bulging of the supraorbital fat pads and increased susceptibility to infection may be present alone or with the signs listed above. Laminitis that is refractory to standard treatment regimens and infertility are the two signs of ECD recognized most commonly in younger horses. These horses do not usually have abnormally long hair, but owners often report that these horses shed their winter coats later in the spring than normal. As these horses grow older, more typical signs of ECD appear.

Diagnosis

Although hirsutism is reported to be pathognomonic for ECD, the diagnosis should be confirmed using clinical pathology. Abnormal clinical pathology results typically occur rather late in ECD and usually include hyperglycemia, hyperlipidemia and a stress leukogram.

A diagnosis of ECD is usually confirmed by testing the pituitary–adrenal axis. Single or multiple measurements of plasma cortisol are not diagnostic for ECD. In fact, cortisol concentrations vary widely in normal horses and the values from horses with *pars intermedia* dysfunction are often within the reference range (Dybdal et al 1994). Additionally, cortisol concentrations may be elevated secondary to exercise, hypoglycemia and stress. Plasma cortisol levels exhibit a diurnal rhythm in equines, with morning values higher than evening values. Horses with ECD appear to lose this pattern of variation but this is not diagnostic for ECD since it can also occur in normal horses (Beech 1987). However, a horse with marked diurnal variation in cortisol concentrations probably does not have ECD.

The dexamethasone suppression test is the best way to evaluate the pituitary–adrenocortical axis function in horses. In normal horses, dexamethasone administration in the late afternoon, by intramuscular (i.m.) injection at a dose rate of $40\,\mu g/kg$ (approximately 20 mg for a 450 kg horse), depresses cortisol production to less than $10\,ng/ml$ ($1\,\mu g/dl$) by the following morning and cortisol levels will remain well below baseline for over 24 h. Cortisol levels are usually slightly depressed after dexamethasone administration to horses with ECD but the degree of suppression is less than in normal horses and plasma cortisol concentrations rebound more quickly.

The measurement of endogenous ACTH concentrations is valuable in the diagnosis of ECD (Sojka & Levy 1995). Plasma samples for ACTH determination require special handling: blood must be collected in chilled disodium ethylenediamine-tetraacetic acid (EDTA) tubes, maintained at 4°C, centrifuged promptly and the plasma stored at −70°C until analysis. The ACTH reference range may vary between laboratories. There can be an overlap in the values of stressed normal horses and early cases of ECD.

Horses with ECD have deranged glucoregulatory mechanisms and are often insulin resistant. Normal horses show an immediate rise in plasma glucose concentrations and a return to a baseline level within 1.5 h of intravenous (i.v.) administration of glucose (0.5 g/kg). Plasma glucose concentrations return to baseline with some delay in horses with ECD. Basal insulin levels are also persistently increased, even in the absence of hyperglycemia. When subjected to an exogenous i.v. insulin tolerance test (0.4 IU/kg), horses with ECD do not show a significant decline in blood glucose (Ralston 2002).

Treatment

The most important aspect of keeping horses with ECD healthy is excellent basic husbandry and vigilance for any intercurrent diseases. In affected horses that are not persistently hyperglycemic, regular dental care, deworming, foot care, responsive nutritional management and close attention to stable cleanliness and hygiene are generally all that is needed. Body clipping (with appropriate blanketing) is recommended for affected horses that have the characteristic heavy hair coat. A combination of hyperhidrosis and/or appropriate sweating means that horses with ECD often end up wet or with heat stress, which can lead to many indirect complications (Schott 2002).

Medical intervention is recommended for horses with ECD that are hyperglycemic, hyperlipemic, infertile or suffering from acute laminitis. There are currently three agents that are recommended for use in horses with ECD (Table 5.1).

Pergolide

Treatment with pergolide, a long-acting, oral dopamine receptor agonist, is currently the most frequently recommended approach. Pergolide is a semisynthetic ergot alkaloid derivative that is a potent agonist at both D_1 and D_2 receptors. Its stimulatory effects on postsynaptic dopamine receptors in the nigrostriatal system are used in the treatment of Parkinson's disease in humans (Beech 1994). It also inhibits the secretion of prolactin (and, as such, has been used to inhibit lactation in humans), produces transient increases in serum growth hormone and decreases in luteinizing hormone concentrations. The actions of pergolide may be decreased if horses are also given phenothiazine tranquilizers or reserpine.

Controlled studies to establish the pharmacokinetics (e.g. plasma concentrations, half-life, bioavailability and metabolism) of this drug have not been performed in horses. This lack of basic data has prevented the rational development of therapeutic plans for the treatment of ECD in horses. The current treatment recommendations are based on information extrapolated from the literature in human medicine and clinical dose–response trials using limited numbers of horses. Pergolide is active and appears to be safe in horses with ECD at the doses used currently (Schott et al 2001). Pergolide is expensive; therefore, it is recommended that treatment of affected horses is started using a total daily dose of 0.5 mg/horse, the lowest effective dose reported to date; some ponies can be successfully maintained on 0.25 mg/pony daily. If normal blood glucose concentrations are not achieved within 4–6 weeks of starting therapy, the daily dose can be increased by 0.25–0.5 mg/horse. This schedule should be repeated until the dose that maintains the horse in euglycemia is reached. Pergolide has been

Table 5.1 Comparison of drugs used to treat equine Cushing's disease

	Pergolide	Cyproheptadine	Bromocriptine
Mechanism of action	D_2 receptor agonist	Antiserotonergic, antihistamine	D_2 receptor agonist
Dose	1 µg/kg daily: for horses 0.5 mg, daily; for ponies 0.25 mg daily	0.25–0.5 mg/kg daily	0.02 mg/kg twice daily
Increase dose over time if needed	Yes, by 0.25 mg/day	Yes, increase dose or give same dose twice daily	Not reported
Route	Oral	Oral	Intramuscular
Assessment of efficacy	Normal blood glucose level, normal endogenous ACTH, dexamethasone suppression test	Improved appetite, improved hair coat, normal blood glucose level	As for pergolide
Precautions	None	High doses may result in depression	Do not give to pregnant or lactating animals

ACTH, adrenocorticotropic hormone

administered safely to pregnant mice and rabbits (Thompson & Montvale 2003).

Based on both subjective and objective criteria, most horses treated to date have shown marked and ongoing clinical improvement. Pergolide is a replacement therapy; therefore, it must be administered for the lifetime of the horse if it is going to have continued therapeutic benefits. In horses that are hyperglycemic, blood glucose levels can be monitored as a surrogate marker of the response to therapy. The reestablishment of euglycemia is evidence of a successful clinical response to therapy. However, establishing euglycemia does not always coincide with a return to normal pituitary function. Repeated evaluation of endogenous ACTH concentrations may also be used to determine the response to therapy. If the ACTH levels are within the reference range, it can be assumed that the dose of pergolide is adequate. If hyperglycemia is not present at the start of therapy or the return to normal pituitary function is the desired clinical end-point, a repeat dexamethasone suppression test should be carried out to confirm the reestablishment of a functional pituitary–adrenal feedback loop.

Cyproheptadine

Cyproheptadine is an antihistaminic and antiserotonergic agent that also has anticholinergic and sedative effects. It is used for its antihistaminic actions in humans. It has been used with limited success in the treatment of *pars intermedia* dysfunction in horses.

Anecdotal evidence indicates that a positive response is achieved in about 35% of the horses with ECD treated. Reed reported successful outcomes in 25 horses treated cyproheptadine (Reed 1998). Objective studies to elucidate the mechanism of action of cyproheptadine have failed to support these clinical findings: no changes were identified in the plasma concentrations of proopiomelanocortin-derived peptides or in the response to dexamethasone administration. Cyproheptadine may have non-pituitary mechanisms of action, since the horses that respond to therapy have normal hair growth and improved 'energy' levels. Cyproheptadine is known to be

an appetite stimulant in humans and some of the improved clinical condition seen in treated horses might be related to an increase in caloric intake and consequent improvement in the condition of the horses. In one pilot study (six horses), weight gain, improved hair coat, a return to or tendency towards normoglycemia and an improved response to the dexamethasone suppression tests were observed. However, these results could not be repeated when horses with ECD were first stabilized clinically and conditioned to their new environment (e.g. dewormed, teeth floated (rasped) and a minimum of 4 weeks at a stable body weight on a high plane of nutrition).

There is no basic information on the pharmacokinetics of cyproheptadine in horses. The recommended starting dose extrapolated from dosage recommendations in humans and corrected for metabolic body size is 0.25 mg/kg once daily (Dybdal & Levy 1997). A daily dose of 0.25 mg/kg twice daily can be given if there is no response to therapy after 6–8 weeks. Higher dose rates produce lethargy and excess drowsiness in horses. Geldings and stallions may develop paraphimosis during treatment. However, cyproheptadine appears to have a wide margin of safety in horses.

Bromocriptine

Bromocriptine is an ergot alkaloid dopamine receptor agonist that activates postsynaptic dopamine receptors. It blocks the release of prolactin from the pituitary gland via effects on D_2 receptors in the tuberoinfundibular system, inhibiting prolactin release and decreasing hyperprolactinemia and the size of some tumors. It is used in human medicine in the treatment of prolactin-secreting tumors and other micro- and macroadenomas of the pituitary gland (Anon. 2002). It is also used in the treatment of menstrual disorders and acromegaly and has been recommended as an adjunct therapy for Parkinson's disease in humans. In the horse, bromocriptine is used much less widely for the treatment of ECD than pergolide and cyproheptadine.

There is no basic information on pharmacokinetics of bromocriptine in horses. Administration of 0.02 mg/kg i.m. twice daily has been reported.

Bromocriptine is also available as an oral formulation, but oral administration to horses has not been reported. This drug should not be used in pregnant or lactating animals because of its effects on prolactin and lactation. Concomitant administration of bromocriptine and the phenothiazine tranquilizers or reserpine is contraindicated.

Mitotane (o,p'-DDD)

The adrenocorticolytic drug mitotane (o,p'-DDD), used in dogs and humans to treat adrenocortical hyperplasia, is of no therapeutic benefit in the treatment of ECD in horses.

Follow-up to treatment

The response to treatment in horses with ECD is usually judged using the subjective improvement in the clinical signs: improvement or resolution of the laminitis, reduction in the frequency of urination, decrease in water intake, shedding of hair and weight gain. Repeating a dexamethasone suppression test (Williams 1995) or reevaluating endogenous ACTH levels would give an objective evaluation of the efficacy of treatment. It is important to follow the overnight test protocol, since full suppression takes an extended period to develop fully and remains low for at least 24 h in normal horses (Beech 1987). A decrease in plasma cortisol concentrations in horses with ECD will not persist for the 17–19 h in which the overnight protocol is performed.

BRAIN

Environmental toxins can affect the brain and its hormone production. Fescue toxicosis is one such disease.

ENDOPHYTE INFECTED FESCUE TOXICOSIS

Tall fescue is a cool season grass that is grown widely throughout the world. It has many characteristics that make it a valuable forage source. Much of the fescue in the USA is infected with the endophytic fungus *Acremonium coenophialum*. It has been proven to be the causative agent of a host of problems in horses, most commonly problems in pregnant and lactating mares. These include an increased incidence of prolonged gestation, stillborn foals, agalactia and thickened placentas. An increased incidence of laminitis has been reported in younger horses. The hormonal changes that occur in mares include decreased serum prolactin and progesterone and increased serum estrogen concentrations (Cross 1994).

Treatment

The toxin acts as a dopamine receptor agonist in the brain. Dopamine antagonists can reverse the effects of the toxin, as do prolactin stimulators, such as TRH and metoclopramide. Treatment is generally accomplished using the D_2 receptor antagonist domperidone. Unlike other D_2 receptor antagonists, domperidone does not cross the blood–brain barrier and, therefore, it does not produce neuroleptic effects (Evans 2002). Rather, it blocks the effect of the fescue toxin on the D_2 receptors in the pituitary gland, which are outside the blood–brain barrier. Domperidone has been administered orally (p.o.), at a dose rate of 1.1 mg/kg once daily, to treat fescue toxicosis in pre- and postpartum mares (Evans 2002). The treated mares remained on the fescue-infected pastures but showed none of the typical signs of fescue exposure and went on to foal and lactate normally. Their prolactin levels were found to be higher than in the untreated control mares and were comparable to normal values. Domperidone also appeared to increase milk production in mares with poor milk production in this study. The phenothiazine tranquilizer perphenazine has also been used to increase prolactin levels in agalactic mares (Cross 1994).

THYROID GLAND

Thyroid disease is one of the most controversial areas in equine medicine. Practitioners run the gamut from those who do not "believe in" thyroid disease to those who diagnose and treat it frequently. Many of the clinical signs often attributed to thyroid deficiency are more commonly signs of ECD. These include obesity, a thickened neck, abnormal fat distribution, infertility and laminitis. If horses demonstrate these clinical signs without ECD, they have recently been characterized as suffering from "metabolic syndrome". Equine metabolic syndrome is analogous to non-insulin-dependent diabetes mellitus in humans. Currently, there are no recommended medications for the treatment of this syndrome. Restricting caloric intake and increasing exercise appear to be the most effective means of correcting the syndrome's effects. It is noteworthy that experimentally induced thyroid deficiency (removal of the thyroid glands) produces none of the "typical" signs of hypothyroidism in horses. Most horses with "thyroid syndrome" have normal thyroid gland function. A large number actually have normal resting thyroid hormone levels but are treated because they are "low normal". Others may have resting values below the normal range but respond normally to stimulation testing. Anecdotal reports state that these horses generally appear to respond to thyroid hormone supplementation (lose weight and regain normal behavior and fertility) despite having no demonstrable thyroid axis problem. It is clear that these horses do not have primary thyroid disease and in most cases have either ECD or equine metabolic syndrome. Why they respond to thyroid supplementation is not known, but the effect may be mediated via alterations in fat metabolism produced by the thyroid supplementation. The term "thyroid hormone responsive syndrome" better describes these horses as it acknowledges the fact that they respond to treatment, without implying that they have primary hypothyroidism.

Following surgical thyroidectomy, horses develop signs including exercise intolerance, decreased body temperature and heart rate, increased cold sensitivity, increased blood cholesterol and thickened facial features. These horses do not become particularly obese or depressed, or develop laminitis. Low resting thyroid hormone levels have also been associated with signs such as infertility, anhidrosis, myositis, abnormal behavior, laminitis, agalactia and infertility.

In adult horses, thyroid gland enlargement is usually caused by adenoma of the thyroid gland. These tumors are benign and do not, in the vast majority of instances, alter thyroid function. These masses should be removed surgically if they obstruct the trachea or esophagus or if hypothyroidism can be documented.

Diagnosis

Diagnosis of thyroid disease is made primarily through the detection of blood thyroxine (T_4) and triiodothyronine (T_3) concentrations and through the use of stimulation tests. An assay for endogenous equine TSH is not yet available commercially. When (and if) this test becomes available for use in diagnostic laboratories, it may help to shed some more light on thyroid disease in adult horses.

Baseline thyroid hormone measurements

There are a large number of factors that affect resting thyroid hormone levels in adult horses. Thyroid hormones set the resting metabolic rate and thus increase at times when the metabolic rate increases and decrease when the metabolic rate decreases. Euthyroid sick syndrome is the name given to the situation where the thyroid gland downregulates in response to debilitating illness or a catabolic state: the body is trying to conserve energy and calories by lowering its basal metabolic rate. In this syndrome, resting thyroid hormone levels are low although the thyroid glands are normal. In human patients with euthyroid sick syndrome, thyroid hormone supplementation is associated with increased mortality rate because of the primary disease process. It is likely that many horses with ECD have a form of euthyroid sick syndrome. Thyroid hormone supplementation is of no help and may be harmful in these animals.

Thyroid hormones are present in the blood in two forms; protein-bound and free hormone. Although the free portion constitutes only approximately 1% of the total hormone, it is the metabolically active form and the one that is transported into cells to exert its effects. Many drugs have been shown to lower the resting thyroid hormone concentrations in humans and other animals. These include phenylbutazone, glucocorticoids, insulin, halothane, diphenylhydantoin (phenytoin), phenobarbital, sulfonamides, furosemide (frusemide) and radioopaque contrast (iodine-containing) dyes (Sojka 1993). In all likelihood, these agents decrease thyroid hormone levels in horses as well, but only the effects of phenylbutazone (Sojka 1993) and glucocorticoids have been documented. Phenylbutazone does not displace T_4 from the protein binding sites but does suppress the circulating concentrations of both free and total T_4 (Sojka 1993). Despite the large numbers of horses on prolonged therapy with potentiated sulfonamides (trimethoprim/pyrimethamine plus a sulfonamide) for the treatment of EPM, side-effects from the action of these agents on thyroid hormone concentrations have not been reported in horses. Any iodine-containing compound (such as i.v. radioopaque contrast media) will temporarily inhibit thyroid hormone secretion. In adult animals with normal thyroid glands, tolerance will develop and thyroid hormone levels in the blood will recover to pretreatment levels even in the face of prolonged iodine administration. The fetus and animals with damaged or diseased thyroid glands will not be able to reestablish normal thyroid function in the face of high iodine ingestion and goiter may result.

Bayly and coworkers reported a survey of resting thyroid hormone concentrations in racing thoroughbreds (Morris & Garcia 1983). Many of these healthy animals with no signs of disease had resting T_4 levels significantly below the published reference ranges for sedentary horses. The conclusion was that T_4 is very susceptible to the effects of a variety of exogenous stimuli and as such is a very unreliable indicator on which to base thyroid status in horses. Concentrations of T_3 appeared to be much more stable. Consequently, if the thyroid status of a horse is to be evaluated using a one-off sample, T_3 should be determined.

Treatment

The effects of thyroid supplementation in horses with normal thyroid function are not known. It is likely that the glands respond in most instances by down regulating their production of T_4 and the normal thyroid axis is maintained. Therefore, when thyroid supplementation is withdrawn, it should be done gradually over a period of several weeks. Horses with low thyroid hormone levels and debilitating disease (euthyroid sick syndrome) should *not* receive thyroid supplementation unless a true thyroid deficiency has been diagnosed definitively.

There is very little published research looking at blood T_4 levels in horses on thyroid supplementation. A single dose of $20 \mu g/kg$ T_4 will maintain blood levels in the reference range for 24 h (Bayly et al 1996). There are several other forms of T_4 available for the treatment of horses. Iodinated casein, orally at $5.0 g/day$, is not readily available currently but has been recommended in the past (Sojka 1995). Concentrated bovine thyroid extract at a dosage of $10.5 g/day$ has been reported to return thyroid hormone serum concentrations to normal (Sojka 1995).

A horse receiving thyroid supplementation should have its serum T_4 and T_3 values monitored every 4–6 weeks and the dosage of the supplement should be adjusted to maintain serum concentrations of thyroid hormone within the reference range. If therapy is discontinued, the horse should be weaned slowly from the medication to allow its thyroid tissue function time to return to normal.

REFERENCES

Anon. 2002 Bromocriptine mesylate. In: Mosby's drug consult. Mosby, St Louis, MO pp. III356–III358

Bayly W, Andrea R, Smith J et al 1996 Thyroid hormone concentrations in racing thoroughbreds. Pferdeheikunde 12:534–538

Beech J 1987 Tumors of the pituitary gland (pars intermedia). In: Robinson N E (ed) Current therapy in equine medicine, 2nd edn. Saunders, Philadelphia, PA, pp. 182–185

Beech J 1994 Treatment of hyophyseal adenomas. Compendium on Continuing Education for the Practicing Veterinarian 16:921–923

Cross D L 1994 Effects and remedial therapy associated with the toxins of fescue in gravid mares. In: Proceedings of the 40th American Association of Equine Practitioners Annual Convention, Vancouver BC, pp. 33–34

Dybdal N O, Levy M 1997 Pituitary pars intermedia dysfunction in the horse Part II. Diagnosis and treatment. In: Proceedings of the 15th American

College of Veterinary Internal Medicine Forum, Lake Buena Vista, FL, pp. 470–472

Dybdal N O, Hargreaves K M, Madigan J E et al 1994 Diagnostic testing for pituitary pars intermedia dysfunction in horses. Journal of the American Veterinary Medical Association 204:627–632

Evans T J 2002 Endocrine alterations associated with ergopeptine alkaloid exposure during equine pregnancy. Veterinary Clinics of North America Equine Practice 18:371–378

Lavoie J P 2003 Heaves (recurrent airway obstruction): practical management of acute episodes and prevention of exacerbations. In: Robinson N E (ed) Current therapy in equine medicine, 5th edn. Saunders, Philadelphia, PA, pp. 417–421

Morris D D, Garcia M 1983 Thyroid-stimulating hormone: response test in healthy horses and effects of phenylbutazone on equine thyroid hormones. American Journal of Veterinary Research 44:503–507

Ralston S L 2002 Insulin and glucose regulation. Veterinary Clinics of North America Equine Practice 18:295–304

Reed S M 1998 Pituitary adenomas: equine Cushing's disease. In: Reed S M, Bayly W M (eds) Equine internal medicine. Saunders, Philadelphia, PA, pp. 912–916

Schott H C 2002 Pituitary pars intermedia dysfunction: equine Cushing's disease. Veterinary Clinics of North America Equine Practice 18:237–270

Schott H C, Coursen C L, Eberhart S W et al 2001 The Michigan Cushing's project. In: Proceedings of the 47th American Association of Equine Practitioners Annual Convention, San Diego, CA, pp. 22–24

Sojka J E 1993 Factors which affect serum T_3 and T_4 levels in the horse. Equine Practice 15:15–19

Sojka J E 1995 Hypothyroidism in horses. Compendium on Continuing Education for the Practicing Veterinarian 17:845–851

Sojka J E, Levy M 1995 Evaluation of endocrine function. Veterinary Clinics of North America Equine Practice 11:415–435

Sojka J E, Johnson M A, Bottoms G D 1993 Serum triiodothyronine, total thyroxine, and free thyroxine concentrations in horses. American Journal of Veterinary Research 54:52–55

Medical Economics Staff, PDR Staff and Physicians 2002 Physician's Desk Reference 2003, 57th edn. Thompson Healthcare, Montrale, NJ, pp. 569–571

Williams P D 1995 Equine Cushing's syndrome: retrospective study to twenty four cases and response to medication. In: Proceedings of the 34th British Equine Veterinary Association Congress, p. 41

CHAPTER CONTENTS

Introduction 85

Overview of gastrointestinal function 86
  Motility 86
  Drugs affecting alimentary tract motility 88
  Secretion and absorption 91
  Summary 95

Esophagus 95
  Drugs used for esophageal relaxation with
  obstruction 95
  Drugs used to treat reflux esophagitis 96

Stomach 97
  Drugs affecting gastric acidity 99
  Drugs acting on gastric mucosal protection 106
  Drugs acting on gastric motility 107

Small and large intestine 108
  Pathophysiology of intestinal motility
  disorders 108
  Clinical conditions with intestinal motility
  disorders 108
  Drugs acting on motility of the small and large
  intestine 109
  Pathophysiology of intestinal secretory
  disorders 113
  Drugs acting on intestinal secretion and
  absorption 113
  Agents promoting digestion and absorption 115
  Drugs acting on intestinal mucosa 115

Antimicrobial agents 115

References 116

6

Drugs acting on the gastrointestinal system

Michael J. Murray

INTRODUCTION

Many of the drugs used in horses in veterinary practice affect the gastrointestinal tract. Some of these effects are intended and may be beneficial for specific disorders, whereas other effects are secondary to the intended effect and are considered to be adverse effects. This chapter will cover those drugs that have a direct effect on segments of the gastrointestinal tract and which may, under certain circumstances, alleviate disease and improve gastrointestinal function. The majority of drugs targeting the gastrointestinal tract in equine practice are intended to affect motility of one or more segments of the alimentary tract, to permit healing of injured mucosa or to influence secretion or absorption. In some cases, these drugs are highly specific and effective. For example, omeprazole blocks gastric acid secretion and permits healing of gastric ulcers. In other circumstances, the drug effect is general and variably effective. Metoclopramide, for instance, affects the motility of much of the gastrointestinal tract but in many disorders, such as postoperative ileus (POI) and duodenitis-proximal jejunitis, the effectiveness of the drug is highly variable and arguable.

Our knowledge of the physiological and pathophysiological mechanisms of the gastrointestinal tract continues to grow rapidly and studies since the mid-1990s have revealed a highly complex interrelationship between the intestinal cells, blood vessels, smooth muscle cells and neurons within bowel segments. The concept of the different layers of the gut (mucosa, lamina propria, submucosa, muscularis, serosa) being anatomically connected yet more or less independent is yielding to the recognition that the cells within the different bowel layers "talk" to each other and to cells in other layers of the intestinal wall via a multitude of cytokines. The enteric microenvironment is a dynamic, responsive system and several cell types should be taken into account when considering adaptive changes in the enteric microenvironment: neurons, enteric glial cells, smooth muscle cells and the interstitial cells of Cajal, which are viewed as the intestinal pacemaker cells (Giaroni et al 1999). Mast cells and mesenchymal cells may also play an important role in the mediation of neuroimmune interactions. These cells and their products regulate normal intestinal function and help the gastrointestinal tissue to respond to various conditions, but they can also initiate and sustain pathophysiological events that can severely compromise intestinal function and viability.

Intestinal mucosal cells also can activate mediators of inflammation. Intestinal epithelial cells express an array of cytokine receptors and produce a spectrum of immune mediators, suggesting that they play an integral role in mucosal innate and acquired immunity (Dwinell et al 1999). Consistent with those functions, human intestinal epithelial cells have been shown to upregulate the expression and secretion of a variety of proinflammatory chemokines in response to infection with enteroinvasive pathogens or stimulation with proinflammatory cytokines. Epithelial cell-derived chemokines appear to act as mediators of intercellular communication between the epithelium and immune and inflammatory cells in the adjacent and underlying mucosa.

The enteric nervous system (ENS) is a frequent target of pharmacological agents; many are intended to improve propulsive motility. The ENS is a highly complex system that not only affects motility of the gastrointestinal tract but also is associated intimately with cells that can release homeostatic and proinflammatory cytokines. Recent evidence suggests possible cross-talk between intestinal smooth muscle cells and dorsal root ganglion cells (Ennes et al 1997), a finding that may affect our understanding of altered visceral sensitivity and reinforce the concept of a brain–gut axis. The interactions of intrinsic and extrinsic afferent and efferent fibers interacting with several cells, cytokines, neuropeptides and growth factors are beginning to be understood. The ability to manipulate these processes in a beneficial manner is in the earliest stages of investigation.

In this light, it is unrealistic to expect many of the pharmacological agents available currently to have their intended effects. Most of these drugs act on the most grossly and readily recognized elements of gastrointestinal function. Given the complexity of normal homeostatic mechanisms and pathophysiological processes, many of our current drugs must be seen as being rather unsophisticated. Nonetheless, many traditional drugs remain effective tools in our therapeutic armentarium and new drugs have arrived recently or are in development for use in gastrointestinal disorders.

OVERVIEW OF GASTROINTESTINAL FUNCTION

The primary function of the digestive tract is the digestion and absorption of nutrients. The small intestine of the horse is presumed to be functionally similar to that of other species, albeit having adapted to an herbivorous diet that is lower in fat and protein than the diets of carnivorous species. The equine digestive system is highly adapted for the microbial digestion of cellulose and absorption of the resulting short-chain fatty acids (SCFA). There are few disorders related to maldigestion or malabsorption in equine species for which there are specific treatments. One example is lactase deficiency in foals, either innate or acquired as a result of enteritis, which can be treated orally (p.o.) with lactase. Most of the disorders of the equine alimentary system relate to motility and secretion/absorption in the different segments of the gut.

MOTILITY

Normal intestinal motility is a complex interplay between central and peripheral nerves, local feedback mechanisms and cells in the target tissue that release an array of cytokines which can promote or inhibit the effects of neural stimulation on the gut. Alimentary motility has typically been studied by measuring changes in pressure within the bowel lumen, changes in tension of strain gauges implanted in the wall, electrical activity (via electrodes implanted in the serosa) and by using scintigraphy to assess transit time of radiolabeled materials. The different segments of the equine alimentary system, esophagus, stomach, small intestine, cecum and large colon and small colon, have distinct motility characteristics, based on their functions.

An important electrophysiological feature of the intestinal tract is the electrical rhythm of the gut, with electrical activity coordinated on a rhythm or pattern of slow waves. It is now thought that the interstitial cells of Cajal, which are electrically coupled to smooth muscle cells and which propagate slow wave activity, control the rhythmicity of intestinal electrical activity (Der-Silaphet et al 1998). The migrating myoelectrical complex (MMC) is a repeating sequence of action potentials in the smooth muscle, which consists of three phases. Phase I is a period of quiescence without action potential activity. During phase II, action potentials are intermittent; this is when most propulsion of ingesta along the intestinal tract occurs. During phase III, action potentials are very active and continuous on slow waves. The periodicity of the MMC in horses is approximately 2 h (Merritt 1999).

The large intestine of the horse is the reservoir in which microbial fermentation of cellulose occurs. The two primary features of motility in the cecum and large colon are propulsive motility and retrograde motility, which retains ingesta in the large colon in order to maximize digestive efficiency (Sellers et al 1982). Electrical activity in the large intestine is characterized by short spike bursts and long spike bursts, with the long spike bursts propagated aborally and associated with contractions of the wall of the colon (Roger et al 1985).

Components of neuromuscular stimuli to the gut include parasympathetic, sympathetic, motilide and non-adrenergic, non-cholinergic (NANC) stimuli and receptors (Merritt 1999). In general,

parasympathetic stimulation promotes motility and secretions in the gut. Parasympathetic stimuli originate in the vagal nucleus and are transmitted via the vagus nerve and pelvic nerves. Presynaptic fibers synapse in the myenteric and submucosal plexuses onto postsynaptic fibers that innervate intestinal smooth muscle, vessels in the submucosa, muscularis mucosa and mucosal cells. Acetylcholine is the neurotransmitter at both the synaptic junction and the neuromuscular junction. The cholinergic receptors in the plexuses are nicotinic receptors and on smooth muscle are muscarinic M_2 receptors.

Sympathetic stimuli are generally inhibitory to gastrointestinal motility and secretion (De Ponti et al 1996). Sympathetic fibers originate in the intermediolateral horn of thoracolumbar segments of spinal cord gray matter. Sympathetic preganglionic fibers synapse onto postganglionic fibers in paravertebral ganglia, from which fibers travel to the intestine and terminate on cholinergic fibers that synapse onto smooth muscle. Gastrointestinal receptors of sympathetic fibers include α_1, α_2 and β_2 adrenoceptors, which are inhibitory to gut motility. Release of norepinephrine (noradrenaline) and binding to α_2 adrenoceptors on the cell bodies of intestinal cholinergic neurons inhibits these neurons.

Motilin is a neuropeptide expressed predominantly in the gastrointestinal tract that stimulates the contraction of gastrointestinal smooth muscle throughout the gut (Tonini 1996). Physiologically, its most characteristic role seems to be the induction of coordinated interdigestive antral and duodenal contractions (phase III of the migrating motor complex). The effects of motilin are both species and dose dependent. Motilin appears to have at least two receptors, one muscular and the other neuronal. Recent studies in vivo have emphasized the importance of the latter pathway and it is currently hypothesized that motilin acts on neurons in the myenteric plexus to release acetylcholine and other excitatory neurotransmitters.

The NANC neurotransmitter system includes several substances that may be inhibitory or excitatory. Inhibitory NANC neurotransmitters include adenosine trisphosphate (ATP), vasoactive intestinal peptide and nitric oxide (NO). These neurotransmitters mediate descending inhibition during peristalsis and receptive relaxation. Substance P is an excitatory NANC transmitter involved in large intestinal contraction through activation of neurokinin 1 receptors. Recent studies have provided evidence that inducible NO may contribute to ileus in various diseases and that inhibitors of NO synthesis may have a role in the future in the treatment of ileus (Kalff et al 2000).

DRUGS AFFECTING ALIMENTARY TRACT MOTILITY

Several drugs are used for alimentary tract motility disorders in humans and there are excellent reviews on their mechanisms of action and clinical use (Longo & Vernava 1993, McCallum 1999, Tonini 1996).

Cholinomimetics

The cholinomimetics act on the neuromuscular junction (muscarinic), either by directly stimulating the acetylcholine receptors on the smooth muscle cells or by increasing the levels of acetylcholine in the neuromuscular junction by blocking cholinesterase activity. Some cholinomimetics, such as bethanechol, can act both at the level of the myenteric plexus (nicotinic) and directly on the intestinal smooth cells.

Bethanechol

Bethanechol is a synthetic derivative of acetylcholine and is not degraded by cholinesterase. Bethanechol has been used in humans to increase lower esophageal sphincter (LES) tone and to enhance gastric emptying. The cholinergic side-effects (salivation, abdominal discomfort) of bethanechol have reduced its use in human medicine since the introduction of metoclopramide and cisapride.

Bethanechol has been shown to stimulate antroduodenal motility in humans and laboratory animals. In one study in humans, bethanechol caused a dose-dependent stimulation of antroduodenal motility and gastropancreatic secretion

(Katschinski et al 1995). High doses of bethanechol increase release of gastrin, cholecystokinin and pancreatic polypeptide. Unlike in other species, bethanechol does not increase gastric acid output in horses (Sandin et al 2000), but it does cause a small but significant increase in gastric fluid collection in cannulated horses (Thompson et al 1994), perhaps reflecting non-parietal secretions derived from the pancreas.

Bethanechol has been shown to increase gastric contractility and hasten the emptying of liquid and solid-phase radiolabeled materials from the stomach of normal horses (Ringger et al 1996). The effects of bethanechol in horses are not restricted to the upper alimentary tract, because bethanechol also significantly enhances the rate of cecal emptying of radiolabeled markers in normal ponies (Lester et al 1998a).

Bethanechol can produce cholinergic side-effects, such as abdominal discomfort, sweating and salivation, but these are seen either when the recommended dose rates (0.02 mg/kg subcutaneous (s.c.) three times a day, or 0.35 mg/kg p.o. three to four times a day) are exceeded or when the drug is administered intravenously (i.v.). Side-effects occur infrequently in horses when the drug is administered at the recommended dose rate.

Benzamides

The primary benzamides used to enhance gastrointestinal motility are metoclopramide and cisapride. Each drug has its benefits and hazards, and recently cisapride was withdrawn from the market because of its potential to cause fatal cardiac arrhythmias in humans.

Metoclopramide

Metoclopramide is a first-generation benzamide. The drug acts presynaptically, mainly as a 5-hydroxytryptamine (5-HT; serotonin) 5-HT$_4$ receptor agonist and 5-HT$_3$ receptor antagonist but it is also an antagonist at dopamine 1 (D$_1$) and 2 (D$_2$) receptors (MacDonald 1991). The net effect of the interactions with these receptors is to facilitate acetylcholine release from enteric neurons and promote smooth muscle contraction. Metoclopramide is used in humans to increase LES tone, improve gastric emptying and minimize the nausea that may accompany several conditions.

Cisapride

Cisapride is a second-generation substituted benzamide that is used to treat a variety of conditions in humans, including gastroesophageal reflux disease, peptic ulcer disease, intestinal pseudo-obstruction and constipation (Washabau & Hall 1995). The drug appears to act as a 5-HT_4 agonist, which enhances release of acetylcholine from neurons in the myenteric plexus. In contrast to metoclopramide, cisapride does not have anti-dopaminergic effects. The density and distribution of 5-HT_4 receptors varies along the gastrointestinal tract and between species; therefore, extrapolation of effects between species should be done with caution. Cisapride has the advantage over metoclopramide in that it affects colon motility and induces defecation in constipated human patients. In addition, it has no central nervous system (CNS) effects because it does not affect dopaminergic receptors.

There are reports that suggest that cisapride is efficacious in the management of intestinal diseases in horses, including persistent large colon impaction, equine grass sickness and to prevent POI after small intestinal surgery. Cisapride is absorbed very poorly when administered p.o. (Steel et al 1998) and is absorbed erratically when administered rectally to horses (Cook et al 1997). This limited its use in equine practice in the USA since the drug was available in tablet form only. However, cisapride was withdrawn from the market in the USA and Europe in 2000 because of infrequent adverse cardiac side-effects in humans, including lengthening of the QT interval and the development of a potentially fatal arrhythmia, torsades de pointes.

Dopamine antagonists

Two sets of dopamine receptor are present in the gut: D_1 receptors are located on effector cells and D_2 receptors predominate on the cell bodies in the myenteric and submucosal plexuses. The result

of stimulation of the D_2 receptors is diminished release of acetylcholine at the neuromuscular junction. The effects of stimulation of dopamine receptors in the alimentary tract include reduction of LES tone, reduction of gastric tone and intragastric pressure and inhibition of antroduodenal coordination.

Metoclopramide

Metoclopramide has inhibitory effects on dopamine D_1 and D_2 receptors, which influences its prokinetic activity and CNS side effects.

Domperidone

Domperidone is a competitive antagonist at peripheral D_2 receptors. It influences the motility of gastric and small intestinal smooth muscle and has been shown to have some effects on the motor function of the esophagus (Barone 1999). It also has antiemetic activity as a result of blockade of dopamine receptors in the chemoreceptor trigger zone. In some controlled clinical trials, domperidone provided better relief of symptoms (anorexia, nausea, vomiting, abdominal pain, early satiety, bloating, distension) than placebo in human patients with symptoms of diabetic gastropathy. However, domperidone has not appeared to offer any advantages over other prokinetic drugs. Very little domperidone crosses the blood–brain barrier; therefore, reports of CNS adverse effects in humans are rare.

Domperidone has recently received attention as a therapeutic agent for agalactia in mares grazing endophyte-infected fescue, principally through its role in enhancing prolactin release (Redmond et al 1994). The dose of domperidone recommended for fescue endophyte-associated agalactia in mares (1.1 mg/kg daily) is considerably greater than that used to treat motility disorders in humans (0.2–0.3 mg/kg). Effects on gastrointestinal motility (increased borborygmi, increased defecation) are not apparent in mares given domperidone to increase milk production. The potential prokinetic effects of domperidone have not been studied extensively in horses; however, Gerring & King (1989) reported modest efficacy of domperidone

(0.2 mg/kg i.v.) in an experimental model of ileus in two ponies. The drug is commercially available in Europe but not in the USA, where it is available through some compounding pharmacies.

Aminoguanidine indoles

Unlike metoclopramide and cisapride, the aminoguanidine indoles have purely 5-HT receptor agonist effects. The molecules are structurally similar to 5-HT, with different substitutions affecting receptor affinity and specificity.

Tegaserod

Tegaserod maleate is a partial agonist that binds with high affinity at human $5\text{-}HT_4$ receptors but has no appreciable affinity for $5\text{-}HT_3$ or dopamine receptors. It has moderate affinity for $5\text{-}HT_1$ receptors. Tegaserod, by acting as an agonist at neuronal $5\text{-}HT_4$ receptors, triggers the release of further neurotransmitters, such as calcitonin gene-related peptide from sensory neurons. The activation of $5\text{-}HT_4$ receptors in the gastrointestinal tract stimulates the peristaltic reflex and intestinal secretion, as well as inhibits visceral sensitivity. The drug has been shown to increase emptying of the stomach, small intestine and large intestine in animals and humans (Degen et al 2001, Nguyen et al 1997). An interesting feature of the drug is its ability to reduce the sensation of colorectal distension (Camilleri 2001), which may have applications in horses. Tegaserod maleate is licensed in Europe, Canada and the USA for use in women with irritable bowel syndrome. In one report, tegaserod maleate was given to four horses at a dose rate of 0.2 mg/kg twice daily for four doses (Lippold et al 2002). There was a significant increase in the transit rate of barium-filled spheres given by nasogastric tube at the time of administration and an increase in fecal output.

Motilides

The motilides interact with motilin receptors on gastrointestinal neurons and smooth muscle, stimulating smooth muscle contraction and gastrointestinal motility. Erythromycin has prokinetic activity in most species studied, including horses. Erythromycin probably exerts its prokinetic effects by enhancing the release of motilin through cholinergic and serotoninergic mechanisms and by direct interaction with motilin receptors (Tonini 1996). Erythromycin binds to motilin receptors readily. There are regional differences in response to erythromycin within the intestine and differences between species, which may correspond to differences in motilin-receptor density. Depending on the dose administered, erythromycin has many effects on motility, including initiating new MMC complexes, increasing gastric fundic tone and increasing antroduodenal motility.

Other macrolide antimicrobials, such as clarithromycin and azithromycin, appear to interact with motilin receptors. Current investigations center on developing motilides that lack antimicrobial activity, thus not disrupting the normal intestinal flora, but have more potent effects on motility. Isolation and purification of motilin receptors will facilitate the development of drugs that have highly specific motilide activity.

Narcotic agonists and antagonists

The narcotic drugs affect the gastrointestinal tract by alleviating pain perception, altering motility and affecting secretion. Narcotics interact with the intestinal tract via opioid μ and κ receptors, which have opposing effects, depressing and promoting propulsive motility, respectively (De Luca & Coupar 1996). The presence of these receptors in the gut implies a functional role for opioids in intestinal function. A recent study found that slowing of intestinal transit by fat in the distal half of the gut depends on an opioid pathway located in the efferent limb of this response (Zhao et al 2000). Additionally, opioid κ receptor agonists that act peripherally have been shown to inhibit spinal cord pathways of visceral nociception (Ness 1999) and such drugs may be useful in treating painful abdominal disorders.

Narcotics are no longer typically used in the management of gastrointestinal disorders in horses because they are controlled substances and other drugs can effectively provide visceral analgesia. Likewise, although the narcotic antagonist naloxone was shown to increase colonic motor activity in experimental ponies (Roger et al 1985), inhibition of μ receptors by naloxone would be expected to augment the horse's perception of visceral pain (Kamerling et al 1990). Advances in targeting specific κ receptors may result in drugs that can both improve motility and provide visceral pain relief.

SECRETION AND ABSORPTION

The different segments of the alimentary tract have specialized secretory and absorptive functions. The initial secretion of the equine alimentary system is saliva, which is produced in copious amounts when horses eat. The equine esophagus has no secretory or absorptive function, although in other species submucosal glands secrete mucins and a variety of polypeptides such as growth factors. The primary secretory product of the stomach is aqueous hydrochloric acid; basal gastric secretions approximately 100– 200 μEq/h per kg for hydrochloric acid and 1 l/h for water (Kitchen et al 1998a). The stomach probably has minimal absorptive functions. There is a large non-parietal (non-acidic) component of the secretion, which has been measured in secretions obtained from the stomachs of cannulated horses; this is thought to come from the duodenum (Kitchen et al 1998b). These secretions have a high pH, high sodium content, are stimulated by pentagastrin infusion and probably originate from the pancreas.

The duodenum and jejunum are capable of both absorption and secretion but absorption usually predominates. Regulation of intestinal secretion and absorption is highly complex and involves extrinsic and intrinsic neural stimuli, numerous receptor types and intercellular and intracellular transport pathways. Intracellular pathways of electrolyte transport involve membrane-associated receptors that activate cyclic nucleotide metabolism, membrane calcium channels and intracellular calcium metabolism, luminal and basal chloride channels and multiple sodium transport channels. Cholinergic stimuli tend to stimulate intestinal chloride secretion and decrease sodium and chloride absorption. Conversely, catecholamines tend to promote increased sodium and chloride absorption in the gut, via α_2 adrenoceptors. The effects of these stimuli are dose dependent and can vary between different segments of intestine. Increased levels of prostaglandins E_1 and E_2 promote intestinal secretion, which is mediated through cyclic nucleotides and intracellular calcium metabolism. Other modulators of intestinal secretion and absorption of fluid and electrolytes include VIP, opioids and NO.

There is active sodium absorption throughout the intestine that is powered by cellular energy derived from the sodium pumps (Na$^+$,K$^+$-ATPase) in the basolateral membrane of intestinal epithelial cells. This energy powers the exit of sodium from the cell against an electrochemical gradient. The movement of virtually all other solutes against their electrochemical gradients occurs by transport processes that are "secondarily active" in that they are coupled, either directly or indirectly, to the movement of sodium ions. Sodium entry into the enterocyte is energetically downhill and is believed to involve three major mechanisms: (i) electrodiffusion, via selective sodium channels; (ii) electroneutral sodium chloride absorption via "coupled" cation (Na$^+$–H$^+$) and anion (Cl$^-$– HCO$_3^-$) exchange; and (iii) electrogenic solute-linked sodium absorption, in which sodium is transported into enterocytes coupled to the absorption of organic solutes, including glucose, amino acids, bile salts, water-soluble vitamins and organic acids.

The movement of water and electrolytes across the mucosa in the cecum and large intestine is linked to the intraluminal production of SCFAs, primarily acetic acid, and their absorption across the mucosa (Argenzio & Stevens 1975). On a daily basis, there is normally net absorption of water and electrolytes in the cecum and large colon. However, there are frequent large fluxes of water and electrolytes into the lumen of the colon, particularly after meal feeding, in horses (Clarke et al 1990). Equine feeding regimens that entail the twice daily feeding of concentrates are associated with episodes of secretion of large volumes of fluid into the intestine, resulting in transient hypovolemia (up to 15% loss of plasma volume) (Clarke et al 1990). Initially, with abundant substrate for fermentation, the concentration of SCFAs increases, which results in a net flux of fluid into the lumen. This fluid tends to neutralize the increase in osmolality created by the SCFAs. As SCFAs are absorbed into the mucosa and their concentration in the lumen decreases, water is reabsorbed into the colonic mucosa. The effects of these large fluid fluxes on the development of large intestinal disorders remains to be fully characterized, but they contrast sharply with the more modest intestinal fluid fluxes that occur when horses are fed small meals frequently. Presumably, the large fluid fluxes that accompany meal feeding in horses are more susceptible to perturbation and disruption of digestive processes.

Passive secretion of water into the lumen of the intestine depends on the semipermeable diffusion characteristics of the mucosa of the intestine and the osmotic and oncotic differences exerted across this semipermeable barrier. The permeability of capillaries in the submucosa and mucosa and the density of intercellular tight junctions in the mucosa determine the permeability of the mucosa. The density of tight junctions is very high in the stomach, relatively low in the small intestine and moderate in the large intestine and small colon.

In diseases of the small intestine, active secretion caused by cyclic nucleotide stimulation can result in a large volume of water and electrolytes moving into the lumen. Additionally, enteric neuron activation of mast cells can increase intestinal capillary permeability and promote passive fluid secretion. Diseases that increase intestinal permeability can result in passive secretion of protein-rich fluid into the intestinal lumen. Active secretion of electrolytes and water is a feature of many diarrheal disorders and can be stimulated by bacterial enterotoxins. Several bacterial enterotoxins interact with intestinal epithelial cell membrane adenylate cyclase or guanylate cyclase, resulting in increased cAMP or cGMP. These, in turn, activate basolateral chloride channels, resulting in an increase in the luminal secretion of chloride, accompanied by sodium and followed by water (Gemmell 1984). Bacterial enterotoxins that stimulate cAMP include cholera toxin, *Escherichia coli*

heat-labile toxin and *Salmonella* heat-labile toxin. *E. coli* heat-stable toxin, which is responsible for most cases of traveler's diarrhea and has been reported in diarrheic foals (Holland et al 1989), induces cGMP. Prostaglandins E_1 and E_2 have a role in intestinal fluid secretion and these mediators have been shown to be associated with both active and passive secretory processes (Eberhart & Dubois 1995).

The role of NO in intestinal fluid and electrolyte secretion depends upon whether the conditions under study are physiological or pathophysiological (Izzo et al 1998). In physiological conditions, constitutive NO seems to promote fluid absorption, based on the findings that NO synthase inhibitors convert net fluid absorption to net secretion in several animal species. This pro-absorptive mode involves the ENS, the suppression of prostaglandin formation and the opening of basolateral potassium channels. However, in some pathophysiological states, NO synthase may be produced at higher concentrations and is capable of evoking net secretion. NO synthase contributes to the diarrheal response to the laxative action in the rat of several intestinal secretogogues, including castor oil, phenolphthalein, bisacodyl, magnesium sulfate, bile salts and cascara.

Drugs affecting gastrointestinal secretion

Few drugs truly decrease the secretion of electrolytes and water from the intestine and the use of antisecretory drugs to treat acute diarrhea in humans has limitations. Also, some drugs that have appeared to have antisecretory effects in experimental animal models have not proven widely useful clinically in humans or horses. For instance, the α_2 adrenoceptor agonist drugs clonidine and lidamidine have demonstrable antisecretory effects in several animal species, but related drugs, such as xylazine and detomidine, do not appear to share these effects in horses. The non-steroidal anti-inflammatory drug (NSAID) indomethacin has shown apparent antisecretory effects in a variety of models of intestinal fluid secretion, including those involving enterotoxin and live enteropathogens. Similar antisecretory effects of NSAIDs, such as flunixin meglumine, have not been apparent in a clinical setting, despite the widespread use of NSAIDs in horses with diarrhea.

Loperamide

Loperamide is a narcotic agonist acting on opioid μ receptors. Loperamide has mild antisecretory effects but its primary effects are to increase segmental intestinal contractions and slow the propulsion of intestinal contents (Ruppin 1987). Loperamide has been associated with reduction in diarrhea in many clinical studies in humans but has minimal impact on the patient's fluid and electrolyte balance because the secreted fluid remains in the bowel lumen. Loperamide can have dose-dependent CNS depressant effects. Loperamide also has been shown to promote intestinal bacterial overgrowth because of promoting the retention of fluid within bowel segments (Duval-Iflah et al 1999), which may favor the proliferation of enteropathogenic bacteria.

Racecadotril

Enkephalins are pentapeptides that bind to opiate receptors. In the gut, enkephalins promote the absorption of sodium, chloride and water (Dobbins et al 1980). Racecadotril is an oral enkephalinase inhibitor used in France and the Philippines for the treatment of acute diarrhea. It prevents the degradation of endogenous opioids (enkephalins) and thus promotes absorption of water and electrolytes from the intestinal lumen (Matheson & Noble 2000). Studies have demonstrated the efficacy of racecadotril in two models of hypersecretory diarrhea: infusion of cholera toxin and castor oil induced diarrhea. Moreover, unlike loperamide, racecadotril did not prolong transit time in the small intestine or colon. Further experiments have shown that racecadotril does not promote bacterial overgrowth in the small intestine (Duval-Iflah et al 1999). There are no reports on the use of racecadotril in horses.

Somatostatin analogs

Cells throughout the gastrointestinal tract release somatostatin. Somatostatin inhibits acid secretion in the stomach and it promotes absorption of sodium, chloride and water in the small intestine and colon (Krejs 1986). The somatostatin analogs octreotide and lanreotide have been shown to decrease intestinal secretion in animal models (Botella et al 1993) and in humans with specific metabolic intestinal secretory disorders; however, these drugs are not used widely in human medicine. In one study in horses, octreotide was shown to decrease gastric acidity (Sojka et al 1992) but its effects on intestinal or colonic secretion in horses have not been reported.

Oral replacement solutions

Oral replacement solutions (ORSs) are used extensively in humans with acute diarrhea, characterized by large losses of water and electrolytes, caused in many cases by enterotoxigenic bacteria. Oral replacement therapy is indicated in many cases of equine diarrhea, particularly in foals. An effective ORS should include carbohydrate as an energy source, sodium, chloride, potassium ions and a base (bicarbonate or citrate); the concentrations of these constituents should be such that the solution is somewhat hypotonic (Table 6.1) (Thillainayagam et al 1998). The standard ORS recommended by the World Health Organization (WHO) contains 90 mEq/l (1 mmol/l) sodium, 20 mEq/l (1 mmol/l) potassium, 80 mEq/l (1 mmol/l) chloride and uses glucose as the carbohydrate source and bicarbonate as the base source. Although standard glucose–electrolyte ORSs have proved highly effective in achieving and maintaining rehydration, it does not reduce stool volume or the duration of the diarrheal illness. Recent ORS formulations used in humans not only replace lost water and electrolytes but may also reduce intestinal secretions. Incorporating rice components into the ORS appears to reduce stool volume and recently a component of rice was shown to decrease cAMP-mediated intestinal secretion (Mathews et al 1999). These approaches to ORS therapy may have utility in

Table 6.1   Commercially available oral rehydrating solutions

	Na⁺ (mEq/l)	K⁺ (mEq/l)	Cl⁻ (mEq/l)	Carbohydrate source	Base source	Base (mEq/l)	% w/v
Rehydrating solutions							
Rehydralite	75	20	65	Glucose	Citrate	30	2.5
WHO formulation	90	20	80	Glucose	Bicarbonate	30	2
Maintenance fluids							
Resol	50	20	50	Glucose	Citrate	34	2
Pedialyte	45	20	35	Glucose	Citrate	30	2.5
Enfalyte	50	20	40	Rice syrup solids	Citrate	34	3

WHO, World Health Organization

equine patients, although introduction of fermentable carbohydrates into the adult equine digestive tract should be done with caution.

Drugs acting on intestinal mucosa

Bismuth subsalicylate

Bismuth subsalicylate (BSS) is used widely in humans for treatment of diarrhea and is specifically recommended for the prevention of traveler's diarrhea. The precise mechanism of action remains undetermined and although the end result of treatment with BSS is reduction in diarrhea (Figueroa-Quintanilla et al 1993), its effect is probably not related to a direct antisecretory mechanism. Salicylates have been shown to stimulate intestinal fluid and electrolyte absorption per se but it is likely that, in many cases of colitis, resolution of inflammation and restoration of a normal surface epithelium is required to restore mucosal function. When used as pretreatment or coadministered, BSS significantly reduced the fluid secretory response to E. coli LT enterotoxin and cholera toxin in intestinal loops of rabbits and pigs (Ericsson et al 1990). However, when administered even 5 min after the enterotoxins, BSS had no significant effect on enterotoxin-stimulated intestinal secretion. These results suggest that BSS adsorbs or neutralizes bacterial enterotoxins but does not alter the effect of enterotoxins once they have bound to intestinal mucosa. BSS also modulates normal colonic bacterial flora growth in vitro. In one study in humans with histological colitis and chronic diarrhea, BSS significantly improved fecal consistency, decreased frequency of defecation and fecal weight in 85% of patients and resolved histological colitis in 75% of patients. After an 8 week course of treatment, clinical remission of diarrhea lasted for as long as 28 months without further treatment (Fine & Lee 1998).

In humans, the absorption of the heavy metal bismuth is negligible (<1%) but salicylate is absorbed readily (Nwokolo et al 1990), with as much as 95% of the administered dose excreted in urine. No data are available on the degree and consequence of absorption of bismuth or salicylate in horses.

Prostaglandin analogs

Damage to the intestinal mucosa is a well-characterized adverse effect of excessive administration of NSAIDs. Mucosal changes include mucosal atrophy, erosion and ulceration throughout the alimentary tract. The prostaglandin E_1 analog misoprostol is used to prevent and treat gastrointestinal mucosal injury in humans taking NSAIDs on a chronic basis (Schoenfeld et al 1999). In one report, the coadministration of phenylbutazone with a prostaglandin E_2 analog significantly attenuated the alimentary mucosal injury associated with the administration of phenylbutazone alone (Collins & Tyler 1985).

SUMMARY

In the following sections the specific alimentary tract segments are described together with drugs having specific effects on these segments.

ESOPHAGUS

Most disorders requiring pharmacological intervention in foals and horses involve obstruction to the passage of ingesta or damage to the stratified squamous mucosal lining of the esophagus secondary to gastroesophageal reflux or motility disorders. In the proximal two-thirds of the equine esophagus, the tunica muscularis comprises striated skeletal muscle, whereas in the distal third the muscular layer is smooth muscle. The upper esophageal sphincter prevents esophagopharyngeal reflux, with subsequent tracheobronchial aspiration and hindrance of air distention of the esophagus during inspiration. The LES is functional smooth muscle located at the gastroesophageal junction. The LES restricts gastroesophageal reflux and permits the passage of ingested material from the esophagus to the stomach during relaxation. Normally, the LES remains closed owing to intrinsic myogenic tone and gastric distention with ingesta.

Motor innervation to the striated muscle of the esophagus includes the pharyngeal and esophageal branches of the vagus nerve, which originate in the nucleus ambiguus of the medulla (Richards & Sugarbaker 1995). Esophageal peristalsis and sphincter function are controlled by the autonomic nervous system, with contributions from parasympathetic, sympathetic and enteric divisions. Proximal portions of the esophagus, including the upper esophageal sphincter, are under direct (cholinergic) control of vagal motor neurons located in the nucleus ambiguus. Intramural enteric nerves, with a contribution from vagal preganglionic fibers arising in the dorsal motor nucleus of the vagus control the distal esophageal regions, including the LES.

DRUGS USED FOR ESOPHAGEAL RELAXATION WITH OBSTRUCTION

Adrenergic agonist drugs

The α_2 adrenergic receptor agonists xylazine and detomidine are used frequently to relax the esophagus in horses with esophageal obstruction. No studies document the utility of this class of drugs in relieving esophageal obstruction per se, although their sedative properties permit the veterinarian to attempt to relieve the obstruction. Also, a horse sedated with an α_2 adrenergic receptor agonist will drop its head below the level of the thorax, which will reduce the opportunity for aspiration of saliva and ingesta. There is indirect evidence that the α_2 adrenoreceptor agonists cause esophageal relaxation and may facilitate relief of esophageal obstruction. Detomidine was shown to alter esophageal transit of barium contrast, including dose-dependent increases in the transit time, the retention of barium within the longitudinal mucosal folds and retrograde peristalsis and pooling of contrast agent within the esophagus at both the thoracic inlet and caudal to the base of the heart (Watson & Sullivan 1991).

Doses of xylazine and detomidine used in the treatment of esophageal obstruction should be sufficient to permit the veterinarian to pass a nasogastric tube or endoscope and attempt to relieve the obstruction while causing minimal trauma to the horse. Xylazine may be preferable during the initial examination because the obstruction may have resolved spontaneously or may be easily relieved by the veterinarian. With more difficult obstructions, detomidine may be preferable because of its longer duration of action (up to 45–60 min), which is desirable to limit aspiration of saliva and ingesta. Xylazine can be administered i.v. at 0.5–0.7 mg/kg and, for more prolonged sedation, detomidine can be administered i.v. or intramuscularly (i.m.) at 0.02 mg/kg.

The β_2 adrenergic agonists are used for bronchodilatory effects in horses and may facilitate esophageal relaxation. In humans, peristaltic amplitude was increased in the distal smooth muscle part of the esophageal body after infusion of the non-selective beta blocker propranolol (Lyrenas

1985). After infusion of the β_2 adrenoceptor agonist terbutaline, a profound decrease in esophageal peristaltic amplitude was reported. Peristaltic velocity in the distal part of the esophagus was decreased by β_2 adrenoceptor stimulation. Clenbuterol, which is used commonly in horses, caused relaxation of rat esophageal smooth muscle (de Boer et al 1993), but it is not known whether drugs such as clenbuterol or terbutaline will similarly affect the equine esophagus.

Oxytocin

It has been suggested that oxytocin would reduce esophageal contractility and be useful in the treatment of esophageal obstruction in horses (Hance et al 1997). In one study in nine horses, intraluminal esophageal pressure was reduced during i.v. infusion of oxytocin at dose rates of 0.11, 0.22 and 0.44 IU/kg (Meyer et al 2000). Increasing the dose increased the duration of the response. Signs of abdominal discomfort were observed in two horses at the lowest dose. Neither the effect of oxytocin on striated or smooth muscle nor its mechanism of action is known. Its clinical efficacy is presumed but has not been documented.

Acepromazine

Acepromazine maleate is advocated for use in the treatment of esophageal obstruction but, aside from its sedative effects, there is no direct evidence that it promotes esophageal relaxation. In one report using barium contrast radiography, acepromazine appeared to cause mild segmental dilatations in the thoracic esophagus (King et al 1990). The duration of effect of acepromazine is 2 to 3 h and it may be useful in the treatment of obstructions that do not resolve quickly. The dose rate is 0.02–0.04 mg/kg i.v. or i.m.

DRUGS USED TO TREAT REFLUX ESOPHAGITIS

Gastroesophageal reflux disease (GERD) is a frequent disorder in humans but is uncommon in horses. The disorder is seen most often in foals and it occurs as a result of gastric outflow impairment. Mucosal injury can range from mild erosions to severe ulceration. Severe gastric ulceration typically accompanies GERD in equine and treatment of the primary problem (gastric emptying disorder) and the secondary GERD includes suppression of gastric acid secretion and promotion of gastric emptying. The drugs used to promote gastric emptying also increase LES tone, further limiting gastroesophageal reflux. Drugs used to suppress gastric acidity are covered in the section on the stomach. Drugs used to promote LES tone include bethanechol, metoclopramide and motilides.

Bethanechol

Bethanechol has been used in humans to improve LES tone and reduce gastroesophageal reflux (Sondheimer & Arnold 1986) but has now been replaced by other treatments that produce fewer side-effects. Bethanechol has been used, in conjunction with acid-suppressing drugs, by the author to treat GERD in foals and adult horses. Treatment was associated with healing of the esophagitis but it is not known whether the responses could be attributed to the effects of bethanechol or reduced acidity. Its effects on the LES in horses have not been examined but bethanechol does accelerate gastric emptying in horses (Ringger et al 1996), which may explain the positive clinical response to treatment with bethanechol in foals and horses with GERD.

Metoclopramide

Metoclopramide increases LES sphincter tone but it is of questionable efficacy in the treatment of GERD in humans (Bellissant et al 1997, Grande et al 1992). Doses as low as 0.1 mg/kg p.o. three times a day have been suggested but no data support the use of metoclopramide in the treatment of GERD in horses or foals. The author has used metoclopramide, at a dose rate of 0.3 mg/kg p.o. four times a day, with apparent success in one foal with GERD but, as has been reported in the human medical literature, adverse neurological effects accompanied treatment. When the dose was reduced to 0.2 mg/kg, GERD and delayed gastric emptying recurred.

Motilides

There are few reports of the effects of motilides on LES tone. Data from these reports, on small numbers of individuals, suggest that erythromycin does increase LES pressure and may prevent gastroesophageal reflux.

STOMACH

The principal functions of the stomach are to serve as a reservoir for ingesta, to deliver small boluses of ingesta to the small intestine, to begin the digestion of proteins and to serve as a first line of defense against enteric pathogens. It is these latter two functions for which the secretion of hydrochloric acid and pepsin are physiologically most relevant. The stomach also has important endocrine activities, such as the release of the hormone gastrin, and influences the physiology of other segments of the intestinal tract via both endocrine and neural pathways. The functions of the stomach that are most often manipulated using pharmacological agents are motility and emptying, secretion of hydrochloric acid and the barrier to hydrochloric acid and pepsin on the surface of the glandular mucosa.

The equine stomach is lined dorsally by a stratified squamous epithelium and ventrally by a glandular epithelium, which have different functions and susceptibility to peptic injury. The squamous portion of the stomach has no secretory or absorptive function and appears to serve as a reservoir for ingesta. The gastric glandular mucosa has an array of secretory and endocrine functions.

Gastric motility is initiated via impulses from the vagus nerve. In horses, the vagus nerve travels along the esophagus, through the diaphragm and, once through the diaphragm, immediately enters the wall of the stomach, whereupon it divides into several branches that in the horse, unlike in humans, lie deep within the wall of the stomach. Smooth muscle in the wall of the stomach becomes progressively thicker towards the antrum and pylorus. Contractions progress from the body to the pylorus, and strong, circumferential propulsive contractions in the antrum result in a golf-ball-sized bolus of ingesta moving into the duodenum. Afferent fibers arising from the vagus nerve and from splanchnic and mesenteric nerves can detect noxious substances (such as hydrochloric acid) and stimulate mucosal arteriolar vasodilation (Holzer 1998). These extrinsic afferent neurons can be stimulated by capsaicin and the effector substance for vasodilation is NO. This system may be an appropriate target for pharmacological intervention in the future.

Hydrochloric acid is secreted by parietal cells via H^+,K^+-ATPase pumps (proton pumps), of which there are more than one million per cell. The H^+,K^+-ATPase pumps utilize the phosphorylation of ATP to exchange water-solvated protons (protonated water, hydroxonium ion, H_3O^+) for potassium ions. In conjunction with parallel potassium and chloride ion conductances, this ATPase is responsible for the secretion of hydrochloric acid into the secretory canaliculus of the parietal cell, the enclosed space reaching a pH of near 1.0 (Rabon & Reuben 1990). In the resting parietal cell, these pumps reside within the membranes of vesicles in the cell cytoplasm. When activated by histamine and gastrin, the parietal cells alter their shape and the vesicles merge with the outer cell membrane to form secretory canaliculi.

The stomach secretes hydrochloric acid under the influences of vagus nerve stimulation, gastrin and histamine. Histamine is the most potent stimulus of gastric acid secretion in some animal species studied, such as the horse (Kitchen et al 1998a). Histamine is released by mast cells and enterochromaffin-like cells that are immediately adjacent to the parietal cells. Histamine interacts with two distinct subsets of histamine H_2 receptors on the parietal cell membrane, initiating a series of reactions that result in the phosphorylation of protein kinases and increased intracellular calcium within the parietal cell. This, in turn, results in transformation and translocation of the coiled tubular vesicles in which the H^+,K^+-ATPase pumps reside to the secretory canaliculi. Gastrin is released into the blood by G cells in the stomach and acts as a true hormone. Gastrin reaches parietal cells via the blood and initiates a series of reactions that result in increased intracellular calcium. Gastrin also interacts with gastric mast cells and enterochromaffin cells, promoting the release of histamine. In addition to stimulating hydrochloric acid secretion by the stomach, gastrin appears to stimulate the secretion of water, sodium, chloride and bicarbonate from the pancreas into the duodenum, some of which normally refluxes into the stomach. The primary physiological inhibitor of gastric acid secretion is somatostatin; prostaglandins E_1 and E_2 and epidermal growth factor appear to modulate acid secretion to a lesser degree.

The equine stomach secretes hydrochloric acid continuously, even when the horse is not eating (Campbell-Thompson & Merritt 1990). Gastric acid secretion is pronounced even in neonatal foals (Sanchez et al 1998). Gastric acidity is lowest when the horse eats, because eating stimulates the secretion of bicarbonate-rich saliva, which can neutralize some gastric acid, and roughage absorbs gastric secretions so they do not contact the mucosal surface. Once a horse stops eating, the gastric acidity can rapidly increase, with the pH falling to below 2.0, and the acidity will remain high for as long as the horse does not eat (Murray & Schusser 1993).

Peptic injury refers to damage to the mucosa of the alimentary tract by hydrochloric acid and pepsin. Bile acids can contribute to peptic injury but both bile acids and pepsin require an acidic milieu to cause injury. The stomach is the predominant site of peptic injury in foals and horses, although gastric secretions may also injure the esophagus and duodenum. Protection of the equine esophageal and gastric squamous mucosae from peptic injury is dependent upon limited exposure to acidic gastric secretions, because there is no surface barrier to hydrochloric acid and these epithelia have limited properties to prevent peptic injury. The esophagus is normally spared exposure to gastric secretions by the LES, although disorders that result in impaired gastric emptying (pyloric ulcers, duodenitis) are frequently accompanied by gastroesophageal reflux and esophagitis. The gastric squamous mucosa is spared from exposure to hydrochloric acid and pepsin by the frequent consumption of roughage by adult horses (Murray & Schusser 1993), or milk by foals (Sanchez et al 1998), which absorbs gastric secretions and is probably accompanied by salivary bicarbonate, which can neutralize hydrochloric acid. The continuous secretion of hydrochloric acid by the equine stomach makes horses particularly susceptible to damage to the gastric squamous mucosa. Periods of prolonged high gastric acidity (pH < 2.0) were created in horses using a protocol of alternating 24 h periods of feed deprivation with free choice Timothy hay, which consistently resulted in erosion and ulceration, often severe, of the gastric squamous epithelial mucosa (Murray & Eichorn 1996). Erosions, sometimes bleeding, were seen after 48 h of cumulative feed deprivation and ulcers were seen consistently after 96 h. The gastric glandular mucosa is less susceptible to direct peptic injury than the squamous mucosa, because it has evolved elaborate mechanisms (mucus/bicarbonate barrier, prostaglandins, mucosal blood flow, cellular restitution) to protect itself from peptic injury (Hojgaard et al 1996). The mucus–bicarbonate barrier consists of a thin (200 μm) mucus layer that has hydrophobic characteristics and into which bicarbonate ion is secreted. Surface-active phospholipids in the mucus repel aqueous hydrochloric acid and the bicarbonate that is trapped within the mucus layer creates a pH gradient from the lumen of the stomach to the surface epithelial cells in the order of magnitude of 100 000. These attributes provide a substantial barrier to the back-diffusion of hydrochloric acid. Mucosal blood flow is probably the most important element of gastric mucosal protection. NO and prostaglandins are key regulators of mucosal blood flow, with NO probably being the primary factor.

In studies in which periods of feed deprivation induced ulcers in the squamous mucosa, no lesions were induced in the glandular mucosa. However, the prevalence of lesions in the glandular mucosa of the antrum was 57% in one report of 162 horses (Murray et al 2001). In humans, most lesions in the gastric mucosa are caused by *Helicobacter pylori*, NSAIDs and alcohol. In most cases, the cause of lesions in the equine gastric glandular mucosa is undetermined. *H. pylori* or similar bacteria have not been identified in equine gastric mucosa. NSAIDs can cause injury to the gastric glandular mucosa at high doses in foals and horses.

The physiological impact of hydrochloric acid on the lining of the stomach, as well as the esophagus and duodenum, is based on the hydrogen ion activity and not how much acid is present. Gastric acidity is measured by pH, which is a logarithmic measurement of hydrogen ion activity ($pH = -\log_{10}[{}^{a}H^{+}]$). Hydrogen ion activity is determined by both the hydrogen ion concentration and the ionic strength of a solution. The greater the ionic strength, the lower the pH of a solution with a given concentration of acid. Another perspective on pH is obtained applying Stewart's strong ion theory, in which the balance of strong ions (sodium, hydroxonium, chloride and hydroxide) determines the acidic activity of a solution. Consequently, when evaluating a report on a drug's effect on gastric acidity, the effect of the drug on pH is probably more relevant, as far as the gastric mucosa is concerned, than data on acid output, which are attractive from physiological and quantitative perspectives.

DRUGS AFFECTING GASTRIC ACIDITY

When considering using acid-suppressive therapy in foals or adult horses, one must bear in mind that the horse is a continuous secretor of hydrochloric acid (Campbell-Thompson & Merritt 1990), there is no diurnal pattern to gastric acidity (Murray & Schusser 1993) and that the mechanism of action of an acid-suppressive agent and the dose administered will affect the potency and duration of acid suppression. Additionally, doses of an acid-suppressive agent that appear to result in improved clinical signs may not result in ulcer healing. Importantly, suppression of gastric acidity does not stimulate ulcer healing but is permissive to ulcer healing. Mechanisms of healing are initiated with the onset of mucosal injury and

removal of the acid allows healing to proceed unimpeded.

Antacids

Antacids reduce gastric acidity by neutralizing existing acid. In an environment with an acidic pH, these compounds exchange cations for hydrogen ions, thus removing hydrogen ion activity from the gastric milieu. Most antacids are based on a combination of aluminum and magnesium hydroxides or calcium carbonate. The aluminum hydroxide/magnesium hydroxide antacids neutralize acid by combining with a water-solvated proton (H_3O^+) to yield water plus a metal ion:

$$\text{Metal (OH)}_2 + 2H_3O^+ \rightarrow \text{Metal}^{2+} + 4H_2O$$

Calcium carbonate interacts with hydrooxonium ions to form carbonic acid and a calcium ion, with carbonic acid yielding CO_2 and water:

$$CaCO_3 + 2H_3O^+ \rightarrow Ca^{2+} + 2H_2O + H_2CO_3$$
$$\rightarrow H_2O + CO_2$$

In these reactions within the acidic gastric milieu, the remaining cations (aluminum, magnesium, calcium) combine principally with chloride ions.

Antacids can effectively reduce gastric acidity but only briefly. The dose and gastric emptying limit the magnitude and duration of the effect of antacids on gastric acidity. In one study examining administration of 180 ml of a combination of aluminum and magnesium hydroxide suspension, gastric pH was increased for 45 min at most (Murray & Grodinsky 1992). In another study, 240 ml of a aluminum plus magnesium hydroxide suspension increased gastric pH for 2 h (Clark et al 1996). Therefore, liquid antacid products must be given both in large volumes (240 ml) and very frequently (6–12 times daily!) to be effective in promoting ulcer healing. Some clinicians believe that clinical signs are relieved at lower doses given less frequently, but these empirical claims have not been confirmed. Feed additives that contain antacids are popularly considered to be helpful in controlling gastric ulcers in horses but there are no supportive data. Also, an acid-neutralizing effect is most desirable when the stomach is empty, not when it is full, because gastric pH is naturally high when horses ingest feed (Murray & Schusser 1993).

In humans, antacids are used primarily to control symptoms of dyspepsia (heartburn, upset stomach) and these agents are not considered primary therapy for the treatment of ulcer disease. Only subjective assessments are available for evaluating the effects of antacids on signs of gastric discomfort in horses and the author has noted a substantial disparity between the effectiveness of antacids reported by owners and trainers and endoscopic findings. The latter observations at least indicate ineffectiveness of antacids in treating peptic lesions in horses.

Histamine H_2 receptor antagonists

The histamine H_2 receptor antagonists (H_2 antagonists) inhibit hydrochloric acid secretion by competing with histamine for receptor sites on the parietal cell (Katz 1991). Histamine is the most potent stimulus for hydrochloric acid secretion and, because occupation of the receptor site is by competitive inhibition, the greater the concentration of H_2 antagonist at the receptor site, the greater and more prolonged the degree of suppression of hydrochloric acid secretion. The H_2 antagonists approved for p.o. use in humans in the USA are cimetidine, ranitidine, famotidine and nizatidine. All are available as generic products and are also available over-the-counter in the USA. The over-the-counter products are sold in lower strengths, usually one-quarter strength, than the prescription forms. Injectable formulations of cimetidine, ranitidine and famotidine are also available.

Several studies have examined the effects of histamine H_2 antagonists on gastric acid secretion and gastric acidity in horses. In the first such study reported, ranitidine administered i.v. to young horses at 0.5 mg/kg inhibited gastric acid output but had no significant effect on gastric acidity (pH) (Campbell-Thompson & Merritt 1987). Comparison of two dosages of ranitidine (4.4 and 6.6 mg/kg), administered by nasogastric tube, on gastric fluid pH revealed that the higher dose rate increased gastric fluid pH to a greater

degree (to 5.3 ± 1.1) than the lower dose rate (4.1 ± 1.2) during the 6 h following administration (Murray & Grodinsky 1992). The effects of famotidine (0.5, 1.0 and 2.0 mg/kg) were also investigated in the same study; gastric fluid pH was >6 for longer during the 6 h after administration of ranitidine than for all doses of famotidine. In a study in which an indwelling pH electrode was used to measure gastric pH in horses fed grass hay, oral ranitidine 6.6 mg/kg three times a day resulted in a median 24 h pH of 4.8, compared with a median pH of 3.2 in horses fed hay without treatment (Murray & Schusser 1993).

Sanchez et al (1998) investigated the effects of i.v. (2.0 mg/kg) and p.o. (6.6 mg/kg) ranitidine on gastric acidity in young foals. Mean intragastric pH significantly increased for 5 h after i.v. administration compared with baseline data. After p.o. administration, gastric pH significantly increased for up to 8 h.

Cimetidine is used widely in equine practice but its effect on gastric acidity has received only limited investigation. In one study, cimetidine was administered p.o. to five horses at 8.8 mg/kg and was reported to have increased gastric pH to >3.6 for 8 h after administration (Sangiah et al 1988). Unlike other studies in which gastric fluid samples were collected at 15 min intervals or gastric pH was measured continuously by pH electrode, gastric samples were only collected every 2 h. Because gastric pH can fluctuate considerably and because high pH recordings can occur spontaneously (Kitchen et al 1998b), the results of this study should, therefore, be interpreted with caution.

An important consideration when evaluating the effect of an acid-suppressive drug is that intragastric pH in an individual animal will tend toward the low (1.0–3.0) or high (5.0–7.0) pH range. These are the ranges of greatest pH stability in the stomach. At low pH, the hydroxonium ion is the predominant cation, whereas at higher pH the sodium ion predominates. In fact, in one report, pH values paralleled the sodium concentration of gastric fluid (Merritt et al 1996). In the pH range 3–5, however, there is a transition between the predominant cation and pH tends rapidly either to decrease to <3.0 or to increase to >5.0. This has been noted in horses that had not been

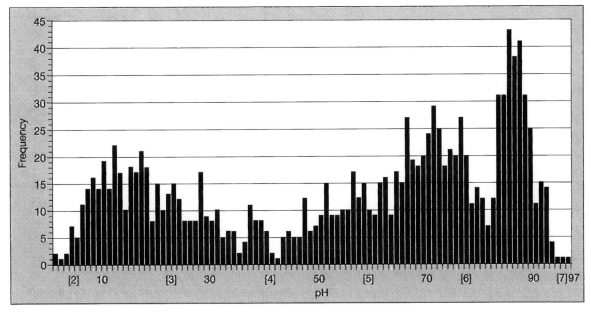

Figure 6.1 Frequency histogram of pH recordings from a horse administered oral ranitidine at 4.4 mg/kg. The horse had Timothy hay available ad libitum. Recordings of pH were made using an indwelling glass pH electrode in the stomach. Notice that the majority of pH recordings are <3.0 or >5.0. Recordings >5.0 reflect the effect of the drug on suppressing gastric acid secretion and pH values rapidly decreased to <3.0 when the effect of the drug subsided.

treated with acid-suppressive drugs and, in the context of measuring gastric pH, as a response to administration of an H_2 antagonist (Fig. 6.1). In the former situation, the increase in pH probably results from reflux of sodium-rich duodenal contents into the stomach, whereas in the latter the increased pH results from suppression of secretion of hydrochloric acid. When an H_2 antagonist, such as ranitidine, is administered into the stomach, the pH of the gastric contents typically increases to >5.0 within 45–60 min. When the effect of the drug wanes, as a result of decreased blood concentrations, pH does not gradually decrease but falls rather precipitously to <3.0.

Horses have individually characteristic gastric pH responses to oral ranitidine and famotidine, with three patterns of response observed (Murray & Grodinsky 1992). A complete response is one where gastric fluid pH increases to 7.0 or greater and remains >6.0 for 4–10 h. An intermediate response is one where there is a biphasic increase in pH (increase, decrease, then increase) and a poor response is one where gastric fluid pH increases

minimally and for a short period (Fig. 6.2). The author has noted that the type of response appears to be both horse and dose dependent. For example, one horse had an attenuated and short-lived increase in gastric fluid pH after p.o. administration of 6.6 mg/kg ranitidine or 2.0 mg/kg famotidine, whereas another had pronounced and prolonged increases in gastric fluid pH (Fig. 6.3).

This variability in response to the H_2 antagonists probably reflects the variable and relatively poor oral bioavailability of these drugs in horses. In one study of five horses, the mean oral bioavailability of cimetidine, ranitidine and famotidine were 30%, 13% and 24%, respectively (Duran & Ravis 1993). In another report, the mean oral bioavailability of cimetidine was 14% (range 7–22%) (Sams et al 1997). When administered p.o. at 3.3 mg/kg, cimetidine could not be detected in plasma (Smyth et al 1990). Pharmacokinetic studies of ranitidine in six foals and six adult horses revealed a mean oral bioavailability of 38% in foals and 27% in adult horses. The half-life of cimetidine ranges from 1 to 2.2 h (Sams et al 1997, Smyth et al

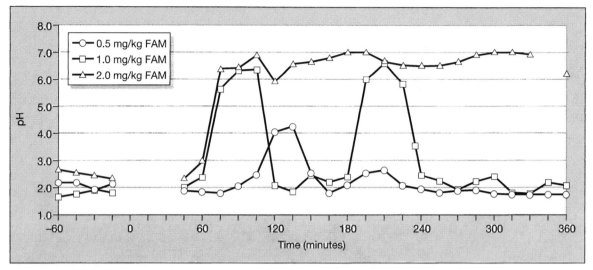

Figure 6.2 Gastric fluid pH measurements after famotidine was administered by nasogastric tube at dose rates of 0.5 (♦), 1.0 (■) and 2.0 mg/kg (▲) to a horse that had not been fed for 18 h. Gastric fluid was aspirated through a weighted nasogastric tube at 15 min intervals for 1 h before and from 45 min after administration. The gastric fluid pH dose–response in this horse typify the poor (0.5 mg/kg), intermediate (1.0 mg/kg) and good (2.0 mg/kg) responses to orally administered H_2 antagonists in horses.

1990). Cimetidine is excreted in the urine of horses as both the parent drug and the sulfoxide (Sams et al 1997).

Administration of H_2 antagonists i.v. is recommended for foals and horses with conditions in which gastric emptying or intestinal absorption is impaired. After i.v. administration of 2.0 mg/kg ranitidine to foals, mean intragastric pH increased significantly to >4.0 for 5 h. The effect of i.v. cimetidine on gastric pH in horses has not been reported, although pharmacokinetic data would support its use (Sams et al 1997, Smyth et al 1990). The author's clinical experience using cimetidine i.v. at a dose rate of 6.6 mg/kg three to four times a day has been consistently positive, with ulcer healing progressing at a rate consistent with excellent suppression of gastric acidity.

There is conflicting evidence regarding the effect of H_2 antagonists on the healing of gastric ulcers in foals and horses. In clinical reports where there were no control horses, p.o. administration of ranitidine at 6.6 mg/kg for 3 weeks was associated with complete ulcer healing in up to 90% of horses (Furr & Murray 1989). Cessation of clinical signs attributed to the gastric ulcers was reported to occur within a few days of beginning treatment. In vehicle-controlled studies in which ulcers were induced experimentally by transendoscopic cautery (MacAllister et al 1994) or flunixin (MacAllister & Sangiah 1993), cimetidine (18 mg/kg p.o. every 12 hours) or ranitidine (4.4 mg/kg p.o. every 8 hours), respectively, failed to enhance healing. In another study, ranitidine 6.6 mg/kg three times a day prevented the induction of ulcers in a feed-deprivation model (Murray & Eichorn 1996).

No large-scale, controlled clinical trial to evaluate the efficacy of H_2 antagonists on ulcer healing in horses have been carried out; yet clinical experience supports the use of these drugs in practice. What is clear from the experimental data is that, to be effective, H_2 antagonists must be administered at doses that can be expected to increase gastric pH for 4–8 h. Ranitidine has been studied most extensively and an oral dosage of 6.6 mg/kg three times a day is supported by several studies (Murray & Eichorn 1996, Murray & Grodinsky 1992, Murray & Schusser 1993, Sanchez et al 1998). Even a 33% reduction in dose, to 4.4 mg/kg, has consistently appeared to have an unpredictable effect on gastric pH increases and was often ineffective altogether (Murray & Grodinsky 1992).

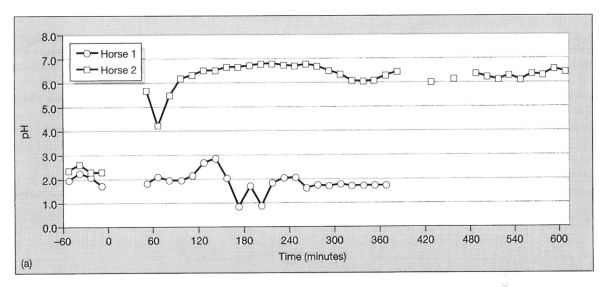

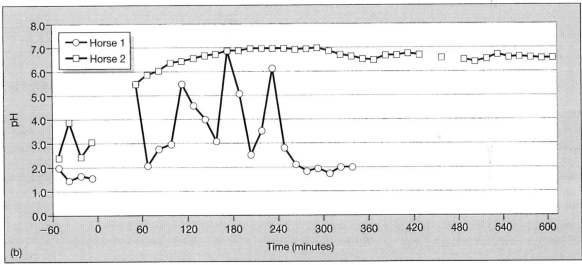

Figure 6.3   Gastric fluid pH in response to the oral administration of famotidine or ranitidine to two horses. (a) Administration of 2 mg/kg famotidine stimulated no response in horse 1 whereas horse 2 has a substantial increase in gastric fluid pH that persisted for more than 10 h. (b) Administration of 6.6 mg/kg ranitidine had an intermediate effect in horse 1, gastric fluid pH intermittently increased and decreased. By comparison, horse 2 showed a substantial increase in gastric fluid pH that persisted for more than 10 h. The pH response in horse 1 may also reflect in part, reflux of duodenal contents into the stomach in addition to, or instead of, a response to ranitidine.

Also, concurrent consumption of roughage appears to enhance the effect of ranitidine on increasing gastric pH (Murray & Schusser 1993).

Cimetidine is used widely in equine veterinary practice but there are sparse data to support its use. Cimetidine at 18 mg/kg p.o. three times a day was no more effective than control in healing electrocautery-induced ulcers in horses

(MacAllister et al 1994). In one published report, cimetidine 20 mg/kg three times a day was ineffective in healing or preventing gastric ulcers in thoroughbred racehorses in training (Nieto et al 2001). The author has administered cimetidine, at doses ranging from 20 to 25 mg/kg p.o. three times a day with variable success. These horses were kept out of work during treatment.

H$^+$,K$^+$-ATPase inhibitors

There are several H$^+$,K$^+$-ATPase systems in mammalian and plant cells and the gastric form of H$^+$,K$^+$-ATPase can be found in a variety of tissues (Scarff et al 1999). However, the H$^+$,K$^+$-ATPase inhibitors, also referred to as proton pump inhibitors, interact specifically with parietal cell H$^+$,K$^+$-ATPase because of their chemical structures and the uniquely highly acidic environment of the secretory domain of the parietal cell H$^+$, K$^+$-ATPase. The H$^+$,K$^+$-ATPase inhibitors available for treatment of peptic disorders (omeprazole, lansoprazole, pantoprazole, rabeprazole) are substituted benzimidazoles that are transferred rapidly from the blood into the acidic secretory canaliculi of the parietal cells (Besancon et al 1997). Substituted benzimidazoles are weak bases, so they become charged within the acidic canaliculi and vesicles of the parietal cells, consequently trapping and accumulating the drug within the parietal cell. These drugs then undergo a series of chemical transformations that require a highly acidic solution, resulting in a cationic sulfenamide; this forms covalent disulfide bonds with sulfhydryl groups of cysteine molecules, which are part of the catalytic subunit of the H$^+$,K$^+$-ATPase and which face the acidic secretory canaliculi. The H$^+$,K$^+$-ATPase inhibitors become bound irreversibly to the catalytic portion of the H$^+$,K$^+$-ATPase enzyme system and block the activity of the enzyme until new enzyme is generated. The magnitude of inhibition of acid secretion is dose dependent, so that at higher doses more catalytic sites are blocked; because of this mechanism of action, these drugs can inhibit acid secretion by up to 99% for 24 h or longer.

Omeprazole, lansoprazole and pantoprazole are highly unstable within the acidic environment of the stomach and lose their activity prior to absorption in the small intestine. The formulations of omeprazole and lansoprazole developed for use in humans utilize an enteric coating to protect the drug as it passes through the stomach. Pantoprazole is available as a delayed-release tablet. The bioavailability of omeprazole, lansoprazole and pantoprazole in humans is 35–60%

(Cederberg et al 1989), 80% (Gerloff et al 1996) and 75% (Huber et al 1996), respectively. The greater bioavailability of lansoprazole and pantoprazole may relate to greater first-pass metabolism of omeprazole.

A paste formulation of omeprazole is approved for use in horses. The bioavailability of the omeprazole is lower from the paste formulation than from the enteric-coated granules. More omeprazole in the paste was absorbed when administered to horses that had feed withheld than when given to horses that were fed (Daurio et al 1999). In humans, approximately 80% of omeprazole and pantoprazole are excreted in urine, with the remainder excreted in feces. Lansoprazole is primarily excreted in feces (up to 70%), indicating substantial hepatic metabolism and biliary excretion.

Omeprazole has been studied extensively in horses. Enteric-coated omeprazole granules, administered to mares at 0.7 mg/kg once daily via nasogastric tube, resulted in significant increases in basal and pentagastrin-stimulated gastric pH after the fifth dose (Andrews et al 1992). However, there was no effect on acid output or gastric pH within 8 h after the first dose. When enteric-coated omeprazole granules were administered at 1.4 mg/kg once daily, the effects on basal and pentagastrin-stimulated acid output and gastric pH were more pronounced and prolonged (Jenkins et al 1992a). On the fifth day of administration, gastric pH was consistently >6.0 and gastric pH remained increased 24 h after the sixth daily dose. As with the 0.7 mg/kg dose, gastric pH was unaffected within 8 h after the first dose of omeprazole. Whereas omeprazole administered as enteric granules did not have an immediate effect to significantly increase gastric pH (Jenkins et al 1992a), within 1 h of administering the second dose (4 mg/kg) of the approved omeprazole paste formulation, gastric pH increased from basal levels to >6.0 (Merritt et al 2002).

Omeprazole administered i.v. (0.5 mg/kg once daily) had a pronounced effect on basal acid output and gastric pH within 2 h of administration, and basal and pentagastrin-stimulated acid output were significantly inhibited 24 h after the fourth consecutive dose (Jenkins et al 1992b).

Omeprazole administered i.m. (0.25 and 1.0 mg/kg) similarly inhibited basal and pentagastrin-stimulated acid output and increased gastric pH, with a greater response to the higher dose rate (Sandin et al 1999). Peak plasma levels of omeprazole were measured 20 min after administration and thereafter plasma levels rapidly declined (half-life of 45 to 60 min). Inhibition of acid secretion persisted for many hours after the plasma levels had declined to barely detectable. The bioavailability of the i.m. administered omeprazole was 75%.

Clearly, the formulation and route of administration of omeprazole in horses strongly influence the onset, magnitude and duration of acid suppression. In one report, the inhibitory effects of different formulations of omeprazole on basal and pentagastrin-stimulated acid secretion were examined (Haven et al 1999). These formulations included an injectable formulation administered i.v. (0.5 mg/kg), acid-stable omeprazole granules given by nasogastric tube (1.5 and 5.0 mg/kg), acid-stable omeprazole granules given p.o. as a paste (1.5 mg/kg) and omeprazole powder given p.o. as a paste (1.5 and 3.0 mg/kg). The i.v. formulation performed as expected, markedly inhibiting acid secretion and increasing gastric fluid pH. The acid-stable omeprazole granules given by nasogastric tube at 5.0 mg/kg once daily also markedly suppressed acid secretion and increased gastric fluid pH; however, this formulation at 1.5 mg/kg had only a moderate effect and less of an effect than reported previously for 1.4 mg/kg (Jenkins et al 1992b). The paste formulations of omeprazole all decreased acid output and increased gastric fluid pH, although to a lesser degree than the i.v. administered omeprazole and the granule formulation given at 5.0 mg/kg by nasogastric tube.

In another report, the paste formulation of omeprazole approved for equine use markedly and equivalently suppressed gastric acid secretion and increased gastric fluid pH at p.o. dosages of 4.0 and 5.0 mg/kg once daily (Daurio et al 1999). Data were collected after the fifth, tenth and fifteenth consecutive daily dosages; acid output (H^+ as μmol/15 min per kg) was 99% suppressed when measured 8 h after the fifth dose, 95% when measured 16 h after the tenth dose and 90% when measured 24 h after the fifteenth dose. Gastric pH was significantly increased, usually to >6.0.

The same paste formulation of omeprazole has been examined in several pre- and postapproval studies. A dose-confirmation trial was conducted in horses in simulated, yet intense, race training that both induced and maintained gastric ulcers (Andrews et al 1999). The study had two 4 week phases: active treatment and prevention of recurrence. During this time, the horses were kept in intensive training. After 4 weeks of treatment with omeprazole paste at 4 mg/kg daily, ulcers were improved (defined as an ulcer score lower than pretreatment) in 92% of the horses receiving omeprazole paste compared with only 32% of the sham-treated horses. Ulcer healing, defined as an ulcer score of zero, occurred in 77% of treated horses compared with 4% of sham-treated horses. In the prevention phase of the study, ulcers did not recur in 84% and 88% of healed horses subsequently treated daily with omeprazole paste at 2 or 4 mg/kg, respectively, whereas ulcers persisted, recurred or became more severe in 92% of sham-treated horses. Field clinical trials have further documented the efficacy of this omeprazole oral paste formulation, at a dose rate of 4 mg/kg once daily, for treatment of gastric ulcers in foals and adult horses. Other studies have shown that this paste formulation is accepted readily by foals and horses and appears not to produce adverse effects, including infertility in stallions.

Other drugs that affect gastric acidity

Misoprostol, an analog of prostaglandin E_1, has acid-suppressive effects in horses when administered p.o. at 5 μg/kg (Sangiah et al 1989). However, it is thought that the primary effect of misoprostol is based on the enhancement of mucosal protection from peptic injury. Misoprostol can cause abdominal cramping and diarrhea in humans and for this reason it may be unsuitable as a treatment for gastric ulcers in equines. In addition, misoprostol offered no advantage over omeprazole in preventing or healing

NSAID- induced gastric or duodenal ulceration in humans (Hawkey et al 1998).

The somatostatin analog octreotide can decrease gastric acid secretion. In one report, octreotide, given s.c. to horses at dose rates of 0.1, 0.5, 1.0 and 5.0 µg/kg, increased gastric pH to >5.0 compared with baseline values (consistently <2.7) (Rabon & Reuben 1990). The duration of effect was dose dependent and ranged from 2.4 to 5.4 h.

DRUGS ACTING ON GASTRIC MUCOSAL PROTECTION

Some agents do not suppress gastric acidity (with the exception of aluminum-containing antacids, which have some mucosal protection properties) but enhance the intrinsic protection of the gastric mucosa against hydrochloric acids and pepsin. Importantly, for the equine stomach, the squamous mucosal lining lacks the surface barriers to peptic injury that are found within the glandular mucosa; therefore, agents that affect mucosal protection will have little to no impact on the glandular mucosa.

Sucralfate

Sucralfate, the major components of which are sucrose octasulfate and aluminum hydroxide, is effective in the treatment of peptic ulcers in humans (McCarthy 1991), although the healing of duodenal ulcers took much longer than with H$_2$ antagonists. Clinical experience suggests that sucralfate can promote the healing of lesions in the gastric glandular mucosa of horses. The mechanism of action probably involves adherence to the ulcerated mucosa, stimulation of mucus secretion and enhanced mucosal blood flow and prostaglandin E synthesis. These are all factors relevant to the glandular mucosa and it is doubtful that sucralfate is effective in treating ulcers in the equine gastric squamous mucosa. In fact, lesions in the squamous mucosa can develop while a horse is undergoing treatment with sucralfate.

No studies have been performed in horses to determine an appropriate dose of sucralfate.

Favorable clinical results have been obtained with p.o. doses of 10–20 mg/kg three times a day. Sucralfate can be administered concurrently with an H$_2$ antagonist. Concurrent administration may reduce the absorption of the H$_2$ antagonist by 10% but this has not appeared to affect efficacy in humans (Mullersman et al 1986). Importantly, sucralfate can substantially interfere with the absorption of other drugs, particularly fluoroquinolones, and thus its use concurrently with other medications should be determined on a case-by-case basis.

Misoprostol

The prostaglandin E$_1$ analog misoprostol enhances mucosal protection by promoting mucosal blood flow and possibly increasing gastric mucus (Dajani & Agrawal 1989). Misoprostol has demonstrated clinical effectiveness in preventing duodenal ulcers in humans, particularly NSAID-induced ulcers (Roth 1990). In one study in horses another prostaglandin E$_1$ analog limited phenylbutazone-induced gastrointestinal mucosal damage (Collins & Tyler 1985).

Aluminum-containing antacids

In addition to their acid-neutralizing properties, antacids containing aluminum appear to have properties that can protect the gastric mucosa from peptic injury. These antacids have been shown to protect the mucosa against NSAID- or ethanol-induced injury by a mechanism that involves the production of NO, which promotes mucosal blood flow (Konturek et al 1992).

NO agonists

Gastric mucosal blood flow is important in maintaining mucosal acid–base balance and in maintaining mucosal barriers to hydrochloric acid. NO is the primary promoter of mucosal perfusion. Inhibitors of NO synthase have been shown to augment gastric mucosal injury and to impair healing of gastric ulcers. Conversely, administration of L-arginine, a substrate of NO synthase, has been shown to enhance gastric mucosal protection and healing in laboratory animals. Positive effects of L-arginine have been demonstrated when it was administered parenterally or p.o. (Brzozowski et al 1997). Aluminum-containing antacids and sucralfate are thought to provide gastric mucosal protection by promoting NO production, resulting in mucosal vasodilation and increased blood flow.

DRUGS ACTING ON GASTRIC MOTILITY

Bethanechol

The cholinergic agonist bethanechol has been used to stimulate gastric emptying in foals and horses with duodenitis, pyloric stenosis and pyloric ulceration. Bethanechol also has been used to facilitate gastroduodenoscopy in foals and horses. In a study in which scintigraphy was used to measure emptying rates of ^{99}Tc-labeled sulfur colloid incorporated into egg albumin administered into the stomach of horses, i.v. administration of 0.025 mg/kg bethanechol increased the rate of gastric emptying significantly (Ringger et al 1996). In saline-treated horses, the average time for emptying of half of the solid gastric contents (T_{50}) was 90 min, compared with a T_{50} of 30 min in bethanechol-treated horses. Excessive salivation was noted in some of the horses administered bethanechol i.v. Clinically, bethanechol is given s.c. at a dose rate of 0.02 mg/kg or p.o. at 0.35 mg/kg three times a day. Cholinergic side-effects are not noted at these doses. Bethanechol has been given to some horses chronically (weeks to months) without apparent adverse effects. It is not known whether the drug remains effective when given chronically or whether horses might become refractory. Indications for chronic administration of bethanechol include pyloric stenosis and chronic ulceration of the pylorus.

Benzamides

Metoclopramide

Metoclopramide has been used effectively in humans to improve gastric emptying and in foals with suspected gastric-emptying disorders. Metoclopramide has the potential to cause severe excitation in foals and horses because of its ability to cross the blood–brain barrier and its inhibitory effects on dopamine receptors. Therefore, the challenge is to administer a dose that effectively stimulates propulsive motility whilst avoiding adverse effects. Foals have been given doses ranging from 0.1 to 0.25 mg/kg three to four times a day. However, there are few data to support the use of metoclopramide to promote gastric emptying in horses. In one report, metoclopramide, given to horses, as a slow infusion at a dose rate of 0.125 mg/kg, was shown to increase gastric emptying in a low-dose endotoxin model (Doherty et al 1999). Bethanechol appears to be preferable to metoclopramide because it is effective and has limited side-effects.

Cisapride

Cisapride is highly effective in increasing gastric emptying in humans. In one report, cisapride given p.o. at 0.4 mg/kg had no effect on gastric emptying in normal horses but improved gastric emptying in horses given low-dose endotoxin (Valk et al 1998). However, other investigators found that the same dose of cisapride was absorbed highly erratically and generally poorly (Steel et al 1998).

Motilides

Similar to other prokinetic drugs, erythromycin has been shown to improve gastric emptying in humans and laboratory animals. In horses, erythromycin lactobionate, at both 0.1 and 1.0 mg/kg, reduced the T_{50} of solid-phase gastric emptying (Ringger et al 1996).

Erythromycin should probably not be the first choice to treat delayed gastric emptying in horses because of its potential adverse effects (clostridial colitis, hyperthermia) even at low doses.

Xylazine and detomidine

Xylazine and detomidine are α_2 adrenoceptor agonists that are commonly used to sedate horses.

Xylazine (0.5 mg/kg i.v.) alone had minimal effects on gastroduodenal motility, but when combined with the narcotic agonist–antagonist butorphanol there is pronounced suppression of antroduodenal myoelectric activity (Merritt et al 1998). Interestingly, butorphanol alone had minimal effects on antroduodenal myoelectric activity. However, detomidine, at 0.0125 mg/kg, markedly depressed duodenal motility and would be expected to affect gastric motility similarly.

SMALL AND LARGE INTESTINE

PATHOPHYSIOLOGY OF INTESTINAL MOTILITY DISORDERS

Disorders that affect intestinal motility, including ileus, peritoneal inflammation, enteritis and obstructive disorders, are frequent problems in horses. Often many of these elements occur concurrently. Gastrointestinal ileus is the functional inhibition of propulsive bowel activity, irrespective of its pathophysiological basis. Ileus accompanies a multitude of intestinal disorders, including strangulating and non-strangulating obstructions, mechanical obstruction with gas distention, enteritis, endotoxemia and peritonitis. There are many pathophysiological mechanisms resulting in disrupted propulsive intestinal motility, many of which are unknown. Disruption of the primary neuromuscular pathways and the intestinal MMCs are well-characterized mechanisms of ileus that result from several causes. For instance, subsequent to large colon volvulus, the neurons in the myenteric plexus undergo degeneration and decrease in number (Schusser & White 1997). Additionally, alterations in smooth muscle mitochondrial morphology have been identified in equine jejunum after low-flow ischemia (Dabareiner et al 1995).

Peritoneal inflammation or irritation can initiate ileus, partly through spinal reflexes (Sjoqvist et al 1985). Afferent fibers from peritoneal surfaces terminate in the dorsal horn of the spinal cord, where they can activate inhibitory sympathetic fibers or synapse directly onto sympathetic ganglia. The efferent limb of the reflex expresses increased sympathetic outflow, primarily mediated through combined stimulation of α_2 adrenoceptors and inhibition of acetylcholine release.

These external neural influences on intestinal motility are common targets for prokinetic drugs, but events within the bowel can have important effects on intestinal motility and cause the bowel to be refractory to traditional prokinetic therapy. Release of cytokines from activated inflammatory cells is probably an important feature of ileus in many cases. Ileus secondary to reperfusion injury is an anticipated response in horses with small intestinal obstruction. However, even apparently mild intestinal injury can initiate cellular responses that lead to impaired motility. Mild intestinal insult by gentle surgical manipulation activated adhesion molecules on leukocytes and increased the expression of P-selectin and intercellular adhesion molecule 1 on endothelial cells within the vasculature of the muscularis layer of the intestine (Kalff et al 1999). Surgical manipulation of the rodent small intestine resulted in substantial extravasation of leukocytes into the intestinal muscularis, consisting mainly of polymorphonuclear neutrophils, monocytes and mast cells and lasting for days. This cellular inflammatory response within the intestinal muscularis externa was associated with a marked decrease in jejunal circular muscle activity (Kalff et al 1998).

CLINICAL CONDITIONS WITH INTESTINAL MOTILITY DISORDERS

Altered gastrointestinal motility can result from many disorders, not all of which primarily affect the gut. For instance, endotoxemia, regardless of its origin, can depress intestinal motility. Motility is also probably affected by diet, subclinical endoparasitism and even exercise.

In neonatal foals, enteritis is associated with the accumulation of fluid in the bowel lumen and either poor propulsive motility or excessive contractions of the bowel. Also, neonatal foals with septicemia often have poor intestinal motility. In these cases, neither enteral feeding nor pharmacological stimulation of intestinal motility is indicated. In older foals, duodenitis is associated with delayed gastric emptying and the prokinetic drugs are useful in some cases.

In adult horses with duodenitis/proximal enteritis (DPE) there are inflammatory changes of variable severity affecting all layers of the proximal small intestine. Most affected horses produce copious volumes of enterogastric reflux and it is presumed that impaired intestinal motility allows the fluid to accumulate within the intestine and that pharmacological enhancement of intestinal motility will reduce the volume of reflux. In most cases, use of prokinetic drugs does not appear to be associated with a reduction in enterogastric reflux. This may reflect an inability of these drugs to stimulate smooth muscle contraction in the inflamed intestine, overriding ENS stimuli that cannot be impacted appreciably by the current roster of prokinetics, and incorrect targeting of pathophysiological processes.

POI is a frequent complication of abdominal surgery in horses. In most cases, the small intestine is the segment of bowel affected primarily and strangulation and distension are the most frequent problems. In both instances, the blood flow to all layers of the intestine is compromised and reperfusion injury is a feature of the postoperative period. Reperfusion injury is a complex process involving mitochondrial and cytosolic changes, activation of a myriad of inflammatory mediators and increased endothelial cell permeability and neutrophil recruitment. Changes can occur throughout much of the intestine, even away from the primary site of injury and the magnitude of injury is often difficult to predict. As mentioned above, simple surgical manipulation of the intestine can promote neutrophil recruitment within the intestine with subsequent impairment of propulsive motility (Kalff et al 1998). Clinical manifestations of POI can include persistent enterogastric reflux, lack of borborygmi and inability to tolerate feeding, for up to 3–5 days.

Cecal dysfunction and cecal impaction occur infrequently but can be very difficult to manage. Many clinicians consider these to be separate entities, with cecal dysfunction characterized by cecal distention with soft to watery contents and cecal impaction characterized by accumulation of doughy, desiccated ingesta. Many clinicians prefer to use a surgical approach to the management of cecal dysfunction. Cecal impactions often require several days until there is complete resolution and feeding can be resumed. Drugs that alter intestinal motility, such as cholinomimetics, benzamides and motilides, may be useful in the management of some cases of cecal impaction or in postoperative management of these cases.

Large-colon impaction is characterized by distention of the large intestine with desiccated digesta. All segments of the large colon can be involved but the pelvic flexure and right dorsal colon are the most frequent sites of impaction. Impactions of the large colon are probably a combination of motility and fluid-balance disorders and most cases are treated with laxatives or hydration solutions.

Impaction of the small colon with meconium occurs in neonatal foals. Typically, these impactions result from an excessive amount of meconium. Small-colon impactions are unusual in older foals and occur infrequently in adult horses. Apparently there is a positive association between small-colon impaction and fecal culture of *Salmonella* spp. (Rhoads et al 1999). Small-colon impactions in adult horses may represent a primary motility disorder secondary to inflammation. Small-colon impactions are often treated conservatively using enemas, although in some cases surgery is required. Drugs that alter motility are typically not used in these cases.

DRUGS ACTING ON MOTILITY OF THE SMALL AND LARGE INTESTINE
Cholinomimetics

Bethanechol

Bethanechol increased electrical activity in the small intestine (Roger & Ruckebusch 1987) and i.v. administration (0.025 mg/kg) was shown to rapidly initiate MMC phase III activity in the ileum of horses, although the effects on transit of digesta through the small intestine were not determined (Lester et al 1998a). Bethanechol also increased the rate of emptying of radiolabeled markers from the cecum, which was associated with an increase in the relative strength and duration of contractions in the cecum and right ventral colon. Bethanechol is not used routinely for treating impactions of the cecum and large colon and its effects may be different in these cases than in normal horses.

Neostigmine

Neostigmine increases receptor levels of acetylcholine by inhibiting the enzyme cholinesterase. Neostigmine (0.02 mg/kg i.v.) increased myoelectrical activity in the jejunum but significantly delayed the emptying of 6 mm beads from the stomach of normal adult horses (Adams & MacHarg 1985). The i.v. infusion of neostigmine was associated with signs of abdominal discomfort. In another report, the i.v. administration of neostigmine (0.025 mg/kg) promoted cecal and colonic contractile activity and hastened the emptying of radiolabeled markers from the cecum but also induced defecation and caused mild abdominal pain (Lester et al 1998a). Neostigmine is used by some clinicians to counteract POI and to promote emptying of the cecum or large colon in cases of impaction. As a cautionary note, it has been suggested that, because of the force of neostigmine-induced activity in the cecum, the drug should probably be avoided in horses with impaction or large intestinal distension (Lester et al 1998a). Other drugs, such as bethanechol or erythromycin, appear to be as effective or more effective in promoting gastrointestinal transit and are associated with fewer adverse effects.

Anticholinergic drugs

Anticholinergic drugs compete with acetylcholine for muscarinic binding sites on smooth muscle, thereby decreasing smooth muscle activity and intestinal motility. In most cases, anticholinergic effects in the intestine are undesirable, often resulting in desiccation and accumulation of digesta within the large intestine (impaction). A useful application of anticholinergic drugs is to relax the rectum, which may be desirable to facilitate palpation of the abdomen per rectum or in rectal tears. In the latter, the evacuation of rectal contents and examination of the rectum may be facilitated by administration of an anticholinergic drug.

Atropine

Atropine is a potent inhibitor of intestinal motility (Adams et al 1984, Roger & Ruckebusch 1987). It is most frequently applied topically to the cornea to promote mydriasis and anecdotal reports suggest that the absorption of atropine from this site may disrupt intestinal motility (see Ch. 13). A single s.c. dose of atropine (0.02 mg/kg) can be given safely to most horses. Dose rates of 0.02–0.04 mg/kg may facilitate evacuation of the rectum in horses with a rectal tear.

Scopolamine (hyoscine)

Scopolamine (hyoscine N-butylbromide) is available as an antispasmodic product (20 mg ampule for injection and 20 mg tablets) for use in humans. In addition, there is a veterinary product that contains scopolamine and dipyrone approved for use as an antispasmodic/analgesic in animals. In addition to blocking the effects of acetylcholine at the muscarinic receptor, scopolamine affects nicotinic receptors in intestinal ganglia and does not affect the CNS. In horses, scopolamine is used as an antispasmodic and to relax the rectum to facilitate abdominal palpation. In one report, 0.2 mg/kg was as effective as 0.2 mg/kg scopolamine plus 2.5 mg/kg dipyrone in relieving discomfort caused by balloon dilatation of the cecum (Roelvink et al 1991). The analgesic effect lasted for 20 min.

Benzamides

Metoclopramide

There are conflicting data on the use of metoclopramide in horses. In some models of POI, metoclopramide appeared effective (Gerring & Hunt 1986), while others found that metoclopramide did not positively affect intestinal motility (Sojka et al 1988). Metoclopramide crosses the blood–brain barrier, where its antagonist properties on central dopamine D_2 receptors can result in extrapyramidal signs, including violent excitation.

These effects, seen with i.v. doses of 0.25 mg/kg and higher, have resulted in poor acceptance of the drug in equine practice. Recently, the use of a low-dose, constant infusion of metoclopramide was examined in 70 horses undergoing small intestinal resection (Dart et al 1996). Constant i.v. infusion of metoclopramide (0.04 mg/h per kg) significantly decreased the volume and duration of gastric reflux postoperatively over that seen in both control and intermittent drug infusion in these clinical cases. The study was not designed in such a way that allows definitive conclusions to be drawn on the efficacy of the treatment; however, the infusion was well tolerated.

Cisapride

Interest in the use of cisapride to improve intestinal motility in horses arose from its use to affect gastrointestinal motility positively without producing the side-effects associated with other prokinetic drugs in humans and other animals. One of the benefits of cisapride over other prokinetic drugs is its effect on promoting motility in the colon. Early studies showed that cisapride administered i.v. (0.05 mg/kg) to horses produced marked and prolonged increases in electrical and mechanical activity in several bowel segments (King & Gerring 1988). In the stomach, there was an increase in total contractile activity with increased contraction amplitude and a slight reduction in contraction rate. In the small intestine, there was an increase in MMC phase II activity with an increase in the number and amplitude of contractions and a decrease in phase III activity. Cisapride increased electrical and contractile activity in the left dorsal colon with increased contraction amplitude and an increase in electrical activity in the small colon. In a report on experimental and clinical use, it was suggested that the i.m. administration of 0.1 mg/kg cisapride was effective in preventing or minimizing POI (Gerring & King 1989).

In the USA, cisapride was only available as an oral formulation, which was poorly absorbed when given by intragastric administration (Steel et al 1998) or per rectum (Cook et al 1997, Steel et al 1999). The use of cisapride in horses has been limited by the erratic absorption of the drug from the intestinal tract and the expense of the parenteral formulation. Cisapride has been withdrawn from the market in the USA and Europe.

Motilides

Erythromycin lactobionate has been shown to promote cecal emptying in normal horses when given as an i.v. bolus dose at 0.1 mg/kg or as a 60 min i.v. infusion at 1.0 mg/kg (Lester et al 1998b). The maximal effect on emptying was seen at 1.0 mg/kg and was greater than that induced by neostigmine or bethanechol. Erythromycin had no effect on ileal myoelectric recordings but induced premature MMC phase III regular spiking activity in the cecum and increased myoelectric activity in the right ventral colon. There are no experimental data on the effects of erythromycin on cecal emptying under clinical conditions, but clinical impressions support its use (i.v. bolus dose of 0.5 mg/kg every 8 h) in the prevention and treatment of cecal impaction. Erythromycin potentially induces clostridial colitis and this must be considered if erythromycin is to be used in adult horses.

Sympathomimetics

α_2 adrenergic agonists

Xylazine and detomidine are α_2 adrenoceptor agonists that are used frequently in horses with colic. They provide temporary analgesia but also have cardiovascular effects that may be counterproductive in horses with already compromised cardiovascular function. Xylazine was reported to induce phase III spiking activity and reset the MMC cycle in the duodenum of horses (Merritt et al 1989) and to increase regular spiking activity in the jejunum (Adams et al 1984). The effect of xylazine on the coordinated propulsion of ingesta through the small intestine is not known and may not be correlated with these myoelectric findings. Xylazine and detomidine have been shown to decrease cecal motility and blood flow and may be risk factors for anesthetic-associated cecal impaction. The α_2 adrenoceptor agonists depressed myoelectric activity and decreased the cecal emptying rate and T_{50} of emptying radiolabeled markers from the cecum (Lester et al 1998a, Rutkowski et al 1991). In ponies in which pelvic flexure fistulas were created and inflation of an intraluminal balloon was used to simulate impaction, xylazine relieved clinical signs of colic for 30 to 60 min and reduced intraluminal pressure in the pelvic flexure (Lowe et al 1980). However, xylazine was also associated with decreased mean arterial blood flow through the colic arteries.

Clearly, the α_2 adrenergic agonists have both benefits and risks. In horses with impaction of the large colon, they can relax the colon and provide pain relief but will also delay the transit of digesta. They are probably best utilized early in treatment, when pain from distention is a problem but the propulsion of the desiccated digesta through the cecum and colon is unlikely until the digesta are better hydrated. Use of the these drugs in horses with more severe intestinal disorders and compromised cardiovascular function should probably be accompanied by supportive treatment (fluid therapy).

β_2 adrenergic agonists

The β_2 adrenoceptor agonists, such as clenbuterol, are used to treat respiratory disorders in horses but they also may impact on gastrointestinal function since they decrease colonic motility (Lyrenas 1985). The β_2 adrenoceptor agonists induced significant decreases in the amplitude and frequency of contraction in equine ileal smooth muscle *in vitro* (Malone et al 1996). The effects of therapeutic doses of β_2 adrenergic agonists used for the treatment of respiratory disease on alimentary function in horses is not known, but the potential for inhibition of intestinal motility should be considered, particularly when administering β_2 adrenergic agonists parenterally.

Sympatholytics

Yohimbine

Activation of presynaptic α_2 adrenoceptors inhibits the release of acetylcholine from cholinergic neurons, resulting in decreased muscular contractions. Disorders such as endotoxemia and peritonitis elicit the release of sympathetic neurotransmitters and increase sympathetic nerve activity, contributing to intestinal ileus. Yohimbine is an α_2 adrenoceptor antagonist that has been shown to affect the equine small intestine and colon (Lester et al 1998a). In normal horses, yohimbine mildly accelerated cecal emptying. In a serosal trauma model of POI, yohimbine restored some electrical–mechanical function to the small intestine (Gerring & Hunt 1986). In an equine endotoxemia model, slow i.v. infusion of 0.075 mg/kg yohimbine attenuated the suppression of the mechanical activity and blood flow in the cecum and large colon (Eades & Moore 1993). The clinical utility of yohimbine to promote intestinal transit has not been examined and this drug does not appear to be used extensively.

Lidocaine (lignocaine)

The i.v. administration of lidocaine has been suggested as a treatment that restores intestinal motility in horses with POI. Lidocaine has been evaluated in both spontaneous and experimental models of intestinal ileus. It does not stimulate bowel motility directly but appears to prevent the inhibition of bowel motility under certain conditions. In rats, epidural administration of lidocaine was associated with a significant recovery in intestinal motility in an intestinal ischemia model (Udassin et al 1994). In humans, i.v. administration of lidocaine reduced POI after non-intestinal abdominal surgery (Rimback et al 1990). This effect appears to be mediated by the suppression of primary afferent neurons from the bowel to spinal segments, thereby limiting reflex sympathetic efferent inhibition of motility. In addition, local anesthetics have anti-inflammatory properties, including inhibiting both granulocyte migration and the release of lysosomal enzymes. In models of myocardial and lung ischemia–reperfusion injury, lidocaine significantly reduced neutrophil recruitment and tissue injury (Vitola et al 1997).

The beneficial effects of i.v. lidocaine in horses with POI have not been confirmed, although the results of a multicenter study suggested that parenteral lidocaine may help to restore intestinal motility in horses with POI (Malone et al 1998). An initial loading dose of 1.3 mg/kg is given followed by a constant i.v. infusion at 0.05 mg/ min per kg. Lidocaine infusion is associated with reversible side-effects including muscle fasciculations, ataxia and seizures.

PATHOPHYSIOLOGY OF INTESTINAL SECRETORY DISORDERS

Disorders that cause increased secretion of fluid and electrolytes into the small intestine of the horse are characterized by abdominal discomfort, distension of the small intestine and enterogastric reflux. In young foals with small intestinal secretory disorders, diarrhea may occur. Increased intestinal secretion can result from the active secretion of electrolytes and water, for example the cyclic nucleotide-stimulated secretion that results from exposure to bacterial enterotoxins. Passive secretion of water can result from increased permeability of the intestine, such as in enteritis, distension or ischemia, or decreased absorption of osmotically active substances, such as with lactose intolerance in foals. Disorders in which there is decreased secretion of fluid into the small intestine are not appreciated, although impactions of ingesta in segments of the small intestine can occur.

Horses with DPE can produce copious volumes of enterogastric reflux. It is generally presumed that this fluid originates as secretion from the inflamed small intestinal mucosa, either as an active, cyclic nucleotide-mediated fluid secretion or as an exudative secretion. Additionally, enteric nerve-mediated secretion, via mast cell degranulation, may contribute to the fluid secretion. Another possible source of the large volume of watery secretions is the pancreas. Endoscopy of a small number of horses with DPE has revealed an almost continuous stream of fluid emanating from the major duodenal papilla. Normally, much of the fluid secreted through the major duodenal papilla, up to 1 l/h, enters the stomach and it is logical to presume that increased pancreatic secretion will result in increased enterogastric reflux.

Disorders that cause increased secretion of fluid and electrolytes in the large intestine of the horse are characterized by diarrhea. Conversely, impactions of ingesta in the large intestine may result, in part, from insufficient secretion of fluid into the large intestine and desiccation of the digesta. Frequently diagnosed causes of diarrhea in foals include infections with rotavirus, *Clostridium difficile, C. perfringens* and *Salmonella* spp. Less- frequent causes of diarrhea in foals include *E. coli, Rhodococcus equi* and endoparasites. Frequently diagnosed causes of diarrhea in adult horses include *Salmonella* spp., *C. difficile, C. perfringens* and *Ehrlichia risticii.* However, the cause of diarrhea in most foals and horses is usually not determined. Mechanisms of fluid secretion include enterotoxin-induced secretion mediated by cyclic nucleotides, mast cell degranulation, cytotoxic effects and increased tissue permeability from damage by the products of inflammatory cells.

Most digesta impactions in foals and horses occur in the large intestine and small colon. Typically an increased volume of desiccated digesta characterizes impactions of the cecum. Other forms of cecal dysfunction are characterized by digesta with a normal to increased proportion of fluid. The former condition may be a combination of disorders of motility and fluid fluxes while the latter is presumed to represent a motility disorder. Impactions of the large colon are typically located in the left ventral colon, pelvic flexure and right dorsal colon. They are characterized by an increased mass of desiccated digesta. Drugs that decrease the motility of the large colon, such as atropine and amitraz, can cause large-colon impactions, but disruptions in fluid fluxes during fermentation of feed may be more relevant in clinical cases.

DRUGS ACTING ON INTESTINAL SECRETION AND ABSORPTION

Laxatives

Lubricants

Mineral oil is used frequently in equines with large intestine impaction to lubricate the impacted digesta and facilitate its passage through the colon. Its effectiveness is limited for large, desiccated impactions because the oil tends to pass around the impaction. Therefore, for mineral oil to be most effective, the digesta must be adequately hydrated. Linseed oil has been compared with mineral oil in normal horses; whereas the administration of mineral oil softened manure and was benign to the horse, linseed oil caused more prolonged stool softening but produced signs of abdominal discomfort in some horses and was associated with increased serum glucose and bilirubin concentrations (Schumacher et al 1997).

Osmotic cathartics

Osmotic cathartics are hypertonic solutions that are absorbed poorly from the lumen of the intestine and draw water into the intestine by passive diffusion. The small intestine has a relatively low density of intercellular tight junctions and consequently should be most responsive to these osmotic agents. The large intestine, a target for osmotic cathartics and a frequent site of impactions of digesta, has a relatively high density of intercellular tight junctions and here the osmotic cathartics should be expected to have less effect.

The osmotic cathartics used frequently in equine veterinary practice are magnesium sulfate and magnesium oxide. The use of these agents has been based on the presumption that they induce a passive secretion of water into the intestine through their osmotic properties. However, this effect may be minimal. Magnesium is absorbed in the intestine and magnesium toxicosis has been reported following the administration of magnesium sulfate (Henninger & Horst 1997). Also, in one report, magnesium sulfate, given at 1.0 g/kg, increased fecal output and fecal water content but in a timeframe that was too short to be explained by an osmotic effect in the large intestine (Freeman et al 1992). An effect of magnesium sulfate was seen by 5 h after administration and preceded the appearance of a concurrently administered liquid transit marker in the feces by many hours, suggesting that this was not a direct osmotic effect but was a result of the secretion of water by the large intestine or small colon giving rise to increased fecal water content and output.

Chemical cathartics

Chemical cathartics stimulate intestinal fluid secretion by activating mucosal secretion. Some chemical cathartics, such as castor oil, also can cause intestinal mucosal injury. Castor oil is used traditionally as a laxative in humans. The active ingredient in castor oil is ricolinoleate. The mechanism of the laxative effect of castor oil may involve an intrinsic afferent reflex, with the afferent limb mediated by tachykinins and with NO as the efferent stimulus to secretion. In addition to inducing fluid secretion, castor oil can induce substantial mucosal damage (Johnson et al 1993). A dose of 60 ml (1 ml/kg) p.o. has been mentioned for treatment of meconium impaction in foals (Madigan 1997). It should be noted that severe colitis has been induced in horses by the administration of 2.5 ml/kg castor oil (Roberts et al 1989).

Surfactants

Dioctyl sodium sulfosuccinate (DSS) is thought to be useful in resolving impactions of the large intestine by acting as a surfactant and facilitating the movement of water into desiccated digesta in the colon. In one study, DSS given at 50 mg/kg in 6 l of water to four normal horses resulted in increased fecal output and fecal water content from 6 to 12 h after administration (Freeman et al 1992). DSS caused mild colic, hyperpnea and diarrhea in one horse 0.3–3 h after administration.

There are many anecdotal reports of DSS toxicosis, which has clinical signs similar to carbohydrate overload (signs of endotoxemia, diarrhea and laminitis). DSS is available as a 5% and 10% solution and the dose should not exceed 25 mg/kg (8.3 ounces (USA) or 250 ml of a 5% solution to a 500 kg horse).

Fiber

Fiber is popularly considered to have a laxative effect and, indeed, in carnivores and omnivores this can be true. In hindgut fermenting herbivores, such as the horse, it seems unlikely that fiber, such as that found in bran, will increase fecal output or water content. Another use of fiber as a laxative is in the management of accumulation of sand in the large intestine. In one study, psyllium administration had no effect on removal of sand from the large intestine in ponies in which sand was placed into the cecum (Hammock et al 1998).

Antisecretory agents

True antisecretory agents, those that block a biochemical process that promotes intestinal fluid secretion, are not available for clinical use in horses. Loperamide can reduce the volume of diarrhea in foals with a primarily small intestinal secretory disorder. However, treated foals may become colicky as a result of fluid distention in the intestines because the mechanism of action is primarily retention of fluid within the intestine. Also, retention of intestinal content may promote the proliferation of enteropathogens. The enkephalinase inhibitor racecadotril appears to have true antisecretory effect in animal models and in humans with diarrhea (Izzo et al 1998). Its safety or effectiveness in foals and horses has not been reported.

AGENTS PROMOTING DIGESTION AND ABSORPTION

Lactase-replacement therapy

Lactose intolerance is an infrequent primary disorder in foals that typically manifests as diarrhea and intermittent abdominal discomfort. Lactose intolerance is more frequently seen in young foals with enteritis. In these foals, ingestion of milk or milk replacer containing lactose is associated with diarrhea and abdominal discomfort. The concurrent administration of lactase (one tablet per hour) concurrently with nursing or feeding a milk replacer appears to be beneficial until the foal's intestinal mucosa heals and endogenous production of lactase becomes sufficient. Different lactase products are available in Europe.

DRUGS ACTING ON INTESTINAL MUCOSA

Bismuth subsalicylate

There are no studies on the effect of bismuth compounds on diarrhea in foals or horses, although such products are used frequently in practice. In a study on the effect of BSS in humans with histologic colitis, patients ingested eight 262 mg tablets per day. Each tablespoon (15 ml) of the BSS suspension available contains 262 mg BSS. An effective dose for horses has not been determined. Empirical doses of 30 ml every 2–4 h have been used in foals. Larger volumes, up to 500 ml every 4 h, have been administered to adult horses with diarrhea. BSS is generally safe (Tillman et al 1996), although adverse effects can include constipation and it may interfere with intestinal absorption of some drugs (Ericsson et al 1982).

Prostaglandin analogs

Right dorsal colitis is a syndrome that results from excessive NSAID administration in horses; it is characterized by ulceration of the mucosa of the right dorsal colon, plasma protein loss and weight loss. Treatment with misoprostol, a prostaglandin E_1 analog has been proposed, but not proven, to result in a positive clinical response in affected horses. In one report, coadministration of phenylbutazone with a prostaglandin E_2 analog significantly attenuated the alimentary mucosal injury compared with phenylbutazone administration alone (Collins & Tyler 1985). Recommended dosages of misoprostol range from 1.5 to 5 µg/kg p.o. three times a day. In clinical cases, the author typically begins treatment at 1.5 µg/kg p.o. three times a day and gradually increases this up to 2.5–3.0 µg/ kg, because higher doses have been associated with abdominal discomfort and diarrhea in clinical cases. Treatment usually lasts for 4–5 weeks.

ANTIMICROBIAL AGENTS

Antimicrobial agents are used frequently in horses with gastrointestinal disorders but in most cases their use is empirical. For some infectious disorders of the alimentary tract, there are specific antimicrobial treatments, including:

- clostridiosis (*C. difficile, C. perfringens*): metronidazole 15 mg/kg p.o. three times a day;

- equine ehrlichial colitis (*E. risticii*): oxytetra-cycline 11 mg/kg i.v., twice daily;
- pylogranulomatous enteritis (*R. equi*): erythromycin phosphate 35 mg/kg p.o. and rifampin 10 mg/kg p.o. both twice a day;
- proliferative enteropathy (*Lawsonia intracellularis*): erythromycin phosphate 35 mg/kg p.o. twice a day; and
- candidiasis (*Candida albicans*): fluconazole 8 mg/kg p.o. three times a day.

The gastrointestinal tract is a frequent site for adverse effects of antimicrobial drugs, primarily because of disruption of normal intestinal microbial populations and proliferation of enteropathogens. Diarrhea, often with accompanying signs of endotoxemia, is the usual clinical manifestation. Antimicrobial agents known to be, or implicated in being, associated with antimicrobial-induced diarrhea include penicillin, ceftiofur, lincomycin, tetracycline, erythromycin and the potentiated sulfonamides. Erythromycin can also promote diarrhea via its motilide activity.

REFERENCES

Adams S B, MacHarg M A 1985 Neostigmine methylsulfate delays gastric emptying of particulate markers in horses. American Journal of Veterinary Research 46:2498–2499

Adams S B, Lamar C H, Masty J 1984 Motility of the distal portion of the jejunum and pelvic flexure in ponies: effects of six drugs. American Journal of Veterinary Research 45:795–799

Andrews F, Jenkins C, Frazier D et al 1992 The effect of oral omeprazole on basal and pentagastrin-stimulated gastric secretion in young female horses. Equine Veterinary Journal Supplement 13:80–83

Andrews F M, Sifferman R L, Bernard W et al 1999 Efficacy of omeprazole paste in the treatment and prevention of gastric ulcers in horses. Equine Veterinary Journal Supplement 29:81–86

Argenzio R A, Stevens C E 1975 Cyclic changes in ionic composition of digesta in the equine intestinal tract. American Journal of Physiology 228:1224–1230

Barone J A 1999 Domperidone: a peripherally acting dopamine 2-receptor antagonist. Annals of Pharmacotherapy 33:429–440

Bellissant E, Duhamel J F, Guillot M et al 1997 The triangular test to assess the efficacy of metoclopramide in gastroesophageal reflux. Clinical Pharmacology and Therapeutics 61:377–384

Besancon M, Simon A, Sachs G et al 1997 Sites of reaction of the gastric H^+,K^+-ATPase with extracytoplasmic thiol reagents. Journal of Biological Chemistry 272:22438–22446

Botella A, Vabre F, Fioramonti J et al 1993 In vivo inhibitory effect of lanreotide (BIM 23014), a new somatostatin analog, on prostaglandin- and cholera toxin-stimulated intestinal fluid in the rat. Peptides 14:297–301

Brzozowski T, Konturek S J, Sliwowski Z et al 1997 Role of L-arginine, a substrate for NO-synthase, in gastroprotection and ulcer healing. Journal of Gastroenterology 32:442–452

Camilleri M 2001 Tegaserod. Alimentary Pharmacology and Therapeutics 15:277–289

Campbell-Thompson M L, Merritt A M 1987 Effect of ranitidine on gastric acid secretion in young male horses. American Journal of Veterinary Research 48:1511–1515

Campbell-Thompson M L, Merritt A M 1990 Basal and pentagastrin-stimulated gastric secretion in young horses. American Journal of Physiology 259:R1259–R1266

Cederberg C, Andersson T, Skanberg I 1989 Omeprazole: pharmacokinetics and metabolism in man. Scandinavian Journal of Gastroenterology Supplement 166:33–42

Clark C K, Merritt A M, Burrow J A et al 1996 Effect of an aluminum–magnesium hydroxide antacid and BSS on gastric pH in horses. Journal of the American Veterinary Medical Association 208:1687–1691

Clarke L L, Argenzio R A, Roberts M C 1990 Effect of meal feeding on plasma volume and urinary electrolyte clearance in ponies. American Journal of Veterinary Research 51:571–576

Collins L G, Tyler D E 1985 Experimentally induced phenylbutazone toxicosis in ponies: description of the syndrome and its prevention with synthetic prostaglandin E_2. American Journal of Veterinary Research 46:1605–1615

Cook G, Papich M G, Roberts M C et al 1997 Pharmacokinetics of cisapride in horses after intravenous and rectal administration. American Journal of Veterinary Research 58:1427–1430

Dabareiner R M, Snyder J R, White N A et al 1995 Microvascular permeability and endothelial cell morphology associated with low-flow ischemia/reperfusion injury in the equine jejunum. American Journal of Veterinary Research 56: 639–648

Dajani E Z, Agrawal N M 1989 Protective effects of prostaglandins against nonsteroidal anti-inflammatory drug-induced gastrointestinal mucosal injury. International Journal of Clinical Pharmacology Research 9:359–369

Dart A J, Peauroi J R, Hodgson D R et al 1996 Efficacy of metoclopramide for treatment of ileus in horses following small intestinal surgery: 70 cases (1989–1992). Australian Veterinary Journal 74:280–284

Daurio C P, Holste J E, Andrews F M et al 1999 Effect of omeprazole paste on gastric acid secretion in horses. Equine Veterinary Journal Supplement 29:59–62

de Boer R E, Brouwer F, Zaagsma J 1993 The beta adrenoceptors mediating relaxation of rat oesophageal muscularis mucosae are predominantly of the beta 3- but also of the beta 2-subtype. British Journal of Pharmacology 110:442–446

Degen L, Matzinger D, Merz M et al 2001 Tegaserod, a 5-HT_4 receptor partial agonist, accelerates gastric emptying and gastrointestinal transit in healthy male subjects. Alimentary Pharmacology and Therapeutics 15:1745–1751

De Luca A, Coupar I M 1996 Insights into opioid action in the intestinal tract. Pharmacology and Therapeutics 69:103–115

De Ponti F, Giaroni C, Cosentino M et al 1996 Adrenergic mechanisms in the control of gastrointestinal motility: from basic science to clinical applications. Pharmacology and Therapeutics 69:59–78

Der-Silaphet T, Malysz J, Hagel S et al 1998 Interstitial cells of Cajal direct normal propulsive contractile activity in the mouse small intestine. Gastroenterology 114:724–736

Dobbins J, Racusen L, Binder H J 1980 Effect of D-alanine methionine enkephalin amide on ion transport in rabbit ileum. Journal of Clinical Investigation 66:19–28

Doherty T J, Andrews F M, Abraha T W et al 1999 Metoclopramide ameliorates the effects of endotoxin on gastric emptying of acetaminophen in horses. Canadian Journal of Veterinary Research 63:37–40

Duran S H, Ravis W R 1993 Comparative pharmacokinetics of H_2 antagonists in horses. In: Proceedings of the 11th American College of Veterinary Internal Medicine Forum, Washington, DC, pp. 687–690

Duval-Iflah Y, Berard H, Baumer P et al 1999 Effects of racecadotril and loperamide on bacterial proliferation and on the central nervous system of the newborn gnotobiotic piglet. Alimentary Pharmacology and Therapeutics 13 (suppl 6):9–14

Dwinell M B, Eckmann L, Leopard J D et al 1999 Chemokine receptor expression by human intestinal epithelial cells. Gastroenterology 117:359–367

Eades S C, Moore J N 1993 Blockade of endotoxin-induced cecal hypoperfusion and ileus with an alpha 2 antagonist in horses. American Journal of Veterinary Research 54:586–590

Eberhart C E, Dubois R N 1995 Eicosanoids and the gastrointestinal tract. Gastroenterology 109:285–301

Ennes H S, Young S H, Raybould H E et al 1997 Intercellular communication between dorsal root ganglion cells and colonic smooth muscle cells in vitro. Neuroreport 8:733–737

Ericsson C D, Feldman S, Pickering L K et al 1982 Influence of subsalicylate bismuth on absorption of doxycycline. Journal of the American Medical Association 247:2266–2267

Ericsson C D, Tannenbaum C, Charles T T 1990 Antisecretory and antiinflammatory properties of bismuth subsalicylate. Reviews of Infectious Diseases 12 (suppl 1):S16–S20

Figueroa-Quintanilla D, Salazar-Lindo E, Sack R B et al 1993 A controlled trial of bismuth subsalicylate in infants with acute watery diarrheal disease. New England Journal of Medicine 328:1653–1658

Fine K D, Lee E L 1998 Efficacy of open-label bismuth subsalicylate for the treatment of microscopic colitis. Gastroenterology 114:29–36

Freeman D E, Ferrante P L, Palmer J E 1992 Comparison of the effects of intragastric infusions of equal volumes of water, dioctyl sodium sulfosuccinate and magnesium sulfate on fecal composition and output in clinically normal horses. American Journal of Veterinary Research 53:1347–1353

Furr M O, Murray M J 1989 Treatment of gastric ulcers in horses with histamine type 2 receptor antagonists. Equine Veterinary Journal Supplement 7:77–79

Gemmell C G 1984 Comparative study of the nature and biological activities of bacterial enterotoxins. Journal of Medical Microbiology 17:217–235

Gerloff J, Mignot A, Barth H et al 1996 Pharmacokinetics and absolute bioavailability of lansoprazole. European Journal of Clinical Pharmacology 50:293–297

Gerring E L, Hunt J M 1986 Pathophysiology of equine postoperative ileus: effect of adrenergic blockade, parasympathetic stimulation and metoclopramide in an experimental model. Equine Veterinary Journal 18:249–255

Gerring E L, King J N 1989 Cisapride in the prophylaxis of equine post operative ileus. Equine Veterinary Journal Supplement 7:52–55

Giaroni C, De Ponti F, Cosentino M et al 1999 Plasticity in the enteric nervous system. Gastroenterology 117:1438–1458

Grande L, Lacima G, Ros E et al 1992 Lack of effect of metoclopramide and domperidone on esophageal peristalsis and esophageal acid clearance in reflux esophagitis. A randomized, double-blind study. Digestive Diseases and Sciences 37:583–588

Hammock P D, Freeman D E, Baker G J 1998 Failure of psyllium mucilloid to hasten evaluation of sand from the equine large intestine. Veterinary Surgery 27:547–554

Hance S R, Noble J, Holcomb S et al 1997 Treating choke with oxytocin. In: Proceedings of the 43rd American Association of Equine Practitioners Annual Convention, Phoenix, AZ, pp. 338–339

Haven M L, Dave K, Burrow J A et al 1999 Comparison of the antisecretory effects of omeprazole when administered intravenously, as acid-stable granules and as an oral paste in horses. Equine Veterinary Journal Supplement 29:54–58

Hawkey C J, Karrasch J A, Szczepanski L et al 1998 Omeprazole compared with misoprostol for ulcers associated with nonsteroidal antiinflammatory drugs. Omeprazole versus Misoprostol for NSAID-induced Ulcer Management (OMNIUM) Study Group. New England Journal of Medicine 338:727–734

Henninger R W, Horst J 1997 Magnesium toxicosis in two horses. Journal of the American Veterinary Medical Association 211:82–85

Hojgaard L, Mertz Nielsen A, Rune S J 1996 Peptic ulcer pathophysiology: acid, bicarbonate and mucosal function. Scandinavian Journal of Gastroenterology Supplement 216:10–15

Holland R E, Sriranganathan N, DuPont L 1989 Isolation of enterotoxigenic Escherichia coli from a foal with diarrhea. Journal of the American Veterinary Medical Association 194:389–391

Holzer P 1998 Neural emergency system in the stomach. Gastroenterology 114:823–839

Huber R, Hartmann M, Bliesath H et al 1996 Pharmacokinetics of pantoprazole in man. International Journal of Clinical Pharmacology and Therapeutics 34(suppl 1):S7–S16

Izzo A A, Mascolo N, Capasso F 1998 NO as a modulator of intestinal water and electrolyte transport. Digestive Diseases and Sciences 43:1605–1620

Jenkins C, Frazier D, Blackford J et al 1992a Duration of anti-secretory effects of omeprazole in horses with chronic gastric cannulae. Equine Veterinary Journal Supplement 13:89–92

Jenkins C C, Frazier D L, Blackford J T et al 1992b Pharmacokinetics and anti-secretory effects of intravenous omeprazole in horses. Equine Veterinary Journal Supplement 13:84–88

Johnson C M, Cullen J M, Roberts M C 1993 Morphologic characterization of castor oil-induced colitis in ponies. Veterinary Pathology 30:248–255

Kalff J C, Schraut W H, Simmons R L et al 1998 Surgical manipulation of the gut elicits an intestinal muscularis inflammatory response resulting in postsurgical ileus. Annals of Surgery 228:652–663

Kalff J C, Carlos T M, Schraut W H et al 1999 Surgically induced leukocytic infiltrates within the rat intestinal muscularis mediate postoperative ileus. Gastroenterology 117:378–387

Kalff J C, Schraut W H, Billiar T R et al 2000 Role of inducible NO synthase in postoperative intestinal smooth muscle dysfunction in rodents. Gastroenterology 118:316–327

Kamerling S G, Hamra J G, Bagwell C A 1990 Naloxone-induced abdominal distress in the horse. Equine Veterinary Journal 22:241–243

Katschinski M, Steinicke C, Reinshagen M et al 1995 Gastrointestinal motor and secretory responses to cholinergic stimulation in humans. Differential modulation by muscarinic and cholecystokinin receptor blockade. European Journal of Clinical Investigation 25:113–122

Katz J 1991 Acid secretion and suppression. Medical Clinics of North America 75:877–887

King J N, Gerring E L 1988 Actions of the novel gastrointestinal prokinetic agent cisapride on equine bowel motility. Journal of Veterinary Pharmacology and Therapeutics 11:314–321

King J N, Davies J V, Gerring E L 1990 Contrast radiography of the equine oesophagus: effect of spasmolytic agents and passage of a nasogastric tube. Equine Veterinary Journal 22:133–135

Kitchen D L, Merritt A M, Burrow J A 1998a Histamine-induced gastric acid secretion in horses. American Journal of Veterinary Research 59:1303–1306

Kitchen D L, Merritt A M, Burrow J A et al 1998b Source of non-parietal component of pentagastrin-stimulated fasting equine gastric contents. In: Proceedings of the 6th Equine Colic Research Symposium, Athens, GA, p. 35

Konturek S J, Brzozowski T, Majka J et al 1992 NO in gastroprotection by aluminum-containing antacids. European Journal of Pharmacology 229:155–162

Krejs G J 1986 Physiological role of somatostatin in the digestive tract: gastric acid secretion, intestinal absorption and motility. Scandinavian Journal of Gastroenterology Supplement 119:47–53

Lester G D, Merritt A M, Neuwirth L et al 1998a Effect of alpha 2 adrenergic, cholinergic and nonsteroidal anti-inflammatory drugs on myoelectric activity of ileum, cecum and right ventral colon and on cecal emptying of radiolabeled markers in clinically normal ponies. American Journal of Veterinary Research 59:320–327

Lester G D, Merritt A M, Neuwirth L et al 1998b Effect of erythromycin lactobionate on myoelectric activity of ileum, cecum and right ventral colon and cecal emptying of radiolabeled markers in clinically normal ponies. American Journal of Veterinary Research 59:328–334

Lippold B S, Weiss R, Mevissen M et al 2002 The properties of a new promotile drug, tegaserod (HTF 919) in equines. In: Proceedings of the 7th International Equine Colic Research Symposium, Birmingham, UK, p. 46

Longo W E, Vernava A M D 1993 Prokinetic agents for lower gastrointestinal motility disorders. Diseases of the Colon and Rectum 36:696–708

Lowe J E, Sellers A F, Brondum J 1980 Equine pelvic flexure impaction. A model used to evaluate motor events and compare drug response. Cornell Veterinarian 70:401–412

Lyrenas E 1985 Beta adrenergic influence on esophageal and colonic motility in man. Scandinavian Journal of Gastroenterology Supplement 116:1–48

MacAllister C G, Lowrey F, Stebbins M et al 1994 Transendoscopic electrocautery-induced gastric ulcers as a model for gastric healing studies in ponies. Equine Veterinary Journal 26:100–103

MacAllister C G, Sangiah S 1993 Effect of ranitidine on healing of experimentally induced gastric ulcers in ponies. American Journal of Veterinary Research 54:1103–1107

MacDonald T M 1991 Metoclopramide, domperidone and dopamine in man: actions and interactions. European Journal of Clinical Pharmacology 40:225–230

Madigan J E 1997 Disorders of the first two weeks of Age. In: Madigan J E (ed.) Manual of equine neonatal medicine, 3rd edn. Live Oak Publishing, Woodland, CA, p. 119

Malone E D, Brown D R, Trent A M et al 1996 Influence of adrenergic and cholinergic mediators on the equine jejunum in vitro. American Journal of Veterinary Research 57:884–890

Malone E D, Turner T A, Wilson J H 1998 Intravenous lidocaine for the treatment of equine ileus. In: Proceedings of the 6th Equine Colic Research Symposium, Athens, GA, p. 42

Matheson A J, Noble S 2000 Racecadotril. Drugs 59:829–837

Mathews C J, MacLeod R J, Zheng S X et al 1999 Characterization of the inhibitory effect of boiled rice on intestinal chloride secretion in guinea pig crypt cells. Gastroenterology 116:1342–1347

McCallum R W 1999 Pharmacologic modulation of motility. Yale Journal of Biology and Medicine 72:173–180

McCarthy D M 1991 Sucralfate. New England Journal of Medicine 325:1017–1025

Merritt A M 1999 Normal equine gastroduodenal secretion and motility. Equine Veterinary Journal Supplement 29:7–13

Merritt A M, Burrow J A, Horbal M J et al 1996 Effect of omeprazole on sodium and potassium output in pentagastrin-stimulated equine gastric contents. American Journal of Veterinary Research 57:1640–1644

Merritt A M, Burrow J A, Hartless C S 1998 Effect of xylazine, detomidine and a combination of xylazine and butorphanol on equine duodenal motility. American Journal of Veterinary Research 59:619–623

Merritt A M, Campbell-Thompson M L, Lowrey S 1989 Effect of xylazine treatment on equine proximal gastrointestinal tract myoelectrical activity. American Journal of Veterinary Research 50:945–949

Merritt A M, Sanchez L S, Burrow J A et al 2002 Bioavailability of "Gastrogard™" vs. three generic compounded omeprazole preparations in mature horses. In: Proceedings of the 7th International Equine Colic Research Symposium, Birmingham, UK, p. 81

Meyer G A, Rashmir-Raven A, Helms R J et al 2000 The effect of oxytocin on contractility of the equine oesophagus: a potential treatment for oesophageal obstruction. Equine Veterinary Journal 32:151–155

Mullersman G, Gotz V P, Russell W L, Derendorf H 1986 Lack of clinically significant in vitro and in vivo interactions between ranitidine and sucralfate. Journal of Pharmaceutical Sciences 75:995–998

Murray M J, Eichorn E S 1996 Effects of intermittent feed deprivation, intermittent feed deprivation with ranitidine administration and stall confinement with ad libitum access to hay on gastric ulceration in horses. American Journal of Veterinary Research 57:1599–1603

Murray M J, Grodinsky C 1992 The effects of famotidine, ranitidine and magnesium hydroxide/aluminum hydroxide on gastric fluid pH in adult horses. Equine Veterinary Journal Supplement 11:52–55

Murray M J, Nout Y S, Ward D L 2001 Endoscopic findings of the gastric antrum and pylorus in horses: 162 cases (1996–2000). Journal of Veterinary Internal Medicine 14:401–406

Murray M J, Schusser G F 1993 Measurement of 24-h gastric pH using an indwelling pH electrode in horses unfed, fed and treated with ranitidine. Equine Veterinary Journal 25:417–421

Ness T J 1999 Kappa opioid receptor agonists differentially inhibit two classes of rat spinal neurons excited by colorectal distention. Gastroenterology 117:388–394

Nguyen A, Camilleri M, Kost L J et al 1997 SDZ HTF 919 stimulates canine colonic motility and transit in vivo. Journal of Pharmacology and Experimental Therapeutics 280:1270–1276

Nieto J E, Spier S J, van Hoogmoed L et al 2001 Comparison of omeprazole and cimetidine in healing of gastric ulcers and prevention of recurrence in horses. Equine Veterinary Education 13:260–264

Nwokolo C U, Mistry P, Pounder R E 1990 The absorption of bismuth and salicylate from oral doses of Pepto-Bismol (bismuth salicylate). Alimentary Pharmacology and Therapeutics 4:163–169

Rabon E C, Reuben M A 1990 The mechanism and structure of the gastric H^+,K^+-ATPase. Annual Review of Physiology 52:321–344

Redmond L M, Cross D L, Strickland J R et al 1994 Efficacy of domperidone and sulpiride as treatments for fescue toxicosis in horses. American Journal of Veterinary Research 55:722–729

Rhoads W S, Barton M H, Parks A H 1999 Comparison of medical and surgical treatment for impaction of the small colon in horses: 84 cases (1986–1996). Journal of the American Veterinary Medical Association 214:1042–1047

Richards W G, Sugarbaker D J 1995 Neuronal control of esophageal function. Chest Surgery Clinics of North America 5:157–171

Rimback G, Cassuto J, Tollesson P O 1990 Treatment of postoperative paralytic ileus by intravenous lidocaine infusion. Anesthesia and Analgesia 70:414–419

Ringger N C, Lester G D, Neuwirth L et al 1996 Effect of bethanechol or erythromycin on gastric emptying in horses. American Journal of Veterinary Research 57:1771–1775

Roberts M C, Clarke L L, Johnson C M 1989 Castor-oil induced diarrhoea in ponies: a model for acute colitis. Equine Veterinary Journal Supplement 7:60–67

Roelvink M E, Goossens L, Kalsbeek H C et al 1991 Analgesic and spasmolytic effects of dipyrone, hyoscine-N-butylbromide and a combination of the two in ponies. Veterinary Record 129:378–380

Roger T, Bardon T, Ruckebusch Y 1985 Colonic motor responses in the pony: relevance of colonic stimulation by opiate antagonists. American Journal of Veterinary Research 46:31–35

Roger T, Ruckebusch Y 1987 Pharmacological modulation of postprandial colonic motor activity in the pony. Journal of Veterinary Pharmacology and Therapeutics 10:273–282

Roth S H 1990 Misoprostol in the prevention of NSAID-induced gastric ulcer: a multicenter, double-blind, placebo-controlled trial. Journal of Rheumatology Supplement 20:20–24

Ruppin H 1987 Loperamide: a potent antidiarrhoeal drug with actions along the alimentary tract. Alimentary Pharmacology and Therapeutics 1:179–190

Rutkowski J A, Eades S C, Moore J N 1991 Effects of xylazine butorphanol on cecal arterial blood flow, cecal mechanical activity and systemic hemodynamics in horses. American Journal of Veterinary Research 52:1153–1158

Sams R A, Gerken D F, Dyke T M et al 1997 Pharmacokinetics of intravenous and intragastric cimetidine in horses. I. Effects of intravenous cimetidine on pharmacokinetics of intravenous phenylbutazone. Journal of Veterinary Pharmacology and Therapeutics 20:355–361

Sanchez L C, Lester G D, Merritt A M 1998 Effect of ranitidine on intragastric pH in clinically normal neonatal foals. Journal of the American Veterinary Medical Association 212:1407–1412

Sandin A, Andrews F M, Nadeau J A et al 1999 Effects of intramuscular omeprazole on gastric acid secretion in horses over a twenty-four hour period. Equine Veterinary Journal Supplement 29:50–53

Sandin A, Andrews F M, Nadeau J A et al 2000 Effect of nervous excitation on acid secretion in horses. Acta Physiologica Scandinavica 168:437–442

Sangiah S, MacAllister C C, Amouzadeh H R 1988 Effects of cimetidine and ranitidine on basal gastric pH, free and total acid contents in horses. Research in Veterinary Science 45:291–295

Sangiah S, MacAllister C C, Amouzadeh H R 1989 Effects of misoprostol and omeprazole on basal gastric pH and free acid content in horses. Research in Veterinary Science 47:350–354

Scarff K L, Judd L M, Toh B H et al 1999 Gastric H(+), K(+)-adenosine triphosphatase beta subunit is required for normal function, development and membrane structure of mouse parietal cells. Gastroenterology 117:605–618

Schoenfeld P, Kimmey M B, Scheiman J et al 1999 Nonsteroidal anti-inflammatory drug-associated gastrointestinal complications: guidelines for prevention and treatment. Alimentary Pharmacology and Therapeutics 13:1273–1285

Schumacher J, DeGraves F J, Spano J S 1997 Clinical and clinicopathologic effects of large doses of raw linseed oil as compared to mineral oil in healthy horses. Journal of Veterinary Internal Medicine 11:296–299

Schusser G E, White N A 1997 Morphologic and quantitative evaluation of the myenteric plexuses and neurons in the large colon of horses. Journal of the American Veterinary Medical Association 210:928–934

Sellers A F, Lowe J E, Rendano V T et al 1982 The reservoir function of the equine cecum and ventral large colon: its relation to chronic non-surgical obstructive disease with colic. Cornell Veterinarian 72:233–241

Sjoqvist A, Hallerback B, Glise H 1985 Reflex adrenergic inhibition of colonic motility in anesthetized rat caused by nociceptive stimuli of peritoneum, Digestive Diseases and Sciences 30:749–754

Smyth G B, Duran S, Ravis W et al 1990 Pharmacokinetic studies of cimetidine hydrochloride in adult horses. Equine Veterinary Journal 22:48–50

Sojka J E, Adams S B, Lamar C H et al 1988 Effect of butorphanol, pentazocine, meperidine, or metoclopramide on intestinal motility in female ponies. American Journal of Veterinary Research 49:527–529

Sojka J E, Weiss J S, Samuels M L et al 1992 Effect of the somatostatin analog octreotide on gastric fluid pH in ponies. American Journal of Veterinary Research 53:1818–1821

Sondheimer J M, Arnold G L 1986 Early effects of bethanechol on the esophageal motor function of infants with gastroesophageal reflux. Journal of Pediatric Gastroenterology and Nutrition 5:47–51

Steel C M, Bolton J R, Preechagoon Y et al 1998 Pharmacokinetics of cisapride in the horse. Journal of Veterinary Pharmacology and Therapeutics 21:433–436

Steel C M, Bolton J R, Preechagoon Y et al 1999 Unreliable rectal absorption of cisapride in horses. Equine Veterinary Journal 31:82–84

Thillainayagam A V, Hunt J B, Farthing M J 1998 Enhancing clinical efficacy of oral rehydration therapy: is low osmolality the key? Gastroenterology 114:197–210

Thompson L P, Burrow J A, Madison J R et al 1994 Effect of bethanechol on equine gastric motility and secretion. In: Proceedings of the 5th Equine Colic Research Symposium, Athens, GA, p. 12

Tillman L A, Drake F M, Dixon J S et al 1996 Safety of bismuth in the treatment of gastrointestinal diseases. Alimentary Pharmacology and Therapeutics 10:459–467

Tonini M 1996 Recent advances in the pharmacology of gastrointestinal prokinetics. Pharmacological Research 33:217–226

Udassin R, Eimerl D, Schiffman J et al 1994 Epidural anesthesia accelerates the recovery of postischemic bowel motility in the rat. Anesthesiology 80:832–836

Valk N, Doherty T J, Blackford J T et al 1998 Effect of cisapride on gastric emptying in horses following endotoxin treatment. Equine Veterinary Journal 30:344–348

Vitola J V, Forman M B, Holsinger J P et al 1997 Reduction of myocardial infarct size in rabbits and inhibition of activation of rabbit and human neutrophils by lidocaine. American Heart Journal 133:315–322

Washabau R J, Hall J A 1995 Cisapride. Journal of the American Veterinary Medical Association 207:1285–1288

Watson T D, Sullivan M 1991 Effects of detomidine on equine oesophageal function as studied by contrast radiography. Veterinary Record 129:67–69

Zhao X T, Wang L, Lin H C 2000 Slowing of intestinal transit by fat depends on naloxone-blockable efferent, opioid pathway. American Journal of Physiology: Gastrointestinal and Liver Physiology 278:G866–G870

CHAPTER CONTENTS

Introduction 121

Anti-inflammatory drugs 121
    Corticosteroids 121
    Hyaluronan 125
    Dimethyl sulfoxide 126

Local anesthetics 127

Antimicrobial agents 128

Synovectomy with radiopharmaceuticals 130

References 131

7

Intraarticular medication

Tom Yarbrough

INTRODUCTION

Selection of intraarticular medication is a daily process for the equine practitioner. This chapter presents some of the literature that exists on the individual drugs described. Wherever possible, studies using horses have been selected to reduce the bias created by species variation and topics have not been included if there is no real consensus opinion; it is hoped that this will present what can be considered as the "industry" accepted opinions.

ANTI-INFLAMMATORY DRUGS

Many drugs that have an anti-inflammatory action may also have other mechanisms of action. Corticosteroids are one of the most commonly administered classes of intraarticular medication in equine medicine. Hyaluronan (sodium hyaluronate, HA) is a natural component of the joint and its intraarticular use has anti-inflammatory actions and may have lubricating effects. Similarly dimethyl sulfoxide is used for both its anti-inflammatory and its antimicrobial actions.

CORTICOSTEROIDS

Safe and effective use of corticosteroids requires at least a cursory understanding of their unique pharmacology and an understanding of the underlying disease process. Corticosteroids are a family of molecules each containing 21 carbon molecules distributed between one 3-carbon and three 6-carbon rings (Axelrod 1993). It should be recognized that all corticosteroids are not effective when used intraarticularly. Cortisone and prednisone would be ineffective since they must be converted in the liver from the inactive 11-keto form to the active 16-betahydroxyl form (Axelrod 1993). Within the corticosteroids, various modifications of the basic molecule are utilized to modify the duration of activity. The most highly water-soluble phosphate and succinate esters are considered the most rapid in onset and have the shortest duration. Duration is felt to be longer in the acetate and acetonide substituted forms, followed by the hexacetonide ester, which is felt to impart the longest duration of action. Structural modification of the ring structure is only one factor in determining the duration of action of particular corticosteroids. Carrier formulations and hydrolysis can each subsequently affect the absorption and activation of these drugs. Although many of the tests used to determine efficacy and duration of action do not take into account variations present in intraarticular use, it still useful for the clinician to have an understanding of the relative potency and duration of action of many of the more commonly used corticosteroid formulations (Table 7.1).

Corticosteroids affect cells through a well-studied series of interactions. All corticosteroid hormones basically act by diffusing through the cell membrane and interacting within the cytoplasm with a specific set of proteins in the corticosteroid receptor superfamily. This is a large class of receptors that contains highly related domains for ligand binding and resultant transcriptional activation. Once the corticosteroid has bound to the receptor, a conformational change in the receptor allows the construct to bind directly to DNA, subsequently modulating gene expression (Cooper 1997, Schimmer & Parker 1996).

The potential mechanisms by which corticosteroids might alter the homeostasis of the joint space proper are numerous. Corticosteroids may benefit any inflammatory condition by modulating the influx of inflammatory cells into the target region. This effect is at least in part a result of their ability to reduce capillary permeability, reduce leukocyte chemotaxis and adhesion and decrease vascular permeability. In addition to modulating the numbers of cells within the region of inflammation, corticosteroids also have the ability to modify the cellular responses as well. Neutrophil function can be ameliorated by reducing phagocytosis and decreasing lysosomal enzyme and prostaglandin release. The most "body wide" effect is created by membrane stabilization and reduced formation of phospholipase A_2, with the subsequent reduction in prostaglandin production in a wide variety of cells (Axelrod 1993, Boumpas et al 1993). Some of the more pertinent research information surrounding the use of corticosteroids in the joint is presented to aid in establishing an opinion as to the benefit and timing of corticosteroid use.

Methylprednisolone acetate

Methylprednisolone acetate (MPA) is a synthetic corticosteroid produced as the 6α-methyl derivative of prednisolone. Pharmacological studies of the esters of MPA show that it is rapidly converted to methylprednisolone, the active form. Reversible metabolism of methylprednis*olone* to methylprednis*one* creates the inactive metabolite. The conversion from the prodrug to the active form of the drug is partially responsible for variations identified in the classification of the duration of MPA activity. High levels of the active product, methylprednisolone, have been identified in synovial fluid within 2 h of MPA injection. Despite the persistence of MPA levels for 5–39 days after injection, the active metabolite was only identifiable for 2–6 days (Auteflage et al 1986).

The potential beneficial and detrimental effects of MPA on articular cartilage and chondrocytes

Table 7.1 Anti-inflammatory potency and duration of action of corticosteroids used commonly for intraarticular administration

Compound	Anti-inflammatory potential (cortisol = 1)	Duration of action (h)
Cortisone	0.8	8–12
6α-Methylprednisolone	5	12–36
Triamcinolone	5	12–36
Betamethasone	25	36–72
Dexamethasone	25	36–72

have been studied in many different systems. Cell culture systems offer an easy cost-effective means to assess some of the basic effects of corticosteroids on cartilage. The primary problem is that chondrocytes devoid of their normal matrix and sheltered from their constant biomechanical stimulation do not perfectly mimic the in vivo state. Maintenance of much of the extracellular matrix in cultured explants is a step towards reconstituting the influence of the intercellular nanostructure, but these systems also vary greatly from what is seen in vivo. Explant samples remain metabolically active and viable but gradually lose proteoglycans. This gradual loss of proteoglycans and a concomitant reduction in proteoglycan synthesis have been discovered after administration of MPA (Jolly et al 1995). It was shown that the aggrecan that is produced was reduced in size and demonstrated increased polydispersity. In the same study, the investigators discovered that MPA induced the synthesis of small non-aggregating proteoglycans. Both of these effects can result in a molecule with a reduced ability to interact with HA, thus reducing proteoglycan retention in the matrix (Todhunter et al 1996). Reduction in the ability of articular cartilage alone would be considered a reason for not using corticosteroids if this were the only factor. Some beneficial effects have been implied from studies demonstrating a MPA-induced reduction in matrix metalloproteinase (MMP) 13 production following stimulation with recombinant human interleukin 1 (IL-1) (Caron et al 1996). Studies assessing the effects on stromelysin, probably the most detrimental MMP, have been less promising (May et al 1988). The general impression with most of these systems is that the anticatabolic effects of MPA on the proteoglycan content of the explants far outweigh any antianabolic or cytotoxic drug effect at clinically important doses (Jolly et al 1995).

Isolated systems are good for answering basic scientific questions but are often difficult to extrapolate to clinical settings, especially when assessing the response of cartilage to the effects of corticosteroids without the influences of the synovium. In vivo modeling allows the study of more clinically relevant situations and reduces the phenotypic changes present with cell culture systems.

With these systems, we have the ability to assess the presence of a time-averaged stable matrix, the sine qua non of healthy articular cartilage. Some of the conflicting realities of the complete biological system were demonstrated in an osteochondral fragment-induced model of middle carpal arthritis/synovitis. The use of MPA, versus a polyionic fluid control, resulted in reduced prostaglandin E_2 concentration in the synovial fluid, improved microscopic scores for intimal hyperplasia and improved vascularity in synovial membrane. However, the occurrence of increased articular cartilage erosion and morphological lesions suggested that the combination of work and corticosteroids was detrimental in active synovitis (Frisbie et al 1998). It should also be noted that the model here required that the animals be exercised with the osteochondral fragment still present in the joint space, a condition most of us would avoid whenever possible. Suggestions have been made that the concomitant administration of HA might be able to ameliorate some of the detrimental effects of corticosteroids on proteoglycan formation and release (Tulamo 1991). A single intraarticular injection of MPA (50 mg) has been shown to decrease type II procollagen and aggrecan mRNA (MacLeod et al 1998). Further evidence of the suppressive effects was seen in ponies, where it was shown that MPA-treated joints had significantly lower glycosaminoglycan content in the articular cartilage than control ponies. This response was not ameliorated by the systemic administration of polysulfated glycosaminoglycans (PSGAGs) (Fubini et al 1993). In an instability model in dogs, created by transection of the anterior cruciate, some overall beneficial effects were seen. MPA was shown to reduce the size of osteophytes, the severity of histological cartilage lesions and the production of the MMP stromelysins (Pelletier et al 1994). The ability to reduce inflammatory mediators and cartilage degeneration is of paramount importance in arthritic conditions. Since most of our patients are not suffering from an instability-induced arthritis and we generally have an articular component to the disease, the ability to eliminate the inflammatory mediators in conditions of traumatic synovitis/arthritis must be weighed up against the effects on the healing of cartilage defects. The use of MPA in the immediate post-operative period has been brought into question by evidence suggesting that it reduces the quantity and quality of healing tissue in experimentally induced cartilage defects (Carter et al 1996).

Other suggested benefits of MPA treatment include improving joint health by increasing lubrication in the joint. Injection of 100 mg into normal carpi has been shown to increase the levels of surface-active phospholipid in the joint, resulting in improved cartilage hydration, promotion of macrophage activity and the ability to scavenge oxygen free radicals (Hills et al 1998).

Triamcinolone

Many of the studies designed to assess corticosteroids ability to affect the anabolic and catabolic effects of inflammatory mediators have been carried out with triamcinolone. In explant cultures, recombinant IL-1α has been shown to increase degradation and reduce the synthesis of proteoglycans, as did triamcinolone. The combination of human recombinant insulin-like growth factor 1 (IGF-1) and corticosteroids was able to normalize collagen production and proteoglycan catabolism and anabolism in this system (Frisbie & Nixon 1997). In a murine model using normal cartilage, IGF-1 resulted in significant enhancement of chondrocyte proteoglycan synthesis. In arthritic cartilage, IGF-1 failed to stimulate proteoglycan synthesis and only proteoglycans with relatively small dimensions were produced in the presence of the corticosteroid triamcinolone acetonide (Verschure et al 1994). Interestingly, in murine patellar cartilage, triamcinolone in combination with IGF-1 was able to stimulate proteoglycan synthesis and maintain the synthesis of hydrodynamically large proteoglycans by chondrocytes (van der Kraan et al 1993). The ability of triamcinolone to protect cartilage against the effects of IL-1-induced catabolism has been shown to vary with the inciting cause in bovine cartilage explants. When the degradation was induced by IL-1α alone, triamcinolone showed no protective effects; however, when the degradation was induced by

IL-1α in the presence of concomitant human plasminogen, glucocorticosteroids statistically significantly inhibited catabolism. The authors felt that the inhibition of cartilage degradation by the glucocorticosteroids might occur through down-regulation of urokinase plasminogen activator (u-PA) activity (Augustine & Oleksyszyn 1997).

Unlike the results described for MPA, triamcinolone acetonide used in another model of exercising horses with carpal osteochondral fragment-induced arthritis resulted in significantly less lameness, lower total protein, higher HA and glycosaminoglycan concentrations in synovial fluid, less inflammatory cell infiltration, subintimal hyperplasia and subintimal fibrosis in the synovial layer, and improved articular cartilage histomorphological parameters (Frisbie et al 1997). Similar results were found in dogs with transection of the anterior cruciate. Triamcinolone significantly reduced the size of osteophytes and the histologic severity of cartilage lesions on the condyles. Microscopic evidence of improved cartilage health included a reduced percentage of immunoreactive chondrocytes for stromelysin, c-Fos and c-Myc (Pelletier et al 1995).

Betamethasone

High doses of intraarticular betamethasone in rabbits have been associated with cellular degeneration (Papachristou et al 1997). In a study using more clinically relevant doses, the chondroprotective effect of betamethasone was examined to determine if it could decrease articular cartilage injury caused by *Staphylococcus aureus* gonioarthritis. Rabbits that received antimicrobial treatment plus parenteral betamethasone demonstrated significantly less articular cartilage proteoglycan loss than rabbits treated with antimicrobial agents alone. Intraarticular betamethasone was somewhat less effective in this regard, possibly reflecting the smaller corticosteroid dosage (Stricker et al 1996).

Any time a needle is placed into the joint, a possibility exists for infection. The most commonly isolated organism following injection is *Staph. aureus* (Schneider et al 1992). There is evidence to suggest that the use of intraarticular corticosteroids reduces the numbers of bacteria required to induce infection (Gustafson et al 1989). A subsequent study suggested that these effects could be blocked by the addition of an aminoglycoside antibiotic to the medication. However, clinical experience would indicate that good patient preparation and situation control provide enough protection against this complication. Depending on the organism involved, the corticosteroid injected and the underlying process being treated, signs of infection may not be evident for some time in corticosteroid-treated animals. Just to be safe, owners should be instructed to watch for any signs of heat, swelling or increased lameness for at least 2 weeks after the injection.

The literature on intraarticular corticosteroids might seem to hold no middle ground for the clinician, but careful assessment helps to identify a logical path for treatment. Ideally, corticosteroids should only be used in low-motion joints, in horses that have had the inciting lesion corrected surgically or in animals that can be rested during the period that the corticosteroids could have reduced the proteoglycan content. It is generally considered ineffective simply to medicate away intraarticular fragmentation. With the accessibility and reliability of arthroscopy, it is generally considered a second option to continue pushing any athlete along by palliating the effusion associated with articular fragments. In these cases, where the owners opt not to remove the offending lesion and simply remove as much of the inflammatory process as possible, the use of HA in conjunction with the corticosteroids might be useful in reducing the rate of deterioration. This is especially important in high-motion joints. Likewise, it is logical to reach for other methods of reducing inflammation, such as non-steroidal anti-inflammatory drugs (NSAIDs, see Ch. 14), intra muscular (i.m.) PSGAG, capsaicin and physical therapy methods rather than using frequent injections. It can be seen that some degree of reduced formation and aggregation of proteoglycans is to be expected with administration of corticosteroids. Whenever possible, this response can be minimized by resting the animal after injection to allow for return of normal levels of aggrecan in the matrix. When rest is again limited by

owner compliance, then the clinician should select a corticosteroid that has as short a duration of action as possible and that produces minimal effects on the cartilage.

HYALURONAN

HA is the most widely used intraarticular medication in horses. The selection of this medication and the route by which it is administered is often decided upon without consideration of the underlying disease process or what is being asked of the drug itself. Naturally occurring HA is a relatively ubiquitous molecule in mammals. It is produced naturally by a membrane-bound enzyme HA synthase. It is often quoted that the HA present in synovial fluid is from the fibroblastic synoviocytes. Recently, it has been demonstrated that there are at least three isoforms of HA synthase and that the enzymes are expressed in cell culture by synovial cells, chondrocytes and osteosarcoma cell lines (Recklies et al 2001). HA itself is a relatively simple molecule of repeating disaccharide units that performs some fairly amazing effects once extruded into the extracellular matrix. It has the ability to confer extraordinary compressive strength to the articular cartilage when functioning as the core molecule for proteoglycan aggregates (Ratcliffe & Mow 1996). It likewise imparts the viscoelastic nature to the synovial fluid (de Smedt et al 1993, Ribitsch et al 1999). With regard to whatever role HA plays in lubrication of the joint surfaces, there is some question as to whether the molecular weight of the molecule has an effect on its action (Kato et al 1995, Mabuchi et al 1999).

While the actions of naturally occurring HA are fairly well characterized, the beneficial effects of the exogenous products are very elusive. In a clinical setting, we often see prolonged benefit in the form of reduced effusion and reduced severity of lameness for prolonged periods. This is very unusual for a product that has a half-life in the synovial space in the order of hours. In an acute inflammatory process, it is thought that at least one possible beneficial mechanism is the return of the steric barrier provided by HA. In support of this idea, HA has been shown to have a protective effect against the invasion of polymorphonuclear cells (Partsch et al 1989). Similar effects have been seen with respect to lymphocyte proliferation and migration. In both cell types, it was felt that the higher molecular weight forms were required to appreciate any benefit (Peluso et al 1990). The actual mechanisms of this effect are yet to be elucidated but it is likely that it is related to cellular interactions with the CD44 molecule (Takeshita et al 1997). Other possible anti-inflammatory benefits have been difficult to identify. The purported induction of endogenous HA and reduction in MMPs have been refuted by some studies (Clegg et al 1998, Lynch et al 1998). It does seem, however, that the intraarticular use of both HA and PSGAG reduces inflammation by modulating the production of prostaglandin E (Frean & Lees 2000).

Extensive research has been undertaken to determine the possible anabolic and anticatabolic benefits of HA on articular cartilage. As mentioned in the section on corticosteroid use, each study must be weighed in the context of how closely it mimics clinical situations. HA has been shown to have a protective effect on cartilage degeneration in a cast confinement model. Repeated injections over a 92 day period were shown to stabilize the catabolic processes associated with atrophy of articular cartilage. It was felt in this situation that downregulation of tumor necrosis factor (TNF) α produced the chondrostabilizing influence on articular cartilage (Comer et al 1996). HA has been shown to stimulated prostaglandin synthesis in both cell and explant cultures (Frean et al 1999). Mixed results have been obtained when using explant cultures for examination of the protective effects of HA. In one study, its use was shown to be beneficial in reducing prostaglandin release induced by human recombinant IL-1β in metacarpal hyaline cartilage, while it had no effect or appeared to increase prostaglandin release in fibrocartilage and navicular hyaline cartilage (Frean et al 2000).

When choosing HA as a therapeutic agent, it is best to have at least some underlying sense of the condition in question. Ideally it is best suited to acute inflammatory conditions where its ability to reduce the influx of white blood cells into the joint proper could modify the disease process by decreasing all of the subsequent steps in the inflammatory cascade. This means that a defined condition of pure synovitis would be the most ideal situation. In a clinical setting, this is rarely the case, since most of the conditions we treat in the equine athlete involve some degree of underlying degenerative joint disease. In these conditions, we might still be able to reduce the rate of degeneration without contributing to the catabolic process already underway in the articular cartilage. It should be noted that HA has little ability to eliminate severe forms of lameness and might even have deleterious effects when put into a joint where inflammation is so overwhelming that the HA is rapidly broken down to its low-molecular-weight fragments (Peloso et al 1993). When using the medication as a protective in conjunction with corticosteroids, it may be possible to select one of the lower cost low-molecular-weight forms. Most clinicians will opt to use the highest-molecular-weight form available when using it as a stand-alone therapy, although this practice has recently again been brought into question (Aviad & Houpt 1994).

DIMETHYL SULFOXIDE

Dimethyl sulfoxide (DMSO) is a clear viscous liquid originally formulated as a solvent. It has gained some medical use as an anti-inflammatory and antimicrobial agent. Its anti-inflammatory properties have been primarily attributed to its ability to scavenge free radicals (Fox & Fox 1983). The potential detrimental effects of DMSO have been studied in both cell culture and *in vivo* systems (Moses et al 2001). DMSO has been shown to have a deleterious effect on the health of synovial membrane cultures; however there were no changes observed in chondrocyte viability after explant incubation with DMSO. The mild effect on proteoglycan metabolism seen in another study was found to be only transient (Smith et al 2000). In horses, injections of 2 ml of a 40% solution of DMSO in lactated Ringer's solution for a total of three injections caused no evidence of cartilage degradation and no alterations in glycosaminoglycan content (Welch et al 1989). Recently, the use of various concentrations of DMSO in balanced polyionic fluids has been advocated for reducing the inflammatory process in the joint (Schneider et al 1992). It has been used in concentrations from 5 to 40% in both traumatic and septic arthritis. Clinically, the use of DMSO in lavage fluids appears to result in reduced edema formation, increased range of motion and better maintenance of arthrotomy portals in conditions of septic arthritis.

LOCAL ANESTHETICS

Intraarticular analgesia is commonly used in the diagnosis of lameness, to enable other invasive procedures involving the joint and as a means of postoperative pain relief. Most commonly used local anesthetics are weak base amide solutions. A cursory understanding of the mechanisms of action of these agents is useful when assessing their effects. The onset and duration of action expected from each drug is a product of their molecular weight, pH, lipid solubility and protein binding. Diffusion across the cell membrane is important in determining the onset of action, since diffusion is inversely related to the square root of the molecular weight of the molecule. As shown in Table 7.2, the molecular weight of the commonly used drugs is so similar as to have a minimal effect within the group. In the body, where the amide local anesthetics exist both in an ionized and a nonionized form, the distribution is a reflection of the pH of the surrounding tissue. As the tissue pH falls, more of the drug is in its ionized form and, since the nonionized portion is the form that has the ability to diffuse through the cell membrane to cause blockade of the sodium channels, efficacy is reduced. If a significant enough

Table 7.2 Features of some commonly used local anesthetics

Agent	Molecular weight	pK_a	Protein binding (%)
Lidocaine (lignocaine)	236	7.9	64
Mepivacaine	246	7.6	77
Bupivacaine	288	8.1	96

fall in pH occurs, as in sepsis, the effect may be completely blocked. It is possible to counter this to some degree by adding sodium bicarbonate to the locale prior to local anesthetic administration. More highly bound anesthetics are less available for diffusion through the cell membrane. The net effect is a prolonged duration of action and a more prolonged onset of action.

It has been shown that injection of lidocaine (lignocaine) or mepivacaine hydrochloride into the equine middle carpal joint increases synovial fluid cellularity. Repeated arthrocentesis by itself caused a moderate increase in cell counts, while injection of local anesthetics caused a greater increase. Alterations in mucin clot quality, HA content, fluid viscosity, total protein and immunoglobulin G were generally of no significance (Kirkham et al 1999). In this study, clear differences between responses to the drugs could not be identified (White et al 1989). An older study determined that mepivacaine was less reactive than lidocaine when assessing synovial fluid parameters (Specht et al 1988). The use of local anesthetics during arthroscopy is a common procedure in veterinary and human orthopedics, although evidence that this is of benefit over NSAIDs is lacking (Sorensen et al 1991).

Morphine

During the 1990s, preclinical investigations in models showed that local injection of small doses of opioid analgesics at sites of inflammation produce potent analgesia (Stein et al 1996). Interestingly, these same low doses given systemically or into the uninflamed site are without effect (Sibinga & Goldstein 1988). Intraarticular opioids have antinociceptive and anti-inflammatory actions in animals (Barber et al 1990, Kolesnikov et al 1996). In humans, intraarticular morphine produces potent inhibition of acute postoperative pain after knee surgery (Kalso et al 1997, Stein & Yassouridis 1997). Both the analgesic and the anti-inflammatory effects are apparently mediated by peripheral opioid receptors, which have been identified on peripheral sensory nerve terminals (Stein et al 1996). Synthesized in the dorsal root ganglia, these receptors are axonally transported towards the nerve terminals, where they can be activated by exogenous agonists as well as by endogenous opioid peptides expressed in inflammatory cells (Khoury et al 1994). Local opioid analgesic effects are more pronounced in inflamed than in non-inflamed tissue. This may be related to an upregulation of peripheral opioid receptors, to their enhanced coupling with G proteins or disruption of the perineural barrier, leading to an improved access for opioid agonists (Shah et al 1997). Analgesia provided by the binding to the opioid receptors is further enhanced by the morphine-induced reduction in substance P release from the nociceptive nerve terminals.

Postoperative analgesia from morphine has been shown to be the most effective if administered at the completion of the procedure (Brandsson et al 2000, Reuben et al 2001, Tetzlaff et al 2000). In these cases, it appears that the postoperative use of morphine allows the clinician to reduce both the level and the duration of other analgesics. This is not to say that the only potential benefit of morphine is in the postoperative patient. Morphine has also been shown to be of equivalent effect to corticosteroid administration in other forms of chronic arthritides (Keates et al 1999, Stein et al 1999). The reductions in inflammatory cell influx, reduced edema formation and analgesia provided with minimal systemic effects make intraarticular morphine a very attractive postoperative therapy. I most commonly use a combination of 5–15 mg morphine with 6 mg lidocaine for postoperative analgesia and have seen no untoward effects. The beneficial effects with respect to improved analgesia and ability to reduce the usage of NSAIDs remains to be proven.

ANTIMICROBIAL AGENTS

Intraarticular agents

Antimicrobial agents are used routinely intraarticularly both for the treatment of established infections and as a preventive measure during administration of other therapeutic and diagnostic medications. Obviously, the use of antibiotics should never be considered as a substitute for adequate preparation and situation control prior to injection. Whenever possible, the selection of the antibiotic should be based on culture and sensitivity results (see Ch. 2). In situations where this is impossible, the clinician should select for the narrowest possible spectrum against the most likely organisms.

The two antimicrobial agents used most commonly intraarticularly are gentamicin and amikacin. Gentamicin offers many advantages from the standpoint of reaching high synovial fluid concentrations with doses as low as 150 mg without inducing significant synovitis (Lloyd et al 1988a). At this dose, peak concentrations in synovial fluid of 1828 µg/ml can be achieved versus 2.53 µg/ml with systemic therapy (Lloyd et al 1988b). The potential to achieve such high levels within the joint allows the clinician to use an antimicrobial agent that might have been seen as moderately effective in the laboratory based solely on the minimum inhibitory concentration (MIC) results. Other considerations when selecting an antimicrobial agent for intraarticular use should include an understanding of the physical properties of the antimicrobial agent, its mechanisms of action, half-life in synovial fluid and potential effects on the synovial membrane and articular cartilage. If possible, a complete synovial fluid analysis, including pH, cell count and total protein, is useful in establishing the possible environmental effects of the fluid on the efficacy of the antimicrobial agent. The various environmental conditions likely to be encountered at a site of infection have been evaluated for their effect on antimicrobial agents. The MIC of gentamicin and amikacin were increased up to five-fold at pH < 6.5. Likewise, magnesium and calcium ion concentrations > 10 mmol/l and ferric iron concentrations of 10 mmol/l increased aminoglycoside MIC values from 3.66- to 8-fold (Nanavaty et al 1998). These results demonstrate the benefit of complete fluid analysis or a good overall knowledge of pathology induced by the inciting agents.

Other antimicrobial agents that have been used intraarticularly include methicillin, ticarcillin–clavulanic acid, ceftiofur and imipenem. Ceftiofur has been shown to develop high synovial fluid concentrations following intraarticular administration. Following administration of 150 mg into the antebrachiocarpal joint, levels peaked at 5825.08 μg/ml at 15 min, compared with 1.43 μg/ml after i.v. administration. The half-life in these normal joints was 5.1 h. Assuming that these results correlate with what would be encountered in an infectious condition, MICs for most organisms would be met with a single injection every 24 h (Mills et al 2000). Imipenem–cilastin usage once daily (500 mg) for 3 days was shown to have minimal inflammatory side-effects (Schneider 1999).

Sustained-release preparations

The use of sustained-release systems for antimicrobial agent delivery offers many advantages to the equine practitioner. The ability to target high, sustained levels of an antimicrobial agent at the site of infection allows us to utilize many antimicrobial agents that would otherwise be prohibited based on cost or systemic side-effects. For a carrier– antimicrobial agent composite to be effective, it must be minimally reactive, provide consistent elution properties and be easy to prepare during procedures or store well if prepared in advance. The most commonly described carrier is polymethylmethacrylate radio opaque bone cement. An understanding of the physical properties of both the antimicrobial agents and the carrier are necessary to utilize this modality to its fullest potential. The elution rates of the antimicrobial agent can be increased by using higher numbers of smaller beads and by making the beads as spherical as possible. These techniques are designed to increase the overall surface area presented to the body since the elution of the antimicrobial agent is from the surface of the beads. The technique described for preparation of the beads involves mixing the antimicrobial agent (powdered or liquid) with the powered PMMA, thoroughly mixing the two and then adding the liquid activator. If a mold is to be used, the composite mixture should be injected immediately and the molds formed. If the beads are to be hand fashioned, care should be taken during the mixing process to avoid beginning to form the beads until the cement is no longer adherent to latex gloves when touched.

The aminoglycosides amikacin and gentamicin are the most commonly studied antimicrobial agents for use in PMMA. The studies have looked at a number of questions including the possibility of altered antimicrobial sensitivity in the presence of PMMA, the elution rates and the ability to incorporate the injectable versus the powered forms into the cement (Arciola et al 2001, Ethell et al 2000). Unlike the ability to use intra-articular injection of antimicrobial agents as a means of achieving high enough levels to overcome microorganisms with borderline sensitivity, care should be taken to select antimicrobial agents described as "sensitive" when choosing one to incorporate into a carrier. Sensitivity to ampicillin, cefamandole, cefazolin, imipenem, amikacin, netilmycin, erythromycin, trimethoprim–sulfamethoxazole, chloramphenicol and vancomycin have all been shown to be reduced following adhesion of bacteria to PMMA (Arciola et al 2001). *In vitro* studies would suggest that either the powdered or the liquid form is appropriate, with sustained release for up to 30 days following doses as low as 150 and 250 mg per 2 g cement. Clinically higher doses, 1–3 g per 10 g cement, are used when maintaining the material properties of the cement are not a concern.

Ceftiofur has been examined as a possible antimicrobial agent for use in PMMA delivery systems (Ethell et al 2000). Results demonstrate that it is also an appropriate antimicrobial agent for combination with PMMA. Its elution profile would suggest that it is released from the carrier rapidly and, therefore, should be placed in such a fashion that removal and replacement of expended beads is possible if prolonged drug levels are to be required.

Other antimicrobial agents that have been incorporated into PMMA beads and shown to have useful elution profiles include penicillin G (benzylpenicillin), ampicillin, amoxicillin, flucloxacillin, amoxicillin–clavulanate, cefamandole, cefazolin, tobramycin, netilmicin, imipenem, erythromycin, ciprofloxacin, trimethoprim–sulfamethoxazole, chloramphenicol and vancomycin (Ethell et al 2000, Mader et al 1997, Veyries et al 2000).

The use of biodegradable materials as vehicles is an appealing alternative. Plaster of Paris (POP), demineralized bone matrix, polylactic acid (PLA) and poly(dl-lactide)-coglycolide (PL:CG) have been examined for possible use (Mader et al 1997, Miclau et al 1993, Santschi 2000). The PLA and PL:CG biodegradable beads have been shown to release high concentrations of antimicrobial agents in vitro for 4–8 weeks (Mader et al 1997). Plaster of Paris and demineralized bone matrix beads elute antimicrobial agents at higher levels over a much shorter period (Bowyer & Cumberland 1994, Miclau et al 1993, Santschi 2000). Unlike PMMA beads, which can be mixed, formed and used in a matter of minutes, POP beads require more prolonged curing. The technique for preparing beads from the powdered POP described by Santschi (2000) is as follows. Mix 5 ml gentamicin sulfate (100 mg/ml) or 4 ml amikacin (250 mg/ml) with 10 ml phosphate-buffered saline then add to 30 g of calcium sulfate hemihydrate. Place the beads in a bead mold (with or without a suture leader) and cure overnight. Gas sterilize before use (Todhunter et al 1996).

Beads can be placed into joints or tendon sheaths as an adjunct therapy in septic conditions. When used within a synovial structure, we most commonly string the beads in series on non-absorbable suture material to allow for removal at the end of treatment. There is little risk of using the beads intraarticularly in most uniaxial, hinged joints in the horse since the sliding action of the apposing articular surfaces is at little risk of damage during times of confinement. This would not be the case if one were to attempt to use beads in the carpus, where the "tight packed" conformation is lost during flexion and extension. In these cases, we prefer to use a bandage cast to reduce the risk of the beads being trapped between the two articular surfaces.

Regional perfusion

Regional perfusion was first assessed in the equine literature as a technique for achieving high levels of antimicrobial agents in the carpus (Whitehair et al 1992). The basic principle involves the saturation of tissues with volume-diluted antimicrobial agent. The antimicrobial agent is maintained in the target region by blocking efflux through the use of pneumatic tourniquets placed at the level of the joint proximad and distad to the site of interest. The antimicrobial agent is further confined to the region of concern by leaving an Esmarch to collapse the superficial vasculature. The basic technique involves isolating a convenient region for placing a cannulated screw into the cortex of the target bone or the palmar, plantar or palmar digital or plantar digital vein for catheter placement. Once the screw or catheter is placed and hooked up to the antimicrobial agent delivery system, the Esmarch is applied to the limb from distal to proximal. After the blood has been expressed from the vasculature, a pneumatic tourniquet is inflated as described previously.

Selection of the appropriate antimicrobial agent, dose, volume and infusion rate are important. Sodium and potassium penicillin, ampicillin, gentamicin and amikacin have all been used successfully (Santschi 2000). Care should be taken when selecting an antimicrobial agent not mentioned on this list. For instance, enrofloxacin will induce an extreme vasculitis following regional perfusion. Wide variations exist in the dose required for high-pressure perfusion; the original descriptions called for using the typical systemic dose for each perfusate. Recent recommendations have cited doses as low as 250–500 mg of amikacin and 100–300 mg of gentamicin for adult horses and 50 mg for foals (Santschi 2000). For adult horses the antimicrobial agent selected is diluted to a volume of 60 ml (30 ml when perfusing the digit); in foals the volume can be reduced to 10–12 ml. Infusion rates vary with the individual clinician's preference. Most commonly, we use 2 ml/min as a standard rate, reduced to 1 ml/min when perfusing the foot.

SYNOVECTOMY WITH RADIOPHARMACEUTICALS

Activation of the synovial membrane has the potential to damage articular cartilage by the liberation of inflammatory mediators and destructive enzymes and the recruitment of inflammatory cells into the joint (Goldberg & Toole 1987, Lukoschek et al 1990). Common treatments for synovitis are directed at reducing one or all of these effects through rest, administration of steroidal and non-steroidal pharmaceuticals or immuno-suppressive drugs, or by synovectomy techniques.

Surgical synovectomy is technically difficult and time consuming and requires general anesthesia. Consequently, less-invasive means of removing the synovial lining, including the intraarticular administration of agents, has been explored. Cartilage damage and the pain associated with the administration of most chemical agents have made radiation synovectomy an attractive alternative (Shortkroff et al 1992, Zalutsky et al 1986, Zuckerman et al 1988).

Samarium-153 hydroxyapatite microspheres ([153]SmM) have been shown to ablate effectively normal and inflamed equine synovium, with minimal radiation hazard to the horse or medical personnel (Yarbrough et al 2000a,b). Within the joint space, the synovial lining primarily absorbs the energy from the [153]Sm emissions, thus allowing the clinician to target the synovium for destruction. When [153]Sm is combined with hydroxyapatite, exposure to other organs or support personnel is minimized.

Within the immediate area of the diarthroidial joint, the endothelium and the synovial lining cells are considered the most radiosensitive tissues. Therefore, radiation-induced synovectomy may produce beneficial effects by direct damage to the synovial lining cells, caused by the ionization and excitation of the tissue atoms and the formation of free radicals, induced by absorbed radiation or by damage to the subintimal vascular supply, as described previously (Johnson & Yanch 1991). The synovial intimal layer and the subintimal vessels were two of the most dramatically affected cell populations in this study. Obstruction of capillaries may occur early in the process of radiation-induced damage, through the swelling of the vascular endothelium or collagenous stroma or perivascular infiltrates. Later, fissuring of the tunica media or loss of the endothelial cells may result in the thrombosis of the affected vessels. Although the actual sensitivity of the endothelial cells to the effects of radiation is in question, it is commonly considered to be one of the central elements involved in radiation-induced tissue damage. The degree of vascular damage, combined with the tissues ability to revascularize, will be important in determining the degree of fibrosis in the area after it recovers from the radiation-induced insult.

In mature cartilage, chondrocytes rarely divide, providing them with a relative degree of resistance to radiation-induced damage. The principal factor in radiation-induced cartilage damage is the damage to the fine vasculature of the perichondrium, with the resultant death of the cells dependent on their nutritional supply. The limited penetration of the carrier particles into the subintimal tissues and the shallow penetration of the beta-radiation generated by the [153]Sm makes it unlikely that the fine vasculature of the perichondrium is at a significant risk of damage even with repeated use of [153]SmM.

The use of [153]SmM in the controlled environment of surgically induced arthritis appears to provide another means of addressing the soft tissue components of arthritis without any extracapsular leakage of radioactivity. Its proposed uses in the horse include the management of preexisting proliferative synovial membranes in long-standing arthritides, the removal of reactive synovia following osteochondral fragment removal, treatment of idiopathic synovitis/tenosynovitis and as a potential ancillary treatment in septic arthritis. It appears to provide a safe, effective means of removing the synovium without inducing histological or histochemical damage to the articular cartilage. Through customized variation in the carrier-isotope construct, the clinician can increase or decrease the level of penetration and duration within the joint space to treat varying degrees of synovial proliferation.

REFERENCES

Arciola C R, Donati M E, Montanaro L 2001 Adhesion to a polymeric biomaterial affects the antibiotic resistance of *Staphylococcus epidermidis*. Microbiologica (Pavia) 24:63–68

Augustine A J, Oleksyszyn J 1997 Glucocorticosteroids inhibit degradation in bovine cartilage explants stimulated with concomitant plasminogen and interleukin-1-alpha. Inflammation Research 46:60–64

Auteflage A, Alvineriere M, Toutain P 1986 Synovial fluid and plasma kinetics of methylprednisolone and methylprednisone acetate in horses following intraarticular administration of methylprednisolone acetate. Equine Veterinary Journal 18:193–198

Aviad A D, Houpt J B 1994 The molecular weight of therapeutic hyaluronan (sodium hyaluronate): how significant is it? Journal of Rheumatology 21:297–301

Axelrod L 1993 Glucocorticoids In: Harris E D, Kelly W N, Ruddy S et al (eds) Textbook of rheumatology, 4th edn. Saunders, Philadelphia, PA, pp. 779–796

Barber A, Gottschlich R, Haase A F 1990 Peripheral effects of various opioid agonists on neurogenic extravasation in skin of the rat hind paw. Society for Neuroscience Abstracts 16:1026–1030

Boumpas D T, Chrousos G P, Wilder R L et al 1993 Glucocorticoid therapy for immune-mediated diseases: basic and clinical correlates. Annals of Internal Medicine 119:1198–1208

Bowyer G W, Cumberland N 1994 Antibiotic release from impregnated pellets and beads. Journal of Trauma 36:331–335

Brandsson S, Karlsson J, Morberg P et al 2000 Intraarticular morphine after arthroscopic ACL reconstruction: a double-blind placebo-controlled study of 40 patients. Acta Orthopaedica Scandinavica 71:280–285

Caron J P, Tardif G, Martel-Pelletier J et al 1996 Modulation of matrix metalloprotease 13 (collagenase 3) gene expression in equine chondrocytes by interleukin 1 and corticosteroids. American Journal of Veterinary Research 57:1631–1634

Carter B G, Bertone A L, Weisbrode S E et al 1996 Influence of methylprednisolone acetate on osteochondral healing in exercised tarsocrural joints of horses. American Journal of Veterinary Research 57:914–922

Clegg P D, Jones M D, Carter S D 1998 The effect of drugs commonly used in the treatment of equine articular disorders on the activity of equine matrix metalloproteinase-2 and -9. Journal of Veterinary Pharmacology and Therapeutics 21:406–413

Comer J S, Kincaid S A, Baird A N et al 1996 Immunolocalization of stromelysin, tumor necrosis factor (TNF) alpha and TNF receptors in atrophied canine articular cartilage treated with hyaluronic acid and transforming growth factor beta. American Journal of Veterinary Research 57:1488–1496

Cooper G M 1997 In: Cooper GM (ed) The cell a molecular approach. American Society for Microbiology Press, Washington DC (and Sinauer, Sunderland, MA), pp. 522–524

de Smedt S C, Dekeyser P, Ribitsch V et al 1993 Viscoelastic and transient network properties of hyaluronic acid as a function of the concentration. Biorheology 30:31–41

Ethell M T, Bennett R A, Brown M P et al 2000 In vitro elution of gentamicin, amikacin and ceftiofur from polymethylmethacrylate and hydroxyapatite cement. Veterinary Surgery 29:375–382

Fox R B, Fox W K 1983 Dimethyl sulfoxide prevents hydroxyl radical-mediated depolymerization of hyaluronic acid. Annals of the New York Academy of Sciences 411:14–18

Frean S P, Lees P 2000 Effects of polysulfated glycosaminoglycan and hyaluronan on prostaglandin E_2

production by cultured equine synoviocytes. American Journal of Veterinary Research 61:499–505

Frean S P, Abraham L A, Lees P 1999 In vitro stimulation of equine articular cartilage proteoglycan synthesis by hyaluronan and carprofen. Research in Veterinary Science 67:183–190

Frean S P, Gettinby G, May S A et al 2000 Influence of interleukin-1beta and hyaluronan on proteoglycan release from equine navicular hyaline cartilage and fibrocartilage. Journal of Veterinary Pharmacology and Therapeutics 23:67–72

Frisbie D D, Nixon A J 1997 Insulin-like growth factor 1 and corticosteroid modulation of chondrocyte metabolic and mitogenic activities in interleukin 1-conditioned equine cartilage. American Journal of Veterinary Research 58:524–530

Frisbie D D, Kawcak C E, Trotter G W et al 1997 Effects of triamcinolone acetonide on an in vivo equine osteochondral fragment exercise model. Equine Veterinary Journal 29:349–359

Frisbie D D, Kawcak C E, Baxter G M et al 1998 Effects of 6alpha-methylprednisolone acetate on an equine osteochondral fragment exercise model. American Journal of Veterinary Research 59:1619–1628

Fubini S L, Boatwright C E, Todhunter R J et al 1993 Effect of i.m. administered polysulfated glycosaminoglycan on articular cartilage from equine joints injected with methylprednisolone acetate. American Journal of Veterinary Research 54:1359–1365

Goldberg R L, Toole B P 1987 Hyaluronate inhibition of cell proliferation. Arthritis and Rheumatism 30:769–778

Gustafson S B, McIlwraith C W, Jones R L 1989 Comparison of the effect of polysulfated glycosaminoglycan, corticosteroids and sodium hyaluronate in the potentiation of a subinfective dose of *Staphylococcus aureus* in the midcarpal joint of horses. American Journal of Veterinary Research 50:2018–2022

Hills B A, Ethell M T, Hodgson D R 1998 Release of lubricating synovial surfactant by intraarticular corticosteroid. British Journal of Rheumatology 37:649–652

Johnson L S, Yanch J C 1991 Absorbed dose profiles for radionuclides of frequent use in radiation synovectomy. Arthritis and Rheumatism 34:1521–1530

Jolly W T, Whittem T, Jolly A C et al 1995 The dose-related effects of phenylbutazone and a methylprednisolone acetate formulation (Depo-Medrol) on cultured explants of equine carpal articular cartilage. Journal of Veterinary Pharmacology and Therapeutics 18:429–437

Kalso E, Tramer M R, Carroll D 1997 Pain relief from intraarticular morphine after knee surgery: a qualitative systematic review. Pain 71:127–134

Kato Y, Mukudai Y, Okimura A et al 1995 Effects of hyaluronic acid on the release of cartilage matrix proteoglycan and fibronectin from the cell matrix layer of chondrocyte cultures: interactions between hyaluronic acid and chondroitin sulfate glycosaminoglycan. Journal of Rheumatology 22(suppl):158–159

Keates H L, Cramond T, Smith M T 1999 Intraarticular and periarticular opioid binding in inflamed tissue in experimental canine arthritis. Anesthesia and Analgesia 89:409–415

Khoury G F, Garland D E, Stein C 1994 Intraarticular opioid–local anesthetic combinations for chronic joint pain. Middle East Journal of Anesthesiology 12:579–585

Kirkham B, Portek I, Lee C S et al 1999 Intraarticular variability of synovial membrane histology, immunohistology and cytokine mRNA expression in patients with rheumatoid arthritis. Journal of Rheumatology 26:777–784

Kolesnikov Y A, Jain S, Wilson R 1996 Peripheral morphine analgesia: synergy with central sites and a target of morphine tolerance. Journal of Pharmacology and Experimental Therapeutics 279:502–506

Lloyd K C, Stover S M, Pascoe J R et al 1988a Plasma and synovial fluid concentrations of gentamicin in horses after intraarticular administration of buffered and unbuffered gentamicin. American Journal of Veterinary Research 49:644–649

Lloyd K C, Stover S M, Pascoe J R et al 1988b Effect of gentamicin sulfate and sodium bicarbonate on the synovium of clinically normal equine antebrachiocarpal joints. American Journal of Veterinary Research 49:650–657

Lukoschek M, Burr D B, Walker E R et al 1990 Synovial membrane and cartilage changes in experimental osteoarthrosis surgical instability and repetitive impulsive loading. Zeitschrift für Orthopaedie und ihre Grenzgebiete 128:437–441

Lynch T M, Caron J P, Arnoczky S P et al 1998 Influence of exogenous hyaluronan on synthesis of hyaluronan and collagenase by equine synoviocytes. American Journal of Veterinary Research 59:888–892

MacLeod J N, Fubini S L, Gu D N et al 1998 Effect of synovitis and corticosteroids on transcription of cartilage matrix proteins. American Journal of Veterinary Research 59:1021–1026

Mabuchi K, Obara T, Ikegami K et al 1999 Molecular weight independence of the effect of additive hyaluronic acid on the lubricating characteristics in synovial joints with experimental deterioration. Clinical Biomechanics 14:352–356

Mader J T, Calhoun J, Cobos J 1997 In vitro evaluation of antibiotic diffusion from antibiotic-impregnated biodegradable beads and polymethylmethacrylate beads. Antimicrobial Agents and Chemotherapy 41:415–418

May S A, Hooke R E, Lees P 1988 The effect of drugs used in the treatment of osteoarthrosis on stromelysin (proteoglycanase) of equine synovial cell origin. Equine Veterinary Journal Supplement 25:28–32

Miclau T, Dahners L E, Lindsey R W 1993 In vitro pharmacokinetics of antibiotic release from locally implantable materials. Journal of Orthopaedic Research 11:627–632

Mills M L, Rush B R, St Jean G et al 2000 Determination of synovial fluid and serum concentrations and morphologic effects of intraarticular ceftiofur sodium in horses. Veterinary Surgery 29:398–406

Moses V S, Hardy J, Bertone A L et al 2001 Effects of anti-inflammatory drugs on lipopolysaccharide-challenged and -unchallenged equine synovial explants. American Journal of Veterinary Research 62:54–60

Nanavaty J, Mortensen J E, Shryock T R 1998 The effects of environmental conditions on the in vitro activity of selected antimicrobial agents against *Escherichia coli*. Current Microbiology 36:212–215

Papachristou G, Anagnostou S, Katsorhis T 1997 The effect of intraarticular hydrocortisone injection on the articular cartilage of rabbits. Acta Orthopaedica Scandinavica 68(suppl):132–134

Partsch G, Schwarzer C, Neumueller J et al 1989 Modulation of the migration and chemotaxis of PMN cells by hyaluronic acid. Zeitschrift für Rheumatologie 48:123–128

Pelletier J, Mineau F, Raynauld J et al 1994 Intraarticular injections with methylprednisolone acetate reduce osteoarthritic lesions in parallel with chondrocyte stromelysin synthesis in experimental osteoarthritis. Arthritis and Rheumatism 37:414–423

Pelletier J, Dibattista J A, Raynauld J et al 1995 The in vivo effects of intraarticular corticosteroid injections on cartilage lesions, stromelysin, interleukin-1 and oncogene protein synthesis in experimental osteoarthritis. Laboratory Investigation 72:578–586

Peloso J G, Stick J A, Caron J P 1993 Effects of hylan on amphotericin-induced carpal lameness in equids. American Journal of Veterinary Research 54:1527–1534

Peluso G F, Perbellini A, Tajana G F 1990 The effect of high and low molecular weight hyaluronic acid on mitogen-induced lymphocyte proliferation. Current Therapeutic Research 47:437–443

Ratcliffe A, Mow V 1996 Articular cartilage. In: Comper W (ed) Extracellular matrix. Harwood, Melbourne, pp. 234–303

Recklies A D, White C, Melching L et al 2001 Differential regulation and expression of hyaluronan synthases in human articular chondrocytes, synovial cells and osteosarcoma cells. Biochemical Journal 354:17–24

Reuben S S, Sklar J, El-Mansouri M 2001 The preemptive analgesic effect of intraarticular bupivacaine and morphine after ambulatory arthroscopic knee surgery. Anesthesia and Analgesia 92:923–926

Ribitsch V, Katzer H, Rainer F 1999 Viscoelastic properties of synovial fluids and their impact on joint lubrication. Biorheology 36:43–44

Santschi E M 2000 Antibiotic delivery for orthopedic conditions. In: Proceedings of the 10th American College of Veterinary Surgery Annual Symposium. Arlington, VA, pp. 147–149

Schimmer B P, Parker K A 1996 Adrenocorticotropic hormone; adrenocortical corticosteroids and their synthetic analogs; inhibitors of the synthesis and actions of adrenocortical hormones. In: Molinoff P B (ed) The pharmacologic basis of therapeutics. McGraw-Hill, New York, pp. 1459–1485

Schneider R K 1999 Orthopedic infections. In: Auer J A, Stick J A (eds) Equine surgery. Saunders, Philadelphia, PA, pp. 727–736

Schneider R K, Bramlage L R, Moore R M et al 1992 A retrospective study of 192 horses affected with septic arthritis-tenosynovitis. Equine Veterinary Journal 24:436–442

Shah S, Breivogel C, Selly D et al 1997 Time-dependent effects of in vivo pertussis toxin on morphine analgesia and G-proteins in mice. Pharmacology Biochemistry and Behavior 565:465–469

Shortkroff S, Mahmood A, Sledge C B et al 1992 Studies on holmium-166-labelled hydroxyapatite: a new agent for radiation synovectomy. Journal of Nuclear Medicine 33:937

Sibinga N E S, Goldstein A 1988 Opioid peptides and opioid receptors in cells of the immune system. Journal of Clinical Investigation 76:219–250

Smith C L, MacDonald M H, Tesch A M et al 2000 In vitro evaluation of the effect of dimethyl sulfoxide on equine articular cartilage matrix metabolism. Veterinary Surgery 29:347–357

Sorensen T S, Sorensen A I, Strange K 1991 The effect of intraarticular instillation of bupivacaine on postarthroscopic morbidity: a placebo-controlled, double-blind trial. Arthroscopy 7:364–367

Specht T E, Nixon A J, Moyer D J 1988 Equine synovia after an intraarticular injection of lidocaine or mepivacaine. Veterinary Surgery 17:42–49

Stein A, Yassouridis A, Szopko C et al 1999 Intraarticular morphine versus dexamethasone in chronic arthritis. Pain 83:525–532

Stein C, Yassouridis A 1997 Peripheral morphine analgesia. Pain 71:119–121

Stein C, Pflueger M, Yassouridis A et al 1996 No tolerance to peripheral morphine analgesia in presence of opioid expression in inflamed synovia. Journal of Clinical Investigation 98:793–799

Stricker S J, Lozman P R, Makowski A et al 1996 Chondroprotective effect of betamethasone in lapine pyogenic arthritis. Journal of Pediatric Orthopedics 16:231–236

Takeshita S, Mizuno S, Kikuchi T et al 1997 The in vitro effect of hyaluronic acid on IL-1-beta production in cultured rheumatoid synovial cells. Biomedical Research (Tokyo) 18:187–194

Tetzlaff J E, Brems J, Dilger J 2000 Intraarticular morphine and bupivacaine reduces postoperative pain after rotator cuff repair. Regional Anesthesia and Pain Medicine 25:611–614

Todhunter R J, Fubini S L, Wootton J A M et al 1996 Effect of methylprednisolone acetate on proteoglycan and collagen metabolism of articular cartilage explants. Journal of Rheumatology 23:1207–1213

Tulamo R M 1991 Comparison of high-performance liquid chromatography with a radiometric assay for determination of the effect of intraarticular administration of corticosteroid and saline solution on synovial fluid hyaluronate concentration in horses. American Journal of Veterinary Research 52:1940–1944

van der Kraan P M, Vitters E L, Postma N S et al 1993 Maintenance of the synthesis of large proteoglycans in anatomically intact murine articular cartilage by corticosteroids and insulin-like growth factor I. Annals of the Rheumatic Diseases 52:734–741

Verschure P J, van der Kraan P M, Vitters E L et al 1994 Stimulation of proteoglycan synthesis by triamcinolone acetonide and insulin-like growth factor 1 in normal and arthritic murine articular cartilage. Journal of Rheumatology 21:920–926

Veyries M, Faurisson F, Joly-Guillou M et al 2000 Control of staphylococcal adhesion to polymethylmethacrylate and enhancement of susceptibility to antibiotics by Poloxamer 407. Antimicrobial Agents and Chemotherapy 44:1093–1096

Welch R D, Debowes R M, Liepold H W 1989 Evaluation of the effects of intraarticular injection of DMSO on normal equine articular tissues. American Journal of Veterinary Research 50:1180–1182

White K K, Hodgson D R, Hancock D et al 1989 Changes in equine carpal joint synovial fluid in response to the injection of two local anesthetic agents. Cornell Veterinarian 79:25–38

Whitehair K J, Bowersock T L, Blevins W E et al 1992 Regional limb perfusion for antibiotic treatment of experimentally induced septic arthritis. Veterinary Surgery 21:367–373

Yarbrough T B, Lee M R, Hornof W J et al 2000a Samarium 153-labeled hydroxyapatite microspheres for radiation synovectomy in the horse: a study of the biokinetics, dosimetry, clinical and morphologic response in normal metacarpophalangeal and metatarsophalangeal joints. Veterinary Surgery 29:191–199

Yarbrough T B, Lee M R, Hornof W J et al 2000b Evaluation of samarium-153 for synovectomy in an osteochondral fragment-induced model of synovitis in horses. Veterinary Surgery 29:252–263

Zalutsky M R, Venkatesan P P, English R J et al 1986 Radiation synovectomy with dysprosium-165 ferric hydroxide macroaggregates: lymph node uptake and radiation dosimetry calculations. International Journal of Nuclear Medicine and Biology 12:457–466

Zuckerman J, Wilson M, Vella M et al 1988 Treatment of pigmented villonodular synovitis by radiation synovectomy: an adjuvant to surgical synovectomy. Arthritis and Rheumatism 31:S102

CHAPTER CONTENTS

Introduction 135
  Intramuscular drug administration 135
  Adverse drug reactions involving skeletal
    muscle 136
  Skeletal muscle disorders 137

Agents that affect skeletal muscle directly 138
  Non-steroidal anti-inflammatory drugs 138
  Tranquillizers 138
  Muscle relaxants 139
  Other drugs affecting skeletal muscle 142

References 144

8

Drugs affecting skeletal muscle

Jennifer M. MacLeay

INTRODUCTION

The interaction of drugs and the muscular system may be approached from two separate angles. Firstly, many drugs are administered to horses by the intramuscular (i.m.) route and, therefore, adverse reactions to treatment involve skeletal muscle. Secondly, primary myopathies involving skeletal muscle include infectious, traumatic and genetic disorders. Typically, these disorders are managed by using medications that target skeletal muscle either directly or indirectly. Drugs that target skeletal muscle directly include the muscle relaxants and anabolic steroids whereas drugs that target skeletal muscle indirectly include antimicrobial and anti-inflammatory agents. This chapter includes a brief discussion of i.m. drug administration and then discusses exertional rhabdomyolysis and agents that directly affect skeletal muscle in greater depth.

INTRAMUSCULAR DRUG ADMINISTRATION

Intramuscular drug administration provides better and more consistent absorption than subcutaneous (s.c.) administration. The rate of absorption is highly dependent upon the blood flow to the site of administration and the solubility of the preparation administered (see Ch. 1). The blood flow to a muscle is dependent upon the cardiovascular status of the animal and the muscle chosen. The capillary density differs between different muscle groups and will increase in fit individuals (Clark et al 1992). Consequently, absorption from the

Table 8.1 Side-effects involving skeletal muscle and the medications associated with each side-effect reported in humans

Side-effect	Drug
Muscle atrophy (loss of muscle mass)	Bupivacaine, corticosteroids
Muscle cramp (painful involuntary contractions of muscles)	Beta blockers, danazol, dyhydroergotamine, lidocaine (lignocaine), nifedipine, spinal/epidural anesthesia
Muscle fibrosis (increased fibrous tissue)	Corticosteroids
Muscle rigidity (decreased ability for relaxation of muscle)	Flunarizine
Muscle weakness (decreased voluntary and involuntary strength)	Botulinum-A toxin, dantrolene, ketoconazole, neuromuscular blocking agents, polymyxins, succinylcholine (suxamethonium), tizanidine
Myalgia (tenderness or pain in muscles)	Albendazole, α_2 interferon, anti-CD5 antibody, azathioprine, dimercaprol, hycanthone, interferon, interleukin 2, iron dextran, ivermectin, ketoconazole, lansoprazole, metoprolol, nalidixic acid, OKT3, pefloxacin, tiabendazole, zidovudine
Myasthenic syndrome (abnormal fatigability or weakness of muscles)	Chloroquine, clarithromycin, erythromycin
Myoclonic encephalopathy (intermittent spasm or twitching of muscles)	Corticotropin
Myoclonus (clonic spasm or twitching of muscles or muscle groups that is persistent or continuous)	Etomidate, maprotiline, metoclopramide, opioids (intrathecally), physostigmine
Myoglobinemia/myoglobinuria (rhabdomyolysis resulting in increased myoglobin in the blood and urine	Succinylcholine (suxamethonium)
Myokymia (wave-like muscle fiber twitching)	Gold salts
Myopathy (generalized abnormal condition of skeletal muscle)	α_2 interferon, aminocaproic acid, amiodarone, beclobrate, butorphenol, carbamazepine, chloroquine, ciclosporin, cimetidine, co-trimoxazole, corticosteroids, dexamethasone, dextropropoxyphene, dihydroemetine, emetine, gemfibrozil, general anesthetics, gemanium, HMG coenzyme-A reductase inhibitors, iopamidol, ipecacuanha, labetalol, nicotinic acid, pentazocine, pravastatin, procainamide, quinine, triamcinolone
Myositis (inflammation of muscle tissue)	Amrinone, cromolyn sodium, gemfibrozil
Myotonia (tonic spasm of a muscle or temporary rigidity after contraction)	Decamethonium

gluteal muscles may be slower in a pastured horse than in a fit racehorse. While these differences in absorption are real, in practice their influence is probably limited.

ADVERSE DRUG REACTIONS INVOLVING SKELETAL MUSCLE

The adverse effects of drugs in skeletal muscle include pain (myalgia), inflammation (myositis), cramp, weakness, myoglobinemia/myoglobinuria, rigidity, atrophy and fibrosis as well as a number of myopathies including myoclonus, myokymia and myotonia or toxic spasm (Table 8.1) (Leuwer & Motsch 1996). These side-effects have been reported primarily in humans; however, similar manifestations may also occur in equines. The origin of the side-effects listed varies and includes receptor blockade, interference with biochemical processes and irritation at the site of administration. In the horse, bacterial infections involving either *Streptococcus* or *Clostridium* spp. or other bacterial organisms at an i.m. injection site is not uncommon. Such bacterial infections may be minor, requiring topical therapy only, to life threatening, requiring vigorous topical and systemic therapy.

SKELETAL MUSCLE DISORDERS

Pathological syndromes may result in muscular spasm, as seen in the exertional myopathies, or weakness, as seen in hyperkalemic periodic paralysis (HYPP). Similarly, infectious diseases may result in muscular rigidity (*C. tetani* infection (tetanus)) or paralysis (*C. botulinum* intoxication (botulism)). Overt rhabdomyolysis may result from the ingestion of the coccidiostats monensin, rumensin and lasalocid, or one of a number of plant mycotoxins. Dietary deficiencies of selenium or vitamin E have also been described as having severe deleterious effects on skeletal muscle health.

Over a 9-year period (1974–1983), 67 horses were referred to one veterinary teaching hospital for muscular problems (Freestone & Carlson 1991). Of these, 68% were referred for exercise-associated myopathy; 11% for infectious myopathy (bacterial, viral or sarcocystis infection); 9% for multiple organ disease occurring within days of high intensity, endurance exercise (postexhaustion syndrome); 6% for purpura hemorrhagica (idiopathic thrombocytopenic purpura); 4.5% for selenium and/or vitamin E deficiency (nutritional myopathy) and 1.5% for HYPP. This is the only published retrospective study of its kind; however, most practitioners would probably agree that it reflects the spectrum of equine muscle diseases that are presented in general practice. No horses were reported to have focal exercise-induced muscle pain/soreness, or exercise- or trauma-induced muscle tearing, which probably reflects the fact that this study was conducted at a referral hospital since minor muscle-related disorders are unlikely to be referred.

HYPP is a heritable myotonia (increased muscular irritability and contractility with decreased power of relaxation), arising from a mutation in the gene for the sodium channel, affecting the skeletal muscle cell membrane. Potassium leakage into the circulation through this dysfunctional sodium channel leads to persistent muscle cell membrane depolarization and hyperkalemia. Consumption of a high potassium diet has been found to exacerbate the disorder. Although to date no drug has been found that acts directly on the muscle cell membrane to counteract the dysfunctional ion channels, horses with HYPP can be managed successfully by maintaining them on a low-potassium diet. In more severe cases, the diuretic acetazolamide may also be used to increase potassium loss in urine. Other congenital myotonias occur rarely and include myotonia congenita and myotonic dystrophy.

The most common muscle disorder is that of muscle cramping in response to exercise, which leads to muscle damage (also known as exertional rhabdomyolysis). Horses that suffer from exercise-induced muscle cramping are commonly thought to fall into one of two categories: those that suffer from a sporadic incident resulting from overexertion and/or a concurrent deficiency of electrolytes, and those that have chronic muscle cramping owing to an underlying myopathy. Pharmaceutical intervention in these cases is aimed at alleviating myalgia, restoring electrolyte and fluid balances and/or preventing future episodes. Overt myoglobinuria and elevated serum creatine kinase and aspartate aminotransferase activities accompany and reflect the severity of muscle damage and can be used to evaluate the success of therapy.

Horses that suffer chronically from episodes of exertional rhabdomyolysis are generally thought to have an underlying myopathy. Several distinct diseases have now been described. These include polysaccharide storage myopathy (PSSM) in Quarter Horses, equine polysaccharide storage myopathy (EPSM) in draft horse breeds, and recurrent exertional rhabdomyolysis (RER) in Thoroughbreds (MacLeay et al 1999a, Valberg et al 1996, Valentine et al 1998). Chronic exertional rhabdomyolysis occurs in other breeds such as the Arabian, Standardbred, warmblood and some breeds of pony, but has not been investigated in any depth.

PSSM is inherited as an autosomal recessive trait and is probably caused by a defect in glucose metabolism within the muscle cell (De La Corte et al 1999a,b). EPSM has similar histological characteristics to PSSM. However, a syndrome of progressive muscular weakness is frequently reported, in addition to the typical clinical signs associated with muscle cramping, in draft horses with EPSM (Valentine 1999). RER in Thoroughbreds is probably inherited as an autosomal dominant trait and may be caused by a defect in calcium regulation within the muscle cell, which is similar but not identical to malignant hyperthermia in swine and humans (Lentz et al 1999, MacLeay et al 1999a, Valberg et al 1999, Ward et al 2000).

Malignant hyperthermia is a frequently fatal condition that involves severe muscle contraction and hyperthermia. Episodes are triggered by stress and/or specific volatile anesthetics, such as halothane, which cause excessive calcium release from the sarcoplasmic reticulum. The disorder is caused by a mutation in the skeletal muscle ryanodine receptor. The physiological mechanism by which stress triggers malignant hyperthermia is not fully understood.

AGENTS THAT AFFECT SKELETAL MUSCLE DIRECTLY

The treatment of acute episodes of exertional rhabdomyolysis is aimed at alleviating pain and muscle contracture, correcting electrolyte and/or body fluid deficiencies and addressing renal dysfunction, if present. Horses with chronic problems typically benefit more from preventative management strategies, such as the combination of a diet low in carbohydrates (concentrates) with increased daily exercise (compared with stall confinement). Supplementation of horses with fats, in the form of corn oil or rice bran, has shown considerable promise.

Few drugs have been evaluated scientifically for their efficacy in preventing episodes of rhabdomyolysis in susceptible horses. Similarly, there are no anecdotal reports of a single therapy that prevents exertional rhabdomyolysis in all horses, and many combinations of pharmaceuticals and nutraceuticals have been employed with varying degrees of efficacy. In a recent survey, 59 thoroughbred racehorse trainers used 27 different

methods (from a total of 117 responses) to reduce the incidence of RER (MacLeay et al 1999b). Dietary change, supplemental vitamin E and/or selenium, dimethylglycine, tranquillizers and the muscle relaxants methocarbamol and dantrolene were cited most commonly. Of the pharmaceutical modalities, only phenytoin has been studied experimentally in a group of horses with chronic exertional rhabdomyolysis and in two horses with myotonia (Beech et al 1998).

NON-STEROIDAL ANTI-INFLAMMATORY DRUGS

The non-steroidal anti-inflammatory drugs (NSAIDs) are covered extensively in Chapter 13 and will not be discussed further here.

TRANQUILLIZERS

This use of tranquillizers is covered in Chapter 15. The effects of acepromazine and diazepam on skeletal muscle are explained further here.

Acepromazine

Acepromazine (acetylpromazine) maleate is a phenothiazine derivative that is commonly referred to as ACE or ACP. It is used as a neuroleptic but it is often also used to treat conditions involving muscle cramping in horses, such as occurs in sporadic exertional rhabdomyolysis, PSSM and RER (Valberg & Hodgson 1996). The phenothiazines block postsynaptic dopamine receptors in the central nervous system and may inhibit the release and/or increase the metabolism of dopamine (Plumb 1995). Phenothiazines also block α adrenoreceptors, muscarinic, histamine H_1 and 5-hydroxytryptamine (serotonin) receptors giving acepromazine some anticholinergic, antihistaminic, antispasmodic and α adrenergic blocking effects (Plumb 1995).

Acepromazine has been shown to reduce the incidence of halothane-induced malignant hyperthermia in susceptible pigs. Its protective action may result from a combination of its tranquillizing, hypothermic and/or antispasmodic effects. There are anecdotal reports that suggest that oral, intravenous (i.v.) or i.m. administration of acepromazine to susceptible horses prior to exercise decreases the incidence of rhabdomyolysis. Acepromazine is also used to help to reduce muscle spasm during episodes of rhabdomyolysis. However, its use is contraindicated in dehydrated horses as it may contribute to acute renal failure through poor renal perfusion. It is administered i.v. or i.m. at dose rates of 0.02–0.1 mg/kg (Plumb 1995). Despite its antispasmodic activity, acepromazine is contraindicated in tetanus because of its extrapyramidal effects.

Acepromazine is either subject to restrictions on its use or is prohibited in many equine disciplines (e.g. FEI Veterinary Regulations, Endurance). It is suggested that tranquillizers of this type should not be administered to horses or ponies within at least 7 days prior to competing. In some horseracing in the USA, low levels of acepromazine are permitted (e.g. a maximum of 25 ng/ml urine); therefore, at least 4 days should elapse between treatment and racing. It should be remembered that these recommendations change periodically and vary between different equestrian disciplines and from country to country.

Diazepam

Diazepam, the most commonly used benzodiazepine in equine medicine, is used as a component of anesthetic protocols (see Ch. 15) and for the treatment of seizures (see Ch. 9) . It induces skeletal muscle relaxation by facilitating the action of the inhibitory neurotransmitter gamma-aminobutyric acid (GABA) within the central nervous system. It acts primarily within the spinal cord and exerts inhibitory effects on polysynaptic reflexes and internuncial neuron transmission.

Diazepam can be used to reduce muscle spasm of any origin including local muscle strain (Miller 1995). The dose rate for the use of diazepam as a minor tranquillizer in horses is 0.01–0.04 mg/kg i.v. (Muir & Hubbell 1989). Diazepam may cause muscle fasciculation, weakness and ataxia in horses when used at doses sufficient to cause sedation, the doses required to produce reduced muscle tone. Doses of greater than 0.2 mg/kg may induce recumbency (Plumb 1995).

MUSCLE RELAXANTS

Skeletal muscle relaxants fall into three major categories: those that reduce spasticity, those that cause neuromuscular blockade and those that work at the cellular level. Spasmolytic agents (e.g. metho-carbamol, guaifenesin) act centrally whereas neuromuscular blockers (e.g. succinylcholine (suxamethonium), pancuronium, atracurium) act at the neuromuscular end plate to produce muscular relaxation. Dantrolene falls into the third category and acts within the muscle cell itself to produce relaxation.

Centrally acting spasmolytics

In humans, spasmolytic agents are used in the treatment of disorders resulting in spasticity (e.g. cerebral palsy, multiple sclerosis and stroke). Agents that interfere with the reflex arc and/or excitation contraction coupling are most useful (Miller 1995). However, these types of disorder are uncommon in horses; instead sporadic episodes of muscle cramping resulting from overexertion, electrolyte depletion or an underlying myopathy are more common. In this group of diseases, the muscle contracture is electrically silent because the cramp arises within the muscle fiber; therefore, centrally acting muscle relaxants are unlikely to provide substantial relief. Muscle relaxants can also be used on a temporary basis, in conjunction with correction of the underlying problem (e.g. an improperly fitted saddle), in the treatment of muscle stiffness and soreness of the back muscles, which may lead to poor performance in horses.

Methocarbamol

Methocarbamol is an aromatic glycerol ether that is a close chemical relative to mephenesin carbamate. Methocarbamol is approved in the USA for parenteral administration to horses as an adjunct to the treatment of acute inflammatory and traumatic conditions of the skeletal muscles and to reduce muscular spasm. Its mechanism of action has not been established, but it may act by central nervous system depression. It has no direct action on the contractile mechanism of striated muscle, the motor end plate or the nerve fiber (Plumb

1995). Methocarbamol also has some antimuscarinic effects.

After i.v. administration to horses, the clearance of methocarbamol from plasma is dose dependent: lower clearance was calculated after higher doses were administered (Plumb 1995). The elimination half-life in horses (30 mg/kg) was 60–90 min. After oral administration, at dose rates of 50 and 100 mg/kg, peak plasma concentrations occurred within 15–45 min and the bioavailability was 51–124% (Muir et al 1984). Methocarbamol is metabolized to a dealkylated and a hydroxylated product. These two metabolites are found primarily as glucuronide and sulfate conjugates. Methocarbamol crosses both the placenta and the blood–brain barrier.

Methocarbamol is effective if administered i.v. at 4.4–22 mg/kg for moderate conditions and 22–55 mg/kg for severe conditions (e.g. tetanus) (Plumb 1995). The dose rate for oral administration should be two to three times the i.v. dose (Cunningham et al 1992): 50–100 mg/kg (Muir et al 1984). Methocarbamol frequently causes sedation in horses and should not be administered to pregnant mares. In addition, because of the presence of polyethylene glycol 300 as the vehicle in the parenteral solution, methocarbamol should not be used in animals with renal failure.

Guaifenesin

Guaifenesin is used primarily as part of anesthetic protocols to produce muscle relaxation, thus allowing decreased amounts of sedatives and general anesthetics to be used and to allow easier intubation (see Ch. 15). The mechanism by which it produces skeletal muscle relaxation is poorly understood. It probably decreases transmission along spinal pathways and/or internuncial neurons, at the level of the subcortical brain, brainstem and spinal cord, which maintain skeletal muscle tone. The diaphragm is apparently unaffected and guaifenesin acts only as a mild sedative and analgesic. Guaifenesin is used primarily in anesthetic protocols to induce recumbency (Plumb 1995). It does not appear to have any direct effect on striated muscle, peripheral nerve fibers or the motor end plate.

After i.v. administration, recumbency and light restraint persists for approximately 6 min. Muscle relaxation persists for approximately 10–20 min and the half-life is longer in males (85 min) than in females (60 min) (Plumb 1995).

Guaifenesin (5% solution) may be administered i.v. at a dose rate of 110 mg/kg, with one-third to one-half of the dose given to induce recumbency and the remainder thereafter unless respiratory or cardiovascular effects are observed (Plumb 1995). Numerous different anesthetic regimens have been described (Muir & Hubbell 1989). Substantial cardiovascular side-effects are rare in the horse. Overdosage is associated with apneusis, nystagmus, hypotension and contradictory muscle rigidity (Plumb 1995).

Neuromuscular blockers

Neuromuscular blocking agents are structurally related to acetylcholine. They either block transmission by simulating an excess of acetylcholine (depolarizing neuromuscular blockers) or prevent depolarization by preventing acetylcholine from binding to its receptor on the motor end plate (non-depolarizing neuromuscular blockers).

Succinylcholine (suxamethonium) chloride

Succinylcholine, a cholinergic antagonist, is the prototype depolarizing blocking agent. Historically in the USA, succinylcholine was used extensively in horses to permit minor surgery such as castration. However, because of its lack of analgesic activity and occasional fatalities, the American Association of Equine Practitioners (AAEP) now discourages its use.

Structurally, succinylcholine is composed of two acetylcholine molecules joined at the acetate methyl (CH_3) group. Succinylcholine binds to the nicotinic receptor and depolarizes the neuromuscular end plate. It is subsequently metabolized more slowly than acetylcholine and the muscle cell membrane remains depolarized and, therefore, unresponsive to additional stimuli. Initially, muscle fasciculation occurs but, without repetitive end plate repolarization to maintain muscle tension, flaccid paralysis follows.

Contrary to their expected action, anti-cholinesterases potentiate the blockade produced by succinylcholine when used with non-depolarizing agents. The continued presence of succinylcholine results in repolarization of the end plate. However, despite repolarization, the end plate remains refractory to stimulation as long as succinylcholine is present. With continued exposure, the end plate begins to respond as it does to non-depolarizing agents, a non-sustained response to tetanic stimulus, which is reversed by anti-cholinesterases.

Succinylcholine is an ultra-short-acting depolarizing skeletal muscle relaxant. The neuromuscular block remains for as long as sufficient quantities of succinylcholine remain. After i.v. administration, the onset of action is typically within 1 min and lasts for 2–3 min. Succinylcholine is metabolized by plasma cholinesterases to choline and the weakly active succinylmonocholine, which is primarily excreted in the urine (Plumb 1995). Succinylcholine should be administered i.v. at a dose rate of 0.088 mg/kg (Plumb 1995). Succinylcholine can also be added to an overdose of barbiturate to produce euthanasia in horses. This is accompanied by a minimal amount of postmortem muscular contraction, making the addition of succinylcholine desirable for use during euthanasia when the client is present.

Succinylcholine exacerbates hyperkalemia and should not be used in horses with HYPP, hyperkalemia resulting from metabolic acidosis, kidney disease or severe rhabdomyolysis. It has been associated with precipitating malignant hyperthermia in other species and should, therefore, be avoided in horses with RER. The AAEP recommend that succinylcholine should not be administered to horses that have been treated within the last 30 days with antimicrobial agents that block acetylcholine release (e.g. the aminoglycosides and tetracyclines), organophosphates, other insecticides or procaine-containing products (inhibitors of acetylcholinesterase).

Pancuronium, vecuronium and atracurium

Pancuronium, vecuronium and atracurium are synthetic non-depolarizing neuromuscular blocking agents that are used to produce muscular relaxation during general anesthesia. Pancuronium is a bis-quaternary steroid and vecuronium is a mono-quaternary homolog of pancuronium. The bulky structure of pancuronium prolongs its duration of action compared with vecuronium and atracurium.

The neuromuscular blocking agents are highly ionized and do not cross membranes well; therefore, they have an apparent volume of distribution similar to the blood volume. They bind to the α subunits of the postsynaptic nicotinic cholinergic receptors, competitively inhibiting the binding of acetylcholine. Depolarization cannot occur and muscle paralysis persists as long as one molecule is attached to an α subunit. At higher doses, they may also physically obstruct ion channel pores to produce blockade. The release of acetylcholine may also be reduced through blockage of the prejunctional sodium channels. The duration of action of pancuronium, vercuronium and atracurium is dependent on competition (acetylcholine, administration of acetylcholinesterase inhibitors) or diffusion away from the receptor.

The onset of neuromuscular blockade typically occurs in 3–5 min of i.v. administration and lasts for 20–35 min. Higher doses will result in a longer duration of blockade. Pancuronium is eliminated primarily in bile and vecuronium undergoes hepatic and renal excretion. The recovery from blockade produced by atracurium is a result of metabolism by non-specific plasma esterases (hydrolysis) and spontaneous Hoffman degradation (spontaneous at body temperature and physiological pH), which is independent of renal or hepatic function and, therefore, unaffected by renal or hepatic disease (Plumb 1995). Atracurium does not accumulate.

Pancuronium can be administered i.v. during general anesthesia at a dose rate of 0.08 mg/kg (Muir & Hubbell 1989). If used appropriately, adverse effects are rare. Pancuronium and vecuronium produce minimal cardiovascular effects, although pancuronium can potentially stimulate the release of norepinephrine (noradrenaline), resulting in increased heart rate and blood pressure. Horses with pre-existing cardiovascular disease may develop hypotension. Atracurium produces minimal cardiovascular effects but may result in slight histamine release at high doses, leading to side-effects such as hypotension, vasodilatation, dyspnea, bronchospasm or urticaria. Systemic alkalosis may shorten the duration of blockade, whereas systemic acidosis may prolong blockade.

Muscle cell relaxants

Dantrolene

Dantrolene is a non-centrally acting spasmolytic that is used to treat and prevent malignant hyperthermia in pigs and humans. It limits the amount of calcium being released from the sarcoplasmic reticulum during malignant hyperthermia (Miller 1995).

Dantrolene is a hydantoin class of anticonvulsant that acts outside the central nervous system to produce skeletal muscle relaxation by interfering with excitation contraction coupling. In normally contracting muscle, activation of the ryanodine receptor within the muscle fiber results in calcium release from the sarcoplasmic reticulum and subsequent muscle contraction. Dantrolene interferes with the release of calcium from the sarcoplasmic reticulum by interfering with the ryanodine receptor. The release of calcium in smooth and cardiac muscle is under different control; consequently, dantrolene primarily affects skeletal muscle.

In Thoroughbred racehorses, dantrolene has been described as having a preventative or limiting role in episodes of exertional rhabdomyolysis, although the ryanodine receptor functions normally in these horses (Klein 1989, Ward et al 2000). It has also been used in draft horse breeds prior to anesthesia to try and reduce the frequency of anesthetic/recumbency-related rhabdomyolysis (Klein 1989).

After oral administration of dantrolene to horses, peak concentrations are reached in 1.5 h and the bioavailability is 39 ± 10% (Court et al 1987). The elimination of dantrolene is rapid: it has a half-life of 2.15 h and a body clearance of 4.16 ml/min per kg.

Slow i.v. administration of dantrolene at 15–25 mg/kg four times a day has been recommended for horses with acute rhabdomyolysis (Robinson

1987). To prevent exertional rhabdomyolysis, dantrolene can be administered orally to horses at 2–5 mg/kg, 60–90 min prior to exercise (Robinson 1987). Dantrolene has also been used to prevent myositis by giving an oral dose of 10 mg/kg 60–90 min prior to the induction of anesthesia. This is sufficient to produce peak concentrations during surgery that will be sufficient for a 2 h surgical procedure. If additional time is needed, an additional dose can be administered i.v. at 1.9–4 mg/kg to provide therapeutic levels for 20 min to 2 h, respectively (Court et al 1987).

In humans, mild side-effects include muscle weakness, sedation, dizziness, nausea, vomiting, constipation, increased urinary frequency and hypotension (Plumb 1995). Dantrolene should not be used in horses with pre-existing liver disease, cardiac dysfunction or pulmonary disease. In the horse, preanesthetic administration of dantrolene has been associated with prolonged postanesthetic recumbency (Valverde et al 1990).

OTHER DRUGS AFFECTING SKELETAL MUSCLE

Phenytoin (diphenylhydantoin) sodium

Phenytoin is a hydantoin derivative like dantrolene and the oldest non-sedative anticonvulsant drug known. It alters sodium, potassium and calcium conductance across cell membranes thereby altering membrane potentials and amino acid and neurotransmitter concentrations (i.e. norepinephrine (noradrenaline), acetylcholine and GABA). Its major mode of action appears to be the blockade of sodium channels and the inhibition of the generation of repetitive action potentials (membrane stabilization) (see Chs 9 and 12).

After oral administration to horses, peak serum concentrations are achieved in 1–4 h. However, phenytoin is poorly absorbed and has a bioavailability of 34.5 ± 8.6%. Its half-life is 8 h (Kowalczyk & Beech 1983).

Phenytoin is not used commonly in horses. It has been used to manage seizures and has been recommended for use in horses with chronic exertional rhabdomyolysis (Beech et al 1998) with variable success. Administration of phenytoin at oral dose rates of 2.83–16.43 mg/kg three times a day produces serum levels of 5–10 µg/ml, which are sufficient for the treatment of seizures (Kowalczyk & Beech 1983; see Ch. 9). Phenytoin is rarely used for the long-term treatment of horses (Plumb 1995). In dogs, chronic use has been associated with anorexia, vomiting, ataxia and sedation. Hepatocellular hypertrophy and necrosis, hepatic lipidosis and extramedullary hematopoiesis have also been reported in dogs. Liver function should be monitored during treatment.

Anabolic steroids

Anabolic steroids are synthetic derivatives of testosterone. All have some androgenic activity depending upon their dosage and length of use and are, therefore, also known as anabolic–androgenic steroids.

Anabolic steroids decrease catabolism and increase skeletal muscle protein synthesis. Whether this results in muscular hypertrophy or hyperplasia, or a combination of these, is unclear and probably depends upon the muscle studied. Different muscle types contain different cytosolic receptor numbers and, therefore, the response to anabolic steroids varies. Anabolic steroids initiate an increase in RNA polymerase activity and the synthesis of either structural or contractile proteins. In some muscles, anabolic steroids may increase the ratio of fast twitch to slow twitch fibers (Nimmo et al 1982, Snow et al 1982). Increased activity of enzymes involved in energy metabolism may also occur. However, the total glycogen content may remain unchanged (Hyyppa et al 1997). The effects are most profound in females and castrated males (Snow 1993).

Anabolic steroids promote muscle development and, therefore, potentially enhance performance. Their use is forbidden or monitored closely in most countries. Sophisticated methodologies exist to detect these substances and their metabolites and to discriminate them from naturally occurring androgenic hormones in the blood and urine. Anabolic steroids may be employed as adjunctive therapy in horses with debilitating conditions or chronic liver disease, anemia and postsurgical

Table 8.2 Dose rate and treatment regimen for anabolic steroids in horses

Steroid	Dosage
Nandrolone phenylpropionate	1.1 mg/kg every 2–4 weeks as required
Nandrolone laurate	1.1 mg/kg every 4 weeks
Boldenone undecyclenate	1.1 mg/kg every 3 weeks by deep intramuscular injection
Stanozolol	0.55 mg/kg once weekly
Methandriol dipropionate	0.75 mg/kg every 2 weeks

catabolism. It has also been suggested that occasional use of anabolic steroids may protect against the catabolic side-effects of chronic corticosteroid therapy in some horses (Snow 1993).

Anabolic steroid are metabolized and conjugated in the liver before excretion. The synthetic anabolic steroids are produced by modifying the basic structure of testosterone, a 19-carbon steroid with methyl groups at C18 and C19. The basic compounds are metabolized relatively quickly. The addition of an ester chain to the 17-hydroxyl group prolongs the activity of the basic compound. Depending on the type of ester group added, the duration of action is increased to several days to several weeks. The compounds employed most commonly in equine practice are nandrolone, boldenone, stanozolol and methandriol. Trenbolone and methandienone (methandrostenolone) are used less frequently. To further slow absorption, preparations are oil based and these are generally administered by deep i.m. injection (Table 8.2).

The adverse effects of anabolic steroids depend upon the total dosage and the frequency of administration. Most commonly androgenic signs are seen. In addition, behavior changes including aggression, increased tendency to bite, flehmen, erection (in males) and mounting of other horses may be seen. Depending on the formulation and product used, these signs may persist for weeks to months after treatment. Long-term use in colts and stallions may reduce testicular size and decrease spermatogenesis, sperm output and sperm quality. In fillies and mares, long-term use may delay the onset of puberty, reduce ovarian size, suppress ovulation, increase the rates of early embryonic death and produce clitoral enlargement. Although most of these signs abate after the withdrawal of treatment, clitoral enlargement may be permanent.

REFERENCES

Beech J, Fletcher J E, Johnston J et al 1998 Effect of phenytoin on the clinical signs and in vitro muscle twitch characteristics of horses with chronic intermittent rhabdomyolysis and myotonia. American Journal of Veterinary Research 49:2130–2133

Clark W G, Brater D C, Johnson A R 1992 Drug absorption and distribution In: Clark W G, Brater D C, Johnson A R (eds) Goth's medical pharmacology, 13th edn. Mosby, St Louis, MO, pp. 33–40

Court M H, Engelking L R, Dodman N H et al 1987 Pharmacokinetics of dantrolene sodium in horses. Journal of Veterinary Pharmacology and Therapeutics 10:218–226

Cunningham F E, Fisher J H, Bevelle C et al 1992 The pharmacokinetics of methocarbamol in the thoroughbred racehorse. Journal of Veterinary Pharmacology and Therapeutics 15:96–100

De La Corte F D, Valberg S J, MacLeay J M et al 1999a Glucose uptake in horses with polysaccharide storage myopathy. American Journal of Veterinary Research 60:458–462

De La Corte F D, Valberg S J, Mickelson J R et al 1999b Blood glucose clearance after feeding and exercise in polysaccharide storage myopathy. Equine Veterinary Journal Supplement 30:324–328

Freestone J F, Carlson G P 1991 Muscle disorders in the horse: a retrospective study. Equine Veterinary Journal 23:86–89

Hyyppa S, Karvonen U, Rasanen L A et al 1997 Androgen receptors and skeletal composition in trotters treated with nandrolone laureate. Zentralblatt für Veterinarmedizin Reihe A 44:481–491

Klein L 1989 Post-anesthetic equine myopathy suggestive of malignant hyperthermia. A case report. Veterinary Surgery 18:479–482

Kowalczyk D F, Beech J 1983 Pharmacokinetics of phenytoin (diphenylhydantoin) in horses. Journal of Veterinary Pharmacology and Therapeutics 6:133–140

Lentz L R, Valberg S J, Balog E M et al 1999 Abnormal regulation of muscle contraction in horses with recurrent exertional rhabdomyolysis. American Journal of Veterinary Reseach 60:992–999

Leuwer M, Motsch P 1996 Neuromuscular blocking agents and skeletal muscle relaxants. In: Dukes M N G (ed), Meyler's side-effects of drugs. Elsevier, Amsterdam, pp. 298–346

MacLeay J M, Valberg S J, Sorum S A et al 1999a Heritability of recurrent exertional rhabdomyolysis in thoroughbred racehorses. American Journal of Veterinary Research 60:250–256

MacLeay J M, Sorum S A, Valberg S J et al 1999b Epidemiologic analysis of factors influencing exertional rhabdomyolysis in thoroughbreds. American Journal of Veterinary Research 60:1562–1566

Miller R D 1995 Skeletal muscle relaxants. In: Katzung B G (ed) Basic and clinical pharmacology. Appleton & Lange, Norwalk, NJ, pp. 404–418

Muir W W, Hubbell J A E 1989 Handbook of veterinary anesthesia. Mosby, Toronto, p. 340

Muir W W, Sams R A, Ashcraft S 1984 Pharmacologic and pharmacokinetic properties of methocarbamol in the horse. American Journal of Veterinary Research 45:2256–2260

Nimmo M A, Snow D H, Munro C D 1982 Effects of nandrolone phenylpropionate in the horse: (3) skeletal muscle composition in the exercising animal. Equine Veterinary Journal 14:229–233

Plumb D C 1995 Veterinary drug handbook, 2nd pocket edn. Iowa State University Press, Ames, IA, p. 790

Robinson N E 1987 Table of common drugs: approximate doses. In: Robinson N E (ed) Current therapy in equine medicine. Saunders, Philadelphia, PA, p. 761

Snow D H 1993 Anabolic steroids. In: Hinchcliff KW, Sams R A (eds), Drug use in performance horses. Saunders, Philadelphia, PA, pp. 563–576

Snow D H, Munro C D, Nimmo M A 1982 Effects of nandrolone phenylpropionate in the horse: (1) resting animal. Equine Veterinary Journal 14:219–223

Valberg S J, Hodgson D R 1996 Diseases of muscle. In: Smith B P (ed) Large animal internal medicine. Mosby, St Louis, MO, pp. 1489–1518

Valberg S J, Geyer C, Sorum S A et al 1996 Familial basis of exertional rhabdomyolysis in quarter horse-related breeds. American Journal of Veterinary Research 57:286–290

Valberg S J, Mickelson J R, Gallant E M et al 1999 Exertional rhabdomyolysis in quarter horses and thoroughbreds: one syndrome, multiple aetiologies. Equine Veterinary Journal Supplement 30:533–538

Valentine B A 1999 Polysaccharide storage myopathy in draft and draft-related horses and ponies. Equine Practice 21:16–19

Valentine B A, Hintz H F, Freels K M et al 1998 Dietary control of exertional rhabdomyolysis in horses. Journal of the American Veterinary Medical Association 212:1588–1593

Valverde A, Boyd C J, Dyson D H et al 1990 Prophylactic use of dantrolene associated with prolonged post-anesthetic recumbency in a horse. Journal of the American Veterinary Medical Association 197:1051–1053

Ward T L, Valberg S J, Gallant E M et al 2000 Calcium regulation by skeletal muscle membranes of horses with recurrent exertional rhabdomyolysis. American Journal of Veterinary Research 61:242–247

CHAPTER CONTENTS

Therapy of infections 145
  Equine protozoal myeloencephalitis 145

Anti-inflammatory therapy in central nervous
system disorders 147

Therapy of seizures 149

Therapy of behavioral disorders 151

References 152

9

Drugs acting on the neurological system and behavior modification

Patricia M. Dowling

THERAPY OF INFECTIONS

EQUINE PROTOZOAL MYELOENCEPHALITIS

Equine protozoal myeloencephalitis (EPM) is a multifocal, progressive disease of the central nervous system (CNS) caused by infection with the protozoal parasite *Sarcocystis neurona*. The parasite biology, pathogenesis, clinical signs, diagnosis and details of treatment are covered in detail in Chapter 3. A short review of the four different classes of drug (or drug combinations) used in treatment of EPM is included here:

- potentiated sulfonamides (pyrimethamine plus sulfadiazine);
- benzeneacetonitriles (diclazuril);
- symmetrical triazinones (toltrazuril, ponazuril); and
- nitrothiazoles (nitazoxanide).

These drugs are considered further in Chapters 2 and 3.

One of the problems with the diagnosis and treatment of EPM is that the sensitivity and specificity of the tests available currently to diagnose this disease continue to be debated and antibodies to *S. neurona* may persist in the cerebrospinal fluid (CSF), making it difficult to evaluate treatment efficacy. A negative result on Western blot of a CSF sample is evidence of absence of infection (Daft et al 2002). It also indicates resolution of infection and is the most reliable predictor that a horse will not relapse if the treatment is discontinued.

Potentiated sulfonamides

A combination of pyrimethamine (1.0 mg/kg orally, once daily) and sulfadiazine (20–30 mg/kg daily orally) is commonly recommended for the treatment of EPM in horses (Fenger 1997). Pyrimethamine is a diaminopyrimidine dihydrofolate reductase (DHFR) inhibitor that has greater activity against protozoa than bacteria but is not approved for use in horses. The combination of pyrimethamine with a sulfonamide has synergistic activity against coccidia (Lindsay & Dubey 1999, Sheffield & Melton 1975). Of the sulfonamides, sulfadiazine is recommended because of its documented synergism with pyrimethamine against *Toxoplasma* spp. and its comparatively higher apparent volume of distribution than other sulfonamides.

In the past, EPM was treated using a trimethoprim-containing potentiated sulfonamide in combination with pyrimethamine, mainly because of the difficulty in finding sulfonamide formulations without trimethoprim. However, trimethoprim adds little to the antisarcocystis activity but is believed to increase the risk of hematological toxicity (Fenger et al 1997). Currently, there are numerous veterinary pharmacies in the USA that will compound pyrimethamine with sulfadiazine for the treatment of horses with EPM.

Pyrimethamine should be administered once daily, as high peak drug levels appear necessary to achieve therapeutic concentrations in the CNS (Clarke et al 1992). Hay and complete grain contain sufficient folic acid to interfere with pyrimethamine absorption, so the dose should be administered on an empty stomach. This is most easily achieved by administering it by dose syringe, which also ensures that underdosing is avoided. Some horses will demonstrate an acute exacerbation of clinical signs after beginning treatment. This "treatment crisis" is thought to result from CNS inflammation occurring in response to dead and dying merozoites; it should be treated with anti-inflammatory drugs.

The recommendations for duration of therapy are controversial. The majority of horses show some response to therapy within 2 weeks. Pyrimethamine plus sulfadiazine is usually administered for at least 3 months but must sometimes continue for 4 months or more to achieve clinical resolution. Clinical signs recur in some horses and it is not clear whether these are relapses or reinfection. When relapses occur, it is presumed that some degree of protozoal resistance has developed to the antimicrobial agents and the duration of treatment should be prolonged. Some horses must remain on therapy for life.

Prolonged therapy with antifolate medication requires biweekly monitoring for signs of bone marrow suppression, such as anemia, thrombocytopenia and neutropenia (Fenger et al 1997). Folic acid deficiency is known to be teratogenic in humans and results in neural tube defects. Supplementation with folate, folinate and yeast are often recommended to prevent the hematological and teratogenic side-effects of chronic pyrimethamine therapy in horses (Brendemuehl et al 1998). Supplementation of mares with oral folic acid (40 mg/day) has been associated with abortions and congenital defects in foals (Toribio et al 1998). Studies in other species suggest that folic acid is not protective against or may even increase pyrimethamine toxicity. However, there was neither a reduction in pregnancy rates nor an increase in embryonic loss in mares receiving pyrimethamine and sulfadiazine with or without folic acid supplementation (Brendemuehl et al 1998). Therefore it is not yet known whether supplementation with 40 mg folic acid per day increases the risk of pyrimethamine toxicity or if this dose is insufficient and should be increased in pregnant mares.

Even if initial therapy is successful, some clinicians recommend periodically placing horses back on treatment following stress, which appears to play a role in the pathogenesis of EPM (Saville et al 2001). Other intermittent treatment regimens have also been used, such as treatment once every 2–4 weeks or daily during the first week of every month. However, such intermittent treatment may increase the risk of the development of resistance in *S. neurona* and is, therefore, not recommended. Poor responses to therapy have led to the use of increased dosages of pyrimethamine and sulfadiazine in horses that do not respond clinically within 30–60 days of commencing treatment.

Increasing the dose of pyrimethamine increases the risk of folic acid deficiency, so complete blood counts should be performed regularly to monitor bone marrow function.

Benzeneacetonitriles and symmetrical triazinones

Recently, triazine-based coccidiocidal drugs have been investigated for their potential efficacy in horses with EPM. Diclazuril is a poultry coccidiostat that is formulated as a premix (5 g/kg feed). Diclazuril has a terminal half-life of 43 h in the horse and steady-state concentrations of 100–250 ng/ml are reached in the CSF during repeated dosing (Dirikolu et al 1999), with concentrations of around 1 ng/ml in the CSF sufficient to produce 95% inhibition of *S. neurona* proliferation (Lindsay & Dubey 2000). Diclazuril has been used in the treatment of EPM in horses (Granstrom et al 1997); however, at the suggested dose rate of 5 mg/kg (2.5 g/450 kg horse), the horse has to consume large volumes of the premix daily. In addition, the poultry premix has to be imported into the USA from Canada. A more concentrated pellet formulation of diclazuril is currently in clinical trials in horses in the USA.

The triazine anticoccidial drugs are absorbed after oral administration in horses and have long plasma half-lives (Tobin et al 1997). Toltrazuril is used to treat coccidiosis in swine. This product is not available in the USA but can be imported from Canada. Ponazuril is an active metabolite of toltrazuril that, at concentrations of 5.0 μg/ml, is 95% effective at inhibiting the production of merozoites by *S. neurona in vitro* (Lindsay et al 2000). Evidence suggests that both toltrazuril and ponazuril are efficacious in some horses with EPM, with a shorter duration of therapy than with pyrimethamine plus sulfadiazine (Furr et al 2001).

Ponazuril formulated as a paste has recently been approved for use in horses in the USA. The elimination half-life of ponazuril in the horse is 4.5 days. Ponazuril administered once daily for 28 days at a dose rate of 5 mg/kg appears to be well tolerated in the horse (Kennedy et al 2001).

Nitrothiazoles

The broad-spectrum anthelmintic nitazoxanide has been undergoing efficacy trials in the USA for the treatment of EPM (Vatistas et al 1999). This drug is currently used to combat intestinal parasites of humans in developing countries and in patients with the acquired immunodeficiency syndrome complicated by secondary protozoal infections. Nitazoxanide is administered daily for 28 days as an oral paste. The side-effects of this drug are more serious than with other medications because it kills other parasites in addition to *S. neurona*. This has led to recommendations for deworming with another anthelmintic prior to starting this treatment (McClure & Palma 1999). Nitazoxanide may also cause colic in treated horses.

ANTI-INFLAMMATORY THERAPY IN CENTRAL NERVOUS SYSTEM DISORDERS

Anti-inflammatory agents are discussed in detail in Chapter 14. Their relevance in the treatment of CNS disorders is discussed further here.

Glucocorticoids

Glucocorticoids are recommended for the treatment of CNS disorders as they stabilize microvascular permeability, reduce edema formation, reduce intracranial pressure, decrease oxygen-derived free radicals and prevent post-traumatic autodestruction of nervous tissue. Their clinical use in equine medicine includes the treatment of brain and spinal cord trauma, cerebral edema associated with neonatal maladjustment syndrome (NMS), endotoxic shock and EPM. This is despite the fact that the safety and efficacy of glucocorticoids in the treatment of many types of nervous system inflammation has not been established and their use and dosing schedules continue to be debated.

In the cat, there is some evidence that supports the efficacy of intravenous (i.v.) methylprednisolone sodium succinate when administered within 1 h of acute spinal cord trauma (Fukaya et al 2003). Other glucocorticoid formulations have been used widely in veterinary medicine for a variety of CNS insults but their clinical efficacy is debatable, especially when therapy is delayed. For emergency treatment of trauma or NMS, rapidly acting succinate or phosphate esters are given intravenously (i.v.). Dexamethasone sodium phosphate, methylprednisolone sodium succinate and prednisolone sodium succinate are available but their cost means that their use is limited to neonatal foals and extremely valuable adult horses. Consequently, free alcohol formulations of dexamethasone or prednisone are used more commonly. These contain the carrier polyethylene glycol, which is associated with adverse CNS effects; therefore, high doses of these formulations are not recommended for i.v. administration.

In the past, glucocorticoids were considered contraindicated in the treatment of bacterial infections of the CNS. The anti-inflammatory effects of glucocorticoids have been studied in animal models of meningitis (Syrogiannopoulos et al 1987). Treatment with methylprednisolone or dexamethasone reduced CSF outflow resistance, brain edema and intracranial pressure. The efficacy of dexamethasone as an adjunct to cephalosporin treatment has been investigated in controlled trials in infants and children (Odio et al 1991). When dexamethasone was administered prior to the antimicrobial agent, patients had lower CSF pressure, less inflammation and lower cytokine concentrations in the CSF. Although the survival rates in the two groups were similar, the dexamethasone-treated patients developed fewer neurological sequelae. Glucocorticoid-associated adverse effects were rare and glucocorticoid use did not delay sterilization of the CSF. The American Academy of Pediatricians now endorses the use of glucocorticoids together with antimicrobial agents for therapy of childhood meningitis.

The timing of glucocorticoid administration is crucial; therefore, their use in the treatment of equine neonatal septicemia may be limited, unless diagnosis is prompt. Glucocorticoids may reduce the efficacy of EPM treatment by inhibiting the immune response of the horse to the sarcocystis parasite. Administration of dexamethasone to horses with EPM is controversial but recommended if a "treatment crisis" occurs.

Non-steroidal anti-inflammatory drugs

Non-steroidal anti-inflammatory drugs (NSAIDs) are more useful than the glucocorticoids in the treatment of CNS inflammation in horses. In animal models of meningitis, NSAIDs effectively reduce the influx of leukocytes and the elevation of protein concentration in the CSF (Tuomanen et al 1987). NSAIDs (e.g. flunixin meglumine, ketoprofen, vedaprofen or phenylbutazone) are recommended routinely for acute treatment of horses with clinical signs of EPM. A large number of studies performed in horses support the use of flunixin meglumine as adjunctive therapy in septicemia and endotoxic shock (Bottoms et al 1981, Dunkle et al 1985, Ewert et al 1985, Templeton et al 1987). Flunixin is superior to phenylbutazone for treating endotoxemia, because of a greater ability of flunixin to inhibit thromboxane A_2 production. In an endotoxemia model in calves, ketoprofen was as effective as flunixin in ameliorating the clinical signs (Semrad 1993).

Dimethyl sulfoxide

The organic solvent dimethyl sulfoxide (DMSO) has a wide range of pharmacological actions (Jacob & Herschler 1986). The intraarticular use of this agent is discussed in Chapter 7. A short discussion on DMSO including its use in the treatment of CNS trauma and cerebral edema in horses is included here.

The benefits of DMSO derive from its anti-inflammatory actions, which largely result from its ability to scavenge hydroxyl radicals that are released from neutrophils and macrophages in inflammatory processes and from cells injured by ischemia or ionizing radiation. The membrane-stabilizing effects of DMSO reduce the release of inflammatory mediators. DMSO also produces analgesia in some kinds of pain by slowing nerve conduction (Evans et al 1993).

DMSO (90%) gel or liquid is approved for topical use in horses in the USA. However, liquid or industrial grade DMSO solutions are commonly used in clinical practice as a 10% solution diluted in saline for i.v. administration to horses at a dose rate of 1 g/kg (Blythe et al 1986). DMSO is distributed widely into all tissues after i.v. administration to horses and is excreted, predominantly unchanged, in urine. Based on its half-life, DMSO should be administered i.v. twice daily for the treatment of increased intracranial pressure and/or cerebral edema in horses (Blythe et al 1986). Foals with NMS caused by birth hypoxia may benefit from treatment with DMSO to relieve cerebral edema (Del Bigio et al 1982). DMSO, once daily for 3 days, either i.v. or via nasogastric tube, is also recommended in the acute treatment of EPM (Green et al 1990).

The administration of DMSO is accompanied by few problems and is relatively safe. However, concentrations higher than 10% administered i.v. may cause intravascular hemolysis, diarrhea, muscle tremors and colic. Ocular toxicity and teratogenicity have been reported in laboratory animals treated with DMSO. In addition, the cutaneous absorption of DMSO may cause sedation, dizziness, headache or nausea in certain individuals. Because of these potential adverse effects, users, especially pregnant women, should take care to avoid contact when applying DMSO. Another major concern is the ability of DMSO to translocate other chemicals (Brayton 1986). Despite this, the i.v. administration of DMSO does not increase the CSF concentrations of trimethoprim or sulfamethoxazole (Green et al 1990).

THERAPY OF SEIZURES

Seizures occur more infrequently in horses than in dogs and cats. Seizures are seen in adult horses from brain trauma, bacterial meningitis, viral encephalitis and, rarely, hepatic encephalopathy or vascular accidents. Convulsions are seen in young neonatal foals with NMS as a result of brain hypoxia and in Arabian foals aged 3–9 months (idiopathic Arabian epilepsy). Anticonvulsant therapy is used to prevent the spread of the seizure focus, increase (raise) the seizure threshold and decrease the electrical excitement of abnormal

neurons without disrupting normal function. The duration of therapy depends on the underlying condition, for example foals with NMS and Arabian foals improve with time.

Phenobarbital

Phenobarbital is the most commonly used anticonvulsant in horses as it has effects at doses lower than those that produce sedation. It potentiates the actions of gamma-aminobutyric acid (GABA), the inhibitory neurotransmitter in the CNS. Neuronal stabilization by GABA in postsynaptic neurons occurs from increased intracellular chloride conductance, which hyperpolarizes the membrane; the overall result is an increase in the seizure threshold and a decrease in the electrical activity of the seizure focus.

Phenobarbital is absorbed rapidly and well after oral administration to horses, with bioavailability approaching 100% (Ravis et al 1987). It is distributed widely into the tissues but, because of its lower lipid solubility, does not distribute into the CNS as rapidly as other barbiturates. After i.v. administration, it may take 15–20 min before therapeutic concentrations of phenobarbital are reached in the CNS. Phenobarbital primarily undergoes hepatic metabolism and only 25% is excreted as unchanged drug. The half-lives reported in horses, around 18–24 h (Duran et al 1987, Knox et al 1982, Ravis et al 1987) and 12 h in foals (Spear et al 1984), are substantially shorter than in other species, meaning that steady-state concentrations can be achieved more rapidly.

In the acute management of seizures in horses, phenobarbital is administered i.v. In foals, it has been recommended that a loading dose of phenobarbital, administered i.v. at a dose rate of 20 mg/kg, is followed by maintenance doses of 9 mg/kg i.v. three times a day (Spear et al 1984). In adult horses, a loading dose of 12 mg/kg i.v. followed by 6.65 mg/kg as a 20 min infusion twice daily has been proposed (Duran et al 1987). Long-term therapy is usually administered by the oral route with a dose rate of 11 mg/kg once every 24 h proposed (Ravis et al 1987).

Therapeutic drug monitoring is necessary to ensure appropriate plasma concentrations of phenobarbital. Initial samples should be taken once steady-state concentrations have been reached, after 4 days in adult horses and 3 days in foals (five to six half-lives have elapsed). Samples are usually taken to assess peak and trough plasma concentrations (i.e. a few hours after a dose is administered and just before the next dose). The suggested therapeutic plasma concentrations, extrapolated from data in other species, are 15–45 μg/ml (70–175 μmol/l).

Phenobarbital stimulates the microsomal enzymes in the liver. This results in increases in liver enzyme concentrations and more rapid metabolism of not only phenobarbital but also other concurrently administered drugs. In the horse, it has been shown that the half-life of phenobarbital decreases (to around 11 h) following repeated oral dosing (Knox et al 1982). Dosage adjustments of phenobarbital may be required to maintain plasma concentrations within the therapeutic window and can be made using the equation:

$$\text{New dose} = \text{Old dose} \times \frac{\left[\begin{array}{c}\text{Target peak plasma}\\ \text{concentration}\end{array}\right]}{\left[\begin{array}{c}\text{Measured peak plasma}\\ \text{concentration}\end{array}\right]}$$

Phenytoin (diphenylhydantoin)

The anticonvulsant phenytoin (diphenylhydantoin) has been used in horses to treat hyperkalemic periodic paralysis and rhabdomyolysis (see Ch. 8) and cardiac arrhythmias (see Ch. 12). It is not usually used as an anticonvulsant in horses.

Potassium bromide

Potassium bromide is the oldest and chemically the simplest of the anticonvulsants. It was first used in 1857 to treat seizures in people. It was the sole effective anticonvulsant drug until the early 1900s when less-sedative drugs became available. Although it is rarely used in humans because of its toxicity, potassium bromide has become popular as a second anticonvulsant drug when seizures continue to occur in dogs and cats despite adequate plasma concentrations of phenobarbital (Dowling 1994).

Potassium bromide appears to stabilize neuronal cell membranes by interfering with chloride ion transport across them. It potentiates the effect of GABA by hyperpolarizing the membrane. Other drugs with GABAergic activity, such as the barbiturates, may act synergistically with potassium bromide to raise the seizure threshold.

Anecdotal evidence suggests that potassium bromide may be useful in horses when phenobarbital therapy is ineffective (J. Bertone, personal communication, 2001). The suggested dose is 35 mg/kg orally every 24 h. The therapeutic range is suggested to be approximately 1–2 mg/ml in combination with phenobarbital and up to 3 mg/ml when used as monotherapy (Trepanier et al 1998).

Diazepam

The use of diazepam in equine anesthesia is covered in Chapter 15. Although all of the benzodiazepines have some anticonvulsant activity, diazepam is the most popular for treatment of status epilepticus because it is distributed rapidly to the CNS after i.v. administration. The limbic, thalamic and hypothalamic areas of the CNS are depressed by diazepam, resulting in its anxiolytic, sedative, skeletal muscle relaxant and anticonvulsant effects.

Diazepam hyperpolarizes neurons and suppresses neuronal activity by binding to a specific GABA-binding site. It may modify the GABA-binding sites and increase the action of GABA on nerve cells. As anticonvulsants, the benzodiazepines act to suppress the presynaptic transmission of seizure activity.

In horses, diazepam is distributed widely to the tissues and metabolized extensively; the values quoted for elimination half-life range from 3 to 22 h (Muir et al 1982). High doses of benzodiazepines cause muscle weakness, facial and neck muscle fasciculations, ataxia and recumbency. In neonatal foals, the i.v. administration of benzodiazepines can cause respiratory depression or arrest, through accumulation (Norman et al 1997), so resuscitation equipment should be available and repeated doses should be administered with extreme care.

In foals that have been overdosed, the benzo-diazepine antagonist flumazenil may be of help (see Ch. 15).

THERAPY OF BEHAVIORAL DISORDERS

Behavioral disorders and stereotypies are common in horses (Waters et al 2002). There are anecdotal reports of the use of the tricyclic antidepressants and buspirone in horses; however, pharmacological intervention is uncommon, partly because of expense. Before prescribing any drug for problem behavior, the clinician should have (i) a reasonable diagnosis; (ii) an appreciation for the mechanism of action of the drug; (iii) a clear understanding of the potential side-effects; (iv) an understanding of how the drug will specifically alter the problem behavior; and (v) an understanding of the potential for abuse (unethical use).

Headshaking behavior (photic headshaking) in horses has been associated with exposure to bright light, in a manner similar to photic sneezing in humans, where light causes an optic–infraorbital nerve summation and pain (Whitman & Packer 1993). The disorder is more common in geldings and appears to be seasonal with onset in the spring (Madigan & Bell 2001). Affected horses typically snort and sneeze and rub their noses on a forelimb when exercised in daylight.

Endogenous opioids may be involved in equine stereotypies. Opioid release is facilitated by a stress-primed system and may sensitize dopaminergic mechanisms involved in the stereo-typic behavior.

Cyproheptadine

Some horses exhibiting signs of photic headshaking respond favorably to treatment with the antihistamine drug cyproheptadine (Wilkins 1997). In addition to antihistaminic action, cyproheptadine has anticholinergic action and is a 5-hydroxytryptamine (serotonin) antagonist, altering proopiomelanocortin peptide metabolism

(see Ch. 5). Cyproheptadine appears to moderate infraorbital nerve sensation but the mechanism is not known. Relief from the behavior is usually seen within 24 h of beginning cyproheptadine therapy and often resumes within 24 h of discontinuing therapy. Mild side-effects, depression, lethargy and anorexia, may be noted. Other antihistamines are not effective at eliminating headshaking.

Hormonal therapy

Some clinicians believe that seasonal increases in follicle-stimulating hormone (FSH) and luteinizing hormone (LH) cause neurochemical instability of the trigeminal ganglion and nerve that may be involved in photic headshaking (Madigan et al 1995). In order to mimic the hormonal status of winter, affected horses can be given 10 mg melatonin orally once daily starting in October. The progestagen altrenogest can be given daily to inhibit FSH and LH production. Horses on this type of therapy will not shed their winter haircoat normally in the spring.

Opioid antagonists

The opioid antagonists naloxone, nalmefene and diprenorphine have been successfully used to control stereotypic behavior, such as self-mutilation and crib-biting, in horses (Dodman et al 1987, 1988). However, these drugs must be administered parenterally and are prohibitively expensive.

Fluphenazine

Short-acting phenothiazine drugs are used commonly in equine practice for sedation and restraint (see Ch. 15), while long-acting phenothiazines are used in human patients as antipyschotic agents.

The phenothiazine drugs act by blocking dopamine receptors in the limbic system. Unfortunately, phenothiazines also block dopamine in the striatum, upsetting the balance between dopamine and acetylcholine and resulting in side-effects known as extrapyramidal motor signs. These signs include bradykinesia, muscle rigidity, involuntary muscle spasms of the head, neck and proximal extremities, and akathisia (motor restlessness causing the patient to pace or rock); they have also been reported in the horse (Brewer et al 1990).

Depot formulations of fluphenazine in humans have an onset of action of 24–72 h and duration of 1–6 weeks (Jann et al 1985). These formulations have been used in horses for a long-lasting sedative effect and as a result may be abused, since plasma and urine concentrations rapidly decline below the limit of detection of the available assays. Fluphenazine can cause dramatic extrapyramidal motor signs in horses within 12 h of administration of the decanoate or enanthate esters (Kauffman et al 1989). Horses exhibiting extrapyramidal motor signs can be extremely dangerous to humans. Restoring the dopamine–acetylcholine balance by the i.v. administration of anticholinergic drugs, such as diphenhydramine hydrochloride, reverses these effects.

Reserpine

Reserpine is a Rauwolfia alkaloid that has been used for centuries to treat insanity, insomnia and hypertension in humans. Reserpine inhibits normal sympathetic activity in both the CNS and the peripheral nervous system by binding to catecholamine storage vesicles, causing catecholamines to leak into the synapse so that they are not available for release when the presynaptic neuron is stimulated. This prevents the normal magnesium and ATP-dependent storage of catecholamines and 5-hydroxytryptamine in nerve cells, the result being catecholamine (norepinephrine (noradrenaline)) depletion. This results in the inhibition of normal sympathetic activity.

Purified reserpine was one of the first of the modern tranquillizers, acting by reducing 5-hydroxytryptamine concentrations, but it was associated with severe side-effects in humans. Low-dose oral reserpine (5 mg) has been used in the treatment of postpartum mares with agalactia caused by fescue toxicosis and resulted in serum reserpine concentrations that were below the limit of detection of a commercial enzyme-linked immunosorbant assay (ELISA) kit (see Ch. 11). Once the latter became widely known, oral reserpine became used widely in performance horses for its sedative effects because of its efficacy at extremely low doses, difficulty of detection (Chapman et al 1991) and long duration of action.

The side-effects of reserpine include hypotension, bradycardia and increased gastrointestinal motility and diarrhea (Lloyd et al 1985), all resulting from decreased sympathetic tone and increased parasympathetic tone. The hypotensive effects of reserpine may take days to several weeks to occur but may persist for 1 to 6 weeks after the withdrawal of the drug. Administration of induction agents, such as xylazine and ketamine, that produce hypotension may be fatal in horses treated with reserpine.

REFERENCES

Blythe L L, Craig A M, Christensen J M et al 1986 Pharmacokinetic disposition of dimethyl sulfoxide administered intravenously to horses. American Journal of Veterinary Research 47:1739–1743

Bottoms G D, Fessler J F, Roesel O F et al 1981 Endotoxin-induced hemodynamic changes in ponies: effects of flunixin meglumine. American Journal of Veterinary Research 42:1514–1518

Brayton C F 1986 Dimethyl sulfoxide (DMSO): a review. Cornell Veterinarian 76:61–90

Brendemuehl J P, Waldridge B M, Bridges E R 1998 Effects of sulfadiazine and pyrimethamine and concurrent folic acid supplementation on pregnancy and embryonic loss rates in mares. In: Proceedings of the 44th American Association of Equine Practitioners Annual Convention, Baltimore, MD, pp. 142–143

Brewer B D, Hines M T, Stewart J T 1990 Fluphenazine induced Parkinson-like syndrome in a horse. Equine Veterinary Journal 22:136–137

Chapman C B, Courage P, Huntington P J 1991 Detection of reserpine in horses by high-performance liquid chromatography. Australian Veterinary Journal 68:296–298

Clarke C R, Burrows G E, MacAllister C G et al 1992 Pharmacokinetics of intravenously and orally administered pyrimethamine in horses. American Journal of Veterinary Research 53:2292–2295

Daft B M, Barr B C, Gardner I A et al 2002 Sensitivity and specificity of Western blot testing of cerebrospinal fluid and serum for diagnosis of equine protozoal myeloencephalitis in horses with and without neurologic abnormalities. Journal of the American Veterinary Medical Association 221:1007–1013

Del Bigio M, James H E, Camp P E et al 1982 Acute dimethyl sulfoxide therapy in brain edema. Part 3: effect of a 3-hour infusion. Neurosurgery 10:86–89

Dirikolu L, Lehner F, Nattrass C et al 1999 Diclazuril in the horse: its identification and detection and preliminary pharmacokinetics. Journal of Veterinary Pharmacology and Therapeutics 22:374–379

Dodman N H, Shuster L, Court M H et al 1987 Investigation into the use of narcotic antagonists in the treatment of a stereotypic behaviour pattern (crib-biting) in the horse. American Journal of Veterinary Research 48:311–319

Dodman N H, Shuster L, Court M H et al 1988 Use of a narcotic antagonist (nalmefene) to suppress self-mutilative behaviour in a stallion. Journal of the American Veterinary Medical Association 192:1585–1586

Dowling P M 1994 Management of canine epilepsy with phenobarbital and potassium bromide. Canadian Veterinary Journal 35:724–725

Dunkle N J, Bottoms G D, Fessler J F et al 1985 Effects of flunixin meglumine on blood pressure and fluid volume compartment changes in ponies given endotoxin. American Journal of Veterinary Research 46:1540–1544

Duran S H, Ravis W R, Pedersoli W M et al 1987 Pharmacokinetics of phenobarbital in the horse. American Journal of Veterinary Research 48:807–810

Evans M S, Reid K H, Sharp J B 1993 Dimethylsulfoxide (DMSO) blocks conduction in peripheral nerve C fibers: a possible mechanism of analgesia. Neuroscience Letters 150:145

Ewert K M, Fessler J F, Templeton C B et al 1985 Endotoxin-induced hematologic and blood chemical changes in ponies: effects of flunixin meglumine, dexamethasone, and prednisolone. American Journal of Veterinary Research 46:24–30

Fenger C K 1997 Pyrimethamine-sulfonamide dosage and treatment duration recommendations for equine protozoal myeloencephalitis: findings from a retrospective. In: Proceedings of the 15th Annual American College of Veterinary Internal Medicine Forum, Lake Buena Vista, FL, pp. 484–485

Fenger C K, Granstrom D E, Langemeier J L et al 1997 Epizootic of equine protozoal myeloencephalitis on a farm. Journal of the American Veterinary Medical Association 210:923–927

Fukaya C, Katayama Y, Kasai M et al 2003 Evaluation of time-dependent spread of tissue damage in experimental spinal cord injury by killed-end evoked potential: effect of high-dose methylprednisolone. Journal of Neurosurgery 98(suppl 1):56–62

Furr M, Kennedy T, MacKay R et al 2001 Efficacy of ponazuril 15% oral paste as a treatment for equine protozoal myeloencephalitis. Veterinary Therapeutics 2:215–222

Granstrom D E, McCrillis S, Wuff-Strobel C et al 1997 Diclazuril and equine protozoal myeloencephalitis. In: Proceedings of the 43rd American Association of Equine Practitioners Annual Convention, Phoenix, AZ, pp. 13–14

Green S L, Mayhew I G, Brown M P et al 1990 Concentrations of trimethoprim and sulfamethoxazole in cerebrospinal fluid and serum of mares with and without a dimethyl sulfoxide pretreatment. Canadian Journal of Veterinary Research 54:215–222

Jacob S W, Herschler R 1986 Pharmacology of DMSO. Cryobiology 23:14–27

Jann M W, Ereshefsky L, Saklad S R 1985 Clinical pharmacokinetics of the depot antipsychotics. Clinical Pharmacokinetics 10:315–333

Kauffman V G, Soma L, Divers T J 1989 Extrapyramidal side-effects caused by fluphenazine decanoate in a horse. Journal of the American Veterinary Medical Association 195:1128–1130

Kennedy T, Campbell J, Selzer V 2001 Safety of ponazuril 15% oral paste in horses. Veterinary Therapeutics 2:223–231

Knox D A, Ravis W R, Pedersoli W M et al 1992 Pharmacokinetics of phenobarbital in horses after single and repeated oral administration of the drug. American Journal of Veterinary Research 53:706–710

Lindsay D S, Dubey J P 1999 Determination of the activity of pyrimethamine, trimethoprim, sulfonamides, and combinations of pyrimethamine and sulfonamides against Sarcocystis neurona in cell cultures. Veterinary Parasitology 82:205–210

Lindsay D S, Dubey J P 2000 Determination of the activity of diclazuril against Sarcocystis neurona and Sarcocystis falcatula in cell cultures. Journal of Parasitology 86:164–166

Lindsay D S, Dubey J P, Kennedy T J 2000 Determination of the activity of ponazuril against Sarcocystis neurona in cell cultures. Veterinary Parasitology 92:165–169

Lloyd K C, Harrison I, Tulleners E 1985 Reserpine toxicosis in a horse. Journal of the American Veterinary Medical Association 186:980–981

Madigan J E, Bell S A 2001 Owner survey of headshaking in horses. Journal of the American Veterinary Medical Association 219:334–337

Madigan J E, Kortz G, Murphy C et al 1995 Photic headshaking in the horse: 7 cases. Equine Veterinary Journal 27:306–311

McClure S R, Palma K G 1999 Treatment of equine protozoal myeloencephalitis with nitazoxanide. Journal of Equine Veterinary Science 19:639–641

Muir W E, Sams R A, Huffman R H et al 1982 Pharmacodynamic and pharmacokinetic properties of diazepam in horses. American Journal of Veterinary Research 43:756–1762

Norman W M, Court M H, Greenblatt D J 1997 Age-related changes in the pharmacokinetic disposition of diazepam in foals. American Journal of Veterinary Research 58:878–880

Odio C M, Faingezicht I, Paris M et al 1991 The beneficial effects of early dexamethasone administration in infants and children with bacterial meningitis. New England Journal of Medicine 324:1525–1531

Ravis W R, Duran S H, Pedersoli W M et al 1987 A pharmacokinetic study of phenobarbital in mature horses after oral dosing. Journal of Veterinary Pharmacology and Therapeutics 10:283–289

Saville W J, Stich R W, Reed S M et al 2001 Utilization of stress in the development of an equine model for equine protozoal myeloencephalitis. Veterinary Parasitology 95:211–222

Semrad S D 1993 Comparative efficacy of flunixin, ketoprofen, and ketorolac for treating endotoxemic neonatal calves. American Journal of Veterinary Research 54:1511–1516

Sheffield H G, Melton M L 1975 Effect of pyrimethamine and sulfadiazine on the fine structure and multiplication of *Toxoplasma gondii* in cell cultures. Journal of Parasitology 61:704–712

Spear A M, Hill M R, Mayhew I G et al 1984 Preliminary study on the pharmacokinetics of phenobarbital in the neonatal foal. Equine Veterinary Journal 16:368–371

Syrogiannopoulos G A, Olsen K D, Reisch J S et al 1987 Dexamethasone in the treatment of experimental *Haemophilus influenzae* type b meningitis. Journal of Infectious Diseases 155:213–219

Templeton C B, Bottoms G D, Fessler J F et al 1987 Endotoxin-induced hemodynamic and prostaglandin changes in ponies: effects of flunixin meglumine, dexamethasone, and prednisolone. Circulatory Shock 23:231–240

Tobin T, Dirikolu L, Harkins J D et al 1997 Preliminary pharmacokinetics of diclazuril and toltrazuril in the horse. In: Proceedings of the 43rd American Association of Equine Practitioners Annual Convention, Phoenix, AZ, pp. 15–16

Toribio R E, Bain F T, Mrad D R et al 1998 Congenital defects in newborn foals of mares treated for equine protozoal myeloencephalitis during pregnancy. Journal of the American Veterinary Medical Association 212:697–701

Trepanier L A, van Schoick A, Schwark W S et al 1998 Therapeutic serum drug concentrations in epileptic dogs treated with potassium bromide alone or in combination with other anticonvulsants: 122 cases (1992–1996). Journal of the American Veterinary Medical Association 213:1449–1453

Tuomanen E, Hengstler B, Rich R et al 1987 Nonsteroidal anti-inflammatory agents in the therapy for experimental pneumococcal meningitis. Journal of Infectious Diseases 155:985–990

Vatistas N, Fenger C, Palma K et al 1999 Initial experiences with the use of nitazoxanide in the treatment of equine protozoal encephalitis in northern California. Equine Practitioner 21:18–21

Waters A J, Nicol C J, French N P 2002 Factors influencing the development of stereotypic and redirected behaviours in young horses: findings of a 4 year prospective epidemiological study. Equine Veterinary Journal 34:572–579

Whitman B W, Packer R J 1993 The photic sneeze reflex: literature review and discussion. Neurology 43:868–871

Wilkins P A 1997 Cyproheptadine: medical treatment for photic headshakers. Compendium of Continuing Education for the Practicing Veterinarian 19:98–99

CHAPTER CONTENTS

Introduction 155

Renal dysfunction 155
  Increasing urine output 155
  Increasing renal blood flow 157
  Increasing glomerular filtration rate 158
  Effectiveness of drug therapy in acute
    renal failure 158

Urine output: diuretic agents 159
  Loop (high ceiling) diuretics 159
  Benzothiadiazides or thiazide-type
    diuretics 163
  Carbonic anhydrase inhibitors 165
  Osmotic diuretics 166
  Potassium-sparing diuretics 167
  Xanthines 168

Polyuria and polydipsia: antidiuretic agents 168

Urine retention and incontinence 169
  Treatment 170

Urolithiasis 172
  Urine acidifying agents 172

Urinary tract infections 172

References 174

10

Drugs acting on the urinary system

Harold C. Schott II

INTRODUCTION

Drugs acting on the urinary system include medications administered to increase renal blood flow (RBF) and urine output during periods of compromised renal function; diuretic agents given to increase urine output for a variety of reasons; antidiuretic agents used in the diagnostic evaluation and management of polyuria; autonomic drugs administered in an attempt to stimulate detrusor function or modulate urethral sphincter tone in cases of urine retention or incontinence; and medications used to decrease urine pH in the management of urolithiasis. Although presented in detail elsewhere in this book (see Ch. 2), antimicrobial therapy for urinary tract infections will also be discussed briefly with specific emphasis on the principles unique to the urinary system.

RENAL DYSFUNCTION

When renal function is compromised, treatment involves the use of drugs to increase RBF, glomerular filtration rate (GFR) and urine output. In equine patients with acute renal failure (ARF), furosemide (frusemide), dopamine and mannitol (Table 10.1) are the most common drugs utilized (Jose-Cunilleras & Hinchcliff 1999).

INCREASING URINE OUTPUT
Furosemide (Frusemide)

Furosemide (frusemide), a loop diuretic (p. 159), is usually the first medication administered in an

Table 10.1   Drugs used to increase renal blood flow and urine output in horses with oliguric acute renal failure

Drug	Mechanism of action	Advantages	Disadvantages
Furosemide (frusemide)	Loop diuretic: inhibits the $Na^+,K^+,2Cl^-$-cotransporter in the thick ascending limb of the loop of Henle	Initially administered as an i.v. bolus Fast acting (response within 1 h after administration) Increases urine excretion of Na^+ and water Few adverse effects Inexpensive	May not reach active site unless high doses are used High doses can precipitate transient vasoconstriction
Dopamine Low dose (0.5–3.0 µg/min per kg body weight)	Stimulation of the dopamine D_1 receptors on intrarenal vessels	Dilatation of renal arterioles leading to a selective increase in RBF Increases urine excretion of Na^+ and water May increase GFR	Constant i.v. infusion required Close patient monitoring required (in hospital treatment) May induce cardiac arrhythmias Greater risk of inducing arrhythmias
Intermediate dose (3–5 µg/min per kg body weight)	Also stimulates cardiac β_1 adrenoceptors	May further increase RBF by increasing cardiac output	
High dose (5–20 µg/min per kg body weight)	Also stimulates peripheral α_1 adrenoceptors	May improve blood pressure in hypotensive patients	Peripheral vasoconstriction may decrease RBF Even greater risk of inducing arrhythmias
Mannitol	Osmotic diuretic	Increases effective circulating volume and RBF May increase GFR May help to flush away debris that may obstruct the tubules May scavenge oxygen radicals	Constant i.v. infusion required May induce hyperosmolality High doses may precipitate acute renal failure

RBF, renal blood flow; GFR, glomerular filtration rate

attempt to increase urine output in oliguric ARF. However, there are several barriers that this drug must overcome in order to be effective. Firstly, the drug must reach the vasculature adjacent to the proximal renal tubules before secretion by organic acid pathways can occur (Hinchcliff & Muir 1991). Therefore, decreased RBF, as well as compromised function of proximal tubular epithelial cells, may limit furosemide (frusemide) entry into the nephron. Secondly, furosemide (frusemide) acts by blocking the sodium ion, potassium ion, chloride ion ($Na^+,K^+,2Cl^-$) cotransporter in the thick ascending limb of the loop of Henle (Hinchcliff & Muir 1991). Tubular obstruction by cellular debris, pigments or crystals can limit tubular flow and thus the amount of furosemide (frusemide) that will reach this segment of the nephron. Thirdly, furosemide (frusemide) is highly bound to albumin in plasma (Hinchcliff & Muir 1991). Increased filtration of protein across the glomerular basement membrane consequent to increased hydraulic pressure in the glomerular capillaries and increased permeability of the basement membrane in some forms of renal disease mean that furosemide (frusemide) may not be active (protein bound) in the renal tubule. For all of these reasons, it should not be surprising that furosemide (frusemide) produces inconsistent increases in urine output in oliguric ARF.

To overcome these limitations, furosemide (frusemide) can be given at higher doses intravenously (i.v.) or as an i.v. infusion (Dishart & Kellum 2000). In normal horses, the i.v. administration of furosemide (frusemide) produces a dose-dependent increase in urine output, up to a maximum dose rate of about 5 mg/kg (Garner et al 1975, Tobin et al 1978). If an increase in urine output is not observed within 1 h of i.v. administration of a standard furosemide (frusemide) dose (1 mg/kg), a larger i.v. dose (5–10 mg/kg) is warranted before it can be concluded that the treatment is ineffective. If urination is observed, the furosemide (frusemide) administration can be continued, at a dose rate of 1–3 mg/kg two to four times a day, or it can be given as a constant i.v. infusion. The latter would, in theory, have the benefit of providing constant drug delivery into the proximal tubules and the active sites in the loop of Henle. However, it produces lower average plasma drug concentrations (and thus a lower rate of entry into the proximal tubules) that may not exceed the threshold needed to produce the diuretic response. The intramuscular (i.m.) administration of furosemide (frusemide) produces higher average plasma concentrations and thus increased delivery to the renal tubules than achieved with constant i.v. infusion (Tobin et al 1978). However, i.m. administration should probably only be used after increased urine output has been demonstrated following i.v. bolus administration of furosemide (frusemide). These factors illustrate the need to monitor closely the diuretic response of animals with oliguric ARF treated with furosemide (frusemide).

Fortunately, furosemide (frusemide) has a relatively wide margin of safety (median lethal dose (LD_{50}) >300 mg/kg following i.v. administration to rats and dogs) and untoward effects (excluding the desired loss of water and electrolytes) have not been observed in normal horses given doses of up to 16 mg/kg i.v. (Garner et al 1975). Transient ototoxicity (as a result of blockade of a transporter involved in the production of endolymph) is a rare adverse effect that occurs in humans and cats given large doses of furosemide (frusemide) i.v. This problem has not been recognized in horses. High doses may also cause convulsions, ataxia and muscle weakness or cramping. Furosemide (frusemide) may occasionally cause arteriolar vasoconstriction and an increase in the systemic blood pressure. This untoward response, which may last for up to 1 h, may result from renin release. Finally, diuretics must always be used in conjunction with judicious fluid therapy and careful monitoring of electrolyte and acid–base status in oliguric ARF.

Although furosemide (frusemide) is administered commonly in oliguric ARF, there is controversy over whether this drug decreases the incidence of ARF in high-risk human patients or enhances recovery (Dishart & Kellum 2000). In fact, there have been few studies that have addressed this question in a prospective, blinded fashion in comparison to placebo treatment. In a recent report that compared furosemide (frusemide, 3 mg/kg i.v. four times a day for 21 days) or torasemide (another loop diuretic) with placebo treatment in 92 humans patients with ARF, the administration of a loop diuretic had a positive effect on urine output during the initial 24 h of treatment but did not shorten the dialysis times or improve the patient outcome (Shilliday et al 1997). Nevertheless, because the adverse effects associated with furosemide (frusemide) use are few, it remains a common treatment in oliguric ARF.

INCREASING RENAL BLOOD FLOW

Dopamine

Dopamine has been used for several decades for the treatment of human patients with oliguric ARF (Denton et al 1996, Dishart & Kellum 2000). A constant low-dose i.v. infusion (0.5 to 3.0 μg/kg/min) produces a dose-dependent increase in the RBF and increases the excretion of sodium and water. Some studies have also reported increases in the GFR but this response is less consistent. A dose-dependent increase in the RBF has also been documented in normal horses (Trim et al 1989). Low doses of dopamine augment the RBF primarily by inducing renal arteriolar vasodilatation by stimulating dopamine D_1 receptors in the intrarenal blood vessels. This effect is typically greater in afferent than in efferent glomerular arterioles and is the mechanism by which dopamine may also promote an increase in the GFR. A secondary role is the stimulation of D_2 receptors on presynaptic sympathetic nerve terminals, which inhibits norepinephrine release. Intermediate doses of dopamine (3–5 μg/min per kg) can also augment renal perfusion by increasing the cardiac output through stimulation of cardiac β_1 adrenoreceptors (Denton et al 1996). However, at higher doses (5–20 μg/kg/min), the beneficial effects of dopamine may be offset by systemic vasoconstriction through stimulation of peripheral α_1 adrenoreceptors (Denton et al 1996). In addition, intermediate or higher doses may also induce cardiac arrhythmias in critically ill patients (Denton et al 1996, Dishart & Kellum 2000) and transient arrhythmias have been observed in normal horses administered dopamine at 5 μg/kg/min for 60 min (Trim et al 1989; see Ch. 12). Therefore, dopamine infusions should only be performed in a hospital setting where patients can be monitored closely. Once initiated, the peak effects of the dopamine infusion usually occur within 8–12 h and the infusion is usually continued for several days until a decrease in serum creatinine concentration has been produced, although tolerance appears to develop within 48 h (Denton et al 1996).

There are few clinical studies that have demonstrated that dopamine is beneficial in human patients with ARF (Dishart & Kellum 2000). In fact, although several recent publications have argued the "pros and cons" of dopamine use, others have suggested that this drug may actually be contraindicated because of its adverse effects in critically ill patients or those with sepsis (Power et al 1999). Recently, in an attempt to decrease the potential negative effects of dopamine, D_1 receptor agonists with no D_2 receptor or α or β adrenoceptor activity (e.g. fenoldopam) have been developed (Singer & Epstein 1998). To date, the latter agents have not been studied in horses.

INCREASING GLOMERULAR FILTRATION RATE

Mannitol

Mannitol is another drug used for the treatment of oliguric ARF. Mannitol administration (1 g/kg i.v. over 30–60 min) increases plasma osmolality and the resultant shift of fluid into the intravascular space effectively increases the circulating volume, RBF and GFR (Dishart & Kellum 2000, Jose-Cunilleras & Hinchcliff 1999). It may also act as a scavenger of oxygen radicals. Mannitol is filtered across the GBM where it continues to exert an osmotic effect, thereby increasing tubular flow within the renal tubule and thus urine output. In theory, mannitol may have a particular advantage when the cause of the decreased GFR is proximal tubular obstruction by pigments and cellular debris. In horses, osmotic diuresis with mannitol along with alkalization of the urine (via concurrent i.v. administration of sodium bicarbonate) has been advocated by some clinicians for the prophylaxis and treatment of pigment nephropathy consequent to rhabdomyolysis. However, the use of mannitol and bicarbonate provided no further renal protection, when compared with saline diuresis alone, in a series of human patients with rhabdomyolysis (Homsi et al 1997). Therefore, there is no strong evidence that mannitol is an effective treatment for oliguric ARF. In fact, high doses of mannitol (>3 g/kg daily or a cumulative dose of >6 g/kg over 48 h) can actually induce or exacerbate ARF (Gadallah et al 1995). Although incompletely understood, renal arteriolar vasoconstriction (mediated via tubuloglomerular feedback) and intraluminal obstruction by edematous epithelial cells are the postulated mechanisms. The risk of mannitol nephrotoxicity appears to be greatest when there is pre-existing subclinical renal disease.

EFFECTIVENESS OF DRUG THERAPY IN ACUTE RENAL FAILURE

Although convincing data for the use of furosemide (frusemide), dopamine and mannitol for prophylaxis and treatment of ARF are lacking (Denton et al 1996, Dishart & Kellum 2000), these drugs remain widely used in at-risk cases. In addition, these medications are often used in combination and have been promoted as having synergistic effects. However, multiple drugs should be used with caution. The outer medulla of the kidney normally operates in a relatively hypoxic environment because it extracts 80–90%

of the delivered oxygen, and the partial pressure of oxygen in this tissue may be less than 20 mmHg (Dishart & Kellum 2000). Vasoactive drugs (dopamine) or agents aimed at increasing GFR (mannitol) potentially increase the workload of the segments of the nephron in the outer medulla, thereby exacerbating tissue hypoxia and precipitating the development of acute tubular necrosis in patients with renal hypoperfusion or ARF. This risk may be even more important in equines that are receiving non-steroidal antiinflammatory drugs (NSAIDs).

Other novel drugs being investigated for the prophylaxis or treatment of oliguric ARF include atrial natriuretic peptide (ANP) analogs and antagonists of calcium, adenosine and endothelin (Dishart & Kellum 2000). Further therapies are also under investigation including several growth factors that may enhance recovery from established ARF. The potential benefits of these medications remain to be established in human patients and there is no information on their use in horses.

URINE OUTPUT: DIURETIC AGENTS

Diuretic agents have been widely used for the treatment of edema and hypertension in human medicine for nearly 50 years. They are also used to manage hypercalcemia, metabolic alkalosis, renal tubular acidosis, diabetes insipidus, hyponatremia (caused by inappropriate secretion of antidiuretic hormone (vasopressin, ADH)) and hypokalemia (caused by primary hyperaldosteronism) (Martinez-Maldonado & Cordova 1990, Rose 1989, 1991, Wilcox 1991). Organic mercurials were the most common diuretic agents in clinical use but these have been replaced by safer and more specifically acting drugs. In horses, the most commonly used of these drugs are the loop diuretics, most notably furosemide (frusemide), for the control of exercise-induced pulmonary hemorrhage (EIPH). In general, all diuretic agents work to increase the renal excretion of sodium and water, although their mechanisms of action differ (Fig. 10.1) (Martinez-Maldonado & Cordova 1990, Rose 1989, 1991, Wilcox 1991).

LOOP (HIGH CEILING) DIURETICS

The loop diuretics include furosemide (frusemide), bumetanide, piretanide, torasemide and etacrynic acid. The pharmacology, renal effects and extrarenal effects of furosemide (frusemide) have been well studied in horses, largely because of this drug's widespread use in racehorses (Garner et al 1975, Hinchcliff & Mitten 1993, Hinchcliff & Muir 1991, Tobin et al 1978). Bumetanide and etacrynic acid have received less attention, although their effects on water and electrolyte excretion in equines have been documented (Alexander 1982). Torasemide, a more recently developed and longer-acting loop diuretic, is used in the management of edema and hypertension in humans with congestive heart failure. In addition to diuretic activity, torasemide also appears to antagonize the effects of angiotensin II, possibly by inhibiting calcium release (Shilliday et al 1997). To the author's knowledge, torasemide has not been used in horses.

Furosemide (Frusemide)

Furosemide (frusemide) is an anthracillic acid derivative (sulfonamide derivative) available as an injectable solution (10 mg/ml or 50 mg/ml) for i.v. or i.m. use, as an oral solution (10 mg/ml) and as tablets (10, 20, 40, 80 and 500 mg). The injectable solutions are unstable in light and are packaged in brown glass bottles and should be kept in the dark when not in use (Hinchcliff & Mitten 1993). As mentioned above, furosemide (frusemide) is a weak organic acid that is highly bound to the plasma protein albumin (>90%). It has a low apparent volume of distribution (241 ml/kg) and is eliminated rapidly via the organic acid pathways in the proximal renal tubules. The majority of a dose is eliminated unchanged in the urine within 4 h of i.v. administration to horses (Hinchcliff & Mitten 1993, Tobin et al 1978).

When administered i.v., furosemide (frusemide) produces a dose-dependent increase in urine output. Administration of a 1 mg/kg dose i.v. typically results in the production of 15–20 ml/kg urine during the initial 60 min after administration. Urine flow peaks within 15–30 min of drug

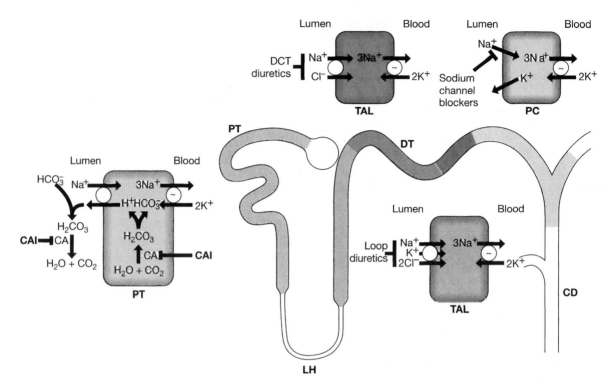

Figure 10.1 Sites and mechanisms of action of diuretics. The location of each cell type along the nephron is indicated by the shading patterns. Spironolactone (not shown) is a competitive aldosterone antagonist and acts primarily in the collecting duct. PT, proximal tubule; LH, loop of Henle; TAL, thick ascending limb; DT, distal tubule; DCT, distal convoluted tubule; CD, collecting duct; PC, principal cell; CA, carbonic anhydrase; CAI, carbonic anhydrase inhibitors; $\sim$, primary active transport. (Adapted with permission from Ellison D H 1991 The physiologic basis of diuretic synergism: its role in treating diuretic resistance. Annals of Internal Medicine 114:886–894.)

administration and the urine concentration (osmolality) decreases to that of plasma ($\sim$300 mOsm/kg). The onset of the diuresis is delayed by several minutes after i.m. dosing but the total urine output (1 mg/kg i.m.) is nearly 30 ml/kg (Tobin et al 1978). This can be explained by the more immediate saturation of the active site after i.v. compared with i.m. administration but a longer period of secretion into the tubule following administration by the latter route.

Although the cellular mechanism of action has not been fully elucidated, furosemide (frusemide) appears to bind competitively to the chloride-binding site of the $Na^+,K^+,2Cl^-$-cotransporter on the luminal surface of the epithelial cells in the thick ascending limb of the loop of Henle, thereby inhibiting the reabsorption of sodium, potassium and chloride ions (Hinchcliff & Muir 1991,

Martinez-Maldonado & Cordova 1990, Rose 1989, 1991, Wilcox 1991). In the absence of a loop diuretic, sodium ions transported into the cell are translocated into the peritubular capillary by the action of the Na^+,K^+-ATPase pump. Chloride ions are translocated out of the cell by two pathways: a selective chloride channel and an electroneutral K^+,Cl^--cotransporter. These processes maintain low intracellular sodium and chloride ion concentrations and favor continued entry of sodium and chloride from the tubular lumen. In contrast, potassium ion concentrations in the tubular fluid and within the cell are lower and higher, respectively, compared with sodium and chloride. Although these potassium ion concentrations would seem to inhibit the action of the $Na^+,K^+,2Cl^-$-cotransporter, this problem is overcome by the recycling of much of the reabsorbed potassium (that does not accompany chloride via the basolateral K^+,Cl^--cotransporter) into the tubular fluid via selective potassium channels in the luminal membrane. The activity of the $Na^+,K^+,2Cl^-$-cotransporter is actually limited by the luminal chloride ion concentration, which progressively decreases because this segment of the nephron is impermeable to water. Back leakage of sodium and chloride ions across the tight junctions between the epithelial cells eventually counterbalances reabsorption by the cotransporter when the luminal chloride ion concentration decreases to approximately 60 mmol/l. There are two additional important consequences of this complex translocation of ions from the tubular lumen to the peritubular capillary. Firstly, the recycling of potassium into the tubular lumen, combined with chloride reabsorption, creates an electrical gradient (tubule positive) that favors the passive reabsorption of sodium, calcium and magnesium ions via the intercellular spaces. Secondly, this electrical gradient allows nearly 50% of the sodium reabsorption in this segment of the nephron to occur passively, thus decreasing the energy requirement (ATP use by the Na^+,K^+-ATPase pump) for sodium reabsorption by one half (Rose 1989, 1991).

As a consequence of the blockade of the $Na^+, K^+,2Cl^-$-cotransporter, the diuresis produced by furosemide (frusemide) results in increased urinary excretion of sodium, potassium, chloride, calcium and magnesium ions. The losses of sodium, potassium and chloride are approximately 1750, 600 and 2150 mmol, respectively, after i.m. administration of furosemide (frusemide) at 1 mg/kg. Although these electrolyte losses are substantial, they are largely replaced (within the 24 h period following furosemide (frusemide) administration) by enhanced renal reabsorption as well increased ion absorption from the intestinal tract. In addition to this primary action, furosemide (frusemide) may have a lesser inhibitory effect on other chloride ion transporters and the drug can also inhibit carbonic anhydrase activity (Martinez-Maldonado & Cordova 1990, Rose 1989, 1991, Wilcox 1991). Finally, some of the renal and extrarenal effects of furosemide (frusemide) appear to be mediated through increased prostaglandin production.

Furosemide (frusemide) produces a rapid decrease in the plasma and blood volumes and a concomitant increase in the total protein concentration. This effect is maximal about 30 min after its i.v. administration but is attenuated, in part, over the next few hours by fluid shifts into the vascular compartment from the intestinal tract and intracellular and interstitial fluid spaces (Hinchcliff & Mitten 1993). The changes in the plasma and blood volumes are accompanied by decreases in the plasma concentrations of potassium, chloride, calcium and hydrogen ions (a mild metabolic alkalosis is produced). In contrast, the sodium ion concentration remains essentially unchanged (Hinchcliff & Mitten 1993). These electrolyte changes can be exacerbated and a mild decrease in the sodium ion concentration may also be observed if horses are allowed to replace water losses by drinking.

The extrarenal effects of furosemide (frusemide) include changes in the function of the cardiovascular and respiratory systems (Hinchcliff 1999, Hinchcliff & Mitten 1993). Decreases in right atrial and pulmonary arterial pressures and an increase in the peripheral resistance accompany the decrease in blood volume consequent to diuresis. Administration of furosemide (frusemide) during exercise also produces a dose-dependent decrease in pulmonary capillary pressure (Hinchcliff 1999). This latter effect is commonly used to explain the touted (but not conclusively demonstrated) beneficial effect of furosemide (frusemide) in ameliorating EIPH in racing horses. Furosemide (frusemide) also has bronchodilatory activity. In ponies with recurrent airway obstruction (heaves), both i.v. and nebulized (inhaled) furosemide (frusemide) decreased pulmonary resistance and improved compliance. In dogs, furosemide (frusemide) has also been demonstrated to have direct vasodilatory activity on the pulmonary veins but this effect was produced by furosemide (frusemide) concentrations that were orders of magnitude higher than those found after i.v. administration of furosemide (frusemide), at a dose rate of 0.5–1.0 mg/kg, to horses (Hinchcliff 1999).

The effects of furosemide (frusemide) on hemodynamics and pulmonary function appear to be mediated, in part, by increased prostaglandin production (both locally in the vessel and airway walls as well as by increased renal prostaglandins escaping into the renal vein). The role of prostaglandins is further supported by the fact that treatment with NSAIDs prior to furosemide (frusemide) administration abolishes many of these extrarenal effects. However, NSAID treatment also attenuated the magnitude of furosemide (frusemide) diuresis by 30–40%, and ligation of the ureters prior to furosemide (frusemide) administration abolished these hemodynamic changes in anesthetized horses (Hinchcliff 1999, Hinchcliff et al 1995). Therefore, it appears that most of the effects of furosemide (frusemide) on the cardiovascular system can be explained as a simple consequence of a decrease in blood volume following the diuretic effect of the drug, although there may be minor effects related to increased prostaglandin production (Hinchcliff 1999). Finally, although beyond the scope of this chapter, the potential performance-enhancing effect of furosemide (frusemide) in racing horses may also be the simple consequence of body weight reduction rather than any effect on the pulmonary vasculature or the severity of EIPH (Hinchcliff 1999).

Bumetanide

Bumetanide is a benzoic acid derivative (also a sulfonamide derivative) that has a mechanism of action similar to furosemide (frusemide). It is highly protein bound (>99%) and after i.v. administration it has a volume of distribution (68 ml/kg) of about one-third of that of furosemide (frusemide). Bumetanide is secreted into the renal tubule via the organic acid pathway and essentially all of an i.v. dose is eliminated in urine within 1 h of administration (Delbeke et al 1986). This drug is 40 times more potent than furosemide (frusemide) (on a weight basis) and induces a similar, rapid-onset diuresis. Standardbred mares produced ~10 ml/kg urine during the 1 h after i.v. administration of 15 μg/kg bumetanide, which is similar to a comparable dose of furosemide (frusemide; 0.6 mg/kg). The magnitude of diuresis was also increased by about 50% after i.m. administration of the same amount of the drug (Hinchcliff et al 1995). In ponies, administration of

bumetanide (200 μg/kg via a nasogastric tube) was nearly as effective at increasing sodium and water excretion in urine as one-sixth of the dose (30 μg/kg) administered i.v. However, the diuretic response to both doses of bumetanide in these ponies was assessed using the 24 h urine output, which was considerably less than that produced by administration of furosemide (frusemide) (2.5 mg/kg i.v.) (Alexander 1982).

Etacrynic acid

Etacrynic acid is an aryloxyacetic acid derivative that is structurally different from the other loop diuretics (not a sulfonamide derivative) (Hinchcliff & Mitten 1993). It appears to have the greatest ototoxic potential in humans; consequently, its use is generally limited to patients that are allergic to one of the other loop diuretics (Rose 1989). In horses, etacrynic acid produces a dose-dependent diuresis, similar to the other loop diuretics, after either i.v. or oral administration. Although the degree of protein binding has not been studies in horses, it is assumed to be relatively high and the drug is also secreted via the organic acid pathway. Oral doses of 1.0 mg/kg produced diuresis that peaked after 1 h and lasted for 3 h (Wilcox 1991). The i.v. administration of sodium ethacrynate (0.5 mg/kg) to ponies produced a modest diuresis in comparison with that of furosemide (frusemide) (2.5 mg/kg i.v.), while administration via a nasogastric tube (2.5 mg/kg) failed to increase either sodium or water excretion over the 24-h collection period. In fact, urinary sodium excretion actually decreased after the oral administration of sodium ethacrynate, leading to speculation that the drug may have interfered with sodium absorption by blocking a similar cotransporter in the ileum (Alexander 1982). Therefore, there is conflicting information on the diuretic effects of oral etacrynic acid, and the pharmacokinetics of this drug in horses has not been published.

Other uses of loop diuretics

In addition to the use of furosemide (frusemide) to induce urine flow in oliguric ARF and in the prophylaxis of EIPH in performance horses, the main clinical use of the loop diuretics is to limit or decrease edema formation consequent to trauma or cardiac or pulmonary disease. In practice, these drugs are not used commonly for this purpose in horses. In fact, many traditional uses of loop diuretics to induce urine flow (e.g. to "flush" myoglobin out of the kidney during a bout of rhabdomyolysis) are no longer recommended because the drugs exacerbate the dehydration associated with many disease processes. In addition, concurrent dehydration is now well recognized as an important risk factor for nephrotoxicity with many medications (e.g. aminoglycosides, tetracyclines and NSAIDs).

Furosemide (frusemide) tablets may occasionally be prescribed for horses with heaves or congestive heart failure accompanied by edema (see Chs 12 and 16). Furosemide (frusemide) has a bioavailability of 50–70% following oral administration to humans (Wilcox 1991) and anecdotal reports suggest that oral furosemide (frusemide) is effective in horses. However, when 50 mg furosemide (frusemide) was administered i.v. or orally to ponies on separate occasions, there was a doubling of 24-h urine output following the i.v. dose but no increase following the oral dose (Alexander 1982). It is not known whether this decreased effect after oral dosing was a consequence of lower bioavailability or of presystemic (hepatic) metabolism of furosemide (frusemide). It is also important to recognize that the loop diuretics will only produce a net loss of sodium for a few days after the initiation of treatment. A new steady-state balance of sodium intake and excretion usually develops within 1 week; however, if a successful response to treatment has occurred, the edema has already largely resolved.

Complications of therapy with loop diuretics

Potential complications of long-term furosemide (frusemide) treatment in humans, in addition to the more obvious problems such as volume depletion and the development of azotemia, are potassium depletion leading to hypokalemia (see p. 353), nephrolithiasis, nephrocalcinosis and hypomagnesemia (Rose 1989, Wilcox 1991). Although a greater dietary supply of potassium in feedstuffs makes the development of hypokalemia less likely in horses, it is prudent to assess the electrolyte and acid–base status at regular intervals during the first 2–3 weeks of diuretic treatment. Nephrolithiasis and nephrocalcinosis have been attributed to increased urinary excretion of calcium produced by the loop diuretics. As discussed above, calcium reabsorption in the loop of Henle is primarily passive; therefore, the blockade of the $Na^+,K^+,2Cl^-$-cotransporter in the thick ascending limb leads to a parallel increase in the excretion of calcium. In humans, this latter effect is clinically important because the loop diuretics are combined with i.v. saline in the treatment of hypercalcemia. The hypercalciuria associated with the use of loop diuretics does not appear to increase the risk of osteopenia because there is a concomitant increase in the absorption of calcium in the intestines. Finally, it is interesting to note that an increased incidence of renal cell carcinoma is recognized in human patients receiving long-term treatment with the loop diuretics. It is not known whether there is a risk of these complications during the repeated use of furosemide (frusemide) in racing horses.

BENZOTHIADIAZIDES OR THIAZIDE-TYPE DIURETICS

The thiazide-type diuretics (chlorothiazide, hydrochlorothiazide, methylchlothiazide, cyclothiazide, hydroflumethiazide and bendrofluazide (bendroflumethiazide)) and other similar drugs (metolazone, chlorthalidone, quinethazone and indapamide) act by competing with the chloride-binding site of the Na^+,Cl^--cotransporter on the luminal surface of the epithelial cells of the distal convoluted tubule and connecting segment (Martinez-Maldonado & Cordova 1990, Rose 1989, 1991, Wilcox 1991). In the absence of these drugs, sodium and chloride are reabsorbed until the luminal chloride ion concentration falls to about 40 mmol/l, at which point back leakage of sodium and chloride ions tends to balance the reabsorption. Because only a relatively small amount of sodium and chloride (about 5% of the filtered load) is normally reabsorbed in the distal tubule and connecting segment, the thiazide-type diuretics produce a more limited diuresis than the loop diuretics. Therefore, they are more commonly used for treatment of hypertension than edema in humans. In addition to blocking the Na^+,Cl^--cotransporter (on which furosemide (frusemide) but not bumetanide also has a lesser effect), the thiazide-type diuretics also modestly impair sodium reabsorption in the proximal tubule by the partial inhibition of carbonic anhydrase (Rose 1989, 1991). The latter effect does not contribute to the diuresis because the excess sodium and water leaving the proximal tubule is reabsorbed in the loop of Henle. In contrast to the loop diuretics, the thiazide-type diuretics increase calcium reabsorption in the distal tubule, thereby decreasing the urinary excretion of calcium. This mechanism is not well understood but is thought to be a consequence of increased permeability of the luminal membrane to calcium ions, perhaps in combination with increased activity of a basolateral Na^+,Ca^{2+}-exchanger (Martinez-Maldonado & Cordova 1990, Rose 1989, 1991, Wilcox 1991). In fact, thiazide-type diuretics decrease the frequency of new urolith formation in humans with idiopathic hypercalciuria (Rose 1989).

Prolonged use of either the loop or thiazide-type diuretics can lead to potassium depletion and hypokalemia (Martinez-Maldonado & Cordova 1990, Rose 1989, 1991, Wilcox 1991). Both groups of diuretics increase potassium excretion by increasing the delivery (flow) of filtrate to the more distal segments of the nephron. This is often more significant with the thiazide-type diuretics than with the loop diuretics. Normally, at low tubular flow rates, the potassium ion concentration in the tubular fluid increases as it approaches the distal tubule and collecting duct. However, with diuretic use, the tubular flow rate increases and the luminal potassium ion concentration falls, producing a cell-to-lumen gradient that favors potassium excretion. Secondly, increased passive reabsorption of sodium ions via selective sodium channels in the collecting ducts produces a more negative lumen potential that enhances the excretion of potassium ions via selective potassium channels. Thirdly, increased sodium reabsorption also increases the activity of the basolateral Na^+,K^+-ATPase pump, which translocates sodium to the adjacent capillaries. Increased pump activity increases potassium entry from the interstitium into the cells and expands the intracellular potassium pool that is available for secretion. Fourthly, the use of these diuretics indirectly stimulates the release of aldosterone and ADH. Aldosterone increases the number of open sodium channels on the luminal border of the principal cells in the collecting ducts, resulting in enhanced sodium reabsorption. It is unclear whether the concomitant increase in potassium excretion is a direct effect of aldosterone (opening more potassium channels) or simply a consequence of increased sodium reabsorption. ADH increases potassium excretion in the collecting ducts by increasing the number of open potassium channels. Finally, both types of diuretic typically increase the distal excretion of hydrogen ions and, less importantly, produce a mild metabolic alkalosis owing to volume contraction. Alkalosis shifts potassium ions into the cells in exchange for hydrogen ions and thereby exacerbates the hypokalemia. As mentioned above, the typically high potassium intake of horses consuming a forage diet makes hypokalemia (and potassium depletion) less of a concern than in other species. Nevertheless, it is prudent to assess serum electrolyte concentrations and acid–base balance regularly during long-term diuretic therapy and potassium supplementation is indicated if the serum potassium concentration falls below 3.0 mmol/l.

In humans, the thiazide-type diuretics are absorbed readily from the gastrointestinal tract, bound extensively to plasma proteins and eliminated in the proximal tubule via the organic acid pathway (Wilcox 1991). Excretion of the more water-soluble drugs (e.g. chlorothiazide and hydrochlorothiazide) is largely in urine while the more lipid-soluble agents (e.g. bendrofluazide (bendroflumethiazide) and polythiazide) are also subjected partly to hepatic metabolism. The more hydrophobic agents also tend to be more potent and have a longer duration of action. Thiazide-type diuretics are generally well tolerated, with the development of hypokalemia and hypomagnesemia being the most common drug-induced electrolyte alterations. Hyponatremia can occasionally develop during long-term treatment because the increased sodium excretion may not be matched by increased water excretion. Unlike the loop diuretics, these drugs act at the distal tubule and do not compromise the medullary interstitial concentration gradient. In contrast, the use of the loop diuretics tends to produce a degree of medullary washout leading to a closer matching of sodium and water excretion.

There are no published reports on the pharmacokinetics of the thiazide-type diuretics in horses. A bolus dose of a combination of dexamethasone (5 mg) and trichlormethiazide (200 mg), a product commonly used for treatment of udder edema in periparturient cattle, is occasionally used to treat edema in horses and there are anecdotal reports that it is efficacious. Hydrochlorothiazide (0.5– 0.7 mg/kg orally twice daily) has also been used to enhance urinary potassium excretion and thereby limit the increase in serum potassium concentrations during an episode of hyperkalemic periodic paralysis in horses (Beech & Lindborg 1996, Spier et al 1990; see Ch. 8). However, hydrochlorothiazide was less effective than acetazolamide (see below) and phenytoin in controlling the clinical signs, but it did limit the increase in the serum potassium ion concentrations during an oral potassium chloride challenge test (Beech & Lindborg 1996).

CARBONIC ANHYDRASE INHIBITORS

The carbonic anhydrase inhibitors include acetazolamide, dichlorphenamide, ethoxzolamide and methazolamide.

Acetazolamide

Acetazolamide is the prototype carbonic anhydrase inhibitor and exerts its effects by decreasing the reabsorption of sodium, chloride and bicarbonate in the proximal tubules (Martinez-Maldonado & Cordova 1990, Rose 1989, 1991, Wilcox 1991). Acetazolamide blocks two isoenzymes of carbonic anhydrase, a soluble form

located in the cell cytosol and a membrane-bound form located in the luminal brush border (Martinez-Maldonado & Cordova 1990). Cytosolic carbonic anhydrase favors the formation of bicarbonate and hydrogen ions from carbon dioxide and water. This results in an increased availability of hydrogen ions for secretion into the tubule and the addition of bicarbonate to the systemic circulation via translocation to the peritubular capillaries. In contrast, the isoenzyme in the brush border favors the dissociation of carbonic acid (formed from filtered bicarbonate and hydrogen ions secreted into the proximal tubule) to carbon dioxide and water, which can diffuse back into the tubular epithelium. Rapid, non-enzymatic production of carbonic acid in the tubular lumen (using the secreted hydrogen ions) also maintains a concentration gradient that favors hydrogen ions entering the lumen. A Na^+,H^+-exchanger secretes hydrogen ions and produces a concentration gradient that further promotes the reabsorption of sodium ions in the proximal tubule. Consequently, the inhibition of the cytosolic and membrane-bound isoenzymes decreases both the secretion of hydrogen ions and the reabsorption of sodium ions. In addition, acetazolamide also decreases the reabsorption of bicarbonate and chloride ions (chloride reabsorption in the proximal tubule is largely passive, down a favorable concentration gradient, across the tight junctions of the paracellular space) (Martinez-Maldonado & Cordova 1990, Rose 1989, 1991, Wilcox 1991).

Around 60–70% of the filtered sodium is usually reabsorbed in the proximal tubule; therefore, acetazolamide could be expected to have a rather potent diuretic effect. However, it produces rather modest diuresis because most of the excess sodium leaving the proximal tubule can be reabsorbed in the more distal segments of the nephron. Furthermore, its diuretic action is progressively diminished by the development of hyperchloremic metabolic acidosis caused by the loss of bicarbonate ions into the urine (Martinez-Maldonado & Cordova 1990, Rose 1989, 1991, Wilcox 1991). In humans, the primary indication for acetazolamide (as a diuretic agent) is the treatment of edema with metabolic alkalosis, where the loss of sodium bicarbonate in urine will correct both problems (Rose 1989, 1991, Wilcox 1991). It is important to remember that acetazolamide does not only inhibit carbonic anhydrase activity in the kidneys. The drug is also used to decrease secretion of aqueous humor in the treatment of glaucoma. In addition, acetazolamide decreases the rate of cerebrospinal fluid formation and its effects on multiple tissues and red blood cells can limit carbon dioxide transport. The latter is used to stimulate ventilation in patients with sleep apnea or acute high-altitude sickness, but it can precipitate more serious acidosis in patients with hypoventilation caused by chronic lung disease (Wilcox 1991).

In humans, acetazolamide is absorbed readily from the gastrointestinal tract, with peak blood concentrations achieved within 2 h of an oral dose. It is eliminated unchanged by tubular secretion into the urine within 24 h. Mild adverse effects are common in humans and include taste alteration, paresthesias, gastrointestinal disturbances (e.g. nausea and vomiting), malaise, polyuria and, less frequently, altered libido. Acetazolamide is teratogenic in laboratory animals and, therefore, is contraindicated in pregnant women (Wilcox 1991). Although the pharmacokinetics of acetazolamide have not been studied in horses, it is used widely in the management of horses with HYPP (Beech & Lindborg 1996, Spier et al 1990). The dose employed for the control of HYPP (2.2–4.4 mg/kg orally twice daily) is substantially lower than that employed commonly in humans or required to induce moderate-to-severe acidosis in equines (30 mg/kg orally twice daily), and adverse effects are uncommon (Schott & Hinchcliff 1998). Acetazolamide has been shown to be more effective than hydrochlorothiazide in controlling the clinical signs of HYPP in horses (Beech & Lindborg 1996).

OSMOTIC DIURETICS

The osmotic diuretics (e.g. mannitol, sucrose, urea and glycerol) are agents that are filtered freely in the glomeruli, reabsorbed poorly in the tubules and pharmacologically inert. As sodium and water are reabsorbed in the proximal tubule and the loop of Henle, the osmotic diuretics are concentrated in the tubular fluid, increasing the osmotic pressure and thus limit fluid reabsorption and promote diuresis. An increased medullary blood flow and a decreased medullary solute gradient resulting in a reduction in the urine osmolality accompany the increased tubular flow. In contrast to other diuretics, the osmotic agents produce a relative water diuresis in which the loss of water exceeds that of sodium (Martinez-Maldonado & Cordova 1990, Wilcox 1991).

Mannitol

Mannitol, the most commonly employed osmotic diuretic, is a large polysaccharide molecule. It is often selected for use in the prophylaxis or treatment of oliguric ARF. It is not absorbed from the gastrointestinal tract and, therefore, is only administered i.v. with its elimination dependent on the GFR (within 30 to 60 min with normal renal function). Mannitol is distributed within the plasma and extracellular fluid spaces and produces an increase in the serum osmolality and expansion of the circulating volume. It is not generally used for the treatment of edema because any mannitol retained in the extracellular fluid can promote further edema formation. Furthermore, acute plasma volume expansion may challenge individuals with poor cardiac contractility and can precipitate pulmonary edema. Mannitol is commonly administered for the treatment of cerebral edema consequent to head trauma or to hypoxic–ischemic encephalopathy in neonatal foals. Because mannitol promotes water excretion, hypernatremia is a potential complication in patients that do not have free access to water (Martinez-Maldonado & Cordova 1990, Wilcox 1991).

Glycerol

Glycerol is a three-carbon metabolic intermediate. In the 1990s, human endurance athletes used it to expand their circulating volumes prior to exercise in an attempt to enhance performance. Glycerol typically ingested in water or saline 1 h or so prior to exercise at a dose rate of 0.5–1.0 g/kg.

Whether it enhances performance in human athletes remains controversial; however, not surprisingly, its ingestion may be accompanied by the development of nausea, diarrhea or headache. In exercising horses, the oral administration of glycerol had no benefits over the administration of electrolytes alone for ameliorating body fluid losses in sweat. Although no adverse effects were observed, the urine output was doubled during this endurance ride-simulating treadmill exercise (Schott et al 1999).

Dimethyl sulfoxide

Dimethyl sulfoxide (DMSO) has also been suggested as a potent osmotic diuretic in horses. However, one study that compared the diuretic effects of DMSO with furosemide (frusemide, 1 mg/kg) and hypertonic saline (5 liters) found that DMSO (1 g/kg administered i.v. diluted in 5 liters of 0.9% sodium chloride) was a relatively weak diuretic agent that doubled 4-h urine production in comparison with that achieved with the same volume of isotonic (0.9%) sodium chloride. The most dramatic diuretic response was produced by the hypertonic saline (7.5%), which resulted in the production of more than 40 ml/kg urine during the first 4-h period after administration (Schott & Black 1995).

POTASSIUM-SPARING DIURETICS

There are two types of distal-acting, potassium-sparing diuretic: (i) those that directly inhibit sodium ion reabsorption by blocking the selective sodium channels on the luminal side of the epithelial cells in the collecting ducts (amiloride and triamterene); and (ii) those that indirectly inhibit sodium ion reabsorption by decreasing the number of open sodium channels through antagonizing the effects of aldosterone (spironolactone). Only 1–2% of the filtered sodium is reabsorbed in the nephron segments where these drugs act (connecting tubules and cortical collecting ducts); therefore, the potassium-sparing agents are relatively weak diuretics. These drugs are most commonly used in combination with the loop or thiazide-type diuretics to limit potassium

loss and increase diuresis in patients with refractory edema. Sodium absorption in this nephron segment is also important for the excretion of potassium and hydrogen ions; consequently, the use of these agents can actually produce hyperkalemia and metabolic acidosis. Amiloride and triamterene are also effective in reducing the increased calcium and magnesium ion excretion that is produced by the loop diuretics (Martinez-Maldonado & Cordova 1990, Rose 1989, 1991, Wilcox 1991).

Amiloride and triamterene

In humans, amiloride is absorbed incompletely after oral administration (bioavailability 15–25%) and is effective for about 18 h. It is eliminated unchanged by the kidneys through both filtration and secretion. In contrast, triamterene is absorbed rapidly from the intestine, has a high bioavailability and is about 50% bound to albumin in the circulation. After absorption, triamterene undergoes partial hepatic metabolism (hydroxylation to less-active metabolites) and the excretion of unchanged drug and metabolites by the kidneys by both filtration and secretion peaks 1–2 h after administration. Amiloride is generally better tolerated than triamterene, but both drugs produce hyperkalemia. Both drugs also accumulate in renal failure (and triamterene can accumulate in liver failure); therefore, they should only be used when renal function is normal. Triamterene can also lead to crystalluria and urolith formation and may also cause ARF when used in conjunction with NSAIDs (Martinez-Maldonado & Cordova 1990, Rose 1989, 1991, Wilcox 1991). There are no published reports on the pharmacokinetics or use of these drugs in horses.

Spironolactone

Aldosterone acts in the connecting segments and collecting ducts to increase the reabsorption of sodium and chloride ions and promote the excretion of potassium and hydrogen ions. As with all steroid hormones, aldosterone acts by diffusing into the tubular cells and attaching to specific cytosolic receptors. These complexes are translocated into the nucleus where they interact with the nuclear chromatin to enhance the transcription of messenger and ribosomal RNA. The end result is an increase in the number of open selective sodium channels on the luminal surface of the cells in these nephron segments.

In humans, spironolactone is absorbed readily and is metabolized in the liver to active compounds called canrenones. It is these metabolites that compete with aldosterone for its cytosolic receptor; therefore, the maximal natriuretic effect is not observed until 24–48 h after treatment has been initiated. Spironolactone is indicated for the treatment of primary hyperaldosteronism but is also used in refractory edema and in secondary hyperaldosteronism consequent to use of loop or thiazide-type diuretics (Martinez-Maldonado & Cordova 1990, Rose 1989, 1991, Wilcox 1991). In one study, the administration of spironolactone via nasogastric tube (1 and 2 mg/kg) to ponies more than doubled the urinary excretion of sodium and reduced the urinary excretion of potassium for a period of 72 h, although there was no difference in the volume of urine produced (Alexander 1982). This suggests that spironolactone is a potassium-sparing agent in horses; however, to date, no pharmacokinetic studies have been published.

XANTHINES

The alkylxanthines (e.g. the methylxanthines aminophylline and theophylline) are rarely employed as diuretic agents but are commonly used as bronchodilators. Aminophylline is metabolized to its active metabolite theophylline after oral administration and increases cytosolic cyclic adenosine monophosphate (cAMP) by the inhibition of phosphodiesterase, the enzyme responsible for the degradation of cAMP. cAMP is an important intracellular messenger involved in the phosphorylation of cytosolic and membrane-bound proteins; however, its effect in the kidneys remains unclear. The diuretic effect of theophylline is modest and appears to be mediated by both an increase in cardiac output, leading to increases in RBF and GFR, and a direct tubular effect, leading to increased sodium and chloride ion excretion (Martinez-Maldonado & Cordova 1990).

POLYURIA AND POLYDIPSIA: ANTIDIURETIC AGENTS

Renal insufficiency, behavior problems and endocrine diseases can all cause polyuria and polydipsia in horses. Diabetes insipidus (DI) is such an endocrine cause; DI is termed central or neurogenic when it is caused by a lack of ADH production and secretion or nephrogenic when it is caused by a failure of the collecting ducts to respond to ADH. ADH, or arginine-vasopressin, acts on V_2 receptors on the basolateral membrane of the collecting duct epithelial cells, leading to the insertion of water channels (transmembrane proteins) in the apical membrane. These channels increase the water permeability of the apical membranes and thereby lead to increased water reabsorption. The action of the V_2 receptors is mediated via activation of adenylate cyclase and a stimulatory transmembrane G protein. However, V_2 receptor activation can be antagonized by the activation of adjacent α_2 adrenoceptors and by a prostaglandin E_2-mediated effect on an inhibitory G protein. Other medications administered commonly to horses may antagonize ADH and lead to polyuria. The effects of these vasopressin receptor antagonists vary depending on the species and have not yet been studied in the horse. It is likely that the diuresis associated with administration of α_2 adrenoceptor agonists to horses may be attributed to ADH antagonism in the collecting duct (Schott 1998).

Water deprivation and exogenous ADH administration are two diagnostic tests that can be used to differentiate neurogenic from nephrogenic DI. The latter test is pursued only after there is a failure to produce concentrated urine in response to the water-deprivation test (Schott 1998). Until recently, the most commonly used form of exogenous ADH was a water-insoluble tannate of arginine vasopressin extracted from the posterior pituitary and suspended in peanut oil. This preparation is no longer available. Currently, there are two approaches to performing an ADH challenge test. Firstly, aqueous synthetic vasopressin (20 U/ml) can be administered either as an i.v. infusion (5 U (0.25 ml) in 1 liter 5% dextrose solution administered at a rate of 2.5 mU/kg over a 60 min period (approximately 250 ml to a 500 kg horse)) or as an i.m. injection (0.5 U/kg). An increase in the urine specific gravity to 1.020 or greater after 60–90 min is the expected response, while no increase in urine concentration supports a diagnosis of nephrogenic DI. Secondly, a synthetic analog of arginine vasopressin, desmopressin acetate (DDAVP), can be used. This vasopressin analog is used most commonly in small animals because it has decreased pressor actions compared with aqueous synthetic vasopressin, produces fewer effects in visceral smooth muscle and has an enhanced antidiuretic effect.

A dose of 1 µg desmopressin acetate has antidiuretic activity that is equivalent to 4 U arginine vasopressin. Desmopressin acetate has recently been evaluated in normal horses. The author and coworkers diluted desmopressin acetate (0.1 mg/ml) nasal spray in sterile water and administered 0.05 µg/kg i.v. (25 µg, equivalent to 100 U of antidiuretic activity in a 500 kg horse) to horses with polyuria induced by repeated nasogastric intubation of water for 3 days. Urine was collected for 8 h after desmopressin acetate administration and there was an increase in urine specific gravity to >1.020 from 2 to 7 h after administration (Fig. 10.2). The drug had no effects on heart rate or systemic blood pressure. These preliminary data demonstrate that the i.v. administration of desmopressin acetate appears to be safe and a useful tool for the evaluation of horses with DI.

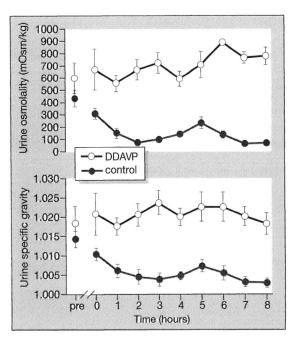

Figure 10.2 Urine osmolality and specific gravity in six horses administered 0.05 µg/kg desmopressin acetate (DDAVP: ○) or placebo (●) i.v. at time 0. The horses had polyuria induced by repeated nasogastric intubation with water (40 ml/kg) twice daily for 3 days preceding DDAVP challenge and again 4 h after administration of DDAVP. Urine was collected for 8 h after treatment and an increase in urine specific gravity to values above >1.020 was observed from 2 to 7 h after DDAVP administration.

URINE RETENTION AND INCONTINENCE

Bladder paralysis leading to urine retention and overflow incontinence can accompany a variety of neurological disorders in horses. With the exception of the bladder paresis accompanying herpes virus myelitis (which generally resolves), the problem is usually frustrating and difficult to treat because it is often long standing before it is recognized clinically (Holt 1997, Schott 1998). In horses with incontinence caused by decreased urethral sphincter tone, medical therapy can be more effective at controlling intermittent incontinence than in horses with altered detrusor function.

The diagnosis and treatment of bladder dysfunction and urinary incontinence in horses is rather primitive compared with that in human patients with these problems (Wise & Cardozo 1994). In humans, the management of these conditions includes a variety of procedures (e.g. exercises, behavioral therapy and surgery) as well as adjunctive drug treatment. Finally, urine scalding is not a problem in human patients with incontinence because they can either wear protective garments or be taught to self-catheterize.

Both women and mares may also develop urine retention in the immediate postpartum period (Groutz et al 2001). This condition is associated with bladder and urethral trauma during delivery and is unlikely to respond well to medication. Early recognition of this complication and temporary placement of an indwelling catheter to decompress the bladder is the treatment of choice. Despite aggressive postpartum management, some affected mares never recover full bladder or urethral sphincter function. When the condition is not recognized immediately, mares may present with end-stage bladder paresis and incontinence months to years later.

Diseases affecting gray matter of the sacral segments of the spinal cord, resulting in the loss of lower motor neuron function, and diseases affecting the lumbar or higher portions of the spinal cord, resulting in the loss of upper motor neuron function, cause bladder dysfunction and associated incontinence. Lower motor neuron damage leads to the loss of detrusor function and overflow incontinence; a large, easily expressed bladder is found on rectal palpation. Increased urethral resistance leading to increased intravesicular pressure before voiding is characteristic in the initial stages of upper motor neuron disease. Short bursts of urine passage with incomplete bladder emptying can be observed and rectal examination may reveal a turgid bladder that is normal to large in size. Although upper motor neuron signs are initially different from those of lower motor neuron disease, incontinence is not usually recognized until overflow incontinence develops as a result of accumulation of urine sediment (sabulous urolithiasis) and progressive loss of detrusor function. The latter also explains why bladder paralysis and overflow incontinence, signs of lower motor neuron disease, are occasionally found in horses with neurological diseases that do not affect the gray matter of the sacral segments of the spinal cord (e.g. cervical stenotic myelopathy, equine degenerative myelopathy and viral encephalomyelitis). Apart from horses with herpes virus myelitis and estrogen-responsive urethral sphincter mechanism incontinence, the prognosis for recovery from incontinence caused by bladder paralysis is generally poor because sabulous concretions and urinary tract infections (UTIs) complicate the problem (Holt 1997, Schott 1998).

The detrusor muscle is innervated by both the parasympathetic and the sympathetic nervous systems and by non-adrenergic, non-cholinergic (NANC) neurons. Stimulation of the parasympathetic neurons, originating from spinal cord segments S1–S4 and traveling to the bladder via the pelvic nerve, leads to detrusor muscle contraction. Sympathetic innervation to the detrusor muscle is via the hypogastric nerve, with preganglionic fibers arriving from L1 to L4 segments and synapsing in the caudal mesenteric ganglion. Postganglionic fibers supply both the detrusor (β_2 adrenoreceptors) and proximal urethra (primarily α_1 and some α_2 adrenoceptors). Stimulation of the sympathetic neurons inhibits detrusor muscle contraction and increases urethral sphincter tone. A branch of the pudendal nerve, which originates from spinal cord segments S1 to S2, primarily provides the somatic innervation to the striated muscle of the urethra (external urethral sphincter) (Holt 1997, Schott 1998).

TREATMENT

The treatment of bladder paralysis and overflow incontinence (lower motor neuron disease) includes the removal of sabulous crystalloid material (via bladder lavage through a catheter or via cystotomy), temporary placement of an indwelling catheter in the bladder, appropriate antimicrobial therapy and the administration of cholinergic drugs to stimulate detrusor muscle function. Bethanechol chloride (2.5–10 mg) is sometimes administered s.c. as a diagnostic test for detrusor underactivity in humans because the drug causes rather rapid detrusor muscle contraction. A positive response supports further treatment.

Bethanechol

Bethanechol is a synthetic cholinergic agonist (β-methyl analog of carbachol) that has parasympathomimetic effects in gastrointestinal smooth muscle and in the detrusor muscle. It has predominantly muscarinic effects (carbachol also has nicotinic effects) and is resistant to hydrolysis by acetylcholinesterase and non-specific cholinesterases. In addition to increasing detrusor activity and increasing intravesicular pressure, bethanechol also increases ureteral peristalsis and relaxes the bladder neck and the external urethral sphincter. Administration (i.v. or i.m.) of this drug results in a loss of muscarinic receptor selectivity and causes serious adverse effects in the cardiovascular and respiratory systems. In humans with bladder paresis, the response to bethanechol treatment is quite variable (Wise & Cardozo 1994).

The pharmacokinetics of bethanechol chloride in horses has not been published. However, the drug has been used subcutaneously (s.c.) at doses of 0.025–0.075 mg/kg two to three times a day. It has also been used (0.025 mg/kg) to stimulate cecal myoelectrical activity. This drug has no effect when the bladder is completely atonic or arreflexic. If the detrusor muscle is capable of generating weak contractions, then bethanechol treatment may be useful (more vigorous voiding activity). Whether or not partial detrusor function remains can be determined using cystometry. Although the oral administration of bethanechol has also been described, a favorable response to treatment has not been reported. Disappointing results are more likely to be a consequence of long-standing detrusor dysfunction rather than poor intestinal absorption of the drug. The dose rates for oral administration should be about 10-fold greater (0.25–0.75 mg/kg two to four times a day) than if it is administered parenterally (Holt 1997, Schott 1998, Wise & Cardozo 1994).

Adrenergic agonists and antagonists

The use of α adrenoceptor blockers (e.g. phenoxybenzamine 0.7 mg/kg orally four times a day, acepromazine 0.02–0.04 mg/kg i.m. or orally four times a day) in combination with bethanechol decreases urethral sphincter tone in horses with bladder paresis (Schott 1998). In theory, partial relaxation of the urethral sphincter could improve bladder emptying at lower intravesicular pressures. In practice, however, horses with bladder paralysis may already have decreased sphincter tone as a result of ascending urethritis and cystitis.

Urethral sphincter tone may actually be increased in upper motor neuron disease, especially in the early stages of disease. In this instance, α adrenergic blockers may be effective in decreasing sphincter tone and urine retention (Schott 1998, Wise & Cardozo 1994). There are anecdotal reports that urine retention and bladder enlargement in sick neonatal foals is responsive to α adrenergic blocking drugs. This condition is probably related to prolonged recumbency but could also be related to hypoxic–ischemic encephalopathy.

Urinary incontinence may also develop in horses with normal detrusor function that have decreased urethral sphincter tone. Similarly, detrusor muscle instability (spontaneous detrusor contractions that develop when the animal is attempting to inhibit micturition) or detrusor-sphincter dyssynergia (lack of coordination between detrusor contraction and urethral relaxation, usually as a result of upper motor neuron disease) may also result in incontinence. In affected cases, the α adrenergic agonist phenylpropanolamine (0.5–1.0 mg/kg orally, one to four times a day) has been used to increase sphincter tone but a successful response has not been reported. As with bethanecol, dosing regimens for most of these autonomic drugs have been extrapolated from other species because the pharmacokinetics of these agents (with the exception of acepromazine) has not been studied in horses.

Estradiol

Administration of estradiol cypionate (4–10 µg/kg i.m. daily for 3 days then every other day) or estradiol benzoate (10–12 µg/kg using a similar dosing schedule) has been reported to improve urinary incontinence in mares (Watson et al 1997). Estrogen receptors are present in the bladder neck and the hormone appears to modulate the effects of norepinephrine on the α adrenoceptors in the urethral sphincter, thereby improving urethral sphincter tone. However, the doses of estrogen employed have often been greater than those typically used for the induction of estrus behavior. Therefore, these mares should be considered as having estrogen-responsive incontinence rather than hypoestrogenism.

Imipramine

There is one report of the use of the tricyclic antidepressant imipramine hydrochloride to control urospermia in a stallion with detrusor dysfunction and decreased urethral sphincter tone (Oristaglio Turner et al 1995; see Ch. 11). Imipramine is a phenothiazine analog and appears to have α adrenergic effects via the blockade of norepinephrine reuptake at nerve terminals. It was administered orally at 0.8 mg/kg to this stallion 2–3 h prior to semen collection and was thought to improve urethral sphincter tone and limit urospermia. However, this improvement was not documented using urethral pressure profilometry and the owner of the stallion was also instructed to collect from the stallion shortly after it was observed to urinate. Consequently, it is not clear whether the imipramine treatment was really of any benefit.

UROLITHIASIS

URINE ACIDIFYING AGENTS

The administration of urine acidifying agents is frequently recommended for the prophylaxis and treatment of recurrent UTIs and urolithiasis. Adding grain to the diet is a simple way of decreasing urine pH, although the decline in pH is modest and the urine pH typically remains greater than 7.0. Oral ammonium chloride (20–40 mg/kg per day) is the agent most commonly chosen; however, this does not produce a consistent decrease in urine pH. Recently, higher oral doses of ammonium chloride (60–520 mg/kg daily), oral methionine (1 g/kg daily), oral ascorbic acid (vitamin C, 1–2 g/kg daily) and oral ammonium sulfate (175 mg/kg daily) have been shown to be more successful in reducing urine pH to <6.0 in horses (Schott 1998). Unfortunately, at these dose rates, these medications are often unpalatable

and have to be administered by nasogastric tube or directly into the mouth (using a syringe).

Other methods used to decrease the recurrence of urolithiasis include dietary modifications that decrease calcium excretion and promote diuresis. Changing the diet from alfalfa to grass or oat hay decreases the calcium intake and should decrease the urinary excretion of calcium, since fecal calcium excretion is relatively constant in horses. Although this dietary change should decrease the total calcium excretion, it may also decrease the urinary excretion of nitrogen and the daily urine volume. The latter changes could enhance the supersaturation of urine. In theory, diuresis could be promoted further by the addition of loose salt (50–75 g per day) to the concentrate portion of the diet. However, in one study where ponies were fed sodium chloride (1, 3 or 5% of the total diet dry matter (1% is approximately 75 g sodium chloride for a 500 kg horse)), there were no differences in water intake, urine production or calcium excretion.

Another factor that affects both the urine pH and urinary calcium excretion is the dietary cation–anion balance (sodium plus potassium ions minus chloride ions plus elemental sulfur). A lower balance has been associated with both a decrease in urine pH and an increase in the urinary excretion of calcium (Schott 1998). Increasing the amount of grain in the diet, switching from alfalfa to grass hay, or adding one or more minerals to the diet (ammonium chloride, calcium chloride or ammonium sulfate) all lower the cation–anion balance. It should not be surprising that the supplements that decrease this balance are familiar urine acidifying agents. A diet low in both calcium and cation–anion balance could result in a negative calcium balance; consequently, one possible long-term effect could be a decreased skeletal calcium ion content.

URINARY TRACT INFECTIONS

The treatment of UTIs in horses consists of proper antimicrobial therapy and, if possible, the correction of the predisposing anatomical or functional problems with urine flow (e.g. outflow obstruction, urolithiasis or bladder paralysis). The selection of the most appropriate antimicrobial agent is described in Chapter 2.

It warrants mention that resistance to a particular antimicrobial agent *in vitro* may not preclude successful treatment with the drug as long as high concentrations are achieved in urine. Similarly, demonstrable susceptibility *in vitro* does not always guarantee a successful response to treatment. For example, *Enterococcus* spp. is often found to be susceptible to the potentiated sulfonamide combinations *in vitro*; however, this pathogen is inherently resistant to these combinations *in vivo* (Jose-Cunilleras & Hinchcliff 1999, Schott 1998). Antimicrobial therapy should be continued for at least 1 week for the treatment of lower UTIs and for 2–6 weeks for upper UTIs in horses. Ideally, a voided, midstream urine sample should be submitted for bacterial culture 2–4 days after the initiation of therapy and again 1–2 weeks after treatment has been discontinued.

If the UTI recurs and the same organism is isolated, a focus of upper UTI should be suspected. Ultrasonographic examination of the kidneys should be considered in such cases to exclude nephroliths or other parenchymal disease. Cystoscopy and ureteral catheterization can also be pursued to evaluate whether the infection is unilateral or bilateral. In contrast, the isolation of a different pathogen from a recurrent UTI suggests that there is an anatomical or functional cause of abnormal urine flow predisposing the animal to recurrent infections. It is not unusual to find highly resistant organisms in the urine of horses with chronic UTIs, especially in those with bladder paralysis that have been repeatedly catheterized and treated with a variety of antimicrobial agents. In such cases, the antimicrobial agent should be selected based on culture and susceptibility reports of serial quantitative urine cultures (Schott 1998).

Penicillins

A single i.m. dose (22 000 IU/kg) of procaine penicillin G (procaine benzylpenicillin) results in urine concentrations exceeding 60 µg/ml for 48 h, well above the minimum inhibitory concentration (MIC) of many organisms. Therefore, the frequency of drug administration could be decreased to once daily or every other day. Although many of the Enterobacteriaceae demonstrate resistance to ampicillin *in vitro*, this drug is concentrated in urine and is often effective against these isolates *in vivo*. The potentiated penicillins (ticarcillin or ticarcillin–clavulanic acid) should be reserved for treatment of horses with UTIs caused by highly resistant organisms (e.g. *Pseudomonas* spp.) and are sometimes selected as an alternative to aminoglycosides in azotemic conditions (Jose-Cunilleras & Hinchcliff 1999).

Aminoglycosides

The aminoglycosides can be nephrotoxic and should be reserved for the treatment of lower UTIs caused by highly resistant organisms or acute, life-threatening upper UTIs caused by aerobic Gram-negative bacteria. Recent pharmacokinetic/pharmacodynamic studies in both adult horses and foals support once daily administration as the preferred dosage schedule because it both improves the bactericidal action (concentration-dependent killing) and lessens the risk of nephrotoxicity (Jose-Cunilleras & Hinchcliff 1999).

Potentiated sulfonamides

Combinations containing the sulfonamide sulfadiazine are preferred for the treatment of UTIs because sulfadiazine is excreted largely unchanged in urine whereas sulfamethoxazole is largely metabolized to inactive products in the liver prior to urinary excretion (Jose-Cunilleras & Hinchcliff 1999).

Other antimicrobial agents

The cephalosporins and tetracyclines are commonly used for treatment of UTIs in other species. However, in horses, the cephalosporins are rarely more advantageous than the penicillins or potentiated sulfonamides. However, ceftiofur has broad-spectrum antimicrobial activity and may be indicated when urinary pathogens are resistant to other drugs. After 48 h of i.m. administration of ceftiofur (2.2 mg/kg twice daily), the urine drug concentrations peaked at 18 μg/ml and had a trough value of 4.6 μg/ml. The tetracyclines are rarely indicated for the treatment of UTIs in horses, and their use is limited to parenteral administration (e.g. of the longer-acting agents). The fluoroquinolones (e.g. enrofloxacin; 2.5–5 mg/kg orally twice daily) may be suitable antimicrobial agents for some chronic or recurrent UTIs where the causative organisms are highly resistant to all of the drugs approved for use in the horse. These agents have the added benefit that they can be administered orally. After oral enrofloxacin 5 mg/kg twice a day, the bioavailability was 60% in horses and the urinary concentrations reached 437–1617 μg/ml. However, the fluoroquinolones are arthrotoxic (particularly in rapidly growing juvenile animals) and their use should, therefore, be limited to adult horses or to foals with urinary pathogens that are not susceptible to other antimicrobial agents (Jose-Cunilleras & Hinchcliff 1999, Schott 1998).

REFERENCES

Alexander F 1982 The effects of ethacrynic acid, bumetanide, furosemide, spironolactone and ADH on electrolyte excretion in ponies. Journal of Veterinary Pharmacology and Therapeutics 5:153–160

Beech J, Lindborg S 1996 Prophylactic effect of phenytoin, acetazolamide and hydrochlorothiazide in horses with hyperkalemic periodic paralysis. Research in Veterinary Science 59:95–101

Delbeke F T, Debackere M, Desmet N et al 1986 Pharmacokinetics and diuretic effect of bumetanide following intravenous and intramuscular administration to horses. Journal of Veterinary Pharmacology and Therapeutics 9:310–317

Denton M D, Chertow G M, Brady H R 1996 "Renal-dose" dopamine for the treatment of acute renal failure: scientific rationale, experimental studies and clinical trials. Kidney International 49:4–14

Dishart M K, Kellum J A 2000 An evaluation of pharmacological strategies for the prevention and treatment of acute renal failure. Drugs 59:79–91

Ellison D H 1991 The physiologic basis of diuretic synergism: its role in treating diuretic resistance. Annals of Internal Medicine 114:886–894

Gadallah M F, Lynn M, Work J 1995 Case report: mannitol nephrotoxicity syndrome. Role of hemodialysis and postulate of mechanisms. American Journal of the Medical Sciences 309:219–222

Garner H E, Hutcheson D P, Coffman J R et al 1975 Urine electrolyte and diuretic responses of horses to seven

dosage levels of Lasix®. In: Proceedings of the 21st American Association of Equine Practitioners Annual Convention, Lexington, KY, pp. 87–90

Groutz A, Gordon D, Wolman I et al 2001 Persistent postpartum urinary retention in contemporary obstetric practice: definition, prevalence and clinical implications. Journal of Reproductive Medicine 46:44–48

Hinchcliff K W 1999 Effects of furosemide on athletic performance and exercise-induced pulmonary hemorrhage in horses. Journal of the American Veterinary Medical Association 215:630–635

Hinchcliff K W, Mitten L A 1993 Furosemide, bumetanide and ethacrynic acid. Veterinary Clinics of North America: Equine Practice 9:511–522

Hinchcliff K W, Muir W W 1991 Pharmacology of furosemide in the horse: a review. Journal of Veterinary Internal Medicine 5:211–218

Hinchcliff K W, McKeever K H, Muir W W et al 1995 Pharmacologic interaction of furosemide and phenylbutazone in horses. American Journal of Veterinary Research 56:1206–1212

Holt P E 1997 Urinary incontinence in mature horses. Equine Veterinary Education 9:85–88

Homsi E, Barreiro M F, Orlando J M et al 1997 Prophylaxis of acute renal failure in patients with rhabdomyolysis. Renal Failure 19:283–288

Jose-Cunilleras E, Hinchcliff K W 1999 Renal pharmacology. Veterinary Clinics of North America: Equine Practice 15:647–664

Martinez-Maldonado M, Cordova H R 1990 Cellular and molecular aspects of the renal effects of diuretic agents. Kidney International 38:632–641

Oristaglio Turner R M, Love C C, McDonnell S M et al 1995 Use of imipramine hydrochloride for treatment of urospermia in a stallion with a dysfunctional bladder. Journal of the American Veterinary Medical Association 207:1602–1606

Power D A, Duggan J, Brady H R 1999 Renal-dose (low-dose) dopamine for the treatment of sepsis-related and other forms of acute renal failure: ineffective and probably dangerous. Clinical and Experimental Pharmacology and Physiology 26(suppl):S23–S28

Rose B D 1989 In: Rose B D (ed) Clinical physiology of acid–base and electrolyte disorders, 3rd edn. McGraw Hill, New York, pp. 389–415

Rose B D 1991 Diuretics. Kidney International 39:336–352

Schott H C 1998 The urinary system. In: Reed S M, Bayly W M (eds) Equine internal medicine. Saunders, Philadelphia, PA, pp. 807–911

Schott H C, Black A 1995 Dimethyl sulfoxide (DMSO) is a relatively weak diuretic agent. Journal of Veterinary Internal Medicine 9:213

Schott H C, Hinchcliff K W 1998 Treatments affecting fluid and electrolyte status during exercise. Veterinary Clinics of North America: Equine Practice 14:175–204

Schott H C, Düsterdieck K F, Eberhart S W et al 1999 Effects of electrolyte and glycerol supplementation on recovery from endurance exercise. Equine Veterinary Journal 30(suppl):384–393

Shilliday I R, Quinn K J, Allison M E 1997 Loop diuretics in the management of acute renal failure: a prospective, double-blind, placebo-controlled, randomized study. Nephrology, Dialysis and Transplantation 12:2592–2596

Singer I, Epstein M 1998 Potential of dopamine A-1 agonists in the management of acute renal failure. American Journal of Kidney Disease 31:743–755

Spier S J, Carlson G P, Holliday T A et al 1990 Hyperkalemic periodic paralysis in horses. Journal of the American Veterinary Medical Association 197:1009–1016

Tobin T, Roberts B L, Swerczek T W et al 1978 The pharmacology of furosemide. III. Dose and time response relationships, effects of repeated dosing and performance effects. Journal of Equine Medicine and Surgery 2:216–226

Trim C M, Moore J N, Clark E S 1989 Renal effects of dopamine infusion in conscious horses. Equine Veterinary Journal 7(suppl):124–128

Watson E D, McGorum B C, Keeling N et al 1997 Oestrogen responsive urinary incontinence in two mares. Equine Veterinary Education 9:81–84

Wilcox C S 1991 Diuretics. In: Brenner B M, Rector F C (eds) The kidney, 4th edn. Saunders, Philadelphia, PA, pp. 2123–2147

Wise B G, Cardozo L 1994 Urinary incontinence. In: Rushton D N (ed) Handbook of neuro-urology. Dekker, New York, pp. 181–207

CHAPTER CONTENTS

Introduction 177

Mares 177
    Induction of ovulation 177
    Infertility 180
    Pregnancy 182
    Parturition 185
    Lactation 186
    Postpartum problems 187

Stallions 187
    Spermatogenesis 187
    Ejaculatory dysfunction 188
    Reproductive tract/performance 189

References 189

11

Drugs acting on the reproductive system

Sally Vivrette

INTRODUCTION

Many different drugs are used to treat horses intended for breeding. These drugs may be administered to enhance fertility or to treat disease. Since the majority of drugs are used as management tools to facilitate equine reproduction this chapter is organized by use rather than by drug class.

MARES

INDUCTION OF OVULATION

Mares are seasonally polyestrous and most experience an anestrous period during the winter months. This is followed in the early spring by a transitional period when there is minimal to moderate follicular development, erratic and sometimes prolonged periods of estrus and unpredictable ovulation. Many commercial breeding operations try to advance the first ovulation in the spring to facilitate the birth of foals earlier in the year.

Induction during the transitional period

Induction of ovulation earlier in the season can be accomplished by increasing the photoperiod beginning in early December or by employing a number of pharmacological approaches.

The oral administration of the synthetic progestagen altrenogest has been shown to time the first ovulation of the breeding season more predictably in transitional mares. This is most effective if it is administered late in the transitional period when there are ovarian follicles of >20–30 mm in diameter. Altrenogest should be administered orally (p.o.) at the recommended dose rate of 0.044 mg/kg for 15 days (Ball 2000a). Rubber gloves should be worn when handling or administering altrenogest to horses as this drug can be absorbed through intact skin. Alternatively, a therapeutic regimen using progesterone (150 mg) and estradiol-17β (10 mg) administered intramuscularly (i.m.) for 10–15 days can be used to induce ovulation in mares in the transitional period.

During progesterone/progestagen therapy, the release of luteinizing hormone (LH) from the anterior pituitary gland is suppressed, while synthesis and storage continues, making increased quantities of LH available for release when the treatment is discontinued. Although LH release is suppressed there is no negative effect on the release of follicle-stimulating hormone (FSH) and follicular development and spontaneous ovulation with corpus luteum development may occur during progestagen treatment. A luteolytic dose of prostaglandin $F_{2\alpha}$ ($PGF_{2\alpha}$) is often administered at the cessation of progestagen treatment (Ball 2000a). Mares typically come into estrus 4–7 days after treatment is discontinued and ovulate 7–12 days later.

Gonadotropin-releasing hormone (GnRH, luteinizing hormone releasing hormone (LHRH) or luliberin) is a hypothalamic hormone that stimulates the synthesis and release of FSH and LH from the gonadotrophs in the anterior pituitary gland. GnRH is transported to the anterior pituitary gland via the hypothalamic–hypophyseal portal veins, veins between the capillary beds in the hypothalamus and the pituitary, where variations in pulse frequency and amplitude differentially stimulate the release of FSH and LH. There are many neuronal, endocrine and environmental factors that stimulate GnRH secretion. Inhibition of GnRH secretion is mainly through dopaminergic neural input (Irvine 1993a). GnRH therapy may be used to hasten ovulation in mares in the transitional period. This may include repeated injections (e.g. every hour to twice daily), the use of controlled-release implants or the administration of deslorelin-containing implants on alternate days

up to a total of six implants. The efficacy of GnRH therapy in the transitional period is enhanced if there is evidence of follicular development (>20 mm in diameter) prior to the start of treatment. Mares ovulate approximately 18 days after the initiation of GnRH therapy (Ball 2000a).

Induction of ovulation in mares may be stimulated by the administration of human chorionic gonadotropin (hCG). This has physiological actions similar to LH but differs structurally in both protein and carbohydrate content. It is produced by the human placenta and is extracted commercially from the urine of pregnant women. hCG may be administered to mares in the transitional period to stimulate ovulation. A dose of 3300 IU administered to mares with a follicle of >40 mm in diameter and signs of estrus that have been present for more than 3 days hastens the first ovulation of the season by approximately 1 week compared with control mares (Ball 2000a). In some states of the USA, hCG is a controlled substance that requires a special license for purchase and use.

The administration of dopamine antagonists is associated with an increase in serum prolactin concentrations, which may have a stimulatory effect on ovarian follicular development. It is also possible that pituitary LH release is stimulated by the feedback produced by the increase in ovarian follicle estrogen production. Some of these drugs may also have an indirect effect, probably the removal of tonic inhibition of endogenous hypothalamic GnRH secretion (Ball 2000a). Treatment with the dopamine antagonists has not been shown to be effective in mares in deep anestrus. The administration of the selective dopamine D_2 receptor antagonists domperidone at 1.1 mg/kg p.o. (Brendemuehl & Cross 1998) or sulpiride at 200 mg/mare i.m. once daily (Besognet et al 1997), has been shown to advance the onset of the first ovulation in mares in the transitional period (see p. 184).

Induction of ovulation in the breeding season

During the physiological breeding season, ovulation may be induced to facilitate ovulation within 24 to 48 h after natural service. When artificial insemination with shipped-cooled or frozen semen is used, the interval between ovulation and insemination must be closely timed. In these situations, the pharmacological stimulation of ovulation may be employed.

Attempts to stimulate ovulation in mares using natural GnRH have been unrewarding because of the short lifespan of this hormone, leading to the need for repeated injections (Perkins 1999). A GnRH analogue, deslorelin acetate, is approved for the induction of ovulation in mares in the USA. This implant is administered subcutaneously (s.c.) and releases the drug over a 2–3 day period. Administration of the implant to a cycling mare with an ovarian follicle ⩾30–35 mm in diameter usually results in ovulation approximately 42 h later (McCue et al 2000). Following the administration of deslorelin acetate, a small proportion of mares that fail to conceive reportedly have reduced follicular development and an increased diestrus period. Occasionally, there may be a complete shutdown of ovarian activity in a small percentage of mares administered the deslorelin acetate implant. These effects may be exaggerated in mares that have been 'short-cycled' with prostaglandins. The longer interovulatory interval results from reduction in the daily concentrations of FSH, the absence of a midcycle FSH surge and a reduced response to FSH following the administration of GnRH midcycle. The cessation of cyclicity may result from prolonged desensitization or down-regulation of the pituitary to GnRH following the administration of GnRH agonists such as deslorelin acetate. It has been suggested that the removal of the deslorelin acetate implant 48 h after administration may stimulate ovulation and result in baseline and midcycle GnRH-stimulated FSH concentrations similar to those found in untreated mares (Johnson et al 2002, McCue et al 2000).

Intravenous (i.v.) or i.m. hCG 2000–3000 IU will induce ovulation within 36–48 h in mares in estrus with a preovulatory follicle of at least 35 mm in diameter (Perkins 1999). Higher doses of hCG (6000 IU) may actually reduce conception rates (Shivola et al 1976). The repeated administration of hCG to mares may result in the formation of anti-hCG antibodies, which can persist for one to several months (Roser et al 1979). Although this has not been found to result in ovulatory refractoriness in clinical settings, it is commonly recommended that hCG be given no more than twice during the same breeding season (Roser et al 1980).

Estrus synchronization

Estrus synchronization may be used in management situations where there is limited stallion availability (e.g. the stallion is often away at horse shows) or the stallion is subfertile. Synchronization may also be used to facilitate the coordination of estrus, ovulation and insemination in mares undergoing artificial insemination or embryo transfer. There are many methods of synchronizing estrus in single mares or in groups of mares.

Progestagen therapy may be used to suppress pituitary LH release and limit ovulation for a specified period during the physiological breeding season. Most often the progesterone/progestagen therapy includes p.o. altrenogest (0.044 mg/kg) once daily or i.m. progesterone (150 mg) daily for 7–10 days. Estrus occurs 4–5 days and ovulation 9–10 days after the progestagen therapy is discontinued. Follicular development may continue during progestagen therapy and spontaneous ovulation with corpus luteum development may occur. It is, therefore, advised that a luteolytic dose of $PGF_{2\alpha}$ is given at the conclusion of the progestagen treatment.

Estradiol-17β (10 mg) may be given at the same time as progestagen therapy to reduce follicular development during treatment; this is thought to reduce the variation in the time to ovulation. Ovulation occurs 10–12 days after combined therapy with progesterone and estradiol is discontinued. The timing of ovulation can be more closely tuned in a group of mares undergoing synchronization, by giving hCG (1500–2500 IU) when an ovarian follicle of >30 mm in diameter is detected and the mare has been in estrus for at least 2 days (Ball 2000b, Bristol 1993).

$PGF_{2\alpha}$ and its analogs cause regression of the corpus luteum, allowing for the resumption of cyclicity. Regression of the corpus luteum occurs both through the direct action on the luteal cells and indirectly via a reduction in the blood flow to the corpus luteum. The corpus luteum develops prostaglandin receptors and is responsive to prostaglandins starting from 5 days after its formation. Following administration of $PGF_{2\alpha}$ to mares, the serum progesterone concentrations fall rapidly; signs of estrus are evident 2–4 days and ovulation occurs 7–12 days after treatment. When a follicle of >40mm in diameter is present at the time of $PGF_{2\alpha}$ administration, the mare may ovulate within 24–72h of treatment. Estrus can be synchronized in a group of mares by giving two injections of prostaglandin 14 days apart. In this situation, 78–92% of the treated mares will show estrus within 6 days of the second injection (Ball 2000b). $PGF_{2\alpha}$ or its analogs are most commonly given i.m. Side effects, including sweating and diarrhea or abdominal discomfort, are observed in a small percentage of mares after standard doses of the prostaglandins are administered. At higher doses or if these drugs are administered i.v., side effects including locomotor incoordination, dragging of the hindlimbs and dyspnea may be observed (Goynings et al 1977, Irvine 1993b). Commercially available prostaglandin analogs appear to have lesser side-effects than the natural form of $PGF_{2\alpha}$. Prostaglandins should be handled with care, especially by pregnant women.

Suppression of estrus in performance mares

During the estrous cycle (and especially during estrus) mares sometimes exhibit undesirable behavioral or physical problems that may interfere with performance. These problems include difficulties in training or riding, back or hindquarter pain and aggressive behavior. A wide variety of treatments have been employed with variable efficacy (Jorgensen et al 1996).

One therapy includes the s.c. administration of pellets containing progesterone (200mg) and estradiol benzoate (20mg). Although the use of 8 to 80 of these pellets has not been found to suppress normal cyclicity or behavioral estrus (McCue et al 1996), approximately 70% of the owners and trainers perceived that this produced an 80% improvement in behavior and approximately 50% perceived that there was an 80%

improvement in performance after therapy. These pellets are marketed for use in cattle and should be used with caution in horses. Another commonly used treatment for estrus-related performance problems in mares is daily oral altrenogest, using the recommended dosage regimen. This treatment may suppress behavioral estrus, and treatment for 60 days does not affect subsequent fertility (Squires 1993). Medroxyprogesterone acetate can be administered by i.m. injection (250–500 mg) once every 2–3 months. This is most commonly used during the luteal phase of the estrous cycle. The overall efficacy of this treatment has not been determined, but it has been suggested that a dose of 250 mg may not effectively suppress estrus behavior (Perkins 1999).

INFERTILITY

Infertility in mares, particularly if they are obese, is sometimes ascribed to hypothyroidism (see Ch. 5). The role of hypothyroidism in equine fertility is unclear. Further research incorporating the evaluation of serum thyroid-stimulating hormone concentrations will help to further elucidate the role of thyroid hormones in equine infertility.

Endometritis and endometriosis

Endometritis in mares may be associated with at least four clinical syndromes. It can be caused by sexually transmitted infections, such as *Taylorella equigenitalis* (contagious equine metritis), *Pseudomonas aeruginosa* and *Klebsiella pneumoniae*. *Pseudomonas* and *Klebsiella* spp. may also be present in the fecal and genital flora. Chronic uterine infection with *Streptococcus equi* subsp. *zooepidemicus* and *Escherichia coli* are often associated with contamination of the uterus by fecal and genital flora.

Endometritis is most common in older multiparous mares and may be associated with impaired uterine defense mechanisms secondary to dysfunctional myometrial electrical activity. Incompetence of the vulva, vestibulo-vaginal sphincter or cervix may also predispose mares to the development of chronic uterine infections.

Table 11.1   Recommended doses for intrauterine antimicrobial agents in uterine bacterial infections in mares

Antimicrobial agent	Dose	Comments
Penicillins		
Penicillin G (benzylpenicillin)	5 million units	Good efficacy against streptococci; cost effective
Ampicillin	3 g	May be irritant: dilute well; sodium salt may leave a persistent precipitate on the endometrium
Carbenicillin	6 g	Reserved for persistent *Pseudomonas* spp. infection; used every 48 h in combination with an aminoglycoside; slightly irritant
Ticarcillin	6 g	
Ticarcillin–clavulanic acid	6 g/200 mg	
Cephalosporins		Broad-spectrum efficacy against Gram-positive and Gram-negative bacteria
Ceftiofur	1 g	
Cefazolin sodium	1 g	
Aminoglycosides		Effective against aerobic Gram-negative bacteria (*E. coli*)
Neomycin sulfate	3–4 g	May be irritant; use postbreeding may lower pregnancy rates in mares
Kanamycin sulfate	1–2 g	May be harmful to spermatozoa: do not use close to breeding
Gentamicin sulfate	0.5–2 g	Buffer with an equal volume of 7.5% bicarbonate
Amikacin sulfate	2 g	Buffer with an equal volume of 7.5% bicarbonate
Others		
Chloramphenicol	2–3 g	May be very irritant; human health risks
Polymyxin B	1 million units	Gram-negative infections especially *Pseudomonas* spp.

Adapted from Blanchard 1998, Robinson 1997, with permission

Persistent mating-induced endometritis, resulting in intraluminal uterine fluid accumulation after breeding, is seen in mares with delayed uterine clearance. Chronic degenerative endometritis (endometriosis) is caused by degenerative changes in the endometrium resulting from repeated episodes of inflammation or from aging (Troedsson 2002).

The treatment of endometritis should include antimicrobial therapy based on culture and susceptibility testing (see Ch. 2). The treatments used commonly for bacterial and fungal uterine infections in horses are included in Tables 11.1 and 11.2. Fungal or yeast infections often result from the extensive use of antimicrobial agents in the uterus. These infections are difficult to treat and may cause permanent damage to the endometrium. An intrinsic problem with uterine yeast or fungal infections is the prolonged and potentially expensive therapy required.

Mares that are susceptible to persistent endometritis should undergo an ultrasonographic examination between 6 and 12 h after mating to identify persistent postbreeding endometritis. Uterine lavage 6–12 h after mating will aid in the clearance of inflammatory products from the uterus without interfering with conception. Following thorough cleansing of the perineum, a sterile catheter (such as a 30 French, 80 cm Bivona catheter with a 75 ml balloon cuff) is inserted through the cervix into the uterine lumen and the cuff inflated. A total of 1–2 liters of sterile buffered saline or lactated Ringers solution should be infused into the uterus. Following brief transrectal uterine massage, to ensure the even distribution of the fluid into both horns, the fluid should be recovered into a clear receptacle to allow visualization of the recovered lavage solution. The uterine lavage should be repeated using further 1 liter portions of sterile fluids until the recovered fluid is clear. Measurement of the recovered fluid or ultrasonographic examination of the uterus will ensure that all of the instilled fluid has been recovered. This is important, since mares undergoing

Table 11.2 Recommended doses for intrauterine administration of antimycotic agents for the therapy of uterine fungal infections in mares

Antimycotic agent	Dose	Comments
Amphotericin B	220–250 mg	Used for *Aspergillus, Candida, Mucor* or *Histoplasma* spp. infections; dilute in 100–250 ml sterile water; treat daily for 1 week
Clotrimazole	500 mg	Used for yeast infections; a number of different formulations are available; tablets are crushed and mixed with 40 ml sterile water; often used after uterine lavage; treat daily for 1 week
Miconazole	200 mg	Most efficacious for yeast infections and used for resistant fungal infections; dilute in 40–60 ml sterile saline; treat daily for up to 10 days
Nystatin	500 000 U	Yeast infections; dilute in 100–250 ml sterile water; treat daily for 7–10 days
Acetic acid	2%	Used as a uterine lavage; 20 ml wine vinegar in 1 litre 0.9% sterile saline

Adapted from Blanchard 1998, Robinson 1997, with permission

this treatment have an impaired ability to clear the uterus spontaneously. To be effective, this treatment regimen should be repeated after each mating (Troedsson 2002).

The use of drugs that stimulate myometrial contraction may assist in the clearance of inflammatory fluid from the uterus. The i.m. administration of oxytocin (20 IU) 4 to 8 h after breeding has been shown to clear the uterus effectively, resulting in improved pregnancy rates. $PGF_{2\alpha}$ and its analogs have also been shown to increase myometrial activity and aid in clearing fluid and inflammatory debris from the uterine lumen. A 20 IU dose of oxytocin causes increased myometrial activity for 1 h and a 10 mg dose of $PGF_{2\alpha}$ causes increased myometrial activity for about 5 h after administration. Both of these drugs also affect the oviductal smooth muscle. Unpublished observations suggest that periovulatory treatment with $PGF_{2\alpha}$ may interfere with the formation and development of a functional corpus luteum and be detrimental to the establishment of normal pregnancy. It is, therefore, advisable to minimize the use of $PGF_{2\alpha}$ postmating (Troedsson 2002).

Alternative treatments reported for chronic endometritis include intrauterine infusion of a variety of disinfectants, irritants, autologous or heterologous blood plasma, colostrums and filtrates of bacterial toxins as well as systemic treatment with immunostimulants. These treatments are controversial since their clinical efficacy and safety have not been tested in controlled studies. It is possible that they may cause

further uterine inflammation, which may be irreversible.

In general, most horses with endometritis benefit from the effective removal of inflammatory debris and tissue-destructive agents along with the causative organism from the uterus rather than from the addition of more potentially damaging chemicals to the uterine lumen. In addition to the antimycotic drugs listed, irrigation of the uterus with a very dilute solution of povidone iodine (1–2%) or acetic acid (vinegar, <5%) has been tried with varying results. The optimal management of endometritis in mares may involve a combination of postmating uterine lavage and oxytocin treatment. In situations where mares have intraluminal uterine fluid prior to mating, uterine lavage and oxytocin administration may be used approximately 6 h prior to insemination.

PREGNANCY

Gestation in horses is usually 320–360 days long with an average length of 345 days. Progesterone secretion by the corpus luteum is very important in the maintenance of early pregnancy. Ideally, mares should have a serum progesterone concentration >4.0 ng/ml by day 12 of pregnancy.

Luteal insufficiency

Luteal insufficiency, as indicated by serum progesterone concentrations of <2.5 ng/ml, is thought to be inadequate for the maintenance of pregnancy and possibly predisposes mares to early embryonic loss.

Progestagen therapy is often used in mares with luteal insufficiency and includes p.o. altrenogest (0.044 mg/kg) once daily. This therapy is usually initiated after luteal insufficiency has been diagnosed and the mare has been confirmed to be pregnant. In mares that habitually abort, progestagen therapy is often started on the day of ovulation and has no known adverse effects on conception or the development of pregnancy (Perkins 1999). Progestagen treatment is usually continued until day 60 of pregnancy, if the mare has a serum progesterone concentration of >4.0 ng/ml, or may be continued until day 120 of pregnancy, when the placenta is capable of producing sufficient progesterone to support pregnancy. In some cases, progestagen supplementation is continued for the duration of pregnancy. Progestagen therapy would be contraindicated in mares with uterine infections as this may impair the uterine defense mechanisms.

Early embryonic loss

Mares in early pregnancy may be susceptible to luteolysis secondary to endotoxin-stimulated prostaglandin release. The non-steroidal anti-inflammatory drugs (NSAIDs), such as flunixin meglumine, have been shown to prevent luteolysis associated with endotoxemia if given prior to or within 2 h of endotoxin exposure. Daily oral altrenogest (0.044 mg/kg), commencing within 12 h of the endotoxemia, may prevent embryonic death (Daels et al 1989).

In one study, repeated doses of hCG between days 24 and 38 of pregnancy resulted in embryonic death but similar doses of hCG after day 39 did not result in pregnancy loss (Allen 1983). A single dose of $PGF_{2\alpha}$ or its analogs between days 12 and 35 of pregnancy has been shown to cause embryonic death. After day 35, repeated injections of $PGF_{2\alpha}$ are required to cause embryonic loss.

Placentitis

Mares with placentitis may exhibit signs of premature lactation, vaginal discharge and fever in late gestation, as a result of ascending infection through the cervix or, less commonly, hematogenous infection. The inflammatory response to placentitis includes prostaglandin production, which leads to abortion. Once placentitis has been diagnosed or is strongly suspected, the treatment usually includes NSAIDs to block endogenous prostaglandin production (see Ch. 14), oral altrenogest to promote uterine quiescence and an appropriate antimicrobial agent (see Ch. 2). In one study investigating the transfer of different antibiotics from mares in late gestation to the fetus, oral trimethoprim 5 mg/kg every 12 h was shown to be present in allantoic and amniotic fluids and in newborn foal serum. In another study, in normal pregnant mares receiving gentamicin and/or penicillin neither drug could be detected in allantoic and amniotic fluid samples or in newborn foal serum. It is possible that penicillin and gentamicin may be transferred to the fetus of mares with placentitis, but at present there are no studies that show this (Sertich & Vaala 1992).

The xanthine phosphodiesterase inhibitor pentoxifylline (oxpentifylline) is sometimes used to promote blood flow in the placental microvasculature and to diminish the production of cytokines, such as tumor necrosis factor (TNF) (see p. 180). Therapy should be continued for as long as the physical, ultrasonographical and clinical pathological findings indicate that there is ongoing infection.

Other therapies during pregnancy

There are very few studies on the effects of different drugs during pregnancy in horses.

The sulfonamides and pyrimethamine (e.g. for equine protozoal myeloencephalitis (EPM) can cause abortion in mares and abnormalities in newborn foals (see Chs 2 and 3) even when the mares received folic acid supplementation. Trimethoprim–sulfamethoxazole given to mares for up to 1 week prior to and after breeding does not appear to potentiate early embryonic death and has not been associated with an increase in birth defects in foals (J. Brendemuehl, personal communication, 2001). Birth defects have not been identified in foals born to mares undergoing treatment during late gestation for placentitis with trimethoprim–sulfamethoxazole.

The quinolone antibiotic enrofloxacin has been found to cause articular cartilage damage in neonatal foals similar to that found in immature animals of other species (Vivrette 2001). Safety studies investigating the effects of enrofloxacin therapy in pregnant mares on the articular cartilage of fetal foals have not been performed; therefore, caution should be exercised in the use of this antibiotic (see Ch. 2).

Certain anthelmintics may be associated with the development of congenital defects or abortion in horses. Cambendazole administration to pregnant pony mares resulted in deformity of foals including short lower jaw, large eyes, deformed legs and constriction of the aorta (Drudge et al 1983). Organophosphate anthelmintics in late gestation may precipitate abortion in mares.

The sedation of pregnant mares using α_2 adrenoceptor agonists (e.g. xylazine, detomidine) may cause bradycardia and decreased movement in fetuses. The fetal cardiac stroke volume cannot be altered significantly and, consequently, fetal cardiac output depends mainly on heart rate (McGladdery & Rossdale 1991). It is, therefore, possible that drug-induced bradycardia may result in a significant decrease in cardiac output in the fetus and eventual fetal hypoxia, especially in a fetus that is compromised. Although detomidine (0.015 mg/kg) given to healthy pregnant mares at 3-week intervals during the last trimester of pregnancy had no measurable detrimental effects on the outcome of pregnancy (Luukkanen et al 1997), pregnant mares should be sedated with caution especially if fetal compromise is suspected.

Clenbuterol, a β_2 adrenoceptor agonist, is sometimes used in pregnant mares with lower airway disease for its bronchodilatory effects. This drug has been found to have minimal effects on fetal heart rate when administered i.v. to mares in the last trimester of pregnancy. The effects on fetal health have not been established.

Oxytocin (1 IU i.v.) given to pony mares in late gestation has been shown to cause an increase in heart rate of 18–50 beats per minute; this 17–50% increase in the baseline heart rate probably relates to the uterine contractions produced in the mares.

Oxytocin can be used to investigate the presence of reduced uterine blood flow and concurrent fetal hypoxia. Following oxytocin administration to mares in late gestation, the anticipated or negative response is acceleration of the fetal heart rate. The positive or abnormal response is a deceleration of the fetal heart rate.

Prolonged gestation (fescue toxicosis)

Consumption of the endophytic fungus *Neotyphodium* (formerly *Acremonium*) *coenophialum* causes reproductive problems in mares, including prolonged gestation, placental thickening, dystocia, delivery of weak or stillborn foals and agalactia. This syndrome, also known as fescue toxicosis, is seen commonly in the USA in pregnant mares consuming fescue pasture or hay. The fungal endophyte acts as a dopamine D_2 receptor agonist and causes a decrease in the serum prolactin concentrations (Cross 1997).

The administration of the D_2 receptor antagonists has been shown to counteract the effects of the endophyte and increase serum prolactin concentrations. The D_2 receptor antagonists may have actions on other hormones that are under the influence of dopamine, such as GnRH and adrenocorticotropic hormone (ACTH). The D_2 receptor antagonist domperidone orally at 1.1 mg/kg once daily has been shown to ameliorate the adverse effects of this endophyte and is most commonly started from 15 days prior to the anticipated foaling date. This dosage regimen has been shown to increase the serum prolactin concentrations within days of the onset of treatment and allows the delivery of the foal around the time of the expected foaling date. Domperidone, unlike the other dopamine antagonists, does not cross the blood–brain barrier to produce adverse neurological signs (e.g. alternating periods of sedation and excitement, behavioral changes and abdominal pain). Reducing or dividing the total daily dose into two doses administered 12 h apart can minimize the premature lactation that may occur as a result of dopamine antagonist treatment. If the treated mare has suboptimal colostral immunoglobulin concentrations at the time of foaling, arrangements should be made to treat the failure of passive transfer in the foal.

Other dopamine antagonists available, but not evaluated in the treatment of prolonged gestation and fescue toxicosis, include perphenazine (administered p.o. at 0.3–0.5 mg/kg every 12 h), sulpiride (1.0 mg/kg every 12 h) and fluphenazine (0.05–0.08 mg/kg i.m. every 2 weeks). The last is available in many formulations including depot injections of the ethanate or deconate esters. Of all these agents, fluphenazine should be used with the most caution as it can produce severe extra-pyramidal signs, including pawing at the air, striking, hypermetric gait, aimless circling, alternating states of severe depression, swinging of the head and rhythmic neck flexion accompanied by extension of the forelimbs leading to injury or (if these side-effects are not recognized as being secondary to drug administration) inappropriate euthanasia. These neurological signs appear to be associated with an imbalance between dopamine and acetylcholine in the striatum. Thus, centrally acting anticholinergic drugs that restore an appropriate dopamine–acetylcholine balance, such as benzatropine, trihexyphenidyl and diphenhydramine hydrochloride (0.5–1.0 mg/kg), may be used to treat these extrapyramidal signs (Brewer et al 1990). The dopamine antagonist reserpine has been found to be ineffective in the treatment of both prolonged gestation and poor prepartum udder development. This drug may be associated with diarrhea and sedation.

Therapy to hasten fetal maturation in late gestation

The horse has a narrow window of fetal maturation relative to gestation length compared with other mammalian species. This may be related to the relatively late rise in cortisol concentrations in the equine fetus compared with other species, e.g. lambs and piglets (Silver et al 1984). Premature foals are at risk of having insufficient lung surfactant to facilitate breathing and oxygen transfer. Additionally, the liver glycogen stores and the immaturity of the gastrointestinal hormones may be inadequate to support homeostasis.

In humans, the exogenous administration of corticosteroids to late-term pregnant women is sometimes used to promote fetal development and enhance the chance of survival of the fetus. In mares, cortisol probably does not cross the placenta. This may be because of the activity of the enzyme 11β-hydroxysteroid dehydrogenase, which converts cortisol to inactive cortisone (Chavette et al 1995).

Intrafetal administration of a synthetic depot $ACTH_{1-24}$ preparation increased maternal plasma progesterone concentrations and significantly reduced gestation length (median 314 days) in equines compared with controls (median 327 days). This is probably mediated via adrenal regulation of fetal maturation and production of maternal progestagens. Abortion was observed in 31% of the treated mares but this did not seem to be associated directly with the injection technique: meconium staining, an indicator of fetal stress, was noted in 50% of the treated foals (Ousey et al 1998). Similarly, administration of depot $ACTH_{1-24}$ to mares on days 300, 301 and 302 of gestation accelerated fetal maturation (Ousey et al 2000). In this study, the gestation length (318 ± 18 days) was significantly shorter in mares bred late in the breeding season (after 1 July in the northern hemisphere) and receiving a high (4–5 mg) dose of $ACTH_{1-24}$ compared with mares that received a low (1 mg) dose (335 ± 3.7 days) or those that received a high dose (340 ± 4.3 days) but were bred prior to 1 July. The clinical application and safety of $ACTH_{1-24}$ in mares in late gestation remains to be determined (Ousey et al 2000).

PARTURITION

Induction

Oxytocin stimulates uterine contractions immediately and also causes the release of endogenous $PGF_{2\alpha}$ (Pashen 1982). In late gestation, the mare is extremely sensitive to the effects of oxytocin and fetal delivery may be induced despite inadequate fetal lung and gastrointestinal tract maturation, thus decreasing the chance of survival. It is, therefore, very important to determine whether the mare is close to spontaneous delivery through evaluation of udder development, presence of colostrum, cervical softening and dilatation, and calculation of an adequate gestation length (>330 days). The evaluation of mammary secretion electrolyte concentrations is also a useful means of determining fetal maturity (Ousey et al 1984).

A number of different dosage regimens and administration routes of oxytocin may be used to induce parturition in mares in late gestation. This may include i.v. or i.m. low (0.5–10 IU) or high (40–120 IU) dose. The induction of parturition using lower doses of oxytocin is very effective and is associated with a lower risk to the fetus and reduced potential for myometrial spasm. Oxytocin may also be diluted (e.g. 60–100 IU in 1 liter sterile normal saline) and administered i.v. through an indwelling jugular catheter.

The prostaglandin analog fluprostenol (250–500 µg i.m.) results in unpredictable delivery times and variability in the time from injection to foaling. In addition, pony mares not close to spontaneous parturition that were treated with fluprostenol delivered premature and weak foals that died shortly after delivery and treatment was associated with dystocia and retained fetal membranes. In contrast, when fluprostenol was given to mares that were close to spontaneous delivery, normal viable foals were born (Bristol 1982).

The glucocorticoids are not as effective at inducing parturition in mares as they are in other species. The repeated administration of dexamethasone, 100 mg daily for 5 days, was found to decrease the mean gestation length significantly and reduce its variability. However, in some mares there was a higher risk of delivery of a weak foal, prolonged parturition and poor milk production following dexamethasone therapy compared with other induction methods (Alm et al 1975).

Retained fetal membranes

Mares usually expel the fetal membranes within 3 h of parturition. If these membranes are retained for longer than 6 h, the mare is at risk of developing metritis, septicemia, endotoxemia, laminitis and possibly death.

The treatment of retained placenta often includes i.m. oxytocin at a low dose (20 IU) every 30 min on six occasions (S. Vivrette, unpublished data, 2001) or a higher dose (up to 120 IU) every 90 to 120 min. Alternatively, oxytocin can be used i.v. at a dose of 10–40 IU every 90 to 120 min or as a slow infusion of 30–100 IU diluted in 1 liter of saline (Perkins 1999).

If the placenta is retained for longer than 6 to 12 h, then treatment directed at the prevention of life-threatening complications should be instituted. This may include broad-spectrum antimicrobial agents, such as a penicillin in combination with the aminoglycoside gentamicin or a potentiated sulfonamide (see Ch. 2). NSAIDs should be used to decrease endotoxin-mediate prostaglandin release (see Ch. 14). The xanthine phosphodiesterase inhibitor pentoxifylline (oxpentifylline) may be administered p.o., at a dose rate of 8 mg/kg every 12 h, to try to increase red blood cell deformability and enhance the circulation in the microvasculature, especially in the feet. Pentoxifylline (oxpentifylline) also decreases the production of TNF by macrophages, which lessens the effects of endotoxin. Oral or i.v. fluid therapy should be used if there is any question of the adequacy of hydration.

Mares undergoing treatment for retained placenta should have been vaccinated against tetanus within the past year. Mares that have been vaccinated adequately against tetanus but not at the time of foaling should be given tetanus toxoid to ensure sufficient protection. The routine administration of tetanus antitoxin to mares at foaling has been associated with the development of fatal hepatic necrosis (Theiler's disease).

LACTATION

Agalactia following parturition may result in failure of passive transfer, hypoglycemia and hypovolemia in foals. This is most commonly, but not exclusively, observed in mares consuming endophyte-infected fescue pastures prior to foaling and which had not been treated with a dopamine antagonist prepartum. Agalactia may be observed in mares known not to have consumed endophyte-infected fescue pasture, and other factors, such as endophyte infection of other pasture grasses or hay or stress, may act as dopamine agonists or stimulate endogenous dopamine secretion.

The p.o. administration of the dopamine antagonists such as domperidone (see p. 184) promotes an increase in milk production within 3 days, most likely through an increase in the serum prolactin concentrations. Alternatively, oral reserpine can be given once daily, at a dose rate of 2.5–5.0 mg/450 kg horse to increase milk production postpartum. The sedation that often occurs as a side-effect of reserpine treatment may be an advantage in mares with a history of foal rejection or in skittish maiden mares. Care must be taken to provide the foal with an alternative source of nutrition (e.g. milk replacer) during the first few days of treatment until the mare's milk production is adequate. Other dopamine antagonists may also be considered (see p. 185).

Oxytocin may be used to facilitate the contraction of the mammary alveolar myoepithelial cells and thus promote milk ejection. After the mammary gland has been emptied manually, i.v. oxytocin (20 IU) will allow the additional collection of milk from lactating mares.

Mastitis may be observed at any stage of lactation and has also been seen in non-lactating, nulliparous mares and in fillies. Mastitis occurs most commonly in the summer months and is often associated with *Strep. equi subsp. zooepidemicus* infection. The treatment of mastitis usually includes the parenteral administration of appropriate antimicrobial agents (see Ch. 2). The udder may also be treated using frequent milking, hydrotherapy and infusion of commercially available intramammary preparations for cattle. A NSAID may be administered to treat both the fever and the discomfort associated with mastitis.

POSTPARTUM PROBLEMS

The middle uterine, utero-ovarian or external iliac arteries may rupture during pregnancy or parturition, leading to signs of shock and colic or to the death of the mare. The therapy of rupture of these major blood vessels is somewhat controversial and may range from drugs that reduce blood pressure to those that increase circulating blood volume and pressure (Vivrette 1997).

Agents that reduce blood pressure, such as the phenothiazine tranquillizer acepromazine maleate (0.04–0.08 mg/kg i.m. every 6 h), are sometimes used, after which the mare and foal should be kept in a quiet, dimly lit stable. Alternatively, mares can be treated with agents that expand the circulating blood volume such as hypertonic saline (1–2 liters 7.4% saline i.v.) followed by an i.v. infusion of a crystalloid such as lactated Ringers or normal saline at 1–2 l/h (for a 500 kg horse).

Some clinicians also advocate i.v. naloxone (an opioid antagonist) at 0.01–0.03 mg/kg for horses with life-threatening hemorrhages. The beneficial mechanisms of action of this therapy are not understood but it may act by increasing cardiac contractility. Aminocaproic acid, 20 g infused i.v. in 1 liter normal saline followed by 10 g in i.v. fluids every 6 h, may be used to inhibit fibrinolysis. Blood transfusions may be indicated, especially in horses with extreme tachycardia or a packed cell volume <15%, which compromises the oxygenation of the myocardium. Following major and minor hemorrhage, cross-matched blood may be administered i.v. at a rate of 1 l/10 min.

Unconventional therapy includes the administration of formalin (10 ml 37% formaldehyde or 30–150 ml 10% buffered formalin) in 1 liter of isotonic fluids. The effects of formalin are not well understood and no difference in clotting parameters can be measured following its i.v. administration to horses. However, it appears to have clinical benefits in horses with massive, life-threatening hemorrhages. Formalin may produce adverse effects, including restlessness, lacrimation, salivation, nasal discharge, frequent defecation, sweating, muscle tremors and abdominal pain, especially at higher doses.

STALLIONS

SPERMATOGENESIS

The effects of GnRH or a GnRH analog have been studied in both normal and subfertile stallions. In normal stallions, GnRH increases plasma LH, FSH and testosterone concentrations during the winter months but has no effects when given during the summer months (Roser & Hughes 1991). The s.c. administration of GnRH (50 µg) 2 h and 1 h before breeding may be used to increase circulating testosterone concentrations and boost libido (McDonnell 1999).

Prolonged, continuous administration of GnRH, a form of "biochemical castration", has been used therapeutically in stallions to decrease stallion-like behavior. In one study, prolonged administration of high doses of GnRH reduced the daily sperm output by more than 50% but had no effects on libido. In another study, GnRH (50 µg or 250 µg s.c. every 2 h for 75 days) did not alter semen parameters (daily sperm output, sperm motility) or FSH concentrations in normal stallions, although there was a significant increase in serum testosterone and LH concentrations compared with controls (Brinsko et al 1998). To date, no study has shown that GnRH or a GnRH analog significantly improves fertility in subfertile stallions.

Therapy with hCG may be used to try to increase serum testosterone concentrations in stallions that are slow to ejaculate or obtain an erection. Long-term use of this therapy may be contraindicated because of the prolonged half-life of hCG, which has a negative feedback effect on endogenous GnRH, leading to a decrease in LH and FSH secretion. Decreased LH concentrations have no significant long-term adverse effects; however, decreased availability of FSH may interfere with spermatogenesis (Amann 1993).

Testosterone or testosterone propionate are sometimes used in stallions with poor libido or problems with ejaculation. Testosterone can be used to boost libido without long-term adverse effects if low doses are used (e.g. 80 mg s.c. of an aqueous preparation of testosterone every 48 h). It may take a few days for the libido to increase and the treatment goal is to have serum testosterone concentrations remaining below 4 ng/ml. However, higher doses or longer-acting exogenous testosterone may exert negative feedback on the hypothalamic secretion of GnRH, leading to reduced serum concentrations of LH and FSH and subsequently reduced serum testosterone concentrations, decreased concentrations of spermatozoa per ejaculate and reduced semen quality. The total scrotal width, daily sperm output and testis weight also decrease, but these parameters return to pre-treatment values within 90 days of the cessation of treatment (Amann 1993). The risks of adverse effects on semen must be weighed against the inability to collect semen from a stallion with poor libido (McDonnell 1999).

Although not approved for use in stallions, anabolic steroids including nandrolone deconate, boldenone undecylenate and stanozolol are sometimes used to increase muscle mass. These drugs have effects on testes and semen similar to those observed with testosterone. These androgenic compounds should not be used in stallions intended for breeding (Amann 1993, Squires 2000). Additionally, the long-term effects and reversibility of the effects of anabolic steroid administration on prepuberal equines have not been well studied.

Progestagens, in particular altrenogest, are sometimes used in performance or racing stallions to reduce sexually aggressive behavior. The effects on behavior and semen quality have been investigated. Normal mature stallions were administered altrenogest p.o., at a dose rate of 0.044 mg/kg (Miller et al 1997) or 0.088 mg/kg (Brady et al 1997), once daily for 30 days. At the lower dose rate, there were no effects on semen quality or quantity and only minor effects on the stallions' behavior. At the higher dose rate, the stallions exhibited significantly decreased sexual behavior (observed during teasing) and poor libido during semen collection. Additionally, there was a reduction in the scrotal circumference, reduced daily sperm output, increased spermatozoal abnormalities and reduced serum testosterone concentrations. In rare instances, stallions receiving p.o. progestagen treatment may have a reduction in libido without adverse affects on breeding performance (McDonnell 2000).

EJACULATORY DYSFUNCTION

Stallions may have problems with penile erection secondary to traumatic injury of the penis. In other stallions, ejaculatory dysfunction, secondary to neurological and musculoskeletal problems that affect the stallion's ability to mount and thrust, may be the primary cause of breeding failure. In these cases, ejaculation in copula or ex copula may be enhanced pharmacologically.

Adrenergic agents and/or tricyclic antidepressants may be used to induce ejaculation ex copula (also known as "chemical ejaculation") in stallions that have inadequate erection prior to or following insertion. Ejaculation is either observed within 3 min of (associated with the onset of sedation) or 15–20 min after (associated with recovery from sedation) the i.v. administration of the α_2 adrenoceptor agonist xylazine (0.66 mg/kg) (McDonnell 1999). Ejaculation typically occurs 10–60 min after the i.v. administration of the tricyclic antidepressant imipramine (2.2 mg/kg) (McDonnell 1999). These two medications may be used in combination: imipramine is administered p.o. at a dose rate of 0.075–2.0 mg/kg followed 1–2 h later by xylazine (0.3 mg/kg i.v.). Ejaculation occurs 3–15 min after the xylazine (McDonnell 1993, McDonnell 2001). $PGF_{2\alpha}$ i.m. at 0.005–0.01 mg/kg results in ejaculation 5–90 min later (McDonnell 1999).

REPRODUCTIVE TRACT/PERFORMANCE

Stallions treated for EPM with drugs that inhibit folic acid synthesis (pyrimethamine, potentiated sulfonamides) (see Chs 2 and 3) have been reported to develop neurological signs including unsteadiness upon mounting, clumsy or weak thrusting, failure to flex the back and thready or inapparent ejaculatory pulses that result in dribbling, rather than forceful, expulsion of semen. These abnormalities developed after approximately 5–6 weeks of treatment and resolved within 60 days of the treatment being discontinued. There were no changes in the semen characteristics, testicular volume, sperm production efficiency, libido and erection nor in the quantitative measures of ejaculatory efficiency. However, stallions that develop neurological signs during treatment with folic acid inhibitors should be used with caution for breeding (Bedford & McDonnell 1998).

Sedation of stallions and geldings with phenothiazine-derivative tranquillizers such as acepromazine causes relaxation and protrusion of the penis. This appears to be secondary to α adrenoceptor blockade, which reduces the motor function of the retractor penis muscles. Penile paralysis or priapism, a morbid engorgement of the corpus cavernosum resulting in intractable erection, may ensue. The precise mechanism of this is not known, but it has been hypothesized that it results from failure of the reciprocal waxing and waning of the cholinergic–adrenergic control of blood flow to the corpus cavernosum. The resultant stasis and sludging of blood in the cavernous spaces and subsequent trabecular fibrosis lead to this condition becoming irreversible. It has been suggested that an i.v. cholinergic blocking agent, benzatropine mesylate (8 mg), may facilitate the removal of blood from the corpus cavernosum and this should be administered as soon as possible (within 24 h) after the onset of priapism (Schumacher & Vaughan 1988). Phenothiazine tranquillizers should be used with caution in male horses. Penile paralysis and priapism need to be distinguished from paraphimosis (inability to retract the penis into the prepuce as a result of preputial injury or disease) because of differences in management techniques and prognoses.

GnRH (500 µg twice daily for 3 weeks) and hCG (2500 IU twice weekly for 4 to 6 weeks) have been used as treatment for cryptorchidism in stallions up to 2 years old. However, there are no publications describing controlled studies using these therapies. hCG (10 000 IU i.v.) may be used to diagnose cryptorchidism in geldings with suspected retained testicular tissue (Silberzahn et al 1989).

REFERENCES

Allen W E 1983 The effect of human chorionic gonadotropin and exogenous progesterone on luteal function during early pregnancy in pony mares. Animal Reproduction Science 6:223–228

Alm C C, Sullivan J J, First N L 1975 The effect of a corticosteroid (dexamethasone), progesterone, oestrogen and prostaglandin $F_{2\alpha}$ on gestation length in normal and ovariectomized mares. Journal of Reproduction and Fertility Supplements 23:637–640

Amann R P 1993 Effects of drugs or toxins on spermatogenesis. In: McKinnon A O, Voss J L (eds) Equine reproduction. Lea & Febiger, Philadelphia, PA pp. 831–839

Ball B A 2000a Hormonal management of transitional estrus. In: Proceedings of the Bluegrass Equine Reproduction Symposium, Lexington, KY, 2000

Ball B A 2000b Estrus synchronization in mares. In: Proceedings of the Bluegrass Equine Reproduction Symposium, Lexington, KY, 2000

Bedford S J, McDonnell S M 1998 Semen, testicular volume, sperm production efficiency, and sexual behavior of stallions treated with trimethoprim–sulfamethoxazole and pyrimethamine. In: Proceedings of the 44th American Association of Equine Practitioners Annual Convention, Baltimore, MD, pp. 1–2

Besognet B, Hansen B, Daels P 1997 Induction of reproductive function in anestrous mares using a dopamine antagonist. Theriogenology 47:467–480

Blanchard T L 1998 Manual of equine reproduction, Mosby, Toronto

Brady H A, Johnson N N, Whisnant C S et al 1997 Effects of oral altrenogest on testicular parameters, steroidal profiles and seminal characteristics in young stallions. In: Proceedings of the 43rd American Association of Equine Practitioners Annual Convention, Phoenix, AZ, pp. 195–196

Brendemuhl J, Cross D 1998 Influence of the dopamine antagonist domperidone on the vernal transition in seasonally anestrus mares. In: Proceedings of the 7th International Symposium on Equine Reproduction, Pretoria, pp. 47–48

Brewer B D, Hines M T, Stewart J T et al 1990 Fluphenazine induced Parkinson-like syndrome in a horse. Equine Veterinary Journal 22:136–137

Brinsko S P, Squires E L, Pickett B W et al 1998 Gonadal and pituitary responsiveness of stallions is not down-regulated by prolonged pulsatile administration of GnRH. Journal of Andrology 19:100–109

Bristol F 1982 Induction of parturition in near-term mares by prostaglandin $F_{2\alpha}$. Journal of Reproduction and Fertility Supplements 32:644

Bristol F 1993 Synchronization of ovulation. In: McKinnon A O, Voss J L (eds) Equine reproduction. Lea & Febiger, Philadelphia, PA, pp. 348–352

Chavette P, Rossdale P D, Tait A D 1995 11-β-hydroxysteroid dehydrogenase (11beta-HSD) in equine placenta. In: Proceedings of the 41st American Association of Equine Practitioners Annual Convention, Lexington, KY, pp. 264–265

Cross D L 1997 Fescue toxicosis in horses. In: Bacon C W, Hill N S (eds) Neotyphodium/grass interactions. Plenum Press, New York, pp. 289–309

Daels P F, Stabenfeldt G H, Kindahl H et al 1989 Prostaglandin release and luteolysis associated with physiological and pathological conditions of the reproductive cycle of the mare: a review. Equine Veterinary Journal Supplement 8:29–34

Drudge J H, Lyons E T, Swerczek T W et al 1983 Cambendazole for strongyle control in a pony band: selection of a drug-resistant population of small strongyles and teratologic implications. American Journal of Veterinary Research 44:110–114

Goynings L S, Lauderdale J W, Geng S et al 1977 Pharmacologic and toxicologic study of prostaglandin $F_{2\alpha}$ in mares. American Journal of Veterinary Research 38:1445–1452

Irvine C H G 1993a GnRH clinical application. In: McKinnon A O, Voss J L (eds) Equine reproduction. Lea & Febiger, Philadelphia, PA, pp. 329–333

Irvine C H G 1993b Prostaglandins. In: McKinnon A O, Voss J L (eds) Equine reproduction. Lea & Febiger, Philadelphia, PA, pp. 319–324

Johnson C A, McMeen S L, Thompson D L 2002 Effects of multiple GnRH analogue (deslorelin acetate) implants on cyclic mares. Theriogenology 58:469–472

Jorgensen J S, Vivrette S L, Correa M et al 1996 Significance of the estrous cycle on athletic performance in mares. In: Proceedings of the 42nd American Association of Equine Practitioners Annual Convention, Denver, CO, pp. 98–100

Luukkanen L, Katila T, Koskinen E 1997 Some effects of multiple administration of detomidine during the last trimester of equine pregnancy. Equine Veterinary Journal 29:400–402

McCue P M, Lemons S S, Squires E L et al 1996 Efficacy of progesterone/estradiol implants for suppression of estrus in the mare. In: Proceedings of the 42nd American Association of Equine Practitioners Annual Convention, Denver, CO, pp. 195–196

McCue P M, Farquhar V J, Squires E L 2000 Effect of the GnRH agonist deslorelin acetate on pituitary function and follicular development in the mare. In: Proceedings of the 46th American Association of Equine Practitioners Annual Convention, San Antonio, TX, pp. 355–356

McDonnell S M 1993 Pharmacologic manipulation of sexual behavior. In: McKinnon A O, Voss J L (eds) Equine reproduction. Lea & Febiger, Philadelphia, PA, pp. 825–830

McDonell S M 1999 Libido, erection and ejaculatory dysfunction in stallions. Compendium on Continuing Education for the Practicing Veterinarian March:263–266

McDonnell S M 2000 Pharmacologic manipulation of sexual behavior in the stallion. In: Proceedings of the Bluegrass Equine Reproduction Symposium, Lexington, KY, 2000

McDonnell S M 2001 Oral imipramine and intravenous xylazine for pharmacologically-induced ex copula ejaculation in stallions. Animal Reproduction Science 68:153–159

McGladdery A J, Rossdale P D 1991 Response of the equine fetus to maternal drug administration and acoustic stimulation. In: Proceedings of the 37th American Association of Equine Practitioners Annual Convention, San Francisco, CA, pp. 223–228

Miller C D, Varner D D, Blanchard T L et al 1997 Effects of altrenogest on behavior and reproductive function of stallions. In: Proceedings of the 43rd American Association of Equine Practitioners Annual Convention, Phoenix, AZ, pp. 197–198

Ousey J C, Dudan F, Rossdale P D 1984 Preliminary studies of mammary secretions in the mare to assess foetal readiness for birth. Equine Veterinary Journal 16:259–263

Ousey J C, Rossdale P D, Dudan F E et al 1998 The effects of intrafetal ACTH administration on the outcome of pregnancy in the mare. Reproduction, Fertility and Development 10:359–367

Ousey J C, Rossdale P D, Palmer L et al 2000 Effects of maternally administered depot ACTH(1–24) on fetal maturation and the timing of parturition in the mare. Equine Veterinary Journal 32:489–496

Pashen R L 1982 Oxytocin: the induction agent of choice in the mare? Journal of Reproduction and Fertility Supplements 32:645

Perkins N R 1999 Equine Reproductive Pharmacology. Veterinary Clinics of North America Equine Practice 15:687–704

Robinson N E (ed) 1997 Current therapy in equine medicine. Saunders, Philadelphia, PA

Roser F J, Hughes J P 1991 Prolonged pulsatile administration of gonadotrophin-releasing hormone (GnRH) to fertile stallions. Journal of Reproduction and Fertility Supplements 44:155–168

Roser J F, Keifer B L, Evans J W et al 1979 The development of antibodies to human chorionic gonadotropin following its repeated injection in the cyclic mare. Journal of Reproduction and Fertility Supplements 27:173–179

Roser J F, Evans J W, Keifer B L et al 1980 Reproductive efficiency in mares with anti-HCG antibodies. In: Proceedings of the 9th International Congress on Animal Reproduction and Artificial Insemination (Madrid) vol 3, p. 194

Schumacher J, Vaughan J T 1988 Surgery of the penis and prepuce. Veterinary Clinics of North America Equine Practice 4:473–491

Sertich P L, Vaala W E 1992 Concentrations of antibiotics in mares, foals, and fetal fluids after antibiotic administration during late pregnancy. In: Proceedings of the 38th American Association of Equine Practitioners Annual Convention, Orlando, FL, pp. 727–733

Shivola A V, Platov E M, Lebendev S G 1976 The use of human chorionic gonadotrophin for ovulation date regulation in mares. In: Proceedings of the 8th International Congress on Animal Reproduction and Artificial Insemination (Crackow) vol. 3, pp. 204–207

Silberzahn P, Pouret E J, Zwain I 1989 Androgen and oestrogen response to a single injection of hCG in cryptorchid horses. Equine Veterinary Journal 21:126–129

Silver M, Ousey J C, Dudan F E et al 1984 Studies on equine prematurity 2: postnatal adrenocortical activity in relation to plasma adrenocorticotrophic hormone and catecholamine levels in term and premature foals. Equine Veterinary Journal 16:278–286

Squires E L 1993 Progestin. In: McKinnon A O, Voss J L (eds) Equine reproduction. Lea & Febiger, Philadelphia, PA, pp. 311–318

Squires E L 2000 Effect of drugs on spermatogenesis and fertility. In: Proceedings of the Bluegrass Equine Reproduction Symposium, Lexington, KY, 2000

Troedsson M 2002 Diagnostic work-up for barren mares and breeding the problem mare. In: Proceedings of the Bluegrass Equine Reproduction Symposium, Lexington, KY, 2000

Vivrette S L 1997 Parturition and postpartum complications. In: Robinson N E (ed) Current therapy in equine medicine, 4th edn. Saunders, Philadelphia, PA, pp. 547–551

Vivrette S L 2001 Fluorquinolone arthropathy in neonatal foals. In: Proceedings of the 47th American Association of Equine Practitioners Annual Convention, San Diego, CA, pp. 376–377

CHAPTER CONTENTS

Introduction 193
    Cardiac rate and rhythm 193
    Stroke volume 194

Antiarryhthmic agents 194
    Class I antiarrhythmic agents 195
    Class Ia antiarrhythmic agents 195
    Class Ib antiarrhythmic agents 200
    Class Ic antiarrhythmic agents 202
    Class II antiarrhythmic agents 202
    Class III antiarrhythmic agents 203
    Class IV antiarrhythmic agents 204
    Other antiarrhythmic drugs 204
    Bradyarrhythmias 205

Therapy to alter stroke volume 205
    Positive inotropes 206
    Novel positive inotropes 207
    Acute inotropes and vasopressors 207
    Diuretics 210
    Vasodilators 210

References 213

12

Drugs acting on the cardiovascular system

*I. Mark Bowen   Celia M. Marr
Jonathan Elliott*

INTRODUCTION

The use of cardiac therapeutic agents in the horse is less developed than in other species and these agents are often used empirically by extrapolation of data from other species. With a few exceptions, there is no difference between the arsenal of cardiac drugs used currently in equine medicine and that used 20 years ago. This chapter describes the current practice in equine cardiac therapeutics and also discusses some newer agents used in other species that are currently under preliminary evaluation in the horse.

The function of the cardiovascular system is to maintain adequate tissue perfusion. Cardiac output is the product of heart rate (rhythm) and cardiac contractility (giving rise to stroke volume). These factors are under neuronal, hormonal and mechanical control systems. Pharmacological manipulation of any of these contributors will result in changes in cardiovascular function and hence peripheral blood flow. In human medicine, the primary goal is to increase life expectancy, while maintenance of performance and quality of life are the main priorities in equine medicine.

CARDIAC RATE AND RHYTHM

The cardiac conduction system of the horse shares many features with other species but also has some important differences. The function of the heart relies upon the presence of cells capable of spontaneous activity; these form the pacemaker areas of the heart. These nodal areas generate the normal cardiac rhythm. The electrical activity of the

Purkinje cells is demonstrated in Figure 12.1 and, like all cardiac myocytes, can be divided into four phases. Phase 4 (pacemaker potential) involves the slow influx of sodium ions, depolarizing the cell until the threshold potential is reached. Once the threshold potential is reached, the fast sodium current is activated, resulting in a rapid influx of sodium ions causing cell depolarization (phase 0; rapid depolarization). Phase 1 (partial repolarization) involves the inactivation of sodium channels and a transient outward current. Phase 2 (plateau phase) results from the slow influx of calcium ions. Repolarization (phase 3) occurs as a result of outflow of potassium ions from the cell and restores the resting potential. There are variations between the different areas of the heart, specifically the nodal tissues do not possess fast sodium channels and slow L-type calcium channels generate phase 0 current (Fig. 12.1). Phase 4 activity varies between nodal areas: the sinoatrial node depolarizes more rapidly than the atrioventricular (AV) node. Automaticity is under autonomic nervous system control. Parasympathetic neurons release acetylcholine, which slows the rate of depolarization (Phase 4 conduction). The AV node has extensive parasympathetic innervation in the horse, so that vagal slowing often results in AV blockade. Sympathetic innervation controls phases 2, 3 and 4, increasing the rate of depolarization and the influx of calcium ions so that more calcium is available for the contraction process, increasing the force of contraction and bringing about more rapid repolarization.

STROKE VOLUME

Several factors, such as preload, afterload, heart rate and contractility, determine normal cardiovascular function. Contractility is affected both by preload and afterload, as well as the inotropic state of the ventricular myocardium. Preload is the diastolic load placed upon the ventricle by the venous return of blood and affects contractility as described by Starling's law of the heart, where increased diastolic volume leads to a greater force of contraction. Preload is affected by the venous tone and by the circulating blood volume. Afterload opposes contraction throughout systole and is determined by the arterial resistance and by the circulating blood volume.

ANTIARRYHTHMIC AGENTS

Arrhythmias can be classified as either physiological or pathological. Physiological arrhythmias are common in horses and several types of arrhythmia are often detected incidentally on electrocardiograms (ECG) taken during ambulatory examinations. Proarrhythmias are arrhythmias that are drug induced or drug aggrevated. Before undertaking any antiarrhythmic therapy, it is important to establish if there is an underlying cause, such as fluid and electrolyte imbalances, and the need for any specific therapy. In the intensive care setting, antiarrhythmic therapy for tachyarrhythmias is generally indicated if:

● the heart rate is greater than 100 beats/min;
● the cardiac rhythm is unstable and likely to progress to a more malignant arrhythmia, such as a multifocal ventricular tachycardia;

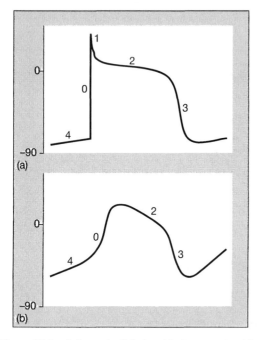

Figure 12.1 Action potential of ventricular myocytes (a) and nodal cells (b), showing four phases of electrical depolarization and repolarization. Note that phase 4 is faster in the nodal tissues, resulting in their increased automaticity compared with myocardial cells.

- a tachyarrhythmia with the R-on-T phenomenon occurs; or
- there are clinical or clinicopathological signs of poor cardiac output, such as weakness, increases in the serum creatinine concentration or reduced urine output.

Bradyarrhythmias are rarely pathological and are discussed separately.

Classically antiarrhythmic agents are divided into four classes (Table 12.1) based upon their actions on ion channels. Although this classification is useful, some agents can be categorized into more than one group.

CLASS I ANTIARRHYTHMIC AGENTS

Class I antiarrhythmic agents block the voltage-sensitive sodium channels of the myocardial cells. They can be further subdivided into classes Ia, Ib and Ic based on their specific effects on these channels. Their actions are mediated mainly through non-nodal tissue; therefore, these drugs affect the propagation of the action potential. These agents are use dependent in that they bind to sodium channels in the open or refractory states so that binding is preferentially to activated sodium channels and drugs dissociate from channels in the closed state. Each subclass of agent possesses

different kinetics for dissociation from the sodium channels.

CLASS Ia ANTIARRHYTHMIC AGENTS

Class Ia antiarrhythmic agents block fast sodium channels and prolong the action potential (class III effect), thereby lengthening the effective refractory period. They can cause QT interval prolongation, which may in turn be proarrhythmic, promoting re-entry. In the horse, they are useful for the treatment of a wide variety of arrhythmias, including both supraventricular and ventricular tachycardias.

Quinidine

Quinidine, the *d*-isomer of quinine, has been used in horses since 1924 (Roos 1924) and has a wide variety of properties. It is currently the drug of choice for the treatment of atrial fibrillation (AF) in horses but can be used for the treatment of a variety of re-entrant and ectopic arrhythmias. Quinidine affects heart rate, cardiac rhythm and vascular tone by a range of mechanisms and also produces a variety of non-cardiac effects. In addition to the class Ia activity, which prolongs the effective refractory period, the drug is vagolytic as a result of its antimuscarinic properties.

Table 12.1 Classification of antidysrrhythmic agents and indications for their use in horses

Class	Pharmacological action	Examples	Clinical indication
I	Sodium channel blocking		
Ia	Prolongs action potential	Quinidine	Atrial fibrillation Ventricular tachycardia
		Procainamide	Ventricular tachycardia
Ib	Rapid kinetics, no effect on action potential	Lignocaine Phenytoin	Ventricular tachycardia Digoxin-induced arrhythmias
Ic	Widen QRS, shortens action potential	Propafenone Flecainide	Ventricular tachycardia
II	Beta blockers	Propanolol	Supraventricular and ventricular tachycardias
III	Potassium channel blocking	Amiodarone Bretylium	Resistant ventricular fibrillation
IV	Calcium channel blocking	Diltiazem	

Quinidine also inhibits α adrenoceptors, causing vasodilatation; the subsequent reflex increase in sympathetic outflow (as a result of hypotension) results in this drug having proarrhythmic effects. Quinidine can be given either via nasogastric tube (quinidine sulfate) or intravenously (i.v.; quinidine gluconate).

Pharmacokinetics

Quinidine is an organic weak base that is 75–80% protein bound (Neff et al 1972). Protein binding is pH dependent, so alkalization promotes protein binding and can be used for the treatment of adverse effects. In horses, there seems to be considerable variation in the time to peak concentrations (mean 146 min, range 60–240 min) and the average bioavailability (48.5 ± 20.4%) after a single oral (p.o.) dose of 10 mg/kg (Mcguirk et al 1981). Feeding reduces the bioavailability by up to 25% (Bouckaert et al 1994). Following i.v. administration to horses, plasma concentrations of quinidine followed a two-compartment model and the elimination half-life was 6.65 ± 3.00 h (Mcguirk et al 1981). Quinidine is metabolized in the liver by hydroxylation; the activity of its metabolites is unknown.

Therapeutic drug monitoring

When quinidine is administered p.o. at a dose rate of 22 mg/kg every 2 h, therapeutic drug monitoring is ideally performed after the fourth to sixth dose, with serum obtained 1 h after the administration of quinidine. The therapeutic range is 2–5 μg/ml (Reef 1999) and signs of toxicity are commonly seen when plasma concentrations exceed 5 μg/ml (Reef et al 1995).

Adverse effects

The adverse effects of quinidine can be divided into cardiac and non-cardiac manifestations. Depression and paraphimosis are seen in many horses treated with quinidine sulfate and resolve once treatment is discontinued. Gastrointestinal effects include flatulence, which is rarely of clinical significance, and colic and diarrhea, both of which are occasionally severe and necessitate the discontinuation of treatment. Nasal mucosal swelling, leading to airway obstruction and ataxia can occur at higher plasma concentrations, whereas colic, diarrhea or tachycardia can occur at any plasma concentration. Hypotension may occur as a result of peripheral vasodilation (α adrenoceptor antagonistic effect) and decreased cardiac contractility; if severe, it can be treated using an i.v. infusion of phenylephrine (Table 12.2). Prolongation of the QRS complex, owing to prolongation of the action potential, is an indicator of potential quinidine toxicity. If the QRS interval exceeds 125% of baseline values, treatment should be discontinued. Supraventricular tachycardia may occur during treatment with quinidine, owing to an increase in the ventricular response rate as a result of the drug's vagolytic activity, such that the AV node cannot limit conduction from the atria to the ventricles. Treatment of supraventricular tachycardia should be commenced if the rate exceeds 100 beats/min (Table 12.2). Ventricular arrhythmias occur as a result of the proarrhythmic affects of quinidine and by QRS prolongation and warrant treatment with specific antiarrhythmic agents (Table 12.2). In the case of life-threatening arrhythmias, bicarbonate should be administered to increase protein binding and reduce the plasma concentrations of quinidine. Torsades de pointes, a bizarre ventricular arrhythmia characterized by wide QRS complexes that rotate around the baseline, can occur following quinidine administration (Fig. 12.2.) Magnesium sulfate is an effective treatment for torsades de pointes in humans (Tzivoni et al 1988) and its antiarrhythmic activity is discussed below.

Clinical indications

Quinidine sulfate is indicated for the treatment of sustained AF while i.v. quinidine gluconate is indicated for treatment of ventricular tachycardia (Fig. 12.3, Table 12.3) and recent onset AF (<7 days duration, Table 12.3) (Gerber et al 1971, Muir et al 1990), although paroxysmal AF can convert spontaneously to sinus rhythm within 48 h in the absence of treatment. The recommended regimen for use of quinidine gluconate is 1.1–2.2 mg/kg i.v.

Table 12.2 Management of the side-effects of quinidine therapy in the horse

Toxic effect	Frequency of effect[a]	Treatment (Reef et al 1995)
Depression	C	None, resolves after cessation of therapy
Paraphimosis	C	None, resolves after cessation of therapy
Urticaria	R	Discontinue treatment; corticosteroids if severe
Upper respiratory tract obstruction (owing to nasal mucosal swelling)	10%	Dexamethasone 0.1 mg/kg i.v.; nasotracheal tube or tracheostomy
Laminitis	R	Discontinue treatment; appropriate laminitis therapy
Ataxia, convulsions	12%	Discontinue treatment; anticonvulsant if severe: diazepam
Diarrhoea	12%	Usually resolves of cessation of therapy, analgesic therapy as required; discontinue treatment if severe
Colic	21%	Usually resolves of cessation of therapy, analgesic therapy as required; discontinue treatment if severe
Supraventricular tachycardia <100 beats/min >100 beats/min >150 beats/min	12%	Monitor for signs of progression Digoxin 2.2 mg/kg i.v. Digoxin 2.2 mg/kg i.v.; sodium bicarbonate 1 mmol/kg. *If unsuccessful or clinical signs of hypotension:* propanolol 0.03 mg/kg i.v.; phenylepherine infusion 0.1–0.2 μg/min i.v. per kg, total does not to exceed 0.01 mg/kg
Ventricular tachycardia	R	Lidocaine infusion 20–50 μg/min per kg or 0.25–0.5 mg/kg *slow* i.v. every 10 min; magnesium sulfate 1–2.5 g/min over 10 min for a 450 kg horse, maximum dose 25 g/450 kg
Congestive heart failure		Digoxin 0.0022 mg/kg i.v.
Hypotension	12%	Treat only if severe; phenylepherine infusion 0.1–0.2 μg/min i.v. per kg; total does not to exceed 0.01 mg/kg

[a]C, common; R, rare or not described; i.v., intravenous

every 10 min until conversion or until a maximum dose of 12 mg/kg has been given (Reef 1999). AF of more than a few days' duration should be treated with quinidine sulfate by nasogastric tube to avoid the development of severe oral ulceration (Reef 1999). An oral quinidine paste has been assessed for use in horses; however, steady-state concentrations were not reached and serum concentrations were highly variable (Bouckaert et al 1994).

The prognosis for conversion to sinus rhythm in horses with sustained AF is dependent on the presence and nature of any underlying cardiac disease and on the duration of the AF. In horses that have developed AF recently, the response to treatment is likely to be good and the recurrence rate is only 15% (Reef et al 1988). It is recommended that continuous ECG is used during the period; if this is not available, a paper trace recording should be obtained prior to each dose to ensure there is no QRS complex prolongation. Some authors recommend a test dose to identify side effects that are not dose dependent, such as urticaria and laminitis (Reef et al 1995); however, this step is considered unnecessary by many clinicians. Quinidine sulfate is given at 22 mg/kg every 2 h until conversion to a normal sinus rhythm, the development of toxic effects or a maximum of five or six doses have been administered. If available, therapeutic drug monitoring should be performed after the fourth to sixth dose. The dosing interval should be extended to every 6 h provided that plasma concentrations exceed 4 μg/ml (Reef et al 1995) and are less than 5 μg/ml. However, if quinidine concentrations cannot be monitored, the dosing interval is generally extended to every 6 h (one half-life) to maintain steady-state plasma concentrations. Potential complications following treatment for AF with quinidine are discussed above and therapeutic options are shown in Table 12.2.

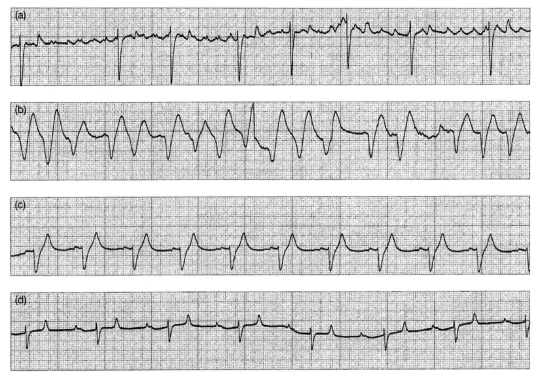

Figure 12.2 Electrocardiograms from a horse undergoing treatment for atrial fibrillation. (a, b) Base-apex (a) and modified base-apex (b) electrocardiograms after treatment with quinidine sulfate (330 mg/kg). Ventricular tachycardia. (torsades de pointes) occurred after 40 h. (c) The horse was treated with five bolus doses of magnesium sulfate, together with intravenous propanolol, which resulted in conversion to normal sinus rhythm with QRS prolongation. (d) Twenty-four hours after conversion, the electrocardiogram showed normal sinus rhythm without QRS prolongation.

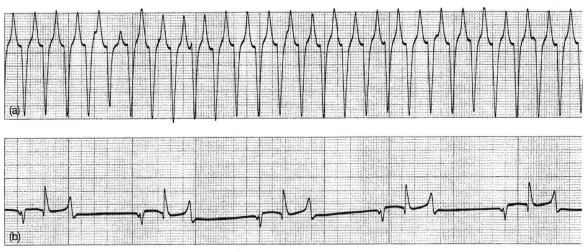

Figure 12.3 Base-apex electrocardiograms from an 11-year-old horse that presented in congestive heart failure. (a) Before treatment, with ventricular tachycardia; (b) Conversion to normal sinus rhythm was achieved with 5 liters 0.64% solution quinidine gluconate, infused at approximately 1 l/h. No specific cause was identified, although echocardiography revealed a segmental area of hypomotile ventricular myocardium, suggestive of ischaemia. The horse was euthanased 3 weeks later after recurrence of the arrhythmia.

Table 12.3   Drug dosages for cardiovascular medicine in the horse

Drug	Indication[a]	Dose
Acepromazine	Vasodilatation in congestive heart failure	1.5 mg/kg p.o., b.i.d. or t.i.d
Atropine	Bradycardia of vagal origin	0.01–0.2 mg/kg i.v. or s.c.
Bretylium	Refractory ventricular fibrillation	3–5 mg/kg i.v.[b]
Digoxin	Congestive heart failure; treatment of atrial fibrillation	2.2 µg/kg i.v., b.i.d. or as required 11 µg/kg p.o., b.i.d.
Dobutamine	Hypotension	1–5 µg/kg/min i.v.
Dopamine	Prerenal renal failure; cardiogenic shock	1–5 µg/kg/min i.v. or 15 µg/kg/min in severe hypotension
Dopexamine	Hypotension in anaesthetized animals	1–5 µg/kg/min i.v.
Enalapril	Vasodilatation in congestive heart failure	0.5 mg/kg p.o. once daily[b]
Furosemide (frusemide)	Congestive heart failure; equine idiopathic pulmonary hypertension	1–3 mg/kg i.v., b.i.d. or t.i.d. 1–3 mg/kg p.o., b.i.d. or t.i.d
Glycopyrrolate	Bradycardia of vagal origin	5 µg/kg i.v.
Hydralazine	Vasodilatation in congestive heart failure	0.5 mg/kg i.v.
Lidocaine (lignocaine)	Ventricular tachycardia	0.25–0.5 mg/kg i.v.; total not to exceed 2 mg/kg
Magnesium sulfate	Torsades des points; refractory ventricular tachycardia	Magnesium sulfate 1–2.5 g/min over 10 min for a 450 kg animal; max. dose 25 g for 450 kg animal
Milrinone	Hypotension	0.5 µg/kg i.v. bolus followed by 1.5–5 µg/kg/min i.v. maintenance
Norepinephrine (noradrenaline)	Severe refractory cardiogenic shock	0.1–0.75 µg/kg/min i.v.
Phenylephrine	Critical maintenance of perfusion	Infusion 0.1–0.2 µg/kg/min i.v.; not to exceed 0.01 mg/kg
Phenytoin	Digoxin-induced ventricular tachycardia	7.5 mg/kg i.v. 10 mg/kg p.o., once daily
Procainamide	Ventricular tachycardia	1 mg/kg/min i.v.; total dose not to exceed 20 mg/kg
Propafenone	Ventricular tachycardia	0.5–1 mg/kg i.v. over 5 min[b]
Propranolol	Refractory ventricular and supraventricular tachycardia (quinidine toxicity)	0.05–0.16 mg/kg i.v., b.i.d. 0.38–0.78 mg/kg p.o., t.i.d.
Quinidine gluconate	Acute-onset atrial fibrillation; ventricular tachycardia	2.2 mg/kg i.v. every 10 min; 12 mg/kg total
Quinidine sulfate	Atrial fibrillation	2.2 mg/kg by nasogastric tube every 2 h for six doses
Scopolamine (hyoscine)	Bradycardia of vagal origin	0.14 mg/kg i.v.

p.o., oral; i.v., intravenous; b.i.d., twice daily; t.i.d., three times a day; kg, body weight in kg
[a] Non-cardiovascular indications not included
[b] No data available for the horse; dosage regimens based upon use in other species

If conversion to normal sinus rhythm has not been achieved by the second day of treatment, digoxin may be coadministered p.o. at 0.011 mg/kg twice daily. This offsets the proarrhythmic effect of quinidine by slowing conduction through the AV node. However, coadministration of digoxin and quinidine will affect serum concentrations of each drug and, therefore, serum digoxin concentration should be monitored if its

coadministration with quinidine continues for more than 48 h (Reef 1999).

Horses with congestive heart failure (CHF) and AF have a poor prognosis for conversion to sinus rhythm (Reef et al 1988). Digitalization is the treatment of choice for horses with AF secondary to CHF to reduce the ventricular response rate and, therefore, to optimize ventricular filling. Propranolol may also be used to reduce the ventricular response rate further. If treatment with quinidine is attempted in these cases, digoxin should be administered from the first day of treatment to offset myocardial depression and reduce the proarrhythmic activity of quinidine.

Drug interactions

Quinidine decreases renal clearance of digoxin and displaces digoxin from skeletal muscle binding sites, resulting in a doubling of plasma digoxin concentrations (Parraga et al 1995). Potential interactions with other antiarrhythmic agents reported in humans are either caused by combined proarrhythmic actions or negative inotropic actions.

Procainamide

Procainamide is a class Ia agent that does not induce QRS complex prolongation and which is a less-potent vagolytic drug than quinidine. Prolongation of the QT interval occurs following i.v. administration (Ellis et al 1994) and may account for its proarrhythmic effect at higher doses. Although mild peripheral vasodilatation occurs (Muir & Mcguirk 1987), the mechanism of this action is through direct inhibition of the sympathetic outflow not direct receptor binding (Rea et al 1991). Procainamide is less effective than quinidine for the treatment of supraventricular arrhythmias (Muir & Mcguirk 1987) but may be more efficacious for the treatment of ventricular arrhythmias. Procainamide has the additional advantage that it is readily available in some countries (e.g. the UK).

Pharmacokinetics

Procainamide undergoes acetylation in plasma to form *N*-acetylprocainamide (NAPA), an active metabolite with class III antiarrhythmic activity (Ellis et al 1994). Procainamide undergoes renal elimination and has a half-life of 3.49 ± 0.6 h following i.v. administration to horses (Ellis et al 1994). The plasma half-life of NAPA is twice that of the parent drug (6.31 ± 1.49 h) with peak NAPA concentrations occurring 5.2 h after administration of a single dose of procainamide (Ellis et al 1994). This results in procainamide having a longer biological half-life.

Adverse effects

Procainamide does not produce serious side-effects like quinidine and lidocaine (lignocaine); however, it is a negative inotrope and may cause hypotension; QRS prolongation and ventricular arrhythmias can occur at high doses (Muir & Mcguirk 1987).

Clinical indications

Procainamide is available for i.v. and p.o. administration. It has been used for the treatment of acute-onset AF in horses (Marr & Reef 1995a), although this requires further investigation. It is used primarily for the treatment of ventricular tachycardias in horses, where its main advantage is the absence of significant side-effects.

Drug interactions

Cimetidine increases plasma concentrations of procainamide in humans. There are no reported drug interactions for procainamide in the horse (Muir & Mcguirk 1987).

CLASS Ib ANTIARRHYTHMIC AGENTS

Class Ib agents rapidly associate with and dissociate from activated sodium channels during a normal cardiac cycle. This means that only premature depolarization is blocked. Furthermore, these agents preferentially bind to refractory sodium channels and thus act primarily on damaged myocardial cells to prevent re-entry pathways. The rapid binding and dissociation kinetics of these agents mean that they are ineffective in controlling atrial arrhythmias since the atrial action potential is very short (Langenfeld et al 1990). These agents do not affect potassium channels and so do not shorten the action potential or cause QT interval prolongation.

Lidocaine (lignocaine)

Lidocaine (lignocaine) is a class Ib antiarrhythmic agent. Its antiarrhythmic action is mediated mainly within the non-nodal tissue of the ventricles and relates to the relatively long ventricular action potential. Electrolyte imbalance should be evaluated and corrected prior to treatment with lidocaine, as the drug is less effective in the presence of hypokalaemia (Singh & Nademanee 1985).

Pharmacokinetics

Lidocaine has a short biological half-life and undergoes de-ethylation by hepatic microsomal enzymes. Its clearance is dependent on hepatic blood flow and may, therefore, be affected by disorders of hepatic blood flow or by the concurrent administration of drugs that reduce hepatic blood flow (Muir & Mcguirk 1987), such as propranolol and halothane. In horses, fasting is known to prolong the hepatic clearance of lidocaine by reducing hepatic blood flow and via intrinsic mechanisms (Engelking et al 1987). Administration of lidocaine p.o. results in a high level of hepatic first-pass metabolism and absorption is variable following intramuscular (i.m.) administration; therefore, only i.v. administration can be recommended.

Adverse effects

The most common adverse effect of lidocaine (lignocaine) is central nervous system (CNS) toxicity: nystagmus, muscle twitching, disorientation,

excitement and convulsions occur if bolus doses of lidocaine exceed 2 mg/kg (Muir & Mcguirk 1987). Although these neurological complications are usually short lived and resolve as plasma concentrations fall, anticonvulsant therapy (i.v. administration of diazepam at 0.05 mg/kg) can be used to control seizures, if necessary. Lidocaine does not produce adverse hemodynamic effects and rarely modifies nodal conduction.

Clinical indications

Lidocaine is indicated for the treatment of ventricular tachycardias (Fig. 12.4). Electrolyte abnormalities should be investigated and corrected prior to lidocaine administration. Lidocaine is administered as i.v. bolus doses of 0.5 mg/kg every 5 min, up to a total dose of 4 mg/kg (Table 12.3) (Muir & Mcguirk 1987). Although lidocaine is used frequently in anaesthetized horses, quinidine gluconate or procainamide are preferred in conscious horses because they do not produce CNS side effects.

Phenytoin (diphenylhydantoin)

Phenytoin is another class Ib antiarrhythmic drug that is used mainly for the treatment of cardiac

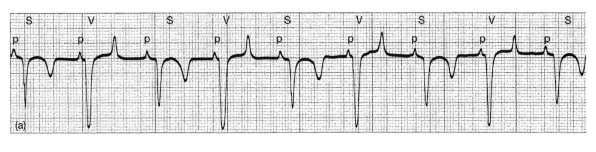

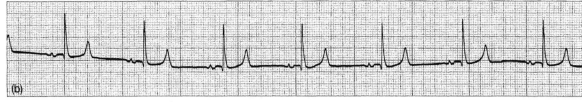

Figure 12.4 Base-apex electrocardiograms from an anaesthetized horse, with endotoxemia caused by a strangulating intestinal lesion. (a) The cardiac rhythm was converted from ventricular tachycardia to the bigeminal rhythm by administration of two bolus doses of lidocaine. Although ventricular complexes (V) are preceded by p waves (p) the p–r distance is shorter than the sinus complexes (S). (b) Magnesium sulfate administered intravenously resulted in conversion to sinus rhythm.

glycoside-induced arrhythmias. Recently, it has been used for the treatment of ventricular ectopy. Phenytoin is also an anticonvulsant drug and is used in the control of recurrent rhabdomyolysis in horses for its membrane stabilizing effect.

Pharmacokinetics

After p.o. administration to horses, phenytoin has poor bioavailability (34.5 ± 8.6%) because of extensive first-pass metabolism. Peak concentrations are achieved after 1–4 h and phenytoin is highly plasma protein bound (73%) (Kowalczyk & Beech 1983). The recommended dose rates are shown in Table 12.3.

Clinical indications

Phenytoin is the drug of choice for the treatment of cardiac glycoside-induced ventricular arrhythmias and has been used successfully by p.o. administration for the management of digitalis toxicity in the horse (Wijnberg et al 1999). Recently phenytoin has been described for the treatment of ventricular ectopy in nine horses (20–22 mg/kg p.o. twice daily) and resulted in resolution of the arrhythmia in all nine after four doses, with plasma concentrations of 9.4 µg/ml (Wijnberg 2001). Sedation may be observed at higher drug concentrations.

Adverse effects

The toxic effects of phenytoin (sedation and depression) occur through its CNS actions.

Other class Ib agents

Other class Ib agents, e.g. tocainide and mexiletine, are administered p.o. for treatment of ventricular arrhythmias in humans and dogs but have not yet been evaluated for use in the horse and appear to offer no significant advantages over procainamide in this species.

CLASS Ic ANTIARRHYTHMIC AGENTS

Class Ic antiarrhythmic agents are powerful inhibitors of the fast sodium channel. They cause differential blockade between the Purkinje fibers and surrounding myocardium, promoting the heterogeneity of action potentials. This effect, together with prolongation of the QRS complex, results in a proarrhythmic effect. The drugs are potent antiarrhythmic agents that are usually reserved for the control ventricular tachyarrhythmias that are resistant to other therapeutic agents. These agents (flecainide, encainide and propafenone) have become unpopular in human medicine after some studies showed an increased incidence of sudden death in human patients receiving treatment for asymptomatic or minimally symptomatic ventricular arrhythmias (Anon. 1989, Siebels et al 1993). Administration of propafenone i.v. at a dose rate of 0.5–1 mg/kg infused over 5–10 min has been described for the treatment of sustained ventricular tachycardia in one horse (Marr & Reef 1995a). The authors have administered propafenone p.o. to a limited number of cases with little success. Flecainide has been successfully used to treat horses with AF induced by right atrial pacing at 1–2 mg/kg i.v. (Ohmura et al 2000). The pharmacokinetics have also been studied following p.o. administration; doses of 4–6 mg/kg resulted in therapeutic concentrations of the drug (Ohmura et al 2001). The toxic effects of flecainide are limited to QRS prolongation; therefore, ventricular arrhythmias may be experienced in clinical use but it is free of the vagolytic, vasodilatory and non-cardiovascular effects of quinidine. At the time of writing, there are no data to support its use in the treatment of sustained, naturally occurring AF.

CLASS II ANTIARRHYTHMIC AGENTS

The β adrenoceptor antagonists (beta blockers) are class II antiarrhythmic agents. They prolong phase 4 of the cardiac action potential (pacemaker potential), slowing the heart rate. There are three subtypes of β adrenoceptors: β_1, β_2 and β_3. Stimulation of β_1 adrenoceptors in the heart increases the force and rate of cardiac contraction, as well as increasing automaticity of the pacemaker sites and conduction through the AV node. The β_2

adrenoceptors are located within the blood vessels and bronchioles and their activation leads to bronchodilation and vasodilatation. These adrenoceptors are also located in the sinoatrial and AV nodes, activation of which causes increased automaticity; this results in an increase in heart rate, such as that seen after the i.v. administration of clenbuterol to horses (Dodam et al 1993, Shapland et al 1981). The β_3 adrenoceptors have been identified in the human heart where they cause a reduction in myocardial contractility, mediated through the activation of nitric oxide synthase (Gauthier et al 1998). To date, β_3 adrenoceptors have not been identified in equine myocardium. Beta blockers are not used frequently in horses.

Propranolol

Propranolol is the prototypical beta blocker that acts at both β_1 and β_2 adrenoceptors. Like all beta blockers, it causes dose-dependent suppression of myocardial contractility, although this is not usually seen at therapeutic doses.

Pharmacokinetics

Propranolol is a lipid-soluble drug that undergoes rapid hepatic metabolism, resulting in a short half-life (2 h). Rapid first-pass metabolism results in a low bioavailability and therapeutic plasma concentrations are rarely achieved in the horse after oral administration (Muir & Mcguirk 1987). The drug can only administered i.v. and plasma concentrations are increased if hepatic blood flow is reduced, e.g. by significant cardiac disease.

Adverse effects

The toxic effects of propranolol are related to its negative inotropic and chronotropic properties, which can lead to sinus bradycardia and hypotension. These complications should be treated with an acute inotrope such as dopamine or dobutamine.

Clinical indications

Propranolol should be reserved for the treatment of supraventricular and ventricular tachycardias

that are refractory to other therapeutic agents, because of its deleterious effects on cardiac performance. It can be used for the treatment of quinidine-induced ventricular tachyarrhythmias (Fig. 12.2), as it has no effect on phase 1 of the cardiac action potential.

Other beta blockers

Atenolol is a selective β_1 adrenoceptor antagonist that undergoes almost no hepatic metabolism. As such, the drug is favored for oral administration to other species but it has not been utilized clinically in the horse. Similarly, esmolol, an ultra-short acting β_1 adrenoceptor-blocking drug that undergoes plasma esterification, has not yet been used in the horse. Esmolol is used in other species for the treatment of supraventricular tachycardias.

CLASS III ANTIARRHYTHMIC AGENTS

Class III antiarrhythmic agents act by suppressing the inward potassium current, slowing phase 3 of the cardiac action potential, prolonging the refractory period and lengthening the duration of the action potential. They are used for the treatment of ventricular tachycardias in humans, where they prevent re-entrant pathways and, therefore, prevent the onset of ventricular fibrillation, which is associated with sudden death in humans receiving class I antiarrhythmic agents (Singh 1993). Prolongation of the action potential and especially of the QT interval is probably caused by potassium channel blockade and may result in a proarrhythmic effect. With the exception of bretylium, these drugs have not been utilized in equine medicine and no data exist on their pharmacokinetics in this species.

Bretylium

Bretylium is used solely for treatment of ventricular fibrillation but it is unique in that it is the only drug that has proven efficacy in this role. In addition to its class III activity, it is classified as a noradrenergic neuron-blocking drug. Bretylium is concentrated in terminal sympathetic neurons of the Purkinje fibers, where it is responsible for the release of stored norepinephrine, although this action is terminated by inhibition of catecholamine release. Its use in human cardiac care is restricted to treatment of ventricular fibrillation following acute myocardial infarction where electroconversion has been unsuccessful. In one study, 27 human patients who had undergone unsuccessful conventional electrical and pharmacological treatment of ventricular fibrillation for 30 min were given a single bolus dose of bretylium: 20 had converted within 9–12 min (Holder et al 1977). Bretylium causes hypotension via the sympathetic nervous system. There are no data to support its use in the horse and its prohibitive cost limits its use to treatment of neonates with ventricular fibrillation, where DC electroconversion is unavailable or unsuccessful. A dosage regimen for horses has not been established but the authors have used it in a limited number of cases at the dose rate recommended for humans (Table 12.3).

Amiodarone

Amiodarone is highly lipophilic with a slow onset of action and long tissue half-life. The drug produces a variety of toxic effects ranging from gastrointestinal to neurological, cardiac and dermatological signs. Sotalol produces fewer side effects, has more predictable pharmacokinetics and is excreted by the kidneys. Both drugs can be given orally.

CLASS IV ANTIARRHYTHMIC AGENTS

Class IV antiarrhythmics (e.g. verapamil and diltiazem) are calcium channel blockers and, therefore, act on phase 2 of the cardiac action potential. These drugs are used for the treatment of supraventricular arrhythmias in humans and dogs but have not been evaluated critically in horses. In dogs, verapamil undergoes rapid first-pass metabolism and so has limited bioavailability (24%); it is therefore only administered i.v. Diltiazem is highly protein bound in the dog. The drug has been proposed as a suitable treatment of digitalis-induced arrhythmias in the dog. It has been proposed to reduce the ventricular response rate in the management of AF in dogs. However, calcium channel blockers depress myocardial contractility and should not be used in animals with CHF. On this basis, they do not appear to be indicated in horses with AF with a rapid ventricular rate since the majority of such horses have CHF caused by underlying organic heart disease.

Drugs that open the potassium channels also block the calcium channels by hypopolarizing the cell membrane. Adenosine causes potassium channel opening by binding to A_1 receptors (purinoceptors), which are linked by a G protein to potassium channels. Adenosine has not been evaluated in horses. Its main indication in human is for the treatment of narrow complex supraventricular tachycardias, such as AV nodal re-entrant tachycardia. It can also be used as a diagnostic aid to distinguish between wide complex tachycardias, which can be either supraventricular with aberrant conduction or ventricular in origin (Camm & Garratt 1991).

OTHER ANTIARRHYTHMIC DRUGS
Magnesium

Magnesium sulfate and magnesium chloride can be effective at terminating refractory ventricular arrhythmias, even in patients with normomagnesemia. Its mechanism of action is not fully understood. However, magnesium acts as a cofactor in the Na^+,K^+-ATPase system and this pump may become inactivated in hypomagnesemia, resulting in hypokalemia, which can predispose to arrhythmias (Wills 1986). In normomagnesemia, the mechanism of action is more complex, partly because of difficulties in determining the magnesium status. The ion occurs mainly in the intracellular fluid; consequently, serum magnesium concentrations may be normal even when the total body magnesium concentration is depleted. In normomagnesemic individuals, magnesium salts may exert their effect through a calcium channel blocking effect (Agus et al 1989). In humans, magnesium salts are the treatment of choice for torsades de pointes, a form of ventricular tachycardia associated with long QT intervals. Torsades de pointes can be induced by quinidine and this potentially fatal complication occurs in approximately 4% of horses treated with quinidine. The authors have used magnesium alone and in combination with propranolol for the treatment of quinidine-induced ventricular tachycardias in three horses (see Fig. 12.2). Magnesium has also been used successfully to treat ventricular tachycardia in hypomagnesemic (Marr & Reef 1991) and normomagnesemic horses (Fig. 12.4).

BRADYARRHYTHMIAS
Anticholinergic agents

In horses, bradyarrhythmias can occur as a result of the normal physiological control of heart rate and from drug administration, derangement of electrolytes or primary myocardial disease. Physiological bradyarrhythmias, which are by far the most common, are mediated by vagal tone and do not require treatment. Primary myocardial disease, such as fibrosis, may result in abnormal nodal conduction and hence AV blockade, whereas hyperkalemia induces bradycardia by partially depolarizing nodal tissue. Drugs, such as the α_2 adrenoceptor agonists (e.g. xylazine, detomidine, romifidine) and inhalational anesthetic agents (e.g. halothane), have both direct actions on the heart and cause bradyarrhythmias by increasing vagal tone.

Pathological bradyarrhythmias that affect cardiac output or peripheral perfusion require appropriate therapy. The primary aim of therapy should be the correction of the underlying disease mechanism; electrolyte abnormalities should be corrected or the depth of anesthesia reduced as appropriate. An α_2 adrenoceptor antagonist (e.g. atipamezole) can be considered in animals sedated with the α_2 adrenoceptor agonists but it should not be administered to animals anaesthetized with ketamine because of the risks of inducing ketamine-related excitement. Corticosteroids are indicated if myocardial inflammation is present.

Anticholinergic agents are only effective in controlling vagal-mediated bradyarrhythmias and, as such, are usually only used to treat or prevent life-threatening bradycardia during anesthesia. Atropine and glycopyrrolate are used most commonly. All anticholinergic agents competitively inhibit the binding of acetylcholine to the postganglionic synapses in the heart, thus blocking vagal-induced slowing of the heart rate. They also produce mydriasis, ileus and decrease salivary secretion.

Atropine

There have been no pharmacological studies of atropine in horses, despite its widespread use since the 1960s. The dose rates used in horses have been extrapolated from human medicine (Table 12.3). In the horse, the gastrointestinal effects of atropine last for up to 12 h (Ducharme & Fubini 1983). Following i.v. administration, there may be a transitory decrease in heart rate. Atropine is a tertiary amine and crosses the blood–brain barrier. It can produce CNS side-effects (e.g. excitement, sedation).

Glycopyrrolate

Glycopyrrolate is a quaternary ammonium compound that does not cross the blood–brain barrier and, therefore, produces far fewer CNS signs. The duration of the effects on gastrointestinal motility is dose dependent, lasting 6.4 h after administration at a dose rate of 5 μg/kg (Singh et al 1997).

Scopolamine (Hyoscine)

Scopolamine is an anticholinergic agent used for the treatment of spasmodic colic; it has been shown to inhibit romifidine-induced bradyarrhythmias (Marques et al 1998). Unlike atropine, scopolamine does not induce an initial bradycardia (Grainger & Smith 1983) and decreased gastrointestinal motility lasts only 20–30 min in horses (Roelvink et al 1991). The use of scopolamine in the face of life-threatening bradycardias in horses has not been established.

THERAPY TO ALTER STROKE VOLUME

Stroke volume can be manipulated pharmacologically through the use of inotropes, to increase the force of contraction of the heart, or the use of diuretics and vasodilators, to reduce the preload and/or afterload.

POSITIVE INOTROPES

All positive inotropes increase the concentration of calcium ions within the cell during systole, the amount of calcium available to the myofibrils and hence the force of muscular contraction. However, positive inotropes can be detrimental both through direct effects and through increasing the myocardial oxygen demand in order to achieve increased cardiac contractility. In animals with myocardial failure, where positive inotropes may increase the workload of the already failing heart; afterload reduction may be more beneficial. In AV valve insufficiency, positive inotropes are particularly controversial since it is argued that they increase regurgitant flow in addition to increasing forward flow.

The cardiac glycosides

Digoxin, the most commonly used cardiac glycoside, is indicated for the treatment of CHF and for the treatment of supraventricular tachyarrhythmias. It possesses positive inotropic and electrophysiological effects resulting from the inhibition of Na^+,K^+-ATPase, which increases intracellular sodium ion concentrations. This increase in intracellular sodium ions slows down calcium extrusion from the cell, resulting in an increase in intracytoplasmic calcium and, thereby, an increase in the contractile force.

Digoxin is a central vasodilator but a peripheral vasoconstrictor. However, it has many additional actions, some of which are mediated via autonomic function. The electrophysiological effects of the cardiac glycosides are mediated through an increase in vagal tone via the baroreceptor reflex. In human patients with CHF, the vasoconstrictive effects of digoxin are offset by the inhibition of renin release, mediated through the renal sodium pump (Ribner et al 1985). Digoxin also possesses mild diuretic effects through the inhibition of the renal sodium pump, inhibiting tubular reabsorption of sodium (Lewis 1990). Digoxin has been shown to be an effective inotrope in the horse,

where a maximal response was achieved with plasma concentrations of 2 ng/ml after i.v. administration of digoxin at a dose rate of 15 μg/kg (Button et al 1980). In equine CHF, digoxin is used to slow the ventricular response rate, especially in the presence of AF (Muir & Mcguirk 1985).

Pharmacokinetics

The pharmacokinetics of digoxin have been established both in normal horses (Brumbaugh et al 1983, Button et al 1980, Francfort & Schatzmann 1976, Pedersoli et al 1981) and those with CHF (Sweeney et al 1993). Digoxin is protein bound and eliminated primarily through the kidneys; therefore, renal function is an important consideration when determining dosing regimens. In the face of renal compromise, digoxin undergoes increased hepatic degradation. Following i.v. administration, plasma digoxin concentrations have been described using a tri-exponential equation in humans, dogs and horses (Button et al 1980, Francfort & Schatzmann 1976) and using a bi-exponential equation in the horse (Pedersoli et al 1978); this difference may result from the frequency of sampling. The half-life of digoxin is highly variable: 16.8 h and 28.8 h have been reported. These differences may reflect large interanimal variation in serum concentrations and demonstrate the importance of therapeutic drug monitoring. Button et al (1980) described the variations that occur after both oral and i.v. administration to horses of different age, sex and disease status.

Following oral administration, digoxin is absorbed rapidly with peak plasma concentrations occurring between 1 h (Button et al 1980) and 2 h (Sweeney et al 1993) after administration. The bioavailability following oral administration is approximately 20% (Button et al 1980, Sweeney et al 1993). Button et al (1980) described two peak plasma concentrations, occurring 9–15 h after administration. This phenomenon has also been reported in humans and probably represents enterohepatic recirculation of the drug.

Therapeutic drug monitoring

Individual variation in absorption, distribution and excretion results in wide interindividual variation in the serum concentrations of digoxin. Therapeutic drug monitoring has been recommended to prevent toxicity and to validate the efficacy of the dose of digoxin. Serum should be obtained 1 h (peak) and 12 h (trough) after dosing. Therapeutic drug monitoring should be performed after 3–6 days (five half-lives, i.e. once steady-state digoxin concentrations have been achieved; Kolibash et al 1989). The therapeutic concentrations should be in the range 0.5–2.0 ng/ml (Button et al 1980). Digoxin-induced arrhythmias should be treated with phenytoin.

Adverse effects

Digoxin toxicity can cause depression, anorexia and cardiac arrhythmias. The cardiac effects of digoxin toxicity are either related to the negative chronotropic actions of the drug or the production of tachyarrhythmias (Francfort & Schatzmann 1976). Tachyarrhythmias often occur when there is hypokalemia, as inhibition of the Na^+,K^+-ATPase exacerbates the hypopolarization of the myocardium.

Drug interactions

Coadministration of quinidine may predispose to digoxin toxicity. However, other antiarrhythmic drugs can also increase serum concentrations of digoxin by modifying either its renal (quinidine) or non-renal (quinidine, verapamil, amiodarone and propafenone) excretion (Muir & Mcguirk 1985).

Clinical indications

In the horse, digoxin is indicated most commonly for the treatment of supraventricular arrhythmias. Slowing the ventricular response rate improves ventricular performance and, therefore, maintains cardiac output. It is most commonly used for treatment of CHF in the presence of AF and can also be used to treat quinidine-induced arrhythmias. Loading doses (digitalizing doses) of digoxin are not recommended in the horse because of the increased chance of digoxin toxicity. However, loading doses of 30 μg/kg have been administered i.v. and p.o. without signs of digoxin toxicity

(Button et al 1980). The recommended dose rates are shown in Table 12.3.

NOVEL POSITIVE INOTROPES

Pimobendan is a new positive inotropic agent that is said to be a calcium-sensitizing agent, which increases the force of contraction at a given prevailing calcium ion concentration. It has been evaluated in dogs but not yet in horses.

ACUTE INOTROPES AND VASOPRESSORS

Inotropes and vasopressors are used in humans for the resuscitation of seriously ill patients and for the treatment of hypotension during surgery. Short-acting inotropes (adrenoceptor agonists) are most commonly used in anesthetized horses to maintain peripheral blood flow. Short-acting inotropes increase contractility whereas vasopressors affect any of the components of cardiac output. Although, many of the pharmacodynamic data available were generated in anaesthetized normal horses, they can also be applied to the critical care setting. However, this use is empirical, since it is not based on clinical research in the horse. The actions of inotropes are mediated through α and β adrenoceptors as well as dopaminergic receptors as summarized in Table 12.4.

Dopamine

Dopamine is a sympathomimetic amine with α and β adrenergic and dopaminergic effects. It is the metabolic precursor of norepinephrine; therefore, some of its adrenergic activity results from norepinephrine release from nerve terminals (Hoffman & Lefkowitz 1996). At low doses, the β adrenergic effects on the myocardium increase contractility, while the peripheral dopaminergic receptors in renal and splanchnic vascular beds result in local vasodilatation. The combination of vasodilatation and increased myocardial contractility may result in arterial blood pressure remaining unchanged while peripheral perfusion increases. High doses of dopamine cause vasoconstriction via α adrenergic stimulation. This

Table 12.4 Acute inotropes and vasopressors: mechanisms of action

Drug	Pharmacological action	Indication	Adverse effects
Digoxin	Na^+,K^+-ATPase inhibition; vagomimetic	Congestive heart failure	Bradycardia, tachyarrhythmia, hypokalemia; increases myocardial oxygen demand
Dobutamine	β adrenergic and weak α effects	Hypotension; cardiogenic shock	Proarrhythmic at high doses; increases myocardial oxygen demand
Dopamine	β adrenergic: ionotropic; doperminergic: vasodilatation; α adrenergic: vasoconstriction (high dose) and chronotropic effects	Prerenal renal failure; cardiogenic shock	Decrease peripheral perfusion at high doses; tachycardia; increase myocardial oxygen demand
Dopexamine	β adrenergic: ionotropic; dopaminergic: vasodilatation, (α adrenergic)	Hypotension in anaesthetized animals[a]	Cardiac arrhythmias; abdominal discomfort; sweating; poor recovery from anesthesia; increase myocardial oxygen demand
Milrinone	Phosphodiesterase inhibitor: vasodilatory and ionotropic; no increase myocardial oxygen demands	Hypotension	
Norepinephrine (noradrenaline)	α adrenergic: vasoconstriction	Severe refractory cardiogenic shock	Increased afterload; decreased peripheral perfusion
Phenylephrine	$α_1$ adrenergic: vasoconstriction; ionotropic effects may occur, via myocardial $α_1$ adrenoceptors	Critical maintenance of perfusion	Increased afterload; decreased peripheral perfusion

[a] Not evaluated for other indications in the horse

increases the heart rate; therefore, the onset of tachycardia and rising blood pressure give an indication that the rate of the infusion should be reduced.

Dopamine is ineffective following oral administration because of its hepatic metabolism and it is usually administered by i.v. infusion at a dose rate of 2.5–5 µg/min per kg. In normal anaesthetized horses, 4 µg/kg has been shown to increase the cardiac output and induce vasodilatation (Young et al 1998). Other studies showed no significant increase in cardiac output at 5 µg/kg (Lee et al 1998), although this dose rate may produce tachycardia (Gasthuys et al 1991).

Dopexamine

Dopexamine is a synthetic analog of dopamine, with β adrenergic and dopaminergic activity. Dopexamine increased cardiac output and heart rate while decreasing systemic vascular resistance

(i.e. vasodilation) in normal anaesthetized horses (Muir 1992). These effects were attenuated both by α and β adrenoceptor blockade (Muir 1992), suggesting that it has a similar mechanism of action to dopamine. Renal blood flow is enhanced through the dopaminergic effects of this drug. Dopexamine has been associated with sweating, poor recovery from anesthesia, colic (Young et al 1997) and cardiac arrhythmias (Lee et al 1998, Muir 1992).

Dobutamine

Dobutamine is structurally similar to dopamine but does not bind to dopamine receptors and is not associated with norepinephrine release from neurons. The drug exists as a racemic mixture, both isomers possesses β adrenergic effects, with the (+) enantiomer (eutomer) being 10 times more potent than the (−) enantiomer (distomer). Furthermore, the eutomer is a potent α adrenergic antagonist while the distomer is a potent

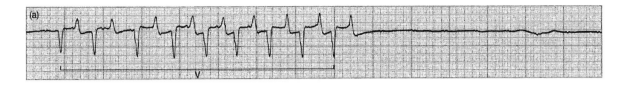

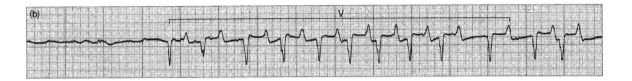

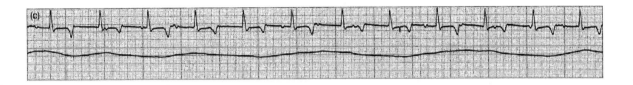

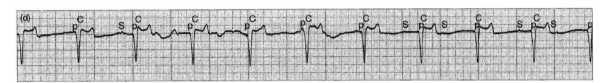

Figure 12.5 Modified base-apex electrocardiograms from a 4-year-old horse with third-degree atrioventricular blockade. (a) and (b) Runs of ventricular ectopy could be identified and the horse was weak and collapsed intermittently. (c) During conscious placement of a unipolar ventricular pacemeker, doubtamine was infused at 2.5 µg/min per kg body weight to increase heart rate. (c). Ventricular pacing was achieved with normal QRS complexes (D) and pacemaker potentials (p). Occasional sinoatrial activity was still present after placement of the pacemaker (S).

α adrenergic agonist. Dobutamine is a more potent inotrope than chronotrope (Ruffolo 1987). If propranolol (β adrenergic antagonist) is coadministered, then vasoconstriction occurs.

Dobutamine is used routinely in anaesthetized horses to increase cardiac output and maintain arterial blood pressure. It is chronotropic at higher doses or after pretreatment with an anticholinergic agent. The drug has a very short half-life (2 min) and undergoes metabolism (conjugation). Steady-state concentrations are usually achieved within 10 min of initiating a constant i.v. infusion. Dobutamine is also used to increase heart rate (Fig. 12.5), through its α adrenergic effects, in horses with pathological bradyarrhythmias (Richardson & Kohn 1983).

Norepinephrine (noradrenaline)

Norepinephrine is a naturally occurring adrenergic agonist, with α, β_1 and weak β_2 adrenoceptor activity. Its primary action is to cause vasoconstriction and administration of norepinephrine (noradrenaline) has, therefore, been advocated for the treatment of cardiogenic shock in human patients that do not respond to dopamine or dobutamine (Anon. 1999). Cardiac contractility increases as a result of the β_1 adrenoceptor action. Initial concerns about the effects of norepinephrine (noradrenaline) on renal blood flow prevented its acceptance in the human critical care setting. Renal blood flow is reduced in normal dogs after the administration of norepinephrine (noradrenaline)

(Arger et al 1999); however, the coadministration of dopamine opposes this effect and increases renal blood flow (Schaer et al 1985). Coadministration of norepinephrine (noradrenaline) and dobutamine to foals with septic shock increased urine production and blood pressure (Corley et al 2000). Norepinephrine (noradrenaline) should be reserved for horses with sepsis and used in conjunction with inotropes and monitoring of urine output. The recommended i.v. dose rates are shown in Table 12.3.

Phenylephrine

Phenylephrine is a selective α_1 adrenergic agonist, with a pharmacological structure similar to norepinephrine (noradrenaline), which causes peripheral vasoconstriction. Stimulation of α_1 adrenoceptors in the myocardium has an inotropic effect. However, phenylephrine produced no increase in cardiac output, increased systemic vascular resistance and mean arterial pressure and reduced muscle blood flow in anaesthetized horses (Lee et al 1998). Phenylephrine should be reserved for critical conditions where the perfusion of essential organs is compromised and inotropes are not effectively maintaining organ function. The recommended infusion rates are shown in Table 12.3.

Milrinone

Milrinone is a phosphodiesterase type III/IV inhibitor that has vasodilatory properties and increases the force of contraction and velocity of relaxation of cardiac muscle. Milrinone has not been evaluated fully in the equine clinical setting. It produces a dose-dependent increase in heart rate, cardiac output, arterial blood pressure and ejection fraction and a reduction in right atrial, pulmonary artery pressures and systemic vascular resistance in normal anesthetized horses (Muir 1995). These changes persisted for 30 min after the termination of a constant i.v. infusion of milrinone.

DIURETICS

Diuretics are used in CHF to offset water and sodium retention and thus reduce preload.

Furosemide (frusemide) is a high-ceiling loop diuretic that inhibits the reabsorption of electrolytes in the thick ascending loop of Henle (Muir & Mcguirk 1985; see Ch. 10). Furosemide (frusemide) is the most commonly used diuretic in the horse and can be given parenterally or orally. In the authors' experience, oral administration of furosemide (frusemide) produces a variable clinical response, perhaps because of interanimal variation in the bioavailability. There are no pharmacokinetic data to support this route of administration in horses. Long-term furosemide (frusemide) administration may lead to hypokalemia, hyponatremia, hypomagnesemia and metabolic alkalosis. Serum electrolyte concentrations should be monitored during long-term furosemide (frusemide) treatment because hypomagnesemia and hypokalemia can result in cardiac arrhythmias. A full description of the actions of furosemide (frusemide) can be found in Chapter 10.

VASODILATORS
Direct acting vasodilators

Hydralazine is a direct-acting arteriodilator. Its mechanism of action is still debated but it is dependent on intact endothelium and is thought to involve calcium channels (Bang et al 1998, Lipe & Moulds 1981, Spokas et al 1983). In normal horses, it produces a sympathetically mediated reflex increase in heart rate (Bertone 1988).

Pharmacokinetics

Hydralazine undergoes hepatic (presystemic) metabolism in most species and so its bioavailability is poor following oral administration despite being well absorbed. It should be administered by i.v. injection, where clinical effects lasting 4 h can be seen (Bertone 1988).

Adverse effects

High doses of hydralazine can induce severe hypotension in humans (Smith et al 1988) and in dogs (Kittleson & Kienle 1998).

Clinical indications

Hydralazine is indicated for the treatment of cardiac valvular insufficiency and ventricular septal defects in humans. It reduces afterload, thus reducing the volume of regurgitant or shunted blood and thereby improving forward flow. There are no data to support the oral administration of hydralazine to horses and it is only useful as an acute vasodilator. Hydralazine has not been critically evaluated in horses with CHF.

Nitrates: nitroglycerin (glyceryl trinitrate)

The nitrates are nitric oxide donors. Their actions depend upon the generation of nitric oxide within vascular smooth muscle, either by enzymatic conversion or by spontaneous decomposition of the drug. Nitric oxide production is the final common pathway of all of these drugs. It binds to and activates the enzyme guanylate cyclase within the myocytes, resulting in the conversion of guanosine monophosphate (GMP) to the cyclic derivative cGMP. cGMP stimulates the phosphorylation of myosin light chains and results in the efflux of calcium, causing myocyte relaxation and hence vasodilatation (Anderson et al 1994).

Nitroglycerin (glyceryl trinitrate) possesses a nitrate ester bond that undergoes biotransformation by unknown mechanisms to form nitric oxide. The drug can be given orally, transdermally, sublingually and i.v.

Pharmacokinetics

Nitroglycerin undergoes rapid hepatic metabolism, to form 1,3-glyceryl dinitrate, 1,2-glyceryl dinitrate and glyceryl monohydrate, resulting in a very short half-life (1–4 min). Although the dinitrate metabolites are pharmacologically active, the parent drug is 10 to 14 times more potent than the principal metabolite. Glyceryl monohydrate is pharmacologically inactive. Transdermal administration of nitroglycerin is often used to limit the hepatic metabolism and prolong the duration of action of the drug. In humans, the absorption from 1 inch (2.5 cm) of a 2% ointment is 0.8 mg/h, with clinical effects starting within 1 h and lasting

for 3–6 h. The absorption of nitroglycerin is affected by the characteristics of the skin and it should be applied to non-hairy skin, such as the inner thigh of the horse. When nitroglycerin was applied to the clipped lateral thorax of normal dogs, there was no change in arterial blood pressure, pulmonary artery pressure or cardiac output (Kittleson & Kienle 1998). The absorption of nitroglycerin has not been established following transdermal administration to horses.

Clinical indications

Nitroglycerin is only marketed for the prevention of *angina pectoris* in humans and the US Food and Drug Administration did not approve its use for the treatment of CHF. If therapeutic plasma concentrations can be achieved in horses, nitroglycerin would be useful for reducing venous return and preload in horses with acute CHF. However, there are no data to support its use in CHF in any veterinary species.

The use of nitroglycerin has been investigated in other equine vascular diseases, including exercise-induced pulmonary hemorrhage and laminitis. Nitroglycerin p.o. (Hackett et al 1999) and i.v. (Manohar & Goetz 1999) failed to reduce pulmonary artery pressures during treadmill exercise tests, although i.v. administration did result in a reduction in pulmonary arterial and right atrial pressures at rest (Manohar & Goetz 1999), indicating that this agent has some pharmacological activity in the horse. In equine laminitis, topical nitroglycerin applied to the pastern area has been shown to increase digital blood flow and reduce systolic blood pressure (Hinckley et al 1996a,b). However, in humans, the use of these products is limited by the development of drug tolerance, which can occur within 24 h of starting treatment (Packer et al 1986). Tolerance develops through depletion of sulfhydryl groups, important in the biotransformation of the drug into nitric oxide. It has been suggested that 10 drug-free hours per day may limit the development of tolerance in humans and that tolerance can be reversed by acetylcysteine. The development and implications of drug tolerance in the long-term management of laminitis in the horse have not been investigated.

Indirectly acting vasodilators

Indirectly acting vasodilators bring about their effects through their actions on α_1 and β_2 adrenoceptors within the vascular smooth muscle. Prazosin is a selective α_1 adrenoceptor antagonist while isoxsuprine is an α adrenoceptor antagonist and a weak β_2 adrenoceptor agonist (Elliott & Soydan 1995). These agents produce vasodilatation in the horse but are not used for the management of equine cardiovascular disease. The phenothiazine tranquilizer acepromazine (see Ch. 15) also is an α adrenoceptor and 5-hydroxytryptamine (serotonin) receptor antagonist, suggesting that it may be a useful and cheap vasodilator for use in the horse (Marr & Reef 1995b).

Angiotensin-converting enzyme inhibitors

Angiotensin-converting enzyme (ACE) inhibitors have been important therapeutic tools in human cardiology since the introduction of captopril in the 1970s. Since that time, their use has become universal in canine and feline medicine, with ever-increasing indications; however, to date, these drugs have received relatively little attention in equine cardiology.

The renin–angiotensin system

The renal juxtaglomerular cells release renin in response to reduced renal perfusion pressure or ischemia, sodium depletion or β adrenergic stimulation. Renin is a protease, which cleaves angiotensinogen to form active angiotensin I (Ang I). ACE, present mainly in the lungs but also in vascular beds, converts Ang I into the vasoconstrictor angiotensin II (Ang II) and inactivates the vasodilator bradykinin (BK). Activation of Ang II receptors within the vascular smooth muscle causes the release of calcium from the sarcoplasmic reticulum. Calcium binds with calmodulin, resulting in smooth muscle contraction and hence vasoconstriction. The glomerular hemodynamics are influenced by Ang II in such a way as to maintain the glomerular filtration rate despite a fall in renal perfusion pressure. This is because

Ang II preferentially constricts the efferent arteriole of the glomerulus, raising glomerular capillary pressure.

ACE inhibitors block the formation of Ang II and the breakdown of BK, resulting in arteriolar vasodilatation. A vagomimetic property has been postulated (Ajayi et al 1985) explaining the lack of tachycardia in the face of peripheral vasodilatation. This, together with potassium retention, caused by inhibition of aldosterone secretion, has been speculated to produce an antiarrhythmic effect in humans (Pahor et al 1994), although this effect may also be a result of inhibition of the local renin–angiotensin system cardiac RAS (Linz et al 1989).

Pharmacokinetics

There are no pharmakinetic data on the ACE inhibitors in the horse. In humans, enalapril is 60% absorbed following oral administration and is de-esterified in the liver to its active form enalaprilat; it undergoes renal clearance. Both the liver and kidneys eliminate the active forms of benazepril (benazeprilat) and ramipril (ramiprilat).

Clinical indications

The ACE inhibition produced by enalapril, enalaprilat and captopril have been determined *in vitro* in the horse (Tillman & Moore 1989). Enalaprilat was effective at inhibiting Ang I-induced hypertension in one horse after i.v. administration (Tillman & Moore 1989). Enalapril has been administered p.o. at 0.5 mg/kg once daily for 2 months to pony stallions without producing any adverse clinical, cardiac or reproductive effects (Sleeper et al 2000). ACE inhibitors have been shown to be effective in humans and dogs with CHF (Anon. 1995, Ettinger et al 1998, Swedberg et al 1999). In humans with asymptomatic heart disease, ACE inhibitors are protective; they slow the progression of the disease (Francis et al 1990). Their use in horses with heart disease has not been evaluated, although it is likely that they will prove to be beneficial in horses with CHF. There is also an increasing body of research to suggest that ACE inhibitors are useful in renal failure (Ruggenenti et al 1999).

There is considerable scope for advances in the field of equine cardiovascular therapeutics as these and other novel approaches, are exploited.

REFERENCES

Agus Z S, Kelepouris E, Dukes I et al 1989 Cytosolic magnesium modulates calcium channel activity in mammalian ventricular cells. American Journal of Physiology 256:C452–C455

Ajayi A A, Campbell B C, Meredith P A et al 1985 The effect of captopril on the reflex control heart rate: possible mechanisms. British Journal of Clinical Pharmacology 20:17–25

Anderson T J, Meredith I T, Ganz P et al 1994 Nitric oxide and nitrovasodilators: similarities, differences and potential interactions. Journal of the American College of Cardiology 24:555–566

Anon. 1989 Preliminary report: effect of encainide and flecainide on mortality in a randomized trial of arrhythmia suppression after myocardial infarction. The Cardiac Arrhythmia Suppression Trial (CAST) Investigators. New England Journal of Medicine 321:406–412

Anon. 1995 Controlled clinical evaluation of enalapril in dogs with heart failure: results of the Cooperative Veterinary Enalapril Study Group. Journal of Veterinary Internal Medicine 9:243–252

Anon. 1999 Practice parameters for hemodynamic support of sepsis in adult patients in sepsis. Task Force of the American College of Critical Care Medicine, Society of Critical Care Medicine. Critical Care Medicine 27:639–660

Arger P H, Sehgal C M, Pugh C R et al 1999 Evaluation of change in blood flow by contrast-enhanced power Doppler imaging during norepinephrine-induced renal vasoconstriction. Journal of Ultrasound in Medicine 18:843–851

Bang L, Nielsen-Kudsk J E, Gruhn N et al 1998 Hydralazine-induced vasodilation involves opening of high conductance Ca^{2+}-activated K^+ channels. European Journal of Pharmacology 361:43–49

Bertone J J 1988 Cardiovascular effects of hydralazine HCl administration in horses. American Journal of Veterinary Research 49:618–621

Bouckaert S, Voorspoels J, Vandenbossche G et al 1994 Effect of drug formulation and feeding on the pharmacokinetics of orally administered quinidine in the horse. Journal of Veterinary Pharmacology and Therapeutics 17:275–278

Brumbaugh G W, Thomas W P, Enos L R et al 1983 A pharmacokinetic study of digoxin in the horse. Journal of Veterinary Pharmacology and Therapeutics 6:163–172

Button C, Gross D R, Johnston J T et al 1980 Digoxin pharmacokinetics, bioavailability, efficacy and dosage regimens in the horse. American Journal of Veterinary Research 41:1388–1395

Camm A J, Garratt C J 1991 Adenosine and supraventricular tachycardia. New England Journal of Medicine 325:1621–1629

Corley K, Mckenzie H, Amoroso L et al 2000 Initial experience with norepinephrine infusion in hypotensive critically ill foals. Journal of Veterinary Emergency and Critical Care 10:267–276

Dodam J R, Moon R E, Olson N C et al 1993 Effects of clenbuterol hydrochloride on pulmonary gas exchange and hemodynamics in anesthetized horses. American Journal of Veterinary Research 54:776–782

Ducharme N G, Fubini S L 1983 Gastrointestinal complications associated with the use of atropine in horses. Journal of the American Veterinary Medical Association 182:229–231

Elliott J, Soydan J 1995 Characterisation of β-adrenoceptors in equine digital veins: implications of the modes of vasodilatory action of isoxsuprine. Equine Veterinary Journal Supplement 19:101–107

Ellis E J, Ravis W R, Malloy M et al 1994 The pharmacokinetics and pharmacodynamics of procainamide in horses after intravenous administration. Journal of Veterinary Pharmacology and Therapeutics 17:265–270

Engelking L R, Blyden G T, Lofstedt J et al 1987 Pharmacokinetics of antipyrine, acetaminophen and lidocaine in fed and fasted horses. Journal of Veterinary Pharmacology and Therapeutics 10:73–82

Ettinger S J, Benitz A M, Ericsson G F et al 1998 Effects of enalapril maleate on survival of dogs with naturally acquired heart failure. The Long-Term Investigation of Veterinary Enalapril (LIVE) Study Group. Journal of the American Veterinary Medical Association 213:1573–1577

Francfort P, Schatzmann H J 1976 Pharmacological experiments as a basis for the administration of digoxin in the horse. Research in Veterinary Science 20:84–89

Francis G S, Benedict C, Johnstone D E et al 1990 Comparison of neuroendocrine activation in patients with left ventricular dysfunction with and without congestive heart failure. A substudy of the Studies of Left Ventricular Dysfunction (SOLVD). Circulation 82:1724–1729

Gasthuys F, de Moor A, Parmentier D 1991 Influence of digoxin followed by dopamine on the cardiovascular depression during a standard halothane anaesthesia in dorsally recumbent, ventilated ponies. Zentralblatt für Veterinarmedizin Reihe A 38:585–593

Gauthier C, Leblais V, Kobzik L et al 1998 The negative inotropic effect of beta3-adrenoceptor stimulation is mediated by activation of a nitric oxide synthase pathway in human ventricle. Journal of Clinical Investigation 102:1377–1384

Gerber H, Chuit P, Schatzmann H J 1971 Treatment of atrial fibrillation in the horse with intravenous dihydroquinidine gluconate. Equine Veterinary Journal 3:110–113

Grainger S L, Smith S E 1983 Dose–response relationships of intravenous hyoscine butylbromide and atropine sulphate on heart rate in healthy volunteers. British Journal of Clinical Pharmacology 16:623–626

Hackett R P, Ducharme N G, Gleed R D et al 1999 Oral nitroglycerin paste did not lower pulmonary capillary pressure during treadmill exercise. Equine Veterinary Journal Supplement 30:153–158

Hinckley K A, Fearn S, Howard B R et al 1996a Glyceryl trinitrate enhances nitric oxide mediated perfusion within the equine hoof. Journal of Endocrinology 151:R1–R8

Hinckley K A, Fearn S, Howard B R et al 1996b Nitric oxide donors as treatment for grass induced acute laminitis in ponies [see comments]. Equine Veterinary Journal 28:17–28

Hoffman B, Lefkowitz R 1996 Catecholamines, sympathomimetic drugs and adrenergic receptor antagonists. In: Hardman J, Limbird L, Molinoff P et al (eds) Goodman & Gilman's the pharmacological basis of therapeutics, 9th edn. McGraw-Hill, New York, pp. 199–248

Holder D A, Sniderman A D, Fraser G et al 1977 Experience with bretylium tosylate by a hospital cardiac arrest team. Circulation 55:541–544

Kittleson M, Kienle R 1998 Management of heart failure. In: Kittleson M, Kienle R (eds) Small animal cardiovascular medicine. Mosby, St Louis, MO, pp. 149–194

Kolibash Jr, A J, Lewis R P, Bourne D W et al 1989 Extension of the serum digoxin concentration–response relationship to patient management. Journal of Clinical Pharmacology 29:300–306

Kowalczyk D F, Beech J 1983 Pharmacokinetics of phenytoin (diphenylhydantoin) in horses. Journal of Veterinary Pharmacology and Therapeutics 6:133–140

Langenfeld H, Weirich J, Kohler C et al 1990 Comparative analysis of the action of class I antiarrhythmic drugs (lidocaine, quinidine and prajmaline) in rabbit atrial and ventricular myocardium. Journal of Cardiovascular Pharmacology 15:338–345

Lee Y H, Clarke K W, Alibhai H I et al 1998 Effects of dopamine, dobutamine, dopexamine, phenylephrine and saline solution on intramuscular blood flow and other cardiopulmonary variables in halothane-anesthetized ponies. American Journal of Veterinary Research 59:1463–1472

Lewis R P 1990 Digitalis: a drug that refuses to die. Critical Care Medicine 18:S5–S13.

Linz W, Scholkens B A, Kaiser J et al 1989 Cardiac arrhythmias are ameliorated by local inhibition of angiotensin formation and bradykinin degradation with the converting-enzyme inhibitor ramipril. Cardiovascular Drugs and Therapy 3:873–882

Lipe S, Moulds R F 1981 In vitro differences between human arteries and veins in their responses to hydralazine. Journal of Pharmacology and Experimental Therapeutics 217:204–208

Manohar M, Goetz T E 1999 Pulmonary vascular pressures of strenuously exercising thoroughbreds during intravenous infusion of nitroglycerin. American Journal of Veterinary Research 60:1436–1440

Marques J A, Teixeira Neto F J, Campebell R C et al 1998 Effects of hyoscine-N-butylbromide given before romifidine in horses. Veterinary Record 142:166–168

Marr C M, Reef V B 1991 ECG of the month. Journal of the American Veterinary Medical Association 198:1533–1534

Marr C M, Reef V B 1995a Cardiac arrhythmias. In: Kobluk C N, Ames T R, Geor R J (eds) The horse: disease

and clinical management. Saunders, Philadelphia, PA, pp. 137–156

Marr C, Reef V 1995b Disturbances of blood flow. In: Kobluk C N, Ames T R, Geor R J (eds) The horse: disease and clinical management. Saunders, Philadelphia, PA, pp. 157–184

Mcguirk S M, Muir W W, Sams R A 1981 Pharmacokinetic analysis of i.v. and p.o. administered quinidine in horses. American Journal of Veterinary Research 42:938–942

Muir W W D 1992 Inotropic mechanisms of dopexamine hydrochloride in horses. American Journal of Veterinary Research 53:1343–1346

Muir W W 1995 The haemodynamic effects of milrinone HCl in halothane anaesthetized horses. Equine Veterinary Journal Supplement 19:108–113

Muir W W, Mcguirk S M 1985 Pharmacology and pharmacokinetics of drugs used to treat cardiac disease in horses. Veterinary Clinics of North America Equine Practice 1:335–352

Muir W W D, Mcguirk S 1987 Cardiovascular drugs. Their pharmacology and use in horses. Veterinary Clinics of North America Equine Practice 3:37–57

Muir W W D, Reed S M, Mcguirk S M 1990 Treatment of atrial fibrillation in horses by intravenous administration of quinidine. Journal of the American Veterinary Medical Association 197:1607–1610

Neff C A, Davis L E, Baggot J D 1972 A comparative study of the pharmacokinetics of quinidine. American Journal of Veterinary Research 33:1521–1525

Ohmura H, Nukada T, Mizuno Y et al 2000 Safe and efficacious dosage of flecainide acetate for treating equine atrial fibrillation. Journal of Veterinary Medical Science 62:711–715

Ohmura H, Hiraga A, Aida H et al 2001 Determination of oral dosage and pharmacokinetic analysis of flecainide in horses. Journal of Veterinary Medical Science 63:511–514

Packer M, Medina N, Yushak M et al 1986 Hemodynamic factors limiting the response to transdermal nitroglycerin in severe chronic congestive heart failure. American Journal of Cardiology 57:260–267

Pahor M, Gambassi G, Carbonin P 1994 Antiarrhythmic effects of ACE inhibitors: a matter of faith or reality? Cardiovascular Research 28:173–182

Parraga M E, Kittleson M D, Drake C M 1995 Quinidine administration increases steady state serum digoxin concentration in horses [see comments]. Equine Veterinary Journal Supplement 19:114–119

Pedersoli W, Belmonte A A, Purohit R C et al 1978 Pharmacokinetic of digoxin in the horse. Journal of Equine Medicine and Surgery 2:384–388

Pedersoli W M, Ravis W R, Belmonte A A et al 1981 Pharmacokinetics of a single p.o. administered dose of digoxin in horses. American Journal of Veterinary Research 42:1412–1414

Rea R F, Hamdan M, Schomer S J et al 1991 Inhibitory effects of procainamide on sympathetic nerve activity in humans. Circulation Research 69:501–508

Reef V 1999 Arrhythmias. In: Marr C (ed) Cardiology of the horse. Saunders, London, pp. 179–209

Reef V B, Levitan C W, Spencer P A 1988 Factors affecting prognosis and conversion in equine atrial fibrillation. Journal of Veterinary Internal Medicine 2:1–6

Reef V B, Reimer J M, Spencer P A 1995 Treatment of atrial fibrillation in horses: new perspectives. Journal of Veterinary Internal Medicine 9:57–67

Ribner H S, Plucinski D A, Hsieh A M et al 1985 Acute effects of digoxin on total systemic vascular resistance in congestive heart failure due to dilated cardiomyopathy: a hemodynamic–hormonal study. American Journal of Cardiology 56:896–904

Richardson D W, Kohn C W 1983 Uroperitoneum in the foal. Journal of the American Veterinary Medical Association 182:267–271

Roelvink M E, Goossens L, Kalsbeek H C et al 1991 Analgesic and spasmolytic effects of dipyrone, hyoscine-N-butylbromide and a combination of the two in ponies. Veterinary Record 129:378–380

Roos J 1924 Auricular fibrillation in domestic animals. Heart 11:1–7

Ruffolo R R Jr 1987 The pharmacology of dobutamine. American Journal of the Medical Sciences 294:244–248

Ruggenenti P, Perna A, Benini R et al 1999 In chronic nephropathies prolonged ACE inhibition can induce remission: dynamics of time-dependent changes in GFR. Investigators of the GISEN Group. Gruppo Italiano Studi Epidemiologici in Nefrologia. Journal of the American Society of Nephrology 10:997–1006

Schaer G L, Fink M P, Parrillo J E 1985 Norepinephrine alone versus norepinephrine plus low-dose dopamine: enhanced renal blood flow with combination pressor therapy. Critical Care Medicine 13:492–496

Shapland J E, Garner H E, Hatfield D G 1981 Cardiopulmonary effects of clenbuterol in the horse. Journal of Veterinary Pharmacology and Therapeutics 4:43–50

Siebels J R, Cappato R, Ruppel R et al 1993 Preliminary results of the Cardiac Arrest Study Hamburg (CASH). CASH Investigators. American Journal of Cardiology 72:109F–113F

Singh B N 1993 Controlling cardiac arrhythmias by lengthening repolarization: historical overview. American Journal of Cardiology 72:18F–24F

Singh B N, Nademanee K 1985 Control of cardiac arrhythmias by selective lengthening of repolarization: theoretic considerations and clinical observations. American Heart Journal 109:421–430

Singh S, McDonell W, Young S et al 1997 The effect of glycopyrrolate on heart rate and intestinal motility in conscious horses. Journal of Veterinary Anaesthesia 24:14–19

Sleeper M, McDonnell S, Reef V 2000 Enalapril therapy in 12 pony stallions. Journal of Veterinary Internal Medicine 14:365

Smith T, Braunwald E, Kelly R 1988 The management of heart failure. In: Braunwald E (ed) A textbook of cardiovascular medicine. Saunders, Philadelphia, PA, p. 485

Spokas E G, Folco G, Quilley J et al 1983 Endothelial mechanism in the vascular action of hydralazine. Hypertension 5:1107–1111

Swedberg K, Kjekshus J, Snapinn S 1999 Long-term survival in severe heart failure in patients treated with enalapril. Ten year follow-up of CONSENSUS I [see comments]. European Heart Journal 20:136–139

Sweeney R W, Reef V B, Reimer J M 1993 Pharmacokinetics of digoxin administered to horses with congestive heart failure. American Journal of Veterinary Research 54:1108–1111

Tillman L G, Moore J N 1989 Serum angiotensin converting enzyme activity and response to angiotensin I in horses. Equine Veterinary Journal Supplement 7:80–83

Tzivoni D, Banai S, Schuger C et al 1988 Treatment of torsade de pointes with magnesium sulfate. Circulation 77:392–397

Wijnberg I D 2001 Phenytoin sodium per os as a treatment for ventricular arrhythmia in the horse. In: Proceedings of the 40th British Equine Veterinary Association Congress, Harrogate, UK, p. 218

Wijnberg I D, van der Kolk J H, Hiddink E G 1999 Use of phenytoin to treat digitalis-induced cardiac arrhythmias in a miniature Shetland pony. Veterinary Record 144:259–261

Wills M R 1986 Magnesium and potassium. Interrelationships in cardiac disorders. Drugs 31 (suppl 4):121–131

Young L E, Blissitt K J, Clutton R E et al 1997 Temporal effects of an infusion of dopexamine hydrochloride in horses anesthetized with halothane. American Journal of Veterinary Research 58:516–523

Young L E, Blissitt K J, Clutton R E et al 1998 Haemodynamic effects of a sixty min infusion of dopamine hydrochloride in horses anaesthetised with halothane. Equine Veterinary Journal 30:310–316

CHAPTER CONTENTS

Introduction 217

Routes of drug delivery 218
  Topical instillation 218
  Periocular injections 220
  Intraocular injections 220
  Parenteral administration 220
  Innovative drug delivery systems 221

Pharmacological principles of ocular
therapeutics 221
  Topically applied drugs 221
  Subconjunctival injections 223
  Parenteral administration 224

Antibacterial therapy 224
  Ocular bacteriology 224
  Routes of delivery 225
  Selection of antibacterial agent 227

Antimycotic therapy 228
  Selection of antimycotic agents 229
  Treatment protocols in keratomycosis 232

Antiviral therapy 233
  Topical antiviral therapy 233

Therapy to control ulceration 234
  Proteinase inhibitors 235

Ocular anti-inflammatory therapy 236

Ocular autonomic drugs 240
  Mydriatics/cycloplegics 240
  Miotics 241

Other ocular medicants 241
  Topical anesthetics 241
  Ocular lubricants 241
  Ocular irrigating solutions and disinfectants 242
  Viscoelastic materials 242
  Intracameral fibrinolytic agents 242
  Topical hyperosmotic agents 242
  Ocular tissue adhesives 242

Medical management of glaucoma 243

References 244

13

Ophthalmic therapeutics

Andrew Matthews

INTRODUCTION

The goal in medical treatment of ophthalmic disease is to achieve therapeutically effective levels of a particular drug or combination of drugs at the targeted anatomical site. While disease of the adnexa and ocular surfaces is readily treated by the topical application of pharmaceuticals, achieving effective intraocular levels of a particular drug can be problematic.

There are three major barriers to the diffusion of drugs into the mammalian eye: the corneal–epithelial barrier, the blood–aqueous barrier and the blood–retinal barrier. The blood–aqueous barrier is created by the tight intercellular junctions and junctional complexes of the non-pigmented ciliary epithelium and iris capillary endothelium, respectively. The blood–retinal barrier is created by the tight intercellular junctions of the vascular endothelium of the end vessels of the paurangiotic equine retina and the retinal pigment epithelium. In addition, there is evidence that the lens–iris barrier may impede diffusion of drugs from the anterior to the vitreous chamber. The facility with which a drug crosses the three major barriers in the healthy eye is determined principally by the drug's lipid solubility and protein binding affinity, and to a lesser extent by its molecular weight. However, the intraocular bioavailability of a particular drug is likely to be increased significantly where these barriers are compromised by injury or disease.

Most studies on ocular pharmacokinetics and drug bioavailability have been carried out in non-equine species, and much of current clinical practice in the horse is based upon extrapolation from other species. This has been modified by common experience into "best practice" protocols, with the inevitable limitations of this approach. In addition to interspecies differences in the pharmacological actions of some drugs (e.g. non-steroidal anti-inflammatory drugs (NSAIDs)), there are likely to be significant differences between species in the ocular pharmacokinetics of any particular drug, resulting from a number of factors:

- relative ocular size and corneoscleral thickness;
- tear production and flow dynamics;
- blink rate;
- presence and motility of the third eyelid;
- presence of ocular pigment; and
- aqueous production and flow.

Each of these factors is potentially able to alter the local bioavailability of a drug, which, in turn, may influence the expected clinical response.

ROUTES OF DRUG DELIVERY

There are four routes open for delivery of drugs to the eye and adnexa:

- topical instillation;
- periocular injection;
- intraocular injection; and
- parenteral administration.

TOPICAL INSTILLATION

Topical instillation is the principal route of ophthalmic drug delivery in the horse. It is used in the treatment of adnexal diseases, such as blepharitis and mebomianitis, and diseases of the ocular surfaces, such as conjunctivitis, superficial keratitis and corneal ulceration. Depending upon their physicochemical formulation, some drugs traverse the intact conjunctival and corneal epithelial barrier. This results in therapeutic levels within the corneal stroma and anterior chamber, facilitating the topical treatment of corneal stromal

infections and anterior uveitis and achieving useful physiological effects such as mydriasis. The bulk flow of aqueous from the posterior to anterior chamber and the physical presence of the lens–iris barrier mean that topically administered drugs do not readily reach therapeutic levels in the posterior segment.

The ability of certain drugs to cross the ocular and nasolacrimal epithelium means that these drugs are to some extent absorbed systemically. The degree to which this occurs in the horse has not been investigated extensively. However, topical atropine has been recognized as causing transient ileus, particularly in foals, and has been implicated in a very small number of fatal colic cases in adult horses (Brooks 1999). Dexamethasone has been detected in the serum of horses 24 h after cessation of administration of a 0.1% ointment three times a day (Speiss et al 1999) and trainers of competition horses should be made aware of the possibility of forensic detection of topically administered ophthalmic drugs.

Topical medication may be achieved in a number of ways:

- direct instillation;
- ocular lavage systems;
- subconjunctival injection; and
- membrane systems.

Direct instillation

Direct instillation is most frequently used in clinical practice. It is cheap and, in most circumstances, relatively easy for handlers to carry out, particularly where ointments are used. However fractiousness or head shyness on the part of the horse may lead to significant compliance problems and therapeutic failure.

Ocular lavage systems

Lavage systems overcome the compliance problems associated with instillation of solutions in some horses. However, they involve increased expense arising from the costs of the system and from the relatively high drug volumes required, much of which may be wasted in the dead space of the system. Dedicated single passage subpalpebral and nasolacrimal systems are commercially available and offer significant advantages over homemade systems in terms of ease of placement, patient tolerance and retention.

Subpalpebral Lavage System

The Subpalpebral Lavage System (Cooks Veterinary Products; MILA International) is easily placed in the standing, sedated horse following perineural anesthesia of the supraorbital nerve in conjunction with topical anesthesia of the ocular surfaces. By inserting a finger under the upper eyelid, the trochar to which the silicone tubing is attached is guided into the central dorsal fornix before being pushed through the eyelid. The tubing is drawn through the lid until the footplate snugly rests in the dorsal fornix, then it is led between the horse's ears and braided into the mane and sutured to the skin on the side of the neck. Alternatively, the tubing may be taped to the head collar. This type of system may be left in place for several weeks, although the manufacturers recommend replacement after 2 to 3 weeks. Cutting the tubing 3–4 cm from the eyelid and inserting a blunt wire guide into the tube before gently dislodging the footplate expedites removal. Placement of the footplate in the ventrolateral fornix has been described.

Subpalpebral lavage systems can be used in conjunction with balloon-type or syringe infusion pumps to provide continuous perfusion of the ocular surface. The indications for continuous ocular perfusion in the horse are probably very few, and any possible advantage is likely to be outweighed by the risks of iatrogenic injury resulting from disruption and damage to the preocular tear film. One situation in which continuous lavage may be beneficial is where proteinase inhibitor solutions are used to control stromal breakdown in corneal ulceration. Where continuous perfusion is used, flow rates of 1–2 ml/h have been recommended (Miller 1992).

Nasolacrimal Lavage System

The Nasolacrimal Lavage System (Brooks 1983; Arnolds Veterinary Products) has a cannula that is passed through a stab incision in the false nostril and introduced into the distal nasolacrimal duct. The cannula is anchored to the skin adjacent to the nasolacrimal orifice and false nostril. Although it is generally well tolerated, retention is a problem and the cannula may kink in the area of the false nostril. Larger volumes of solution are required than in the subpalpebral system and iatrogenic corneal injury, caused by the jet exiting from the lacrimal punctae, may arise. However, this system has the potential advantage of increasing the retention time of the drug solution in the external eye as a result of the partial occlusion of the nasolacrimal duct.

Subconjunctival injection

Injection of soluble drug under the dorsal bulbar conjunctiva results in transient leakage of the drug from the injection port onto the ocular surface. However, the bioavailability on the ocular surface of subconjunctivally injected drugs is likely to be highly unpredictable in the horse and this route should not be used alone as a means of delivering topical medication. In general, where used to supplement direct topical instillation, subconjunctival injections require to be repeated every 12–36 h.

Membrane delivery systems

Membrane systems are a range of drug delivery devices designed to facilitate prolonged topical medication via a reservoir effect at the ocular surface. These devices include ocular inserts, hydrophilic soft contact lenses and collagen shields, which after presoaking in drug solution are applied onto the ocular surface. However, the bioavailability of drugs delivered to the ocular surface using these systems in the horse is largely unknown and this, along with technical difficulties with retention and problems with corneal hypoxia, has been responsible for limiting their development in this species. In the case of collagen shields, accelerated hydrolysis has been recognized as a problem in some horses (Miller 1992).

PERIOCULAR INJECTIONS

Periocular injections physically bypass the external ocular epithelial barriers. Three techniques may be used:

- subconjunctival injection;
- sub-Tenon's injection; and
- retrobulbar injection.

Subconjunctival injection

Injection of hydrophilic drugs under the bulbar conjunctiva results in direct diffusion of relatively high levels of the drug into the anterior chamber, corneal stroma, posterior chamber and anterior vitreous. In the horse, the route is used most frequently to manage acute anterior segment disease or, using depot corticosteroid preparations, in the management of anterior uveitis uncomplicated by corneal ulceration.

The technique is relatively easy and safe to perform on standing sedated horses after topical anesthesia of the ocular surface. Adequate eyelid akinesia is usually achieved following α_2 adrenergic agonist/opiate sedation and palpebral nerve blockade is unnecessary. The injection is usually performed in the dorsolateral quadrant. However, since local drug levels are highest in the immediate vicinity of the injection site, locating the injection adjacent to the targeted lesion may have some therapeutic advantage. In some heavy draught breeds, with relatively small palpebral apertures, the injection is easier to perform in the ventrolateral quadrant. The injection is best performed using a ⅝ inch (15.9 mm) 25 gauge needle with a 1 or 2 ml syringe, and volumes of up to 1 ml are tolerated at any one site.

Drugs injected intrapalpebrally or under the palpebral conjunctiva will largely be lost via the periorbital vascular plexuses, and these techniques offer no therapeutic advantage.

Sub-Tenon's injection

Placement of drug more rostrally than achieved by subconjunctival injection (i.e. under the outer fascial coat of the globe (Tenon's capsule)) in theory facilitates transscleral diffusion of drug into the posterior segment. However, the technique is difficult to perform, requiring general anesthesia, and carries a significant risk of penetration of the globe. Based upon pharmacokinetic studies in other species, this route probably offers no significant advantage over subconjunctival injection used in conjunction with parenteral administration (Mindel 1998a).

Retrobulbar injection

Retrobulbar injection probably offers little therapeutic advantage over the combined subconjunctival and parenteral routes. This route is recommended only for regional anesthesia of the orbit, particularly to supplement general anesthesia (Miller 1992).

INTRAOCULAR INJECTIONS

The paurangiotic equine fundus and the presence of the blood–retinal barrier make intravitreal injection probably the only reliable method of achieving therapeutic levels of most drugs in the equine vitreous. However, the inherent ocular toxicity of most drugs and the empirical nature of dose selection mean that elective intravitreal injections are essentially salvage procedures in the horse, used to preserve the globe in endophthalmitis and in glaucoma. However, early therapeutic intervention with intravitreal antibiotics in some horses with postperforation endophthalmitis could be beneficial in attempting to preserve vision.

Intracameral injection of tissue plasminogen activator (tPA) has been used to disperse fibrin clot in the anterior chamber of the horse (Martin et al 1993). Intracameral viscoelastic preparations facilitate repair of full-thickness corneal lacerations by maintaining an inflated anterior chamber (Wilkie & Willis 1999).

All intraocular injections should be carried out under general anesthesia.

PARENTERAL ADMINISTRATION

Parenterally administered drugs are used to treat adnexal and retrobulbar diseases, such as blepharitis and orbital cellulitis. This route is also used to treat posterior uveitis and to supplement the topical and subconjunctival routes in some anterior segment diseases. In general, intravenous (i.v.) administration is preferred over other routes since peak plasma concentrations are likely to promote passage of the drug into the eye.

INNOVATIVE DRUG DELIVERY SYSTEMS

Intravitreal implants impregnated with ciclosporin (cyclosporin A, cyclosporine) deliver protracted and controlled intraocular drug release and have been successfully used in the management of some cases of equine recurrent uveitis (ERU) (Gilger & Allen 1998, Gilger et al 2000).

Subconjunctivally implanted microosmotic pumps have been shown to be effective and well-tolerated short-term delivery devices in the horse but are not yet in routine clinical use.

PHARMACOLOGICAL PRINCIPLES OF OCULAR THERAPEUTICS

Drug therapy for ocular conditions involves factors of access that are distinct from those for most other areas of the body (Mindel 1998a,b).

TOPICALLY APPLIED DRUGS

Intraocular penetration

Topically applied drugs penetrate the cornea by diffusion. To enter the anterior structures of the eye, a drug must traverse the lipid barriers of the preocular tear film, corneal epithelium and endothelium and the hydrous barrier of the corneal stroma. To do so, a drug must possess biphasic polarity, being both lipid and water soluble, so-called differential solubility. The epithelial barrier largely excludes highly polar hydrophilic drugs, such as the beta-lactam and aminoglycoside antibiotics, whereas more lipophilic drugs, such as fluoroquinolones, readily penetrate the cornea and enter the anterior segment. Within the

cornea, a drug is distributed according to its oil–water partition coefficient. The stroma may act as a reservoir for the hydrophilic or ionized fraction of a drug, resulting in protracted release of the drug into the anterior chamber (Mindel 1998a). Where the epithelial barrier is removed, as in corneal ulceration, much higher levels of topically applied hydrophilic drugs are reached in the anterior segment.

The differential solubility of a drug may be manipulated by altering the pH and chemical formulation. A drug with optimal corneal penetration at a higher pH may be buffered to reduce the discomfort of topical application but at the expense of reduced intraocular penetration. Acidic salts of most drugs are highly polar and have limited transcorneal penetration, whereas the more lipophilic esters of the same drugs readily penetrate the cornea. This is utilized in commercial formulations of the glucocorticoids, where the relative lipid solubility and corneal penetration is: phosphate ≪ free alcohol < acetate.

The rate of diffusion of a drug through the cornea is concentration dependent and this process cannot be saturated. Hence the higher the concentration of drug applied topically, the higher the levels achieved in the anterior segment. However, the concentrations that may be used are limited by the irritant effect of increasing tonicity, with consequent loss of drug by reflex tearing and blepharospasm.

Molecular weight does not appear to be a significant factor in transcorneal diffusion of drugs with molecular weights <500. Most drugs in current veterinary use fall below this threshold.

Bioavailability and pharmacokinetics

The ocular bioavailability of a topically applied drug (i.e. the percentage of effective drug available at the ocular surface or in the anterior segment) depends upon a number of factors. The acidic dissociation constant (pK_a) of the drug and the pH of the vehicle determine the differential solubility of the drug on the ocular surface and its intraocular bioavailability. Increasing the concentration of buffer in ophthalmic solutions extends the time taken for the tear film to return to physiological pH and prolongs the duration of dissociation of a drug, potentially increasing its bioavailability.

Drug preparation

Marked deviation of pH and tonicity from that of tears provokes reflex lacrimation, diluting the drug and accelerating its elution from the eye. Hypertonic solutions may be further diluted by fluid drawn from subconjunctival tissues. Animals will tolerate a pH range of 3.5–10.5 and tonicity from 0.5% to 2% sodium chloride concentration equivalents (Miller 1992).

A major cause of loss of dissolved drug is rapid wash out into the nasolacrimal system. Increasing the viscosity of a preparation increases corneal contact time and ocular bioavailability by retarding nasolacrimal drainage. This is usually achieved by the addition of excipients, such as hydroxypropyl methylcellulose or high-viscosity carbomer gel, to the formulation. However, some high-viscosity solutions may cause shearing of the tear film and accelerated drug loss.

The inclusion of amphipathic detergents (i.e. agents with both hydrophobic and hydrophilic regions) and chelating agents as excipients in drug preparations will enhance corneal penetration by transiently disrupting the integrity of the epithelial barrier. Cyclodextrins have been included in topical formulations as a means of increasing both corneal permeability and drug solubility.

Loss of efficacy associated with prolonged or incorrect storage is a potential problem both with commercial ophthalmic preparations and "fortified" solutions prepared in the clinic. The latter must be handled carefully.

The physical characteristics of the preparation influence ocular bioavailability.

Solutions Drugs in solution have a high bioavailability but a short ocular surface contact time. In primates, over 90% of drug in aqueous solution is eluted from the eye within 5 min of instillation. In the horse, the contact time is likely to be more prolonged because the eye is relatively large and there is a protective nictitans lid. Simultaneous administration of two or more preparations can result in inactivation, dilution or accelerated washout of the drugs.

Gels The use of high-viscosity, water-soluble gel as a drug vehicle will prolong the therapeutic effect and enhance ocular penetration, reducing the frequency of application. However, only a limited number of drugs are available as gel preparations (e.g. fusidic acid) and their use in equine practice is limited.

Suspensions Drugs in topical suspensions are made available by dissolution from the surface of solid particles. Larger particles have a relatively smaller surface area for drug dissolution, with a consequent lower availability. Smaller particles ($<10 \mu m$) result in greater drug availability but more rapid elution from the ocular surface.

Ointments As the melting ointment is brought into the tear interface by the shearing action of blinking, only drug on the surface of the ointment mass is available for dissolution, resulting in relatively poor availability but prolonged retention. However, therapeutic levels of highly lipid-soluble antibiotics (e.g. chloramphenicol) can be achieved in the anterior ocular segment in laboratory animals.

Tissue conditions

The pharmacokinetic influence of the patient's ocular tissues significantly influences the therapeutic response to topical drugs. Increased tearing and blink rate associated with painful anterior segment disease will increase the rate of loss of drug via the nasolacrimal system and simple overflow. Protein binding in the presence of inflammatory or purulent exudate on the ocular surface may inactivate certain drugs (e.g. aminoglycosides). Paradoxically, occlusion of the proximal nasolacrimal system by mucin debris may enhance penetration by increasing retention time on the ocular surface. Temporary tarsorrhaphy is likely to increase drug retention time by inhibition of the blink-driven lacrimal flow.

Corneal edema and endothelial dysfunction will alter the dynamics of diffusion of topically applied drugs into the eye, although the clinical importance of this in the horse is unknown.

Best practice guidelines for topical ocular medication

- This route should be used in the treatment of adnexal and anterior segment disease.
- Select the physicochemical formulation of a particular drug according to whether the ocular surface or anterior segment structures are targeted.
- Solutions are awkward to administer in some horses and are easiest instilled using a small syringe.
- Solutions should be instilled at intervals of no more than 1–2 h. Consider reducing this interval in acute anterior segment disease or where marked epiphora is present.
- The frequency of instillation may be reduced if using viscous preparations or where concurrent subconjunctival injections are used.
- Using solutions, instill sufficient only to fill the lower conjunctival fornix. Excess is wasteful and may accelerate elution of the drug from the eye by capillary action.
- Where two or more preparations are being used, an interval of 15 min should be left between instillations to avoid losses by inadvertent elution, dilution or inactivation. Failure to do so is a common cause of therapeutic failure.
- Inflammatory debris should be flushed from the external eye prior to instilling a drug. Observe a 15 min interval between flushing and instilling the medication.
- Ointments should be applied, in general, every 3–4 h.
- Ointments should not be used in cases of corneal laceration, corneal perforation and where corneal surgery is contemplated.
- "Fortified" solutions made up from parenteral preparations in balanced salt solution (BSS) should be stored in the dark and for short periods only.
- Topically administered ophthalmic medications are potentially epitheliotoxic and may delay corneal repair. The clinician must balance the therapeutic benefits achieved by their use against any possible injurious effects and should be prepared to amend the treatment regimen according to the clinical response.

SUBCONJUNCTIVAL INJECTIONS

Bioavailability and pharmacokinetics

Subconjunctival injections will result in higher levels of drug in the anterior segment than are likely to be achieved by parenteral administration but may not reach the levels achieved by frequent topical instillation. Although more prolonged drug exposure is achieved by subconjunctival injection than by single-dose topical application, most drugs injected subconjunctivally are absorbed rapidly into the systemic circulation and high local drug concentrations are only maintained for short periods. Exceptions are the sustained-release repository formulations prepared from poorly water-soluble esters of the glucocorticoids. Since the lipid-epithelial barrier is bypassed, the entry of relatively hydrophilic drugs with low lipid solubility (e.g. aminoglycosides) into the anterior segment is readily achieved.

The duration of therapeutically effective levels of drug in the anterior segment following subconjunctival injection is determined by its physicochemical formulation and by a number of pharmacokinetic factors. Transscleral diffusion of fluid from the eye may retard diffusion of drug into the eye. This may be particularly relevant in the horse with its extensive uveoscleral-aqueous outflow pathway. Drug is inevitably lost onto the ocular surface via the injection port and is likely to be lost in significant amounts into the conjunctival and episcleral circulation where inflammatory hyperemia is present.

Best practice guidelines for subconjunctival injection

- Subconjunctival injection of drug should not be used as a sole route of medication but should be used to supplement topical administration in anterior segment disease and parenteral administration in posterior segment disease.
- Inject under the bulbar conjunctiva; do not use intrapalpebral techniques.

- Inject volumes of <1 ml, using water-soluble parenteral preparations.
- The duration of effective levels of drug at the injection site is unpredictable. Conventionally, non-repository injections are repeated at 24–36 h intervals, but consider using a shorter interval in acute anterior segment disease.
- Use repository corticosteroid preparations with great care. They are irrecoverable once injected and cause protracted local immunosuppression. They are potentially disastrous if corneal ulceration supervenes.
- Repeated injections cause significant local trauma and injections cannot be continued indefinitely. Some drug formulations are not suitable for subconjunctival injection (e.g. parenteral preparations of NSAIDs).

PARENTERAL ADMINISTRATION

Ocular bioavailability and pharmacokinetics

The blood–ocular barriers present a formidable obstacle to the penetration of parenterally administered drugs, and the selection of highly lipophilic, unionized preparations with low protein binding is generally necessary. However, since in practice the main indication for parenteral therapy is infectious or inflammatory intraocular disease, the blood–ocular barriers are in any event compromised and concerns over restricted drug passage are largely overridden.

Even in the inflamed eye, drug levels achieved in the anterior segment following parenteral administration alone using routine dosages are likely to be lower than those achieved by combined topical and subconjunctival administration. However, parenteral medication in combination with subconjunctival injection is necessary to achieve therapeutic levels of drug in the chorioretina.

The fenestrated nature of the ciliary and anterior episcleral vasculature means that some parenterally administered antibiotics may reach therapeutic levels in the peripheral cornea, and this may be a useful adjunct in the treatment of perilimbal stromal abscesses.

Some of the unionized unbound fraction of parenterally administered drugs will be secreted in the tears. However, the concentrations of drug reached in tears are unlikely to deliver any significant therapeutic effects at the ocular surface.

ANTIBACTERIAL THERAPY

Antibacterial agents are probably the most commonly used ophthalmic therapeutic agents in the horse (Regnier 1999). Overuse or inappropriate use is common in veterinary practice and has been implicated as a risk factor in keratomycosis (Andrew et al 1998), possibly by disrupting commensal population dynamics in the healthy external eye.

Good clinical practice in ocular antibiotherapy demands an accurate diagnosis, selection of an antibiotic with an appropriate spectrum of activity and diffusion to the targeted site, and delivery of adequate levels of the antibiotic for a sufficient time to ensure optimal efficacy (Regnier 1999).

OCULAR BACTERIOLOGY

The microbial population of the conjunctival fornices and proximal nasolacrimal drainage system of the healthy equine eye comprises mainly non-pathogenic or potentially pathogenic Gram-positive cocci and bacilli, along with small numbers of Gram-negative organisms and varying numbers of filamentous fungi (Brooks 1999). The prevalence of the individual species constituting the microbial population of the healthy equine eye is subject to geographical variation, although the identity of the organisms present is relatively constant. With the exception of conjunctivitis and orbital cellulitis, which usually follows penetrating injury of the periorbita, primary bacterial disease of the adnexa is relatively rare in the horse. However, bacterial keratitis, particularly ulcerative disease, is a common clinical presentation. In affected corneas, the prevalence of Gram-negative bacilli, including *Pseudomonas* and *Acinetobacter* spp. and Enterobacteriaceae, markedly increases, although Gram-positive isolates still tend to predominate

(Hamor & Whelan 1999, Moore et al 1995). *Pseudomonas* spp. in particular is typically associated with rapidly progressive, "melting" corneal ulceration. However, beta-hemolytic *Streptococcus (Strep.) equi* subspp. *zooepidemicus* and *equi* (Brooks et al 2000a) and *Bacillus cereus* have been implicated in aggressive ulcerative disease. Gram-positive cocci and Enterobacteriaceae are isolated commonly from corneal abscesses.

Bacterial uveitis or endophthalmitis is rare in horses and most usually follows perforating trauma of the globe. Presumptively hematogenous bacterial uveitis has been described in systemic *Strep. equi* and *Rhodococcus equi* infections and in neonatal septicemia. Leptospires have been isolated from the anterior vitreous of horses with ERU (Brem et al 1998) and uveitis has been reported in *Borrelia burgdorferi* infection (Lyme disease) in the horse. However, with the exception of postperforation endophthalmitis, it is not clear whether bacteria play a direct role in the genesis of intraocular disease or are indirectly involved, precipitating a local immunogenic uveitis.

There is anecdotal evidence implicating *Chlamydia* spp. in some cases of follicular conjunctivitis, and both *Moraxella equi* some *Mycoplasma* spp. may be involved in external ocular disease in the horse (Lavach 1990). The role of anaerobes in equine ocular disease has not been investigated extensively, although *Clostridium perfringens* has been isolated from corneal ulcers in two horses (Rebhun et al 1999).

ROUTES OF DELIVERY

Topical therapy

The therapeutic objectives in treating bacterial keratitis are the rapid elimination of the pathogen from the external eye and gaining control of the inflammatory response. Optimally, broad-spectrum, antibacterial solutions should be used for topical antibiosis. The rapid elution of topical solutions from the ocular surface demands that high-concentration aqueous preparations of antibiotics be administered at 30–60 min intervals. The drug selected should exhibit concentration-dependent, bactericidal activity: that is, the rate

of killing increases as the drug concentration increases above the minimum inhibitory concentration (MIC) for that bacterial pathogen, such as found with the aminoglycosides and fluoroquinolones (see Ch. 2).

In the ulcerated cornea, the epithelial barrier is absent and hydrophilic antibiotics, such as the aminoglycosides and beta-lactams (penicillins and cephalosporins), will rapidly reach high concentrations in the corneal stroma. Where the epithelial barrier is intact, as in stromal abscessation, only highly lipophilic antibiotics, such as fluoroquinolones and chloramphenicol, are likely to achieve therapeutic levels in the cornea after direct topical instillation. In these cases, physically removing the epithelium, by superficial keratectomy, will extend the range of usable antibiotics and will markedly enhance antibiotic penetration. Multiple antibiotic therapy may be considered as a therapeutic option. In particular, the synergy between the cephalosporins and aminoglycoside antibiotics can be usefully exploited in ophthalmic treatment regimens.

High-concentration, "fortified" antibiotic solutions are made up from aqueous formulations for parenteral administration in BSS or artificial tears. These may be instilled directly onto the ocular surface or added to a commercial formulation to reach the required final concentration. The recommended concentrations of fortified antibiotic solutions for topical use are shown in Table 13.1.

Table 13.1 Dosages of antibiotics for topical use in fortified solutions and for subconjunctival injection

	Fortified solution (mg/ml)	Subconjunctival injection (mg) (in <1 ml volume)
Beta-lactams		
Ampicillin	12	100
Ticarcillin–clavulanate	6	100
Carbenicillin	4–8	100
Cefazolin	50	100
Aminoglycosides		
Amikacin	5–15	25
Gentamicin	5–15	20
Tobramycin	15	20–40
Fluoroquinolones		
Ciprofloxacin	Commercial strength 0.3%	
Ofloxacin	Commercial strength 0.3%	
Chloramphenicol	5–10	50–100

Solutions made up in the clinic should be considered unstable and, although some may retain potency for relatively long periods, as a rule should not be stored for more than 3–4 days. Concentrated antibiotic preparations are likely to retard corneal re-epithelialization and their use should be curtailed once the infection is under control. Commercial strength ophthalmic drops can then be introduced. In general, the frequency of topical antibiotic administration should be reduced once the infection is under control, based upon the clinical appearance of the corneal lesion.

Subconjunctival therapy

Although evidence from laboratory animals indicates that concurrent subconjunctival injection of antibiotics adds little therapeutic advantage to aggressive direct topical antibiosis in the treatment of bacterial keratitis (Bazra & Baum 1998), this technique is commonly used to augment topical treatment in the initial management of bacterial keratitis and stromal abscessation in the horse. Antibiotics of low lipophilicity, such as the cephalosporins and aminoglycosides, are generally selected since the epithelial barrier is bypassed. Subconjunctival injections are potentially of greatest benefit when using beta-lactams. The beta-lactams exhibit time-dependent killing characteristics (i.e. the rate of killing is determined by duration of exposure to supra-MIC levels of the drug; see Ch. 2), and combined topical and subconjunctival administration are likely to maximize exposure to the antibiotic.

Subconjunctival antibiotic injections will result in local tissue necrosis and clinicians must use their discretion in assessing the therapeutic benefits against continued treatment. Water-soluble parenteral preparations should be used; the recommended doses of antibiotics for subconjunctival injection are shown in Table 13.1.

Parenteral therapy

There are no published data on the ocular bioavailability of parenterally administered antibiotics in the horse. Based upon recommendations in other species, the antibiotics of choice for parenteral use in the horse are the fluorquinolones, such as enrofloxacin, tetracyclines and potentiated sulfonamides. In humans, cephalosporins are used routinely in the treatment and prophylaxis of postsurgical endophthalmitis because of their ability to penetrate the intraocular fluids and experience in the horse points to the usefulness of ceftiofur sodium in the management of intraocular infection. This probably reflects inflammation-driven breakdown of the blood–ocular barriers in most clinical situations where parenteral antibiosis is indicated. Parenterally administered antibiotics, in particular the penicillins and cephalosporins, may be of some therapeutic value when used to augment topical treatment of perilimbal corneal stromal abscesses.

Intravitreal therapy

Intravitreal injection is believed to be the most reliable means of achieving therapeutic levels of antibiotics within the vitreous in most species. There are no definitive guidelines for the use of intravitreal antibiotics in the horse, nor any information on their retinotoxicity in this species. However, because of their long intravitreal half-life in other species and broad spectrum of activity, the aminoglycosides are probably the drugs of choice. All antibiotics injected intravitreally have the potential to produce significant local toxicity, and they should only be used therapeutically in attempting to salvage ocular integrity in endophthalmitis, where the alternative is enucleation. The dosages for antibiotics injected intravitreally in endophthalmitis in humans are shown in Table 13.2 and some extrapolation for use in the horse may be possible at the discretion of the individual clinician.

Table 13.2 Dosages of intravitreal antibiotics in humans (injection volume 0.1 ml)

Antibiotic	Dosage (mg in 0.1 ml)
Tobramycin	0.2
Gentamicin	0.1–0.2
Amikacin	0.4
Cefazolin	2.5

It is recommended that injections be made through the pars plana into the anterior vitreous, with the bevel of the needle directed towards the posterior face of the lens.

SELECTION OF ANTIBACTERIAL AGENT

Empirical selection of an antibiotic based upon clinical experience is common in initial therapy, since any delay in effective therapy militates against a successful outcome. The antibiotics of choice for topical use in bacterial keratitis in the UK are gentamicin or ciprofloxacin. Ciprofloxacin has a broad spectrum of activity against both Gram-positive and Gram-negative organisms, including *Pseudomonas* spp., and excellent corneal penetration. "Triple antibiotic" (neomycin, polymixin, gramicidin) is a useful empirical alternative in ulcerative disease, having a broad spectrum of bactericidal activity but poor corneal penetration. The antibiotic susceptibility of *Pseudomonas* spp. is unpredictable. However, where infection is suspected, alternative empirical selections are ticarcillin–clavulanate, amikacin or tobramycin.

Gram's stains of smears prepared from superficial corneal lesions can provide some guidance in selecting antibiotics pending the result of culture and sensitivity (Table 13.3). Mixed infections are common and combination therapy employing synergistic pairings, such as cefazolin and gentamicin, should be considered.

Culture and sensitivity testing in cases of bacterial keratitis is good clinical practice. However, the concentration of antibiotics at the ocular surface achieved by topical medication will substantially exceed the levels used in standard antimicrobial susceptibility tests, and organisms deemed resistant or intermediately sensitive using qualitative tests may, in practice, be killed by high local levels of antibiotics in the external eye. Underestimation of the therapeutic efficacy of topical treatments by conventional sensitivity testing procedures suggests that the therapeutic response may be a more valid test of antibiotic efficacy. In making such an assumption, affected eyes must be monitored stringently to assess resolution or deterioration. In all events, careful clinical monitoring of infected eyes is essential since the primary pathogen may change over the course of antibiotic therapy, necessitating change in the antibacterial agents used (Moore et al 1995).

There is increasing concern among ophthalmologists treating humans and small animals over emerging resistance to fluoroquinolones among Gram-positive pathogens, prompting the recommendation that these drugs should not be used in minor infections or for routine topical prophylaxis. Resistance problems have not been reported in the horse; however, this recommendation should be adhered to as good clinical practice.

Fusidic acid, a steroidal antibiotic with good corneal penetration, is effective against a range of Gram-positive pathogens. It is available as a 1% carbomer-based gel formulation and the requirement for once or twice daily application makes it attractive to equine practitioners. However, it should be used with caution because of its relatively limited spectrum of activity.

Chlortetracycline ointment (1%) is indicated for conjunctivitis or keratoconjunctivitis where *Chlamydia* or *Mycoplasma* spp. are the suspected primary pathogens. Topical chloramphenicol is reported to be effective against clostridial infections of the cornea (Rebhun et al 1999).

Table 13.3 Antibiotic selection based upon Gram's staining characteristic

Staining	Antibiotic
Gram-positive cocci	Ciprofloxacin, ampicillin, cefazolin, ticarcillin–clavulanate, chloramphenicol
Gram-positive bacilli	Ciprofloxacin, ampicillin, gentamicin, ticarcillin–clavulanate
Gram-negative cocci	Ciprofloxacin, tobramycin, gentamicin
Gram-negative bacilli	Ciprofloxacin, gentamicin, tobramycin, amikacin

Ulcerative keratitis

Apparent failure of therapy

Ulcerative keratitis in the horse may fail to respond to aggressive antibiotic therapy for several reasons.

1. The ulcer may be sterile. Stromal breakdown and progressive ulceration is largely driven by matrix metalloproteinases (MMPs) and serine proteases derived from local corneal cells and from leukocytes sequestered in the cornea in response to the initial injury (Fig. 13.1). Inoculation and replication of pathogenic bacteria at the site of minor epithelial injury releases exotoxins and microbial proteases that potentiate the initial processes of corneal breakdown and amplify endogenous stromal hydrolysis. However, once started, an ulcer can evolve its own biochemical momentum based upon the host response and may continue to progress in the absence of bacterial pathogens.

2. The selected antibiotic has an inappropriate pharmacokinetic profile.

3. The pathogen involved is resistant to the selected antibacterial agent.

4. The primary pathogen changes during the course of therapy.

5. Inappropriate treatment regimen, e.g. excessively prolonged intervals between treatments or simultaneous administration of two or more topical preparations.

6. Keratomycosis is present. This should be considered in all cases where combined antibacterial and enzyme inhibitor therapy has failed to halt the progression of the ulcer within 2 to 3 days or sooner where the clinical presentation suggests fungal involvement.

Adjunctive therapy in bacterial keratitis

In all cases of ulcerative keratitis, proteinase inhibitor therapy is of primary importance in controlling stromal breakdown and allowing repair to supervene (see p. 235). The use of topical mydriatics/cycloplegics to relieve pupillary spasm is important both for their analgesic effect and in preventing the development of synechiae. Parenteral NSAIDs are useful analgesics and have some benefit in stabilizing the blood–aqueous barrier and ameliorating the effects of reflex uveitis. Topical NSAIDs should be used with caution (p. 238).

Despite aggressive medical therapy, some eyes will inevitably require surgical intervention. The object of surgical intervention is to introduce a blood supply to the ulcer site. Although this may accelerate the repair of the ulcer, it does so at the expense of creating a dense and permanent fibrovascular leukoma. Ultimately, successful medical therapy will produce a cosmetically better end result.

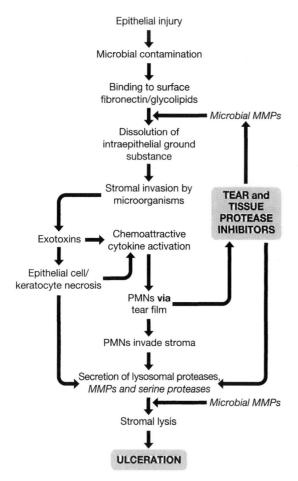

Figure 13.1 Scheme of events leading to corneal ulceration. MMP, matrix metalloproteinase; PMN, polymorphonuclear leukocyte.

ANTIMYCOTIC THERAPY

Fungi are eukaryotic organisms found ubiquitously in the environment within stables. They exist as saprophytes, parasites or symbiotes and are broadly divided into filamentous and diamorphic forms and yeasts (Regnier 1999). Varying numbers of mainly filamentous fungi are usually found amongst the normal microbial population of the ocular surface in the horse. Fungi are probably opportunistic corneal pathogens, and keratomycosis follows minor superficial trauma or, less frequently, preexisting superficial disease. However, recent work has suggested that in some instances fungi can act as primary keratopathogens (Brooks et al 2000b).

Ocular mycoses

Mycotic disease of the ocular adnexa and proximal nasolacrimal system occurs only very rarely in the horse (Brooks 1999). However, mycotic keratitis is a potentially devastating disease and presents a formidable clinical challenge if a visual eye is to be retained. The disease most commonly presents as a deep ulcerative keratitis but may occur as superficial ulceration, interstitial keratitis or frank stromal abscessation. Corneal perforation and iris prolapse are infrequent complications of keratomycosis, and exogenous endophthalmitis is a possible, though rare, sequela of deep mycotic lesions. As in the case of bacterial keratitis, ulceration is a manifestation of corneal degradation driven primarily by the host response to fungal inoculation and mediated by proteases derived from leukocytes, native keratocytes and the fungi themselves. The severity and speed of progression of the lesion reflects the intensity of the host response and the keratopathogenicity of the fungal pathogen involved. The horse appears to be particularly susceptible to keratomycosis, possibly reflecting the high risk of opportunistic infection of the relatively large and exposed cornea. However horses may also have an inherent deficiency in the surface defenses based around the tear film and anterior corneal surface (Brooks 1999).

There are several recognized risk factors in the development of keratomycosis, including inappropriate topical antibiosis and protracted topical corticosteroid therapy. Topical corticosteroids are likely to diminish both cell-mediated immune responses and local innate immune responses in the external eye, creating an immunosuppressed environment in which opportunistic fungi are able to proliferate. Geographic influences play a role in the distribution of keratomycosis, with the disease being relatively common and aggressive in the southern states of the USA but rare in the UK.

The fungi most commonly isolated in keratomycosis are *Aspergillus* and *Fusarium* spp.; *Penicillium, Alternaria* and *Mucor* spp. are implicated less frequently. Of the yeasts, only *Candida* and *Torulopsis* spp. are isolated with any frequency in ulcerative keratitis, although the overall incidence is less than 10% (Hamor & Whelan 1999). In the horse, filamentous fungi appear to have a particular predilection for Descemet's membrane (Grahn et al 1993), resulting in deep stromal infiltration of hyphae, creating problems in both diagnosis and treatment. The diagnosis of keratomycosis depends on the demonstration of fungal elements in corneal scrapings, keratectomy specimens or in cultures of the corneal lesion (Brooks 1999). Samples for diagnosis must be taken from deep within the lesion and repeated sampling may be necessary to demonstrate the organism. Even a single colony isolated from a suspect lesion should be considered significant.

SELECTION OF ANTIMYCOTIC AGENTS

Successful medical therapy in keratomycosis demands early and aggressive treatment with topical antimycotics, in some cases supplemented by deep keratectomy or surgical debulking of infectious material (Brooks 1999). The antimycotic drugs used in topical ophthalmic formulations are fungistatic at the concentrations likely to be routinely achieved on the ocular surface or in the corneal stroma. However, *in vitro* observations suggest that some antimycotic agents, notably amphotericin B and miconazole, may be fungicidal where relatively high local tissue levels can be achieved (Brinser 1998). Intact corneal epithelium impedes the penetration of topical antimycotic drugs and keratectomy performed for diagnosis or for surgical debridement will significantly increase corneal penetration and dissemination of drug and may help to concentrate the drug within the cornea. Early surgical intervention is, therefore, likely to be major factor in the successful resolution of some keratomycosis cases, in particular where there is stromal abscessation or fungal infiltration extending under the peripheral epithelium.

Fungal culture and sensitivity testing of corneal samples can be done (Brooks et al 1998) but is time consuming and has questionable clinical value (Brinser 1998). However, it may be useful in establishing susceptibility patterns amongst potentially pathogenic fungi in specific geographic locations (Brooks et al 1998). In practice, antifungal agents are usually selected empirically and the choice may be limited by the local availability of products capable of being adapted for ophthalmic use. Only one antimycotic agent, natamycin, is available in a specific topical ophthalmic formulation and this may be difficult to access outside the USA. Other drugs may be available as parenteral solutions or as water-miscible dermatological or vaginal preparations, both of which can be used topically in affected eyes. Care should be taken to avoid alcohol-based, lotion type preparations, which are too irritant for ophthalmic use.

Three classes of antimycotic antibiotic are available: polyenes, azoles and nucleoside analogs. In addition, non-specific antimicrobial agents such as povidone iodine, chlorhexidine and silver sulfadiazine can be adapted for ophthalmic use.

Polyenes

Polyenes are *Streptomyces* spp. derivatives whose primary mode of action is to bind preferentially to ergosterol in the fungal cell membrane, disabling the organism by increasing membrane permeability and causing cell leakage. Polyenes also bind to cholesterol in mammalian cell membranes and this mechanism is probably responsible for their cytotoxicity.

Amphotericin B

Amphotericin B has a broad spectrum of antifungal activity but is more effective against yeasts, in particular *Candida* and *Cryptococcus* spp., than

filamentous fungi. In general, it is likely to be only moderately effective against *Aspergillus* spp. It is relatively water insoluble and highly tissue bound, giving it a poor pharmacokinetic profile when used topically, particularly in the presence of an intact corneal epithelium. This, combined with its relative toxicity, has led to its relegation to a reserve position in treating equine keratomycosis. It may be commercially available as a powder for reconstitution for i.v. use. For topical ophthalmic use, the powder should be diluted in water for injection to a concentration of 0.15%. The diluted preparation should be kept in the dark to avoid photodegradation and will retain its potency for 5 to 7 days. Although amphotericin B can be administered subconjunctivally, the injections are painful and may lead to necrosis. The corneal bioavailability of the drug given by this route has been shown to be poor in animal models (O'Day & Head 1998) and this form of treatment cannot be recommended.

Natamycin (pimaricin)

Natamycin may be available as a 5% topical ophthalmic suspension. It is most effective against filamentous fungi, in particular *Aspergillus* and *Fusarium* spp. but is less effective against yeasts. The drug is poorly water soluble and a high degree of tissue binding restricts its bioactivity. Frequent administration is necessary to ensure therapeutic levels are achieved in the cornea. It does not penetrate intact epithelium but is well tolerated topically, although with prolonged use there is a minor risk of epithelial toxicity. It is not suitable for subconjunctival administration. Overall, if available, this drug is a first-choice therapy for keratomycosis caused by filamentous fungi (Bazra & Baum 1998, Brooke 1999). The ophthalmic preparation should be stored in the dark.

Azoles

The principal action of the azole group is to destabilize the fungal cell wall by inhibiting ergosterol synthesis in the cell membrane. In addition, they variably bind to and inhibit mitochondrial cytochrome P450, causing the intracellular accumulation of toxic metabolites. They are divided according to their relative affinities for the fungal and mammalian cytochrome P450 enzymes. The triazoles (fluconazole and itraconazole) have a lower affinity for mammalian cytochrome P450 than the imidazoles (miconazole, ketoconazole and clotrimazole), making them systemically less toxic. Although fungistatic at the levels likely to be achieved within tissues, some of the azoles exhibit fungicidal activity at higher concentrations *in vitro*. This activity is independent of the inhibition of ergosterol synthesis and may have some clinical application when intensive topical administration is used in conjunction with keratectomy.

Miconazole

Miconazole has a broad spectrum of activity against both filamentous fungi and yeasts, as well as against some Gram-positive cocci and anaerobes. It is a first-choice treatment in equine keratomycosis. It may be available as a 1% i.v. preparation and a 2% water-miscible vaginal cream, both of which can be applied topically. Although the corneal epithelium impedes drug penetration, miconazole readily disseminates through the cornea once the epithelium is removed. It is relatively highly tissue bound and it is estimated that, in animal models, only 30% of the drug present in the cornea is bioactive.

In the horse, 5–10 mg miconazole is well tolerated when injected subconjunctivally. However, results assessing the clinical efficacy of subconjunctivally administered miconazole in animal models are equivocal, although the route is thought to have some therapeutic advantage in the horse (Hamor & Whelan 1999).

Ketoconazole

Ketoconazole has a pharmacokinetic profile similar to that of miconazole but it is generally less effective against filamentous fungi, in particular *Fusarium* spp. It is usually only available in tablet form, and adapting the drug to a 1% formulation suitable for topical ophthalmic use may be problematic.

Clotrimazole

Clotrimazole is more effective against *Aspergillus* spp. than miconazole but *Fusarium* spp. are often resistant. It may be available as a 1% water miscible dermatological cream, which is well tolerated for topical ophthalmic use. Care should be taken to avoid using combined clotrimazole–corticosteroid formulations.

Itraconazole

Itraconazole is a triazole with a broad spectrum of activity against filamentous fungi; it is particularly effective against *Aspergillus* spp. Lack of availability of a formulation suitable for topical ophthalmic use may be a problem. A noncommercial, 1% itraconazole–30% dimethyl sulfoxide ointment preparation used topically in trials in the northeastern USA was found to be effective in 8 out of 10 horses with keratomycosis (Ball et al 1997). It may be given orally, at 3 mg/kg twice daily, in conjunction with topical administration, but it is expensive.

Fluconazole

Fluconazole may be available as a 2% solution suitable for topical ophthalmic use. However, its efficacy in treating equine keratomycosis has not been reported. In Florida, fungal isolates from horses with keratomycosis were found to significantly less susceptible to fluconazole than to natamycin or the imidazoles (Brooks et al 1998), although some geographic variation in susceptibility patterns are likely.

Nucleoside analogs

Flucytosine

Flucytosine is a fluorinated pyrimidine that is transported across the fungal cell wall by a permease, where it is deaminated to the cytotoxic principal fluorouracil. Some fungi may lack the permease and are resistant to the drug and its clinical use is usually restricted to treating *Candida* spp. infection, although even here resistance may arise. It is synergistic with amphotericin B and the two may be used in combination. The 1% parenteral solution is well tolerated for topical ophthalmic use.

Other preparations

Topical 2% povidone iodine solution and 0.2% chlorhexidine gluconate solution have broad antimicrobial profiles and may be used as cheap spectrum and effective antifungal agents in equine ketomycosis, particularly where *Fusarium* spp. are involved. A 1% dermatological cream formulation of silver sulfadiazine has both antifungal and antibacterial properties and is reasonably well tolerated topically in the horse eye. Its use is advocated where cost restraints exist or for prophylaxis in corneal injuries involving embedded plant material (Hamor & Whelan 1999).

Lufenuron is a benzoylurea compound with chitin synthetase inhibitory activity that is used principally as a systemic insecticide. Given orally to horses, at a dose rate of 5 mg/kg once daily, lufenuron may be beneficial when used in combination with topical antifungal agents. The potential toxicity of this compound in the horse has not been investigated.

TREATMENT PROTOCOLS IN KERATOMYCOSIS

The poor pharmacokinetic profiles of most topical antifungal agents mean that conventional treatment protocols have been based upon an aggressive loading dose approach. Initially, this involves administration of the antifungal agent every 1–2 h until clinical improvement is observed, after which the frequency of administration is reduced to every 4–6 h until the cornea has healed. However, it has been observed that initial intensive therapy may be associated with apparent clinical deterioration, possibly as a result of an intense anterior uveitis provoked by the sudden death of fungal hyphae in the stroma (Brooks 1999). To prevent this, it has been recommended that initial topical therapy should be reduced to administration three or four times a day for 2 to 3 days before increasing the frequency of application to six times daily (Brooks 1999). Alternatively,

the higher frequency loading dose regimen can be accompanied by more aggressive NSAID medication to control uveitis (Hamor & Whelan 1999), although this may have the disadvantage of suppressing neovascularization and possibly impeding endogenous corneal repair processes.

In addition to topical antimycotic therapy, systemic NSAIDs and topical atropine sulfate are used to the control pain and ameliorate the effects of anterior segment injury associated with the iridocyclitis that inevitably accompanies keratomycosis. Topical proteinase inhibitor therapy is of significant clinical benefit in controlling stromal breakdown and, since potentially pathogenic bacteria contaminate most mycotic lesions, concurrent broad-spectrum, topical antibacterial agents should be used.

Early surgical debridement or keratectomy of all but the most superficial ulcers will improve the therapeutic outcome significantly (Grahn et al 1993). Other surgical options may be considered depending upon the clinical progress of the lesion (Brooks 1999). In particular, posterior lamellar keratoplasty is likely to markedly improve the clinical outcome of deep mycotic abscesses (Andrew et al 2000).

Controlled studies of intracameral administration of antifungal antibiotics in the horse have not been reported and in mycotic endophthalmitis enucleation is generally indicated.

Treatment of equine keratomycosis is inevitably protracted and should continue until corneal healing is complete. Treatment periods of between 24 and 54 days are quoted (Ball et al 1997, Hamor & Whelan 1999). This places a considerable financial burden on owners, who must give informed consent prior to beginning treatment. Owners must also be made aware of the guarded prognosis in keratomycosis. The prognosis is improved significantly where an early diagnosis is made and effective medical and surgical treatment are implemented; however, between 10 and 50% of affected eyes will require enucleation (Brooks 1999). *Aspergillus* spp. infection is particularly difficult to treat successfully in the horse. In all cases where the eye is preserved there will inevitably be dense and permanent corneal scarring.

ANTIVIRAL THERAPY

Viral ocular disease

Keratitis and keratoconjunctivitis in association with equine herpes virus (EHV) respiratory disease has been recorded in foals. In adult horses, putative viral superficial keratitis, unassociated with systemic disease, is commonly seen in practice in the UK and may occur sporadically in the USA and mainland Europe. No specific virus has been isolated consistently from affected eyes and the suspected viral etiology is based largely upon the response to topical antiviral treatment. The disease is characterized by acute ocular pain and focal epitheliopathy. Two specific forms of the disease are encountered. Type 1 is characterized by epithelial fissuring, which occasionally results in dendritic or, rarely, frankly ulcerative lesions. Type 2 is characterized by shallow punctate ulceration.

TOPICAL ANTIVIRAL THERAPY

Ocular antiviral chemotherapy in the horse is adapted from that used in herpes simplex virus (HSV) and varicella zoster keratitis in humans. The agents used are nucleotide analogs capable of inhibiting viral replication by competitive inhibition of the uptake of the nucleotide into the viral genome. These agents are virustatic and require an intact immune system to suppress or eliminate the virus from the eye. They probably do not eradicate any latent infection. The antiviral drugs available currently do not penetrate intact corneal epithelium and are poorly disseminated within the corneal stroma. The availability of these drugs will vary in different countries and some may only be obtained from hospital pharmacies.

Idoxuridine

Idoxuridine is a thymidine analog and is converted into the trisphosphate form by a host cell- or viral-encoded thymidine kinase before being incorporated into the viral DNA. Some incorporation into epithelial cell DNA occurs and, as a result, idoxuridine is relatively epitheliotoxic and may retard the closure of epithelial defects. It may

be available as a 0.1% solution or as a 0.5% ointment for topical ophthalmic use; it is effective against both the type 1 and type 2 forms of putative viral keratitis in the horse. It should be used initially every 2–4h until the epithelial defects are healed; thereafter, the frequency of application may be reduced to 4 to 6 hourly for a further 3 to 4 days. Where affected eyes are treated with idoxuridine during the first episode of the disease, the disease does not generally recur. Epithelial toxicity has not been recognized in treated horses. Topical idoxuridine is known to be teratogenic in rabbits and its use should be avoided in pregnant mares.

Trifluridine

Like idoxuridine, trifluridine is a thymidine analog that requires conversion to the trisphosphate form before incorporation into viral DNA. The trisphosphate form is less readily incorporated into host cell DNA than is the idoxuridine form and, consequently, trifluridine is potentially less toxic. It is relatively soluble and can be used topically as a 1% solution and is effective against both types of putative viral keratitis in the horse. The treatment protocols are the same as described for idoxuridine.

Aciclovir

Aciclovir is a guanosine analog that is converted to the active trisphosphate form by a viral-encoded thymidine kinase which is present only in infected cells. Aciclovir trisphosphate inhibits DNA polymerase but has much greater affinity for the viral enzyme than for the host cell enzyme. As a result, aciclovir is relatively non-toxic to uninfected host cells. Its efficacy in putative viral keratitis in the horse is unpredictable but, in general, it is effective in type 2 but not type 1 disease. It may be commercially available as a 3% ointment for topical ophthalmic use and should be applied every 3–4h.

Other agents

Interferon is a non-specific inhibitor of viral protein synthesis and has both antiproliferative and immunomodulatory effects. Recombinant human interferon α (20–50 IU/ml in BSS four times a day) has been used topically to treat herpes viral keratitis in cats, with equivocal results. There are anecdotal reports of its successful use in treating viral keratitis in the horse.

Topical corticosteroids usually result in some clinical improvement in putative viral keratitis in the horse. However, subsequent recrudescence and worsening of the clinical signs can be a problem, and their use during the acute stages of the disease is not recommended. They can be used with caution in conjunction with the antiviral agent once epithelial repair is complete, when they may promote stromal clearing. There is anecdotal evidence that topical ciclosporin has some therapeutic benefit in type 2 keratitis in the horse (see p. 239).

THERAPY TO CONTROL ULCERATION

Proteinase inhibitor therapy is an adjunctive treatment in ulcerative keratitis to control stromal breakdown and allow tissue repair to occur (Woesner 1999). Corneal ulceration is the result of an amplifying biochemical degradation of stromal collagen and extracellular matrix glycosaminoglycans by host-derived proteinases, principally MMPs and neutrophil serine proteinases (including neutrophil elastase), and by exogenous microbial hydrolases (Fig. 13.1). MMPs are a highly homogenous family of zinc metalloproteinases, divided into four main classes: collagenases (MMP1, MMP8 and MMP13), gelatinases (MMP2 and MMP9), stromelysins (MMP3, MMP10 and MMP11) and membrane type (MT-MMPs). They play a fundamental role in tissue repair and are ubiquitously involved in the inflammatory and autolytic pathologies associated with a range of disease processes. MMPs are produced by a broad spectrum of mammalian cell types, including corneal epithelial cells, keratocytes and polymorphonuclear leukocytes (PMNs), and their synthesis and secretion is controlled by local cytokines. They are secreted as inactive proenzymes and activation is dependent upon cleavage of the zymogen

molecule by enzymes such as neutrophil elastase, tissue kallikrein, plasmin and other heterogeneous MMPs, including some microbial MMPs.

Neutrophil lysosomal serine proteinases are released from cells sequestered at the site of tissue injury and include both collagenases and an elastase capable of degrading basement membrane. Bacteria and fungi produce a range of proteinases, including some MMPs. Of these, the collagenolytic MMPs and MMP-activating proteinases produced by *Pseudomonas* spp. and a serine endopeptidase produced by *Aspergillus* spp. may be of particular importance in the equine eye.

Local tissue inhibitors (TIMPs), a neutrophil-derived inhibitor and systemic inhibitors, such as α₂-macroglobulin and the lower-molecular-weight prealbumin proteinase inhibitor, variably inhibit endogenous MMPs and neutrophil serine proteinases. Inhibitors are present in the mammalian cornea and in the tear film, where they maintain a dynamic equilibrium with endogenously or exogenously derived proteinases as part of the normal molecular homeostasis of the ocular surface. Where this equilibrium is deranged, either by local overexpression of enzyme or by reduction in inhibitory capacity, then keratolysis and ulceration are the probable results.

Re-epithelialization of corneal defects appears to depend in part upon the interaction of MMPs with matrix adhesion proteins on the exposed stromal surface to form the scaffolding for migrating basal epithelial cells (Fini et al 1996). Relative overexpression of MMPs may be a significant factor in refractory or indolent ulceration and in chronic superficial erosion in the horse.

Clearly, inhibition of enzymatic degradation is fundamental to the medical management of corneal ulceration. The ocular surface is openly accessible to topical proteinase inhibitor therapy, administered by direct instillation or via a subpalpebral lavage system. Inhibitor therapy is of most value in acute frank ulceration where it is used in conjunction with antimicrobial agents, but it may also be useful in promoting healing of refractory ulcers and chronic superficial erosions. Antiproteinases may be used prophylactically along with antibiotics in superficial injury where ulceration threatens.

The clinician should be aware that, although overexpression of proteinases appears to be integral to ulcerative pathology, proteinase activity is also integral to restorative repair of the corneal defect, and overuse of inhibitor preparations once the degradative processes are under control may potentially compromise repair.

Several inhibitor preparations may be used topically in the horse. These are likely to vary in their activity against specific proteinases. Some, such as chelating agents, may be principally effective against host cell MMPs and serine proteinases. Others, such as plasma α_2-macroglobulin, have a broader spectrum of activity, inhibiting both microbial and host cell proteinases and some of the proteolytic activators of MMP zymogens. In acute ulcerative disease, inhibitor preparations should be instilled hourly until healing is underway, indicated by decreasing size and rounding of the epithelial margins of the lesion. Once healing is underway the frequency of administration should be reduced to two or three times a day or withdrawn completely at the discretion of the clinician. Continuous perfusion of the ocular surface via a subpalpebral lavage system may be advantageous in rapidly progressive ulcerative disease. In refractory ulceration or chronic superficial erosion, topical administration five to six times daily is necessary and should continue until re-epithelialization is complete. In these cases, if there is no significant re-epithelialization within 10 days, inhibitor therapy alone is unlikely to be curative.

PROTEINASE INHIBITORS

Chelating agents

Ethylenediaminetetraacetic acid (EDTA)

A 0.2–1.0% (w/v) dipotassium or disodium ethylenediaminetetraacetic acid (EDTA) solution may impair or otherwise delay epithelialization and should be withdrawn once significant repair is evident.

Acetylcysteine

Acetylcysteine (5%) has an additional mucinolytic action and prolonged use may retard epithelial repair by degrading tear film mucins. It appears to be most beneficial in the first 2 to 3 days of treatment.

Tetracycline antibiotics

The tetracyclines, in particular doxycycline, have been used in some instances as proteinase inhibitors.

Systemic inhibitors

Isologous or homologous plasma or serum can be harvested and used topically. Plasma or serum may be stored at 0–4°C for up to 36 h. It should be divided into aliquots before storage and returned to physiological temperature before being instilled into the eye. Serum or plasma can be used in combination with EDTA and acetylcysteine to provide a broader spectrum proteinase inhibitor formulation.

Other inhibitors

Heparin

Heparin (1000 IU/ml) has been used to promote re-epithelialization in chronic refractory ulceration in the horse. Its mode of action is unknown but it may have an indirect antiproteinase activity by impeding the extravasation of leukocytes into the tear film.

Ilomastat

Ilomastat or GM60001 is a synthetic hydroxamate inhibitor of endogenous MMPs and *Pseudomonas* spp. proteinases that has been used experimentally to control stromal enzymolysis in laboratory animals. Its clinical use in the horse has not been documented, although workers in Florida have successfully used an ilomastat formulation (800 μg/ml in citrate buffer) to control stromal breakdown in cases of ulcerative keratitis.

Synthetic polysulfated glycosaminoglycans

Synthetic polysulfated glycosaminoglycans have antiproteinase activity, some of which is directed against MMP zymogen activators. A 5% solution in artificial tears may be used as a topical ophthalmic antiproteinase preparation and has been reported to be useful in managing chronic superficial erosions in adult horses.

OCULAR ANTI-INFLAMMATORY THERAPY

Inflammation is integral to eliminating microbial pathogens or autoantigens from the eye and in initiating tissue repair. However, the eye has a low tolerance to inflammatory injury and persistent inflammatory insult can threaten iridopupillary and neurosensory retinal function and the optical clarity of the refractive media. Anti-inflammatory agents downregulate the inflammatory response and can spare the eye from functional loss, but do so at the cost of impaired protective responses and delayed or disrupted tissue repair. The clinician must, therefore, balance the potential therapeutic and vision-sparing benefits of anti-inflammatory therapy against the perceived risks.

Glucocorticoids

The therapeutic properties of the glucocorticoids derive from their facility to modify gene transcription in susceptible cells towards downregulation of the complex molecular and cellular events leading to inflammation (Regnier 1999). This includes promoting lipocortin production leading to the inhibition of phospholipase A and the inflammatory cascade driven by cyclooxygenase (COX) and lipoxygenase. Glucocorticoids suppress expression of proinflammatory and angiogenic molecules such as cytokines, MMPs and nitric oxide synthetase and reduce the influx of PMNs into inflamed tissues by blocking the expression of adhesion molecules on the surface of vascular endothelial cells. Glucocorticoids suppress fibrovascular proliferation within inflamed tissue. In the equine eye, this can be used to limit the extent of vascularization and scarring in the healing cornea and the proliferation of post-inflammatory fibrovascular tissue and synechiae within the anterior chamber and anterior vitreous.

The ophthalmic indications for glucocorticoids in the horse are:

- allergic blepharitis or blepharoconjunctivitis;
- eyelid contusion;
- allergic conjunctivitis and chemosis;
- dacryocystitis;
- adnexal habronemiasis;
- some non-ulcerative superficial keratides;
- endotheliitis;
- eosinophilic keratitis/keratoconjunctivitis;
- limbal keratopathy (peripheral ulceration);
- multiple focal keratopathy;
- non-ulcerative keratouveitis;
- onchocerciasis;
- traumatic keratouveitis;
- endogenous anterior uveitis and panuveitis;
- ERU;
- traumatic optic neuritis;
- glaucoma; and
- promotion end-stage clarity in the healing cornea.

The ocular bioavailability of topical glucocorticoid formulations varies significantly. Lipid-soluble alcohol and ester preparations penetrate intact conjunctival and corneal epithelium readily and rapidly reach therapeutic levels in the anterior chamber of the normal eye. Water-soluble phosphate preparations are retarded by intact corneal epithelium in the normal eye and are generally used in the management of ocular surface disease. However, it has been shown in experimental animals that the intraocular levels of topically applied prednisolone phosphate exceed that of the acetate preparation in the acutely inflamed eye.

The anti-inflammatory potencies of betamethasone and dexamethasone exceed that of prednisolone. However, because of the facility with which prednisolone acetate crosses the cornea, a 1% solution is generally regarded as the drug of choice for the topical treatment of anterior uveitis in the horse, although comparable clinical results can be achieved using 0.1% dexamethasone in alcohol preparations. The frequency of application of topical glucocorticoids is largely determined by the severity and the nature of the clinical problem under treatment. It may be necessary to maintain some animals with chronic superficial keratitis on single alternate day therapy for protracted periods. Conversely, in acute anterior uveitis, maximal clinical benefit is achieved by hourly instillation during the initial stages of treatment, subsequently reducing the frequency of application once the inflammatory reaction is under control. Where aggressive topical treatment is extended over a protracted period, such as in ERU or eosinophilic keratoconjunctivitis, it is good clinical practice to taper withdrawal of the drug over 4 to 5 days once the clinical signs have resolved.

Topically administered glucocorticoids are more effective clinically than subconjunctivally injected drug, although combined therapy is advantageous where high intraocular levels are required or where disease extends beyond the anterior segment. Subconjunctivally injected water-soluble sodium phosphate preparations are likely to have a therapeutic benefit lasting no more than 24–36 h. However, sustained-release (repository) formulations of acetate or acetonamide salts last significantly longer when given subconjunctivally, and these are often used in the horse to reduce the requirement for topical medication. However, it is unlikely that the therapeutic efficacy of subconjunctivally injected sustained-release preparations approaches that of frequent topical administration. Subconjunctival injections of sustained-release preparations should be used with great caution since the drug cannot be recovered once injected. Their use can leave a white precipitate at the injection site, which may cause local conjunctival ulceration or granuloma formation. The doses of glucocorticoids for subconjunctival injection and their predicted duration of action are shown in Table 13.4.

Table 13.4 Doses and predicted duration of action of subconjunctivally injected glucocorticoids

Agent	Dose (mg)	Duration of action
Methylprednisolone acetate	40	7–21 days
Triamcinolone acetonide	40	5–10 days
Dexamethasone sodium phosphate	2	24–36 h
Betamethasone phosphate	2	24–26 h

Parenteral dexamethasone used in conjunction with topical administration can be of considerable therapeutic benefit in managing ERU and traumatic keratouveitis. In these cases, the potential vision-sparing benefits of the parenteral glucocorticoids outweighs the risks incurred, in particular the development of laminitis. Dimethyl sulfoxide administered i.v. in combination with high doses of dexamethasone (2 mg/kg) may be beneficial in the very early management of amaurosis and traumatic optic neuritis following head injury.

There are no reports of direct ocular toxicity of topically administered glucocorticoids in the horse, which may reflect the tendency toward short-term use of these drugs in this species. However, there are significant risks incurred with their use in the eye. They are believed to potentiate the collagenolytic activity of endogenous hydrolases in the ulcerating cornea and are known to impair local innate antimicrobial defenses by suppressing macrophage phagocytosis. As a result, their use in microbial ulceration or where microbial ulceration threatens is absolutely contraindicated. There is some rationale for their very early use in conjunction with bactericidal antibiotics in corneal injury, to limit the influx of PMNs into the damaged cornea, with the aim of suppressing ulcerogenesis. However, there is a significant risk of fungal superinfection once the glucocorticoids are withdrawn and their use in this way is not recommended. In geographic areas where the risk of keratomycosis is high, some clinicians have reservations over the use of ophthalmic corticosteroids under any circumstances. Concern has been expressed that topical glucocorticoid therapy in traumatic keratouveitis may prolong the time to resolution of the uveitis by delaying corneal healing (Moore et al 1998), consequently increasing the possibility of functional compromise of the eye.

Immunogenic corneal ulceration is rare in the horse but has been reported in both limbal keratopathy and in eosinophilic keratoconjunctivitis (Brooks 1999). Topical glucocorticoids are curative in these conditions but may have to be used for up to 9 to 10 weeks in some horses with eosinophilic keratoconjunctivitis. In these circumstances, the concurrent use of topical bactericidal antibiotics should be considered.

Topical glucocorticoids are effective in promoting end-stage clarity in the healing cornea by suppressing local angiogenesis and fibroblast proliferation. Their introduction into the therapeutic regimen is wholly at the discretion of the individual clinician; however, in general, they should not be used until the injured cornea is covered by migrating epithelium and stromal repair is established. Angiogenesis and fibroplasia are integral to corneal healing, and glucocorticoid use during the regenerative stages of corneal repair carries a theoretical risk of inducing structural weakness within the healed cornea.

Non-steroidal anti-inflammatory drugs

NSAIDs are a heterogeneous group of weak acids with a common structural origin (Regnier 1999). Their anti-inflammatory action derives principally from the inhibition of the COX2 isoform of cell membrane COX (see Ch. 14). However, the therapeutic efficacy of individual NSAIDs tends not to correlate with their anti-COX2 activity and other pharmacological actions are attributed variably to these drugs. These include inhibition of PMN activation, scavenging of reactive oxygen species and T cell immunomodulation. The pharmacological actions of the individual NSAIDs are to some extent dose dependent and show significant interspecies variation. At supratherapeutic doses of some NSAIDs, which may be achievable in the external eye using frequent topical administration, some inhibition of the lipoxygenase pathway may occur (see Ch. 14). In humans, their principal ophthalmic uses are in the treatment of hypersensitivity conjunctivitis and in perioperative anti-inflammatory prophylaxis for intraocular surgery.

Topical use

The pharmacokinetics and ocular bioavailability of topical NSAIDs in the horse are unknown. In other species, topical NSAIDs readily penetrate and disseminate within the eye, reaching peak intraocular levels within 2 h. In general, the levels achieved by topical administration exceed those achieved by the oral or parenteral routes. Subconjunctivally injected NSAIDs are likely to reach therapeutic intraocular levels rapidly in the horse, but the parenteral formulations currently available are potentially highly irritant and this route of administration is not recommended. Several topical ophthalmic formulations of NSAIDs are manufactured (1% indometacin, 1% suprofen, 0.03% flurbiprofen, 0.1% diclofenac, 0.5% ketorolac) but local availability will vary.

In general the efficacy of topically administered NSAIDs in suppressing intraocular inflammation is likely to be poorer than that achieved using topical glucocorticoids. In the horse, topical NSAIDs are used in conjunction with the parenteral drug in the management of anterior uveitis and ERU and in traumatic and other nonulcerative keratides and keratouveitides. They are of particular value where circumstances militate against the use of topical corticosteroids. Topical NSAIDs have been used prophylactically prior to intraocular surgery in the horse.

Topical NSAIDs should be used with caution in ulcerative keratitis since their effects on corneal microbial infections and enzymolysis are not known and there is anecdotal evidence of corneal "melting" associated with their use. It should be noted that carprofen, an arylpropionic acid NSAID, has been shown to increase the expression of MMP9 zymogen in equine chondrocytes *in vitro*. Suppression of corneal angiogenesis by topical NSAIDs is likely to impede local corneal defense mechanisms and subsequently delay repair, particularly in deep stromal injury. Concurrent topical bactericidal antibiotics should always be used in conjunction with topical NSAIDs in ulcerative disease; in all cases, the therapeutic benefits of topical NSAID therapy should be weighed against the possibility of any untoward effects.

The comparative anti-inflammatory efficacy of the various topical NSAID formulations in the horse is not known and optimal therapeutic protocols have not been established. In general, the frequency of topical administration is determined by the severity and nature of the clinical problem and by the response to treatment. In acute anterior uveitis or ERU or for presurgical anti-inflammatory prophylaxis, hourly administration may be necessary initially, subsequently reducing the frequency of administration according to the clinical response in anterior uveitis. In ulcerative keratouveitis, topical administration two to four times a day in conjunction with parenteral administration may be adequate.

Parenteral use

Parenteral NSAIDs are used widely in the management of keratouveitis, anterior uveitis and ERU and for the provision of analgesia in ocular pain irrespective of its origin. They are useful in reducing swelling in adnexal trauma and allergic blepharoconjunctivitis and for anti-inflammatory prophylaxis prior to adnexal surgery. Comparative studies of the efficacy of systemic NSAIDs in ocular disease in the horse have not been published, but the potent analgesic and anti-inflammatory effects of flunixin meglumine make this the drug of first choice. Long-term oral aspirin 30 mg/kg has been advocated for maintenance therapy in ERU (Lavach 1990), although its efficacy in preventing further episodes of the disease has not been established. Systemic NSAIDs should be used with caution in very young, very old, debilitated and hypovolemic animals. Topical administration alone may be implemented in these groups, although some systemic absorption is likely.

Ciclosporin

Ciclosporin (Gilger & Allen 1998, Gilger et al 2000), a derivative of the fungus *Tolypocladium inflatum*, is a potent inhibitor of early lymphocyte activation and proliferation. Its immunosuppressive effects are mediated principally via T cell interaction. The drug binds to the immunophilin ligand cyclophilin within the lymphocyte cytosol, subsequently blocking mRNA transcription mechanisms encoding the lymphokines interleukin 2 and 4, tumor necrosis factor and interferon γ. In addition to its immunomodulatory activity, ciclosporin exerts a lacrimogenic effect in many species, including the horse, which appears to be independent of its action on immunocytes. Ciclosporin also has weak antibacterial and antifungal properties.

Ciclosporin is a highly lipophilic molecule that enters the intact cornea readily, reaching high levels within the stroma and creating a reservoir of the drug. The evidence for transcorneal penetration of topical ciclosporin into the anterior chamber in both normal and inflamed eyes in laboratory animals is equivocal, and penetration may vary depending on the dose of the drug and the vehicle used. There are no published studies on the ocular bioavailability of topically applied ciclosporin in the horse; however, it is unlikely that therapeutic levels of the drug are reached in the anterior chamber using the currently available formulations. Ciclosporin is commercially available in some countries as a 0.2% ophthalmic ointment. Alternatively, a 2% preparation for ophthalmic use can be made up from the parenteral formulation in corn oil or olive oil. However, the use of a 2% preparation in olive oil has been associated with worsening of the clinical signs in some horses with chronic non-infectious keratitis. Topical ciclosporin should be administered two to three times a day in the horse.

The use of intravitreal ciclosporin sustained-release devices to manage ERU has been reported (Gilger & Allen 1998, Gilger et al 2000). These are placed via sclerotomy performed under general anesthesia; implants delivering 4 μg/day have shown significant therapeutic potential. However, preexisting cataracts are a contraindication of this type of therapy and care is required in case selection.

The major indication for the use of topical ciclosporin in the horse is in the treatment of non-ulcerative, non-infectious keratitis and keratouveitis. This is a heterogeneous group of poorly understood diseases, some or all of which are likely to be of immunogenic origin, with no direct parallel in other species; they may be unresponsive to topical corticosteroids alone. In some of these cases, topical ciclosporin can very effectively suppress the inflammatory reaction and promote corneal clearing, but treatment may need to be prolonged to maintain the therapeutic response, incurring significant costs. Combining topical ciclosporin with corticosteroids has been reported to improve the clinical response in some horses with keratouveitis, possibly through specific corticosteroid suppression of the iridocyclitis.

Keratoconjunctivitis sicca (KCS) is rare in the horse. It most commonly results from disruption of the parasympathetic nerve supply to the lacrimal gland following fracture of the stylohyoid bone or vertical ramus of the mandible, in vestibular disease or in temporohyoid osteoarthropathy. Other, non-neurogenic, causes include locoweed (*Astragulus hornii*) poisoning and eosinophilic granulomatous dacryoadenitis. Topical ciclosporin may increase tear production in some horses with KCS but the results are unpredictable and treatment may need to be continued for up to 3 months before significant tear production is established. Long-term maintenance therapy is likely to be necessary in instances where ciclosporin is successful in increasing tear production but is so expensive as to be prohibitive for many owners.

Topical ciclosporin may be useful in treating bullous keratopathy (idiopathic primary edema) in the horse and can be effective in the management of type 2 viral keratitis.

OCULAR AUTONOMIC DRUGS

MYDRIATICS/CYCLOPLEGICS

In the horse, mydriasis and cycloplegia (Gelatt et al 1995) are routinely achieved by pharmacological parasympatholysis of the iris sphincter and ciliary muscles, principally using the muscarinic antagonist drugs atropine and tropicamide. Iridocycloplegia is useful in facilitating ophthalmoscopic examination of the posterior segment and, in uveitis, to relieve pain associated with ciliary spasm and to prevent posterior synechiae formation and pupillary restriction.

Atropine

Atropine is a naturally occurring agent with dual solubility that penetrates the cornea relatively well after topical instillation. In the normal horse eye, mydriasis begins within 30–60 min of topical instillation, reaching a maximum after 10–12 h. Atropine-induced mydriasis can last up to 10 to 14 days or longer in normal eyes, possibly through a reservoir effect resulting from binding of the drug to melanin in the heavily pigmented equine iris. For topical ophthalmic use, atropine may be used in 1 to 4% solutions or as a 1% ointment. The higher concentration solutions may not be commercially available and may have to be compounded by a pharmacist. Atropine is the mydriatic/cycloplegic of choice for therapeutic use in anterior uveitis as it appears to have an additional stabilizing effect on the blood–aqueous barrier. However, inflammation reduces the sensitivity of the anterior uvea to atropine and topical solutions require to be instilled into the uveitic eye hourly until maximal mydriasis is achieved, after which time application can be reduced to two to four times a day, or less, to maintain pupillary dilatation. In some instances, instillation of the higher concentration solutions at 30 min intervals may be necessary to achieve mydriasis. To supplement topical instillation, 2 mg parenteral atropine sulfate can be injected subconjunctivally. Ophthalmic preparations of atropine are not suitable for subconjunctival injection.

Ileus is a potential side-effect of the systemic absorption of ophthalmic atropine in the horse. This may be an idiosyncratic response affecting only a few individual horses but all atropine-treated horses should be monitored for signs of colic.

Tropicamide

Tropicamide is a synthetic agent that readily penetrates the cornea after topical instillation since it occurs primarily in the unionized form at physiological pH. It has a less-potent muscarinic blocking action than atropine and is of little value in the treatment of uveitis. However, a 1% solution is used routinely to achieve mydriasis for ophthalmic examination. Mydriasis is usually evident within 20–30 min of instillation, reaching a maximum after 1 h and lasting 8–12 h.

Phenylephrine

Phenylephrine is a sympathomimetic α_1 adrenoceptor agonist capable of producing mydriasis in some species by iris dilator muscle contraction. In the horse, topical application of a 10% solution has been shown to have no effect on the pupil diameter in the normal eye. However, 10% phenylephrine in combination with topical atropine is reported to be useful in reversing pupillary spasm in some stubborn cases of anterior uveitis, although there is no pharmacological evidence to support any additive mydriatic effect when the two agents are used together.

In Horner's syndrome in the horse, topically instilled 10% phenylephrine produces periorbital sweating but its effects on pupil diameter and ptosis reversal are unpredictable.

MIOTICS

There are few, if any, indications for the therapeutic use of miotics in the horse. However, a 2% solution of the parasympathomimetic agent pilocarpine can induce miosis in normal eyes after repeated topical application (van der Woerdt et al 1998). The cholinesterase inhibitor topical miotics, including demecarium bromide and echothiophate iodide, appear to be potentially uveitogenic in the horse and should not be used.

In theory, topical 2% pilocarpine could be used to stimulate tear production in KCS where a functional lacrimal gland is present. However, there are no reports of its successful therapeutic use in the horse.

OTHER OCULAR MEDICANTS

TOPICAL ANESTHETICS

Topical anesthesia of the ocular surface is used to facilitate diagnostic techniques, such as corneal scraping, conjunctival biopsy, ocular ultrasonography and tonography, and is necessary when placing subpalpebral lavage systems or performing subconjunctival injections. Examination of the bulbar surface of the third eyelid or retrieval of foreign bodies from the conjunctival fornices in standing sedated horses requires topical anesthesia. Most topical anaesthetic formulations contain antibacterial preservatives and should, therefore, not be used prior to taking samples from the external eye for microbial culture.

The topical anesthetics in general use in the horse are 0.5% proxymetacaine (proparacaine) and 0.5% tetracaine (amethocaine). The rate of onset and duration of clinical anesthesia of the ocular surfaces using these agents in the horse is not known. However, in general, repeated instillations at 30–60 s intervals over a 5 min period will superficially desensitize the normal eye for around 15 min. In the presence of conjunctival hyperemia, there is likely to be accelerated loss of the drug into the systemic circulation and instillation of the anaesthetic agent at shorter intervals for a longer period may be necessary to desensitize the ocular surfaces effectively.

All topical anaesthetic agents delay corneal re-epithelialization and mask the presence of a fornix-based foreign body or ectopic cilia. They should not be used in the routine management of ocular pain.

OCULAR LUBRICANTS

Topical ocular lubricants are used routinely to manage the ocular surface desiccation that occurs typically in KCS or exposure keratitis and during prolonged general anesthesia. Artificial tear solutions are prepared using viscosity-increasing agents, such methylcellulose or carbomer liquid gels, and are very effective in protecting the ocular surfaces. However, they require instillation every 2–3 h, often for protracted periods, and owner compliance becomes a major problem.

Petrolatum- or lanolin-based lubricant ointments require application every three to four hours and are more generally used in clinical practice. It should be noted that lubricant ointments can harbor pathogenic bacteria, including *Pseudomonas* spp., and partly used tubes should be considered potentially contaminated and should not be stored for further use at a later date.

OCULAR IRRIGATING SOLUTIONS AND DISINFECTANTS

Irrigation of the external eye is necessary in chemical injury or for removal of blood or mucus debris from the conjunctival fornices. BSS or any isotonic solution is suitable; in an emergency, tap water can be used where no alternative is available.

Disinfection of the ocular surface prior to surgery is recommended. A 2% solution of povidone iodine is non-irritant and will reduce the microbial burden of the external eye significantly for up to 1 h after presurgical preparation. A 0.2% chlorhexidine gluconate solution can be used with similar effect, although this may be irritant in some horses. In either case, scrub preparations must not be used.

VISCOELASTIC MATERIALS

The principal uses of viscoelastics, such as sodium hyaluronate, in equine ophthalmology are in the management of full-thickness corneal or corneoscleral wounds and, to a lesser extent, the facilitation of cataract surgery (Wilkie & Willis 1999). In full-thickness corneal injuries, intracameral viscoelastics reform the anterior chamber and reposition the anteriorly prolapsed iris, elevating the corneal wound margins to allow accurate closure. During reflation of the anterior chamber, the viscoelastic substance can help physically to dissect and break down synechiae and will tamponade any bleeding that results. Viscoelastics appear to have a protective influence on the corneal endothelium as well as a more general intraocular anti-inflammatory effect.

Preparations of sodium hyaluronate formulated specifically for intraocular use in humans are commercially available. Individual formulations vary principally in the molecular weight of the polysaccharide component, which affects their rheological properties and determines their specific advantages in a particular surgical situation. In the horse, intraarticular preparations of sodium hyaluronate have been used successfully in ophthalmic surgery for several years and have a significant cost advantage over dedicated ophthalmic preparations. The higher-molecular-weight intraarticular preparations, although more expensive, should be selected since less-viscous lower-molecular-weight preparations tend to egress from the corneal wound and may fail to maintain the anterior chamber. The viscoelastic substance can be left in the anterior chamber following surgical closure.

INTRACAMERAL FIBRINOLYTIC AGENTS

Recombinant tPA may be used intracamerally to break down accumulations of fibrin and organizing hemorrhage in traumatic anterior uveitis (Martin et al 1993). In these cases, 50–150 µg reconstituted tPA as a 250 µg/ml solution in BSS may be injected under general anesthesia into the anterior chamber via the limbus using a 27 gauge needle. The process of intracameral injection will result in some iatrogenic injury to the blood–aqueous barrier and tPA should not be used where the hemorrhage is of less than 48 h duration. Care is necessary in maintaining sterility during the preparation of the tPA solution. Samples of the reconstituted tPA solution may be stored at −70°C.

TOPICAL HYPEROSMOTIC AGENTS

In some cases, topical hyperosmotic preparations may achieve temporary clearing of an edematous cornea and can facilitate examination of the anterior chamber. They may be irritating in some eyes, particularly with repeated or prolonged use. Preparations suitable for use are:

- 2–5% hypertonic saline, hourly;
- 5% sodium chloride ointment, every 2–4 h; and
- 10% glycerin, every 2 h.

OCULAR TISSUE ADHESIVES

Cyanoacrylate tissue adhesives, in particular iso- or *n*-butyl-cyanoacrylate preparations, are suitable for use in the repair of small ulcers and partial-thickness corneal wounds where there is epithelial loss. They will prevent the entry of neutrophils into the wound area and may accelerate healing. The cornea must be thoroughly dried, possibly using photographers' aerosolized air, prior to application and any necrotic or underrun epithelium should be removed. Infection at the ulcer site is a contraindication to their use. Only a thin local application of the adhesive is necessary and this will slough as the cornea heals and epithelium covers the defect.

MEDICAL MANAGEMENT OF GLAUCOMA

Congenital and primary glaucoma is associated with anterior segment dysgenesis or dysfunction; both forms are relatively rare conditions in the horse (Brooks 1999). However, secondary glaucoma is increasingly recognized as a sequel to intraocular inflammatory diseases, including ERU. Horses also suffer from an episodic and progressive form of glaucoma, manifesting in the early stages as glucocorticoid-responsive corneal edema and hydrophthalmos. As the disease progresses, signs of anterior segment inflammatory disease, such as iris heterochromia and anterior cataracts, accompany the episodes of hydrophthalmos, which become increasingly refractory to medical treatment. The precise pathophysiology of glaucoma in the horse is unknown. However, it will differ from other species in that the horse has an open and robust drainage angle and the low-resistance unconventional or uveoscleral aqueous outflow has functional primacy over the high-resistance conventional outflow via the drainage angle.

Medical management of glaucoma is difficult to rationalize in any one horse. The effects of the various therapeutic options are unpredictable and, even where successful, any benefits are frequently difficult to sustain. Several therapeutic options are available.

Topical mydriatics

Topical mydriatics should, in theory, increase aqueous egress from the eye via the uveoscleral outflow. However, although topical atropine sulfate causes a small fall in intraocular pressure (IOP) in normal eyes, in practice it has very little therapeutic value in glaucoma management. Furthermore, caution is necessary when using atropine in glaucomatous eyes since lens luxation may be present, particularly in Appaloosas. In these horses, mydriasis may further compromise the eye by allowing displacement of the lens and anterior vitreous into the anterior chamber.

Pilocarpine

Pilocarpine-induced miosis has very little value in managing glaucoma in the horse and may increase IOP (van der Woerdt et al 1998). Miotics may also potentiate the clinical signs of uveitis where these are present.

Carbonic anhydrase inhibitors

Carbonic anhydrase inhibitors reduce aqueous humor formation. Topical carbonic anhydrase inhibitors, such as 2% dorzolamide two to four times a day, appear to significantly reduce IOP in some glaucomatous eyes. However, this treatment has not been critically evaluated for efficacy or safety in the horse and cost militates against its long-term use. Carbonic anhydrase inhibitors, such as acetazolamide and dichlorphenamide, can be used orally in conjunction with topical therapy.

β adrenergic antagonists

Topical non-selective β adrenoceptor antagonists, such as 0.5% timolol maleate, used two to four times a day, reduce IOP in horses by reducing aqueous humor formation and can be used in conjunction with topical or oral carbonic anhydrase inhibitors.

Latanoprost

Latanoprost, a topical prostaglandin, is used in humans and in small animals to reduce IOP by increasing uveoscleral outflow. In the horse, a topical ophthalmic preparation of 0.005% latanoprost reduces IOP in treated eyes; however, limited experience indicates that this drug is potently uveitogenic in glaucomatous eyes.

Dexamethasone

Topical dexamethasone acetate is probably the single most effective therapeutic agent in most cases of equine glaucoma, presumably acting by suppressing uveitic activity in the affected eye. However, long-term therapy gives rise to local immunosuppression problems. Also owners may assume that any sudden worsening of the ocular signs indicates a recurrence of hydrophthalmos and may inadvertently medicate a lacerated or ulcerated cornea with disastrous consequences. Dexamethasone can be used in conjunction with topical carbonic anhydrase inhibitors or β adrenergic antagonists.

Gentamicin

High doses of gentamicin administered intravitreally are potently cyclodestructive and injection of 1–2 ml of a solution containing 25 mg/ml gentamicin and 1 mg/ml dexamethasone into a glaucomatous eye reduces aqueous production irreversibly and can result in a blind normotonic eye. There are no controlled studies of the efficacy and safety of this procedure in the horse.

REFERENCES

Andrew S E, Brooks D E, Smith P J et al 1998 Equine ulcerative keratomycosis: visual outcome and ocular survival in 39 cases (1987–1996). Equine Veterinary Journal 30:109–116

Andrew S E, Brooks D E, Biros D J et al 2000 Posterior lamellar keratoplasty for treatment of deep stromal abscesses in nine horses. Veterinary Ophthalmology 3:99–104

Ball M A, Rebhun W C, Gaarder J E et al 1997 Evaluation of itraconazole–dimethylsulphoxide ointment for treatment of keratomycosis in nine horses. Journal of the American Veterinary Medical Association 211:199–203

Bazra M, Baum J 1998 Ocular pharmacology of antibiotics. In: Tasman W, Jaeger E A (eds) Duane's foundations of clinical ophthalmology, vol. 2. Lippincott Williams & Wilkins, Philadelphia, PA, Ch. 61

Brem S, Gerhards H, Wollanke B et al 1998 Demonstration of intraocular Leptospira in 4 horses suffering from equine recurrent uveitis. Berlin und Munchen Tierarztliche Wochenschrift 111:415–417

Brinser J 1998 Principles of ocular mycology. In: Tasman W, Jaeger E A (eds) Duane's foundations of clinical

ophthalmology, vol. 2. Lippincott Williams & Wilkins, Philadelphia, PA, Ch. 54

Brooks D E 1983 Use of an indwelling nasolacrimal cannula for the administration of medication to the eye. Equine Veterinary Journal Supplement 2:135–137

Brooks D E 1999 Equine ophthalmology. In: Gelatt K N (ed) Veterinary ophthalmology, 3rd edn. Lippincott Williams & Wilkins, Philadelphia, PA, pp. 1053–1116

Brooks D E, Andrew S E, Dillavou C L et al 1998 Antimicrobial susceptibility patterns of fungi isolated from horses with ulcerative keratomycosis. American Journal of Veterinary Research 59:138–142

Brooks D E, Andrew S E, Biros D J et al 2000a Ulcerative keratitis caused by beta haemolytic Streptococcus equi in 11 horses. Veterinary Ophthalmology 3:121–126

Brooks D E, Andrew S E, Denis H M et al 2000b Rose Bengal positive epithelial microerosions as a manifestation of equine keratomycosis. Veterinary Ophthalmology 3:83–86

Fini M E, Parks W C, Rinehart W B et al 1996. Role of matrix metalloproteinases in failure to re-epithelialize after corneal injury. American Journal of Pathology 149:1287–1302

Gelatt K N, Gum G G, MacKay E O 1995 Evaluation of mydriatics in horses. Veterinary and Comparative Ophthalmology 5:104–108

Gilger B C, Allen J B 1998 Cyclosporine A in veterinary ophthalmology. Veterinary Ophthalmology 1:181–188

Gilger B C, Malok E, Stewart T et al 2000 Long term effect on the equine eye of an intravitreal device used for sustained release of cyclosporine A. Veterinary Ophthalmology 3:105–110

Grahn B, Wolfer J, Keller C et al 1993 Equine keratomycosis: clinical and laboratory findings in 23 cases. Veterinary and Comparative Ophthalmology 13:2–8

Hamor R E, Whelan N C 1999 Equine infectious keratitis. Veterinary Clinics of North America Equine Practice 15:623–646

Lavach J D 1990 Large animal ophthalmology. Mosby, St Louis, MO,

Martin C, Kaswan R, Gratzek A et al 1993 Ocular use of tissue plasminogen activator in companion animals. Veterinary and Comparative Ophthalmology 3:29–36

Miller T R 1992 Principles of therapeutics. Veterinary Clinics of North America Equine Practice 8:479–497

Mindel J S 1998a Pharmacokinetics. In: Tasman W, Jaeger E A (eds) Duane's foundations of clinical ophthalmology, vol. 3. Lippincott Williams & Wilkins, Philadelphia, PA, Ch. 23

Mindel J S 1998b Bioavailability. In: Tasman W, Jaeger E A (eds) Duane's foundations of clinical ophthalmology, vol. 3. Lippincott Williams & Wilkins, Philadelphia, PA, Ch. 22

Moore C P, Collins B K, Fales W H 1995 Antibacterial susceptibility patterns for microbial isolates associated with infectious keratitis in horses: 63 cases (1986–1994). Journal of the American Veterinary Medical Association 207:928–933

Moore C P, Halenda R M, Grevan V L et al 1998 Post traumatic keratouveitis in horses. Equine Veterinary Journal 30:366–373

O'Day D M, Head W S 1998 Ocular pharmacology of antifungal drugs. In: Tasman W, Jaeger E A (eds)

Duane's foundations of clinical ophthalmology, vol. 2. Lippincott Williams & Wilkins, Philadelphia, PA, Ch. 62

Rebhun W C, Cho J O, Gaarder J E et al 1999 Presumed clostridial and aerobic bacterial infection of the cornea in two horses. Journal of the American Veterinary Medical Association 214:1519–1522

Regnier A 1999 Antimicrobials, anti-inflammatory agents and antiglaucoma drugs. In: Gelatt K N (ed) Veterinary ophthalmology, 3rd edn. Lippincott Williams & Wilkins, Philadelphia, PA, pp. 297–336

Speiss B M, Nyikos S, Stummer E et al 1999 Systemic dexamethasone concentration in horses after topical treatment with an ophthalmic preparation of dexamethasone. American Journal of Veterinary Research 60:571–576

van der Woerdt A, Gilger B C, Wilkie D A et al 1998 Normal variation in and effect of 2% pilocarpine on, intraocular pressure and pupil size in female horses. American Journal of Veterinary Research 59:1459–1462

Wilkie D A, Willis A M 1999 Viscoelastic materials in veterinary ophthalmology. Veterinary Ophthalmology 2:147–154

Woesner J F 1999 Matrix metalloproteinase inhibition. From the Jurassic to the third millennium. Annals of the New York Academy of Sciences 878:388–403

CHAPTER CONTENTS

Inflammation, pain and fever 247

Mode of action 248

Indications for use in horses 250

Pharmacokinetics 250

Side-effects in horses 251

Specific agents 254

References 263

14

Non-steroidal anti-inflammatory drugs

Cynthia Kollias-Baker   Karina Cox

INFLAMMATION, PAIN AND FEVER

The inflammatory response is a complex process that occurs following cellular injury. The injury results in the formation and release of a myriad of cell mediators that are responsible for producing early inflammatory events. These include increased microvascular permeability, followed by the leakage of blood components and migration of leukocytes into the interstitial space. These physiological events are responsible for the five cardinal signs of inflammation: erythema, edema, pain, heat and loss of use.

The family of compounds referred to as eicosanoids, which includes the prostaglandins (PGs), leukotrienes (LTs) and thromboxanes (TXs), have been shown to play key roles in the inflammatory process (Flower et al 1985). Eicosanoids are derived from 20-carbon essential fatty acids, with arachidonic acid being the most common precursor. Perturbations of cell membranes, whether chemical, physical or immune-mediated, release phospholipids, which are rapidly converted to arachidonic acid by phospholipase A_2 and other acylhydrolases. Once released, arachidonic acid and its congeners form the substrates for a number of enzyme systems (Fig. 14.1). Products that contain ring structures (PGs and TXs) are the result of metabolism by the cyclooxygenase (COX) enzymes, while the hydroxylated derivatives of straight-chain fatty acids (LTs) result from the action of various lipoxygenases (Flower et al 1985).

In many organ systems, PGs and TXs are produced constitutively and serve numerous homeostatic roles. For example, in the gastrointestinal

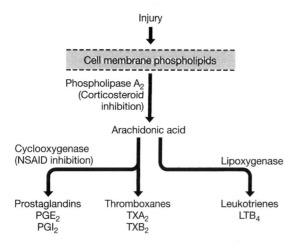

Figure 14.1 Pathway of formation of eicosanoid mediators following cellular injury. NSAID, non-steroidal anti-inflammatory drug.

tract, PGs of the E series, primarily PGE_2, have been shown to protect the gastric mucosa from damage secondary to a multitude of insults, including acids, alcohol and hypertonic solutions (Guth et al 1979). In the kidney, PGs serve a similar protective role (DiBona 1986). PGs and TXs also serve important functions in the process of homeostasis. It has been proposed that a balance between the production of PGI_2, which inhibits platelet aggregation, and TXA_2, which induces platelet aggregation, regulates platelet–vessel wall interactions and the formation of hemostatic plugs and thrombi (Moncada et al 1985).

In addition to homeostatic functions, PGs produce effects that are key to the development of the inflammatory response. PGE_2, for example, produces long-lasting vasodilation, which can counteract the vasoconstrictor effects of norepinephrine and angiotensin II (Campbell & Halushka 1996). In addition, PGE_1, PGE_2 and PGA_2 increase vascular permeability and can produce edema in the absence of other mediators (Flower et al 1985). There is also evidence that PGs act synergistically with other mediators, such as bradykinin, to produce inflammatory responses. PGs are also important mediators of the pain associated with injury or inflammation.

PGs are important in the regulation of body temperature and the development of an elevated temperature or fever. There is evidence that bacterial endotoxins induce fevers by stimulating the biosynthesis and release of endogenous pyrogens from leukocytes (Campbell & Halushka 1996). PGs are thought to be the primary mediators of this elevation in temperature, in part because inhibitors of PG synthesis, such as aspirin, prevent the fever caused by the administration of endogenous pyrogens (Insel 1996).

PGs and TXs are crucial mediators in the development of inflammation, pain and fever. Consequently, non-steroidal anti-inflammatory drugs (NSAIDs), which block the synthesis of PGs and TXs, have become the mainstay of therapies aimed at preventing or minimizing inflammation and fever. In the treatment of pain not associated with inflammation, opiates, rather than NSAIDs, have traditionally been used. However, new evidence indicates that NSAIDs are more effective than previously thought at inducing analgesia independent of their anti-inflammatory effects (McCormack 1994). Furthermore, there is evidence that NSAIDs may work synergistically with opiates to induce analgesia. Therefore, NSAIDs will continue to be one of the most commonly prescribed classes of drugs in veterinary medicine.

MODE OF ACTION

All NSAIDs, by definition, inhibit COX enzymes to some degree. This prevents the metabolism of arachidonic acid to the unstable endoperoxide intermediate PGG_2 (Ziel & Krupp 1975). Currently two isoforms of the COX enzyme, known as COX1 and COX2, have been described (Vane & Botting 1995). The COX1 enzyme is produced constitutively in many tissues and it has been proposed that it is this isoform that is responsible for the production of PGs involved in the homeostatic functions in platelets, the gastrointestinal mucosa and kidneys (Fig. 14.2) (Mitchell et al 1993). In contrast, the constitutive production of the COX2 enzyme in most tissues is extremely limited. COX2 production, however, can be induced in many cells, including those primarily associated with the inflammatory process (Fig. 14.2). For example, in quiescent unstimulated rat macrophages, COX1,

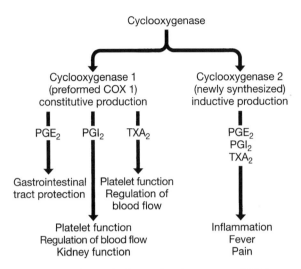

Figure 14.2 The two isoforms of cyclooxygenase (COX1 and COX2) produce identical products but different effects. COX1 is constitutively produced in many tissues, such as the kidney and the gastrointestinal tract, whereas COX2 is an inducible enzyme produced primarily in inflammatory settings. The two isoforms are involved in production of eicosanoids that have various roles. PG, prostaglandin; TX, thromboxane.

but not COX2, can be detected readily (Lee et al 1992). COX2 expression is dramatically increased when the macrophages are exposed *in vitro* to bacterial lipopolysaccharides, while COX1 levels remain unchanged (Lee et al 1992). Many NSAIDs, such as aspirin and indometacin, are more effective at inhibiting COX1 than COX2 (Meade et al 1993, Mitchell et al 1993). Other NSAIDs, such as ibuprofen and meclofenamic acid, are equipotent at inhibiting the COX1 and COX2 isoforms (Meade et al 1993, Mitchell et al 1993). It has been proposed that this inhibition of the constitutively produced COX1 isoform is responsible for many of the adverse effects of NSAIDs, including gastric ulceration, renal function impairment and platelet dysfunction (Vane & Botting 1995).

In an attempt to decrease the side-effects associated with NSAID therapy, new compounds that selectively inhibit the COX2 isoform have been developed (Insel 1996). Although numerous COX2-selective products are available for use in humans, few of these compounds have been studied in veterinary species. Further complicating the issue, it appears that enzyme selectivity is very

species dependent, so a COX2-selective agent in one species may not be selective in another. For example, carprofen has been reported to be a selective COX2 inhibitor in the dog but this selectivity has not been confirmed in other species, such as the horse (Ricketts et al 1998, Vane & Botting 1995). In a similar manner, etodolac has been shown to be a selective COX2 inhibitor in humans (Glaser et al 1995). In the dog, however, etodolac also appears to inhibit the COX1 isoform to some extent, as side-effects commonly associated with COX1 inhibition (gastrointestinal irritation and ulcer formation) are occasionally observed in dogs administered therapeutic doses of this NSAID (Reimer et al 1999). Currently no NSAID has been shown to be a selective COX2 inhibitor in the horse.

There is some evidence that the COX2 isoform may have homeostatic functions, in addition to the inducible role it plays in inflammation. For example, the COX2 isoform is expressed at low levels in the kidneys of normal dogs but its expression is increased significantly in salt-depleted dogs (Venturini et al 1998). Therefore, it is possible that COX2-selective agents may cause renal side-effects in animals with underlying renal disease.

It is also important to remember that most NSAIDs do not affect the metabolism of arachidonic acid by lipoxygenases. This can be important because when NSAIDs block the COX pathway, theoretically, more arachidonic acid substrate is available for lipoxygenase-mediated production of LTs. LTs like PGs, have numerous roles in the inflammatory process. For example, LTB_4 is a potent chemotactic agent for white blood cells. The results of numerous *in vivo* studies in horses using various models of acute, non-immune inflammation confirm that NSAIDs do not affect leukocyte chemotaxis (Lees & Higgins 1986, Lees et al 1994, Owens et al 1996). These results are consistent with the lack of effect of NSAIDs on lipoxygenases. The enhanced production of LTs in the presence of NSAIDs may account for the therapeutic failure of these agents in some inflammatory conditions.

There is limited evidence that a few NSAIDs, such as meclofenamic acid and ketoprofen, have some inhibitory effects on lipoxygenase. For example, meclofenamic acid has been shown to inhibit 5-lipoxygenase and 15-lipoxygenase activities in models using plant-derived enzymes and to inhibit the production of LTs and PGs in human lymphocytes (Stadler et al 1994). In the same study, meclofenamic acid was also shown to inhibit the LT-induced contraction of guinea pig lung parenchymal strips. This latter finding may indicate that meclofenamic acid also has LT receptor antagonist activity (Stadler et al 1994). Ketoprofen was also shown to inhibit rabbit neutrophil and human lung lipoxygenase activity (Williams & Upton 1988) but this has not been confirmed in other species such as the horse (Jackman et al 1994, Landoni & Lees 1995a, Owens et al 1996).

Although the primary mode of action for NSAIDs is the inhibition of the COX enzymes, there now exists ample evidence that some of the effects of NSAIDs are not mediated by inhibition of PG formation at the site of inflammation. For example, for a number of NSAIDs, there is poor correlation between their analgesic potency and their capacity to inhibit PG production (McCormack 1994). This poor correlation between analgesic and anti-inflammatory effects can also be seen for enantiomers of some chiral NSAIDs. For example, the enantiomers of the NSAID flurbiprofen were shown to produce equipotent analgesia but the (R)-enantiomer possessed very little anti-inflammatory activity compared with the (S)-enantiomer (Brune et al 1992). It has been proposed that this differential analgesic activity is mediated by inhibition of PG synthesis within the CNS, as opposed to at the site of inflammation (Brune et al 1992). There is also some evidence that a unique CNS isoform of the COX enzyme exists (Flower et al 1985).

INDICATIONS FOR USE IN HORSES

The NSAIDs are amongst the most commonly prescribed agents for use in horses. Musculoskeletal pain and inflammation are the most common indications for chronic administration of NSAIDs to horses, with phenylbutazone being the NSAID used most frequently for that purpose. Flunixin meglumine is most commonly administered for relief of acute gastrointestinal distress or colic, fever and soft-tissue inflammation. In addition,

flunixin meglumine is the NSAID used most frequently to treat clinical signs of endotoxemia, although there is some experimental evidence that other NSAIDs (such as ketoprofen and phenylbutazone) may also possess antiendotoxic properties (Jackman et al 1994, King & Gerring 1989, Sigurdsson & Youssef 1994).

Comparisons of the efficacy of one agent with another using experimental models of pain or inflammation are common in the literature (Hamm et al 1997, Jackman et al 1994, Landoni & Lees 1995a, Owens et al 1995a,b, 1996). The results of these studies, however, do not support the conclusion that any one of the NSAIDs commonly used in horses is significantly more or less effective than another. The agent that appears most efficacious in a particular study depends, to a great extent, on which model was used to study inflammation or pain.

There is the clinical impression that some NSAIDs are more effective than others against pain or inflammation in particular tissues. This has led to the practice of administering two different NSAIDs to an animal suffering from two different diseases (e.g. back soreness and osteoarthritis). There is little real evidence, however, that the administration of two different NSAIDs is any more effective than a larger dose of one. There is evidence, however, that the duration of effect can be prolonged with concurrent administration of two different NSAIDs. For example, in one study, concurrent administration of flunixin meglumine and phenylbutazone did not alter the pharmacokinetics of either agent but the combination of the two inhibited serum TXB_2 production for a significantly longer period (24 h) than either flunixin meglumine (12 h) or phenylbutazone (8 h) alone (Semrad et al 1993a). Although there is evidence to suggest that the risk of side-effects increase in humans when multiple NSAIDs are administered, there are few studies evaluating the risks of concurrent NSAID administration in horses (Insel 1996).

PHARMACOKINETICS

Although NSAIDs are a large and structurally diverse group of compounds, they share a number of common features. For example, most NSAIDs are administered either intravenously (i.v.) or orally (p.o.). Occasionally they are administered intramuscularly (i.m.) but necrotizing myositis has been associated with this route of administration (Kahn & Styrt 1997). In addition, some formulations can be extremely irritating when administered i.m. and should only be administered i.v. Although most, but not all, NSAIDs are well absorbed following oral administration to horses, there is a considerable amount of variation in the bioavailability of NSAIDs between different animals (Sullivan & Snow 1982). In addition, the presence of ingesta in the proximal gastrointestinal tract has been shown to decrease the rate and the extent of absorption of NSAIDs, such as flunixin meglumine, meclofenamic acid and phenylbutazone, following oral administration (Sullivan & Snow 1982).

In general, NSAIDs share a number of different pharmacokinetic properties. For example, most, but not all, have relatively short plasma half-lives. Meclofenamic acid and ketoprofen, for example, have plasma half-lives of 1–2 h in the horse (Owens et al 1995a, Snow et al 1981). Phenylbutazone has a more variable plasma half-life but it is usually determined to be less than 8 h (Lees & Higgins 1985). In contrast, the plasma half-life of carprofen is between 18 and 21 h in the horse (Lees et al 1994, McKellar et al 1991).

Despite the finding that many NSAIDs have short plasma half-lives, their duration of effect can be very long. For example, ketoprofen has been shown to be an effective NSAID in horses when administered only once per day, although, as discussed above, its half-life is very short (Higgins et al 1987, Landoni & Lees 1995b, Sams et al 1995). This may result in part from the tendency of most NSAIDs to bind with very high avidity to the COX enzyme (Lees & Higgins 1985). In addition, many NSAIDs appear to concentrate in inflammatory sites and their clearance from inflamed tissue is much slower than clearance from plasma (Landoni & Lees 1995a, Owens et al 1995a). For example, 1 h after an i.v. administration of ketoprofen, the synovial fluid concentration of the NSAID was 6.5 times higher in horses with carrageenan-induced synovitis compared with that in saline-treated control horses (Owens et al 1995a). In a similar manner, the half-life of flunixin in carrageenan-induced inflammatory exudates collected from subcutaneously (s.c.) implanted tissue cages was approximately 16 h, whereas the plasma half-life of the NSAID in the same horses was only 4 h (Landoni & Lees 1995a).

Another characteristic pharmacokinetic parameter shared by many NSAIDs is a small apparent volume of distribution (V_d). For many NSAIDs the V_d is often <0.21/kg (Landoni & Lees 1995b, Owens et al 1995a). This small V_d is, at least partially, a direct result of the high degree of plasma protein binding typical of most NSAIDs.

In the presence of inflammation, the pharmacokinetics of NSAIDs may be altered. For example, in one study comparing with normal horses, the clearance and V_d of phenylbutazone were increased in horses with experimentally induced inflammatory loci (Mills et al 1996). Horses with experimentally induced inflammation also cleared ketoprofen faster than normal horses (Owens et al 1995a).

SIDE-EFFECTS IN HORSES

Gastrointestinal effects

In the horse, the most frequently reported side-effect of NSAID therapy is gastrointestinal ulceration, which appears to result primarily from the inhibition of cytoprotective PG production (Boothe 1995). For example, ponies administered phenylbutazone alone developed multifocal gastrointestinal ulceration, while those administered PGE_2 along with the phenylbutazone did not develop significant gastrointestinal lesions (Collins & Tyler 1985). In the gastrointestinal tract, PGs protect the integrity of the gastric mucosa by a number of different mechanisms. For example, they inhibit gastric acid secretion stimulated by feeding, gastrin or histamine and they increase blood flow to the gastric mucosa. PGs also induce mucus and electrolyte secretion into the gastrointestinal lumen. In addition to inhibiting the production of cytoprotective PGs, most NSAIDs can directly irritate the gastric mucosa following oral administration because of their acidic nature (Lichtenberger et al 1995).

The erosive effects of NSAIDs in the gastrointestinal tract are dose related, with higher doses increasing the likelihood that ulceration will develop. For example, horses given flunixin (1.1 mg/kg), ketoprofen (2.2 mg/kg) and phenylbutazone (4.4 mg/kg) three times a day for 12 days all developed significant gastrointestinal ulceration, with the glandular portion of the stomach being the most severely affected (MacAllister et al 1993). Ponies appear to be more susceptible to the erosive effects of NSAIDs, with signs of toxicity occurring at doses usually well tolerated by horses (Tobin et al 1986). In the horse, the right dorsal colon also appears to be particularly susceptible to the ulcerogenic effects of NSAIDs (Karcher et al 1990). Both prolonged treatment with even moderate doses of phenylbutazone and the use of any NSAID in the presence of concurrent hypovolemia appear to predispose the horse to development of ulceration of the right dorsal colon. It has not been determined why the right dorsal colon is more susceptible to the effects of NSAIDs, although it is hypothesized that blood flow to this area is more dependent on PG-mediated vasodilatation than other regions of the colon (MacAllister et al 1993, Murray 1985).

Renal effects

In normal horses, therapeutics doses of NSAIDs have little effect on renal function or blood flow. The administration of high doses of NSAIDs to normal animals, however, can cause acute renal failure (Forrester & Troy 1999). Even therapeutic doses of NSAIDs can result in the development of acute renal failure in patients who are volume depleted, hypotensive or have pre-existing renal disease (Patrono & Dunn 1987, Stillman & Schlesinger 1990).

As in the gastrointestinal tract, the negative effects of NSAIDs on the kidneys are thought to result from inhibition of the production of protective PGs. Several different PG subtypes appear to serve homeostatic functions in the kidney (Dunn 1984, Dunn et al 1988, Stillman & Schlesinger 1990). For example, PGI_2 is the predominant PG produced in the renal cortex, glomeruli, arteries and cortical collecting tubes. In contrast, in the

renal medulla collecting tubules and interstitial cells, PGE_2 production predominates (Campbell & Halushka 1996). During periods of hypovolemia or hypotension, PGI_2 and PGE_2 cause afferent arteriolar dilatation, which acts to maintain renal blood flow and glomerular filtration rate (DiBona 1986). The PGs also counteract the effects of systemic vasoconstrictor agents, such as angiotensin II and antidiuretic hormone (vasopressin). There is also evidence that PGs help to maintain blood flow and glomerular filtration in the surviving nephrons in human patients suffering from chronic renal failure (Dunn 1984).

In addition to vasodilatory responses, PGs have a number of other effects in the kidney. For example, PGs stimulate adenylate cyclase in juxtaglomerular cells, resulting in an increase in cAMP production; this, in turn, increases renin release. Renin stimulates the release of aldosterone, which increases renal tubular secretion of potassium (Stillman & Schlesinger 1990). PGs also enhance tubular excretion of sodium and water (Patrono & Dunn 1987). By causing these effects in the kidneys, PGs can alter electrolyte homeostasis. Therefore, other renal side-effects of NSAID therapy can include hyperkalemia, hypernatremia and edema. Often these metabolic changes are not observed in individuals with normal renal function, but in the presence of pre-existing disease they can become clinically significant.

In the horse, renal papillary necrosis can be a sequela to NSAID therapy (Gunson 1983, MacKay et al 1983, Ramirez et al 1998). It is, however, less common than gastrointestinal ulceration and most commonly occurs when NSAIDs are administered to animals that are dehydrated or have decreased renal perfusion. There is some disagreement as to the clinical importance of renal papillary necrosis. For example, one report indicates that renal papillary necrosis is most often an incidental finding not associated with clinical renal disease (Gunson 1983). However, another study, in which large doses of phenylbutazone were given to normal horses, indicated that renal papillary necrosis was associated with clinical renal failure, as evidenced by the progressive increases in serum creatinine, blood urea nitrogen and phosphorus and decreases in serum calcium concentrations

(MacKay et al 1983). It has been hypothesized that blood flow to the renal pelvis is marginal in the horse and, in the presence of even mild dehydration or hypotension, maintaining adequate blood flow may require PG-mediated vasodilation. Under these conditions, the renal pelvis of the horse may be exquisitely sensitive to ischemic necrosis induced by the anti-PG effects of NSAIDs (Gunson 1983).

In summary, PGs play important roles in maintaining renal blood flow, potassium homeostasis and water and sodium balance in the kidney. The inhibition of these responses by NSAIDs can have significant effects on renal function and viability during periods of hypoperfusion or concurrent renal damage. The risk of developing analgesic nephropathy is highest in geriatric cases, patients and in those with pre-existing renal, cardiac or liver disease, dehydration, shock or undergoing concurrent therapy with nephrotoxic drugs.

Plasma protein binding

Most NSAIDs are highly bound to plasma proteins, with the bound fraction approaching 99% for some agents. Therefore, care should be taken when administering NSAIDs concurrently with other compounds that are also highly protein bound, such as other NSAIDs, sulfonamides, warfarin and gentamicin, because NSAIDs can displace these drugs from their binding sites (Boothe 1995). The ultimate effect of this displacement is difficult to predict. As it is the unbound fraction (or free drug) in the plasma that is responsible for the drug's activity, this displacement can result in an increase in the drug's observed clinical effect. For example, in humans, the anticoagulant activity of warfarin, which is highly protein bound in serum, was significantly increased by the concurrent administration of phenylbutazone (Schary et al 1975). In contrast, an increase in the unbound fraction can also result in an increase in the rate at which the drug is eliminated from the body. For example, when phenylbutazone and gentamicin were concurrently administered to horses the plasma half-life and the V_d for gentamicin decreased by 23 and 26%, respectively, while the kinetic parameters of phenylbutazone were

unaffected (Whittem et al 1996). Because the end result can vary significantly when NSAIDs have to be given concurrently with other highly protein bound drugs, relevant pharmacokinetic or pharmacodynamic parameters should be monitored. For example, when an aminoglycoside and an NSAID are administered, serum concentrations of the aminoglycoside should be determined to ensure that they within the desired therapeutic range. Prothrombin time should be monitored in patients treated with warfarin and phenylbutazone. Doses should be adjusted based on changes in the monitored parameters and not on hypothetically predicted sequela.

Hepatic effects

Nearly all NSAIDs have the potential to induce hepatic injury, although this effect has not been documented in the horse. In other species, hepatic injury associated with most NSAIDs is an idiosyncratic reaction with a low incidence of occurrence. The hepatotoxicity of carprofen in dogs, for example, was not observed until the NSAID was in widespread use in the USA (MacPhail et al 1998). The heptatoxicity of a few compounds, such as aspirin and acetaminophen (paracetamol), however, is a dose-dependent side-effect that is well described (Fry & Seeff 1995).

Although the horse appears to be refractory to the hepatic effects of most NSAIDs, their hepatotoxic potential should be considered, especially when they are concomitantly administered with other potentially hepatotoxic agents, such as fluoroquinolones, potentiated sulfonamides or anabolic steroids. In addition, many herbal preparations are potential hepatotoxic agents and clients may administer these compounds concurrently with prescribed NSAIDs without consulting their veterinarian. Echinacea and kava kava products, for example, are reported to be potential hepatotoxins and both are used in herbal remedy products that claim to produce calming or sedating effects in horses (Abebe 2002).

Coagulation effects

Because of their inhibition of COX activity, NSAIDs can inhibit platelet aggregation. The extent and the duration of this inhibition, and thus its clinical relevancy, varies with the NSAID. For example, aspirin induces an irreversible inactivation of platelet COX, making it a very effective antithrombotic agent in horses despite it short elimination half-life (Kopp et al 1985). In contrast, neither flunixin meglumine nor phenylbutazone had any significant effect on bleeding times in horses (Kopp et al 1985). The effect of other commonly used NSAIDs on coagulation in horses is less clear. For example, in dogs, ketoprofen has been shown to prolong the bleeding time significantly in some studies, but not in others (Grisneaux et al 1999, Mathews et al 2001). In contrast, multiple studies on carprofen in dogs have failed to detect any clinically significant effects on coagulation profiles (Grisneaux et al 1999, Hickford et al 2001). Nevertheless, because the effects of these NSAIDs on bleeding parameters in horses have not been evaluated, if the use of an NSAID prior to surgery cannot be avoided, flunixin meglumine or phenylbutazone would be recommended.

Chondroprotection/ chondrodestruction

Recently the effect of NSAIDs on the pathological process of degenerative joint disease has been an area of intense interest. Numerous studies have been carried out *in vitro* evaluating the effects of NSAIDs on the release of cytokines known to be involved in arthritis and on the production of cartilage proteoglycans. At this time, no clear picture has emerged for the role of NSAIDs in healthy or osteoarthritic joints. Some studies have indicated that NSAIDs could have potentially beneficial effects, while others have supported a detrimental role for these compounds. For example, the NSAIDs ketoprofen, flunixin meglumine and tolfenamic acid were shown in one study, carried out in isolated equine synoviocytes, to decrease the production of β-glucuronidase activity, which would tend to decrease the rate of proteoglycan destruction (Landoni et al 1996). These same compounds, however, also caused an increase in interleukin 1 production, which would result in an increase in proteoglycan degradation.

In other studies, NSAIDs, such as carprofen and benoxaprofen, have been reported to increase proteoglycan synthesis in cartilage explants and chondrocytes (McIlwraith 1996, Palmoski & Brandt 1983). Obviously, more work is needed to determine the effects of NSAIDs on normal and arthritic joints.

SPECIFIC AGENTS

Aspirin

Aspirin or acetylsalicylic acid, an ester of acetic acid, is the oldest known NSAID and the prototype of the salicylate drugs (Collier 1971, Rogstad & Yndestad 1981). In addition to inhibition of COX, salicylates inhibit the formation and release of kinins, stabilize lysosomes and uncouple oxidative phosphorylation (Boothe 1995). In horses, the half-life of aspirin is very short. For example, in ponies, the elimination half-life of aspirin administered i.v. at a dose rate of 19 mg/kg was determined to be approximately 7 min (Lees et al 1987a).

Despite its rapid clearance, aspirin can be very effective as an antithrombotic agent, because relatively small doses can significantly prolong bleeding times. For example, in one study where aspirin (17 mg/kg), phenylbutazone (2 mg/kg) and flunixin meglumine (0.5 mg/kg) were administered p.o. once daily for 3 days, aspirin was significantly more effective at prolonging the bleeding time and inhibiting TXB_2 production than the other two NSAIDs (Kopp et al 1985). In addition, the effects of aspirin on TX production lasted longer, with effects noted 6 days after the last dose was administered. In contrast, neither phenylbutazone nor flunixin meglumine significantly increased bleeding times.

The effect of aspirin on bleeding times has been shown to be dose dependent in the horse (Cambridge et al 1991). For example, 4 mg/kg aspirin i.v. significantly increased the bleeding time for up to 4 h post administration. However, when aspirin was administered i.v. at 12 mg/kg, the bleeding time was significantly prolonged for up to 48 h (Cambridge et al 1991). These effects

Table 14.1 Recommended doses of non-steroidal anti-inflammatory drugs

Drug	Route	Formulation(s)	Dose rate
Aspirin	i.v.	Injectable	19 mg/kg (Lees et al 1987a) (antiplatelet activity)
	p.o.	Bolus	10–100 mg/kg (Tobin 1979) once daily or every other day
Phenylbutazone	i.v.	Injectable	4.4 mg/kg (Lees et al 1987b, Owens et al 1996, Toutain et al 1994); 4.4 mg/kg then 2.2 mg/kg (Raekallio et al 1997)
	p.o.	Tablets, powder, paste	4.4 mg/kg b.i.d. for 1 day, 2.2 mg/kg b.i.d. for 4 days; 2.2 mg/kg once daily for 7 days (Lees & Higgins 1986, Taylor et al 1983)
Meclofenamic acid	i.v.	Injectable	2 mg/kg (Snow et al 1981); 2.2 mg/kg (Johansson et al 1991)
	p.o.	Granules	2.2 mg/kg daily for 10 days (Johansson et al 1991, May & Lees 1999)
Flunixin meglumine	i.v., i.m.	Injectable	1.1 mg/kg (Landoni & Lees 1995a, Soma et al 1988); 0.5–2.0 mg/kg (Toutain et al 1994)
	p.o.	Granules or paste	1.1 mg/kg (Landoni & Lees 1995a, Welsh et al 1992)
Naproxen	p.o.	Granules	4 g (Jones & Hamm 1978); 10 mg/kg twice a day for up to 14 days (package insert, equine-approved product)
Carprofen	i.v.	Injectable	0.7 mg/kg (Lees et al 1994, McKellar et al 1991)
	i.m.	Injectable	0.7 mg/kg (McKellar et al 1991)
	p.o.	Paste	0.7 mg/kg once daily for 14 days (McKellar et al 1991)
Ketoprofen	i.v.	Injectable	2.2 mg/kg once daily for 5 days (Owens et al 1995a)
Vedaprofen	i.v.	Injectable	2 mg/kg (package insert: European Medicines Evaluation Agency 2003a)
	p.o.	Gel	2 mg/kg initially then 1 mg/kg b.i.d. for a maximum treatment period of 14 days (package insert: European Medicines Evaluation Agency 2003b)
Eltenac	i.v.	Injectable	0.5–1.0 mg/kg once daily for 3 days (Hamm et al 1997); 0.5 mg/kg once daily for 5 days (Dyke et al 1998)

i.v., intravenous; i.m., intramuscular; p.o., oral; b.i.d., twice daily

probably result from the irreversible inhibition of COX by aspirin and to the inability of platelets to synthesize new COX.

As an analgesic or anti-inflammatory agent, aspirin must be administered to horses in large doses (10–100 mg/kg) because of its very short half-life; therefore, it is rarely used for these purposes (Tobin 1979). However, aspirin can be useful in horses as an antithrombotic agent. For this purpose, it is generally administered at the low end of the dose range (17 mg/kg) and given daily or every other day (Table 14.1). It is usually given orally but a parenteral product for i.v. administration is available in some countries.

Phenylbutazone

Phenylbutazone is an enolic acid derivative in the pyrazolone class of NSAIDs. The pharmacokinetics and pharmacodynamics of phenylbutazone, the most commonly prescribed NSAID for use in horses, have been well studied. In the horse, the plasma half-life of phenylbutazone ranges from 3 to 8 h. The plasma half-life in an individual horse is dependent on the dose administered and the metabolic capacity of that animal. For example, when a single dose of phenylbutazone was administered i.v. at a dose rate of 4.4 mg/kg, the plasma half-life was 5.5 h (Lees et al 1987b). In a different study, a single higher dose of phenylbutazone (4 g i.v.; approximately 8.8 mg/kg) had a plasma half-life of approximately 7 h (Landuyt et al 1993). When that same dose of phenylbutazone was administered i.m., a plasma half-life closer to 8 h was obtained (Landuyt et al 1993). Still other studies have found the half-life of phenylbutazone to be much shorter, ranging from 3.5 h with a dose of 4.4 mg/kg to 6 h when 17.8 mg/kg was administered (Gerring et al 1981). Nevertheless, the general trend in the horse and in most species in fact, is that the higher the administered dose, the longer the elimination half-life.

This dose-dependent increase in plasma half-life can also be demonstrated when the same dose of phenylbutazone is administered repeatedly. For example, in one study, phenylbutazone (8.8 mg/kg) was administered p.o. once daily for 4 days (Soma et al 1983). The serum concentration 24 h after the first dose was less than 2 µg/ml but the serum concentration 24 h after the second, third and fourth oral doses were 4.2, 4.8 and 5.3 µg/ml, respectively.

The dose-dependent or zero-order pharmacokinetics of phenylbutazone may result from a combination of several different mechanisms. In the horse, phenylbutazone is metabolized extensively in the liver, with very little parent compound excreted unchanged in the urine. Oxyphenbutazone is the primary active metabolite and gammahydroxyphenylbutazone is the primary inactive metabolite (Tobin et al 1986). It is likely that saturation of the hepatic microsomal enzymes responsible for phenylbutazone metabolism accounts for a significant portion of the observed dose-dependent pharmacokinetics of this agent. In addition, enterohepatic recirculation (biliary excretion followed by reabsorption) may also occur (Gerring et al 1981). It is interesting to note that in one study the metabolism of phenylbutazone was not altered by pretreatment with chloramphenicol or quinidine, agents known to inhibit hepatic microsomal enzymes (Tobin et al 1977). However, the rate of metabolism of phenylbutazone was decreased by the administration of its primary active metabolite oxyphenbutazone (Tobin et al 1977). In light of the zero-order kinetics of phenylbutazone in the horse, care should be taken when dosing very young or very old animals or those with impaired liver function even when therapeutic doses are administered. Bioaccumulation can be extensive and can lead to the development of toxic plasma concentrations.

Both the parent phenylbutazone and its active metabolite oxyphenbutazone are so highly bound to plasma proteins that they may displace other protein-bound compounds (Chay et al 1982, Lees & Higgins 1985). Therefore, phenylbutazone should be used judiciously with other highly protein-bound drugs, such as warfarin, gentamicin and the sulfonamides. As discussed previously, phenylbutazone has been shown to decrease the plasma half-life and the V_d of gentamicin in horses and, therefore, therapeutic drug monitoring for aminoglycosides is recommended when these agents are administered concurrently (Whittem et al 1996). The high degree of plasma protein binding is also to some extent responsible for the small V_d (0.15 l/kg) of phenylbutazone (Soma et al 1983).

The physiological mechanisms by which phenylbutazone is cleared from the body in the horse have not been well described. In one study, renal clearance accounted for only 25% of the total drug administered (Lees et al 1985). It has been hypothesized that biliary excretion with subsequent fecal elimination represents the primary clearance mechanism of phenylbutazone in the horse (Lees et al 1985). Renal excretion, of an as yet unidentified phenylbutazone metabolite, may also account for a proportion of total body clearance of the compound.

Excretion of phenylbutazone into the urine can vary depending on the pH of the urine. Because phenylbutazone is a weak acid, in alkaline urine more of the compound will be in the ionized form and the excretion rate will be increased, a process referred to as ion trapping (Moss & Haywood 1973). In contrast, more of the compound will tend to be in the unionized form in acidic urine, thereby favoring the re-absorption of the compound and prolonging the clearance. It is important to note that most horses not in training produce alkaline urine, but after intense exercise, such as a race, performance horses will produce acidic urine (Wood et al 1990).

Phenylbutazone can be administered i.v., and rarely i.m., but is most commonly given orally for chronic therapy. The bioavailability of phenylbutazone following i.m. and oral administration is generally good but can vary extensively. In one study, phenylbutazone was absorbed rapidly after oral administration with a bioavailability of approximately 92% (Soma et al 1983). Feedstuffs, especially hay, can delay the absorption of orally administered phenylbutazone but the bioavailability is unaffected. In addition, a second peak of absorption from the colon and/or rectum may be apparent in the presence of ingesta (Maitho et al 1986). Following i.m. administration, the bioavailability of one phenylbutazone formulation was also excellent, at approximately 90% (Landuyt et al 1993). In addition, in this same study, there was no significant tissue reaction or elevations in plasma creatine kinase activity. Previous studies with i.m. phenylbutazone found significant local tissue reactions and elevations in creatine kinase activity in the plasma (Sullivan & Snow 1982). Most available parenteral formulations of phenylbutazone are extremely irritating and can cause severe perivascular inflammation and sloughing if inadvertently injected extravascularly. Therefore, unless the product label indicates that i.m. injections are safe, it is best to avoid that mode of administration of phenylbutazone in horses and it is, in fact, rarely used.

In humans, phenylbutazone therapy has been associated with bone marrow dyscrasias, such as agranulocytosis and aplastic anemia (Flower et al 1985). Care should be taken when handling the product to prevent human exposure. The use of phenylbutazone in horses has been banned in many European countries because of concerns for human health and because the horse is considered a food animal under European law. Nevertheless, it is still prescribed very commonly for musculoskeletal conditions in the USA and the UK. It is interesting to note that there is only one report in the literature of bone marrow suppression occurring with phenylbutazone therapy in a horse and in that case very high doses of the agent had been administered (Murray 1985).

In general, phenylbutazone has a narrow therapeutic index in horses. Although doses of 2–4 g

phenylbutazone for a 450 kg horse (4.4–8.8 mg/kg) are administered commonly, the high end of the dose range should only be used for short periods. In one study in which six horses were given 15 and 30 mg/kg daily, i.v. or p.o., all of the animals died or required euthanasia within 8 days of beginning treatment (MacKay et al 1983). Marked gastrointestinal lesions and hematological changes were also observed in one horse given 8 mg/kg daily; and doses as small as 3.6 g for 7 to 14 days have been reported to cause toxicity and death in horses (MacKay et al 1983, Tobin et al 1986). The signs of toxicity are typical of most NSAIDs. Clinically, the horses may be depressed, colicky, anorexic and febrile and may occasionally have diarrhea (MacKay et al 1983). Physical and/or postmortem findings often include oral and gastrointestinal erosions and ulcers, low serum protein concentrations, renal necrosis and neutropenia with a toxic left shift (MacKay et al 1983). Together, the data from these studies indicate that the recommended doses of phenylbutazone should never be exceeded and that the highest recommended dose (4.4 mg/kg twice daily) should be administered only for very short periods.

Despite its narrow safety margin, phenylbutazone is an extremely effective and very commonly used NSAID in horses when administered at recommended doses (Table 14.1). Clinical experience and published studies indicate that chronic administration of the lowest recommended dose rate (2.2 mg/kg twice daily) is safe and effective in most normal horses (Lees & Higgins 1986, Taylor et al 1983). In addition, the results of one published study demonstrated that the maximum effects of phenylbutazone are achieved at 2 mg/kg and that higher doses did not increase the efficacy but did increase the duration of effect from 8 h at a dose rate of 2 mg/kg to 24 h at 8 mg/kg (Toutain et al 1994). The results of this study also predicted that doses of phenylbutazone >1 mg/kg are unlikely to have any significant anti-inflammatory effect (Toutain et al 1994). There are numerous studies demonstrating the efficacy of phenylbutazone in various models of pain and inflammation in the horse (Hardee et al 1986, Lees et al 1986, 1987a,b, Moore et al 1986, Owens et al 1995b, 1996, Raekallio et al 1997, Sabate et al 1997, Taylor et al 1983, Toutain et al 1994). None of the results of these studies indicate definitively that phenylbutazone is more effective than other NSAIDs commonly used in horses. Nevertheless, in most situations, phenylbutazone is by far the most economical NSAID to administer to horses requiring chronic anti-inflammatory therapy.

Suxibuzone

Suxibuzone, which is a member of the pyrazolone group of NSAIDs, is a derivative of phenylbutazone. Although its efficacy appears to be indistinguishable from phenylbutazone, there is some evidence that it causes fewer gastrointestinal ulcers (Homedes et al 1997, Sabate et al 1997).

Meclofenamic acid

Meclofenamic acid is an anthranilic acid derivative that is typically administered orally to horses. The pharmacokinetics of this NSAID in horses has been well defined. For example, the plasma half-life in horses has been determined in several studies and varies between 0.7 and 1.4 h (Johansson et al 1991, Snow et al 1981). Absorption is variable after oral dosing with estimates of bioavailability ranging from 60 to 90% and peak plasma concentrations occurring 1–3 h after administration (Johansson et al 1991). The effect of ingesta on the absorption of meclofenamic acid from the gastrointestinal tract has not been determined definitively. In one study, the absorption rate of the NSAID was the same in ponies whether they were fasted or fed (Snow et al 1981). However, another study found that absorption of meclofenamic acid was delayed in horses allowed free access to hay (May & Lees 1999). In horses, the liver metabolizes meclofenamic acid primarily by oxidation to an active hydroxymethyl metabolite, which may be further oxidized to an inactive carboxyl metabolite (Plumb 1999).

The therapeutic index of meclofenamic acid in horses is not well defined. For example, ponies treated with meclofenamic acid at the recommended dosage (2.2 mg/kg) for 10 days had decreased plasma protein concentrations but no other untoward effects (May & Lees 1999). In a different study, mares and stallions treated with the same dose for up to 5 months demonstrated no ill effects (Lees & Higgins 1985).

The efficacy of meclofenamic acid as an anti-inflammatory agent in horses has been determined in a number of studies using the recommended doses (Table 14.1) (Galbraith & McKellar 1996, Johansson et al 1991, Tobin 1979). It is known for its slow onset of action, requiring 36–96 h of therapy before clinical effects are evident (Boothe 1995). It has also been proposed to be particularly effective in the treatment of acute and chronic laminitis, although its superiority over other NSAIDs in the treatment of these conditions has not been definitively proven (Lees & Higgins 1985). In one study, meclofenamic acid was shown to decrease the accumulation of lactate and increase the lactate threshold in an exercise tolerance test carried out in seven standardbred horses (Johansson et al 1991).

Flunixin meglumine

Flunixin meglumine, a nicotinic acid derivative, is a potent analgesic commonly used to control severe intestinal pain or colic in the horse. In this setting, it has effects comparable to opioid analgesics without inducing the unwanted side-effects commonly observed with opiates in horses, such as CNS excitation and ileus (Boothe 1995). In addition, flunixin meglumine has been shown in several experimental models to produce antiendotoxic effects at doses lower than those used for anti-inflammatory effects (Jackman et al 1994, Moore et al 1986, Templeton et al 1987).

In horses, the pharmacokinetics of flunixin meglumine has been well defined. Flunixin meglumine, at the recommended dose of 1.1 mg/kg, has a short plasma half-life of approximately 1.5–3 h. It persists in inflammatory exudates for much longer, however, with an exudate half-life of approximately 16 h (Landoni & Lees 1995a, Soma et al 1988). Renal excretion of the parent compound seems to be the primary mode of elimination of flunixin meglumine in horses (Lees & Higgins 1985).

The pharmacokinetics of flunixin meglumine has also been studied in foals. In neonatal foals, the plasma half-life of flunixin meglumine was longer than 5 h, much longer than that reported in adults (Semrad et al 1993b). However, by 1 month of age, the plasma half-life was similar to adult values, between 2 and 3 h (Landoni & Lees 1995a, Soma et al 1988). As expected, the total body clearance of flunixin meglumine in neonatal foals (29 ml/h per kg) was approximately one-third of the value reported in adult horses (92 ml/h per kg; Semrad et al 1993b, Soma et al 1988). The V_d of flunixin meglumine in foals (223 ml/kg) was larger than that reported in adult horses (145 ml/kg) (Semrad et al 1993b, Soma et al 1988). Therefore, flunixin meglumine appears to be cleared more slowly and have a larger V_d in neonatal animals than in adults. No clinical signs of toxicity were observed in normal, healthy foals given typical adult doses (1.1 mg/kg) of flunixin meglumine, and only mild gastrointestinal ulceration was caused by high doses (6.6 mg/kg) (Semrad et al 1993b). The effect of concurrent disease on the pharmacokinetics of flunixin meglumine has not been determined. Based on the increased V_d and the decreased clearance of flunixin meglumine in neonatal foals, it would seem prudent to give a larger initial dose but to increase the dosing interval for ill foals of this age group.

The pharmacokinetics of flunixin meglumine may also be altered in older horses. In one study, in older horses (>9 years of age) the plasma half-life of flunixin meglumine (approximately 4 h) was significantly longer than in younger horses (<2 h) (Jensen et al 1990). Similarly, the total clearance of flunixin meglumine was lower in the older horses (25 l/h) than in younger horses (>40 l/h) (Jensen et al 1990). Although these changes were not of the magnitude to require dose rate or dosing interval adjustments, similar determinations have not been made in geriatric horses (>20 years), where dosage adjustments might be necessary if clearance continues to decrease with age.

Flunixin meglumine is available in both parenteral and oral formulations. The bioavailability of the oral products is generally reported to be good. In one study, when flunixin meglumine granules were administered via a nasogastric tube, the bioavailability was 85.8% (Soma et al 1988).

In another study carried out in fasted ponies, the oral administration of a flunixin meglumine paste (1.1 mg/kg) resulted in peak plasma concentrations >2 µg/ml less than 1 h after administration (Welsh et al 1992). In ponies with free access to hay, the peak plasma concentration decreased to approximately 1.3 µg/ml and the peak concentration was not reached until 7.6 h after administration (Welsh et al 1992). Nevertheless, the mean area under the plasma concentration–time curve (AUC) was not significantly different whether the ponies had been fasted or fed. The parenteral preparation of flunixin meglumine can be administered i.m.; however, necrotizing soft-tissue infections have been reported following i.m. administration (Kahn & Styrt 1997) and so aseptic preparation of the injection site is advisable.

While flunixin meglumine has a better therapeutic index than phenylbutazone, gastrointestinal ulceration has been reported when moderately high doses (1.1 mg/kg three times a day) were administered i.v. for 12 days (MacAllister et al 1993). In a case report, a pony was administered six times the recommended dose rate of flunixin meglumine for 5 days (Trillo et al 1984). Postmortem findings were consistent with the toxicosis produced by other NSAIDs, most strikingly severe gastrointestinal ulceration. In addition, twice the recommended dose of flunixin meglumine was shown to cause a decrease in plasma protein concentrations after a total dosing period of 10 days (May & Lees 1999).

The pharmacodynamics of flunixin meglumine has been well defined in horses and it is an effective NSAID when used at recommended doses (Table 14.1). For example, in a non-immune acute inflammatory model, flunixin meglumine inhibited serum TXB_2 and PGE_2 production for up to 24 h and 30 h, respectively (Landoni & Lees 1995a). In this same study, flunixin meglumine decreased bradykinin-induced swelling for approximately 25 h (Landoni & Lees 1995a). The pharmacokinetic/pharmacodynamic modeling of flunixin meglumine in horses was studied using a Freund's adjuvant-induced model of carpal arthritis. This study predicted that doses of flunixin meglumine <0.5 mg/kg are unlikely to have any significant anti-inflammatory effect (Toutain et al 1994). In addition, the maximum effects of flunixin meglumine were achieved at 1 mg/kg; higher doses did not increase the efficacy but did increase the duration of effect from 16 h at a dose rate of 1 mg/kg to 24 h at a 2 mg/kg (Toutain et al 1994).

Naproxen

Naproxen is a propionic acid derivative that has a structure similar to ibuprofen and ketoprofen. It can be administered either i.v. or p.o. to horses, even though it is poorly absorbed with a bioavailability of approximately 50% (Pasargiklian & Bianco 1986). It has a relatively short half-life in plasma (4 h) (Tobin 1979). There is little information available on the therapeutic index of naproxen in the horse.

When used at recommended doses, naproxen appears to be an effective NSAID in horses but the clinical effects are slow to develop, often requiring a number of days of therapy (Table 14.1) (Plumb 1999). In one study, naproxen was shown to be more efficacious than either placebo or phenylbutazone in the treatment of experimentally induced myositis (Jones & Hamm 1978). Although the evidence is not compelling, anecdotal reports indicate that naproxen may be particularly effective in the treatment of soft-tissue injuries and myositis.

Carprofen

Carprofen, a propionic acid derivative, is an effective analgesic and weak anti-inflammatory agent. Carprofen contains a chiral center at the C2 of the propionic moiety and, therefore, exists in two stereoisomeric forms, the $S(+)$- and $R(-)$-enantiomers. The approved product for the horse is a racemic mixture of the two antipodes. In the horse the $S(+)$-form has more rapid clearance, as a result of selective glucuronidation and subsequent biliary excretion of that enantiomer (Soraci et al 1995). Unlike many NSAIDs in the horse, the half-life of carprofen is long, with estimates ranging from 14 to 31 h (Lees et al 1994, McKellar et al 1991). Despite the slow clearance, there was no evidence of accumulation of carprofen in plasma when

0.7 mg/kg carprofen was given orally once a day for 14 days (McKellar et al 1991). In this study, the bioavailability of carprofen was estimated to be approximately 70%.

Carprofen appears to have a favorable therapeutic index in the horse. For example, carprofen as a single i.v. dose at five times the recommended dose rate (3.5 mg/kg) or orally for 14 days at twice the recommended dose rate (1.4 mg/kg), was well tolerated with no observable sign of toxicity (McKellar et al 1991). In addition, i.m. carprofen (0.7 mg/kg) did not cause obvious signs of swelling or inflammation but was associated with significant increases in creatine kinase, suggesting muscle cell damage. More studies are needed to determine the safety of i.m. administration of carprofen in the horse.

The exact mechanisms of action of carprofen are unclear; as in many species, it is a more efficacious analgesic agent than its anti-inflammatory effects would predict. In various laboratory animals, however, carprofen was found to be an effective analgesic only when the pain was associated with inflammation (Strub et al 1982). The favorable safety profile of carprofen in the horse may result from selective inhibition of the COX2 enzyme. Although carprofen has been shown to inhibit the COX2 enzyme selectively in dogs, this has not been demonstrated in the horse (Ricketts et al 1998). Typical side-effects of NSAID therapy, such as gastrointestinal ulceration, are not very commonly observed following carprofen administration to dogs. An idiosyncratic reaction involving mild to fatal, severe hepatocellular damage has been reported in the dog but not, to the authors' knowledge, in the horse.

There is some evidence that carprofen is an effective NSAID when used in horses at recommended doses (Table 14.1). For example, using an in vivo model of non-immune acute inflammation, carprofen was found to decrease swelling significantly and to decrease the production of TXB_2 moderately (Lees et al 1994). As expected, there was no effect on the leukocyte numbers in the exudates but, somewhat surprisingly, there was not a correlation between the antiedematous effects of carprofen and its concentration in plasma or exudate. In this study, the authors concluded that the antiedematous effects of carprofen were not caused by inhibition of COX (Lees et al 1994).

Ketoprofen

Ketoprofen is a propionic acid derivative that, like carprofen, exists as two enantiomers. In horses, ketoprofen, like most NSAIDs, has a short plasma half-life of approximately 1–1.5 h (Landoni & Lees 1995a). There is also evidence that in the horse the $R(-)$-enantiomer is cleared slightly faster than the $S(+)$-enantiomer, with half-lives of 1.1 and 1.5 h, respectively.

The pharmacokinetics of ketoprofen in the horse may be altered in the presence of inflammation. For example, in one study, the mean half-life of a single dose of ketoprofen (2.2 mg/kg i.v.) was significantly shorter in horses with experimentally induced synovitis than in normal horses: 0.55 h versus 0.88 h, respectively (Owens et al 1995a). Also in this study, the concentrations of ketoprofen in synovial fluid of horses with synovitis, at 1 h after administration, were six times higher than those of normal horses. In another study, ketoprofen was shown to persist in inflammatory exudates for much longer than in plasma, with an exudate half-life of approximately 21 h (Landoni & Lees 1995a). Together, the results of these studies indicate that inflammatory loci serve as sites of sequestration for ketoprofen and that this may alter the pharmacokinetics of the NSAID in plasma.

The pharmacokinetics of ketoprofen has also been studied in neonatal foals. Neonatal foals clear ketoprofen more slowly and have a larger V_d than adult horses (Wilcke et al 1998). It is important to note that these studies were carried out in healthy normal foals and that pharmacokinetic parameters could be altered in sick or compromised foals. Nevertheless, the results of these studies suggest that the initial dose of ketoprofen may need to be increased in neonatal foals and the subsequent dosing interval increased in order to produce plasma concentrations comparable to adults (Wilcke et al 1998).

Although ketoprofen is highly bound to plasma proteins, one recent study indicated that it did not alter the coagulation cascade parameters or prothrombin time in humans treated concurrently with the anticoagulant warfarin (Mieszczak & Winther 1993). Although there is some evidence that in dogs ketoprofen can increase mucosal bleeding time, it is unknown whether this is also the case in horses (Grisneaux et al 1999).

When ketoprofen is administered orally, it is well absorbed in humans and dogs but several studies suggest that bioavailability is very poor when it is given orally or rectally to horses (Corveleyn et al 1996, Landoni & Lees 1995a). In contrast, it had excellent bioavailability when administered i.m. and the lysine salt formulation was well tolerated, causing no obvious signs of tissue damage (Anfossi et al 1997). Most commonly, however, ketoprofen is administered i.v. to horses (Table 14.1).

Ketoprofen appears to have a high therapeutic index in horses. In one study that compared high doses of phenylbutazone, flunixin meglumine and ketoprofen in horses, ketoprofen was considered to be the least toxic (MacAllister et al 1993), although the doses of both flunixin meglumine and phenylbutazone used in this study were higher than the dose rates typically used in clinical settings. High doses of ketoprofen can cause gastrointestinal and oral ulceration but these lesions develop rarely when therapeutic doses are administered.

The mechanisms of action of ketoprofen have not been definitively proven in the horse, although ketoprofen has been shown to inhibit COX enzymes. Several studies carried out in horses have shown that ketoprofen, administered at doses that significantly inhibited PG production, had no effect on LT production (Landoni & Lees 1995a, Owens et al 1995a) and, therefore, appears not to have any significant effect on lipoxygenase activity.

Ketoprofen has been shown to be a potent analgesic with effects equivalent to pentazocine and meperidine (pethidine) in the treatment of postoperative pain in humans (Avouac & Teule 1988). In horses, ketoprofen has also been shown to be an effective analgesic and anti-inflammatory agent. In one study, the pharmacodynamics of ketoprofen (2.2 mg/kg) were studied in a non-immune acute inflammatory model (Landoni & Lees 1995a). In this study, ketoprofen inhibited serum TXB_2 and PGE_2 production for up to 24 h and 12 h, respectively and also reduced bradykinin-induced swelling for approximately 10 h.

The efficacy of ketoprofen compared with other NSAIDs, such as phenylbutazone and flunixin meglumine, in relieving pain and/or inflammation is very much dependent on the model used in the study. For example, phenylbutazone was found to be more effective in relieving signs of inflammation in an experimentally induced carpal synovitis model (Owens et al 1996). However, ketoprofen was more effective than phenylbutazone at relieving pain and decreasing lameness in a chronic hoof pain model (Owens et al 1995b). In clinical case studies of horse suffering from various musculoskeletal injuries and inflammatory conditions, ketoprofen was found to be equivalent to flunixin meglumine in its ability to decrease the signs of pain and inflammation (Foreman et al 1994). Ketoprofen was also shown to be equivalent to flunixin meglumine in the relief of pain associated with colic in horses (Betley et al 1991) and to have significant antiendotoxic effects in horses (Jackman et al 1994).

Vedaprofen

Vedaprofen is a propionic acid derivative that, like carprofen and ketoprofen, exists as two enantiomers with different pharmacokinetic profiles in the horse. For example, the plasma disposition of $S(+)$-vedaprofen is characterized by a very rapid decline with a plasma half-life of less than 1 h while $R(-)$-vedaprofen has a more prolonged elimination phase with a plasma half-life of over 2 h (Lees et al 1999). Both enantiomers also accumulate in and exhibit a delayed elimination from inflammatory exudates. In horses, vedaprofen appears to be slightly selective for the COX1 enzyme. For example, the median effective concentration for inhibition of serum TXB_2 production, which is assumed to be a reflection of COX1 activity, was much lower than that for inhibition of inflammatory infiltrate PGE_2 production, which is assumed to be a reflection of COX2 activity. Although the results of these studies are promising, there are no published data on the clinical effectiveness and safety of vedaprofen in horses, although it is approved for i.v. and p.o. use in horses in Europe and for p.o. use in Canada.

Ketorolac

Ketorolac is a propionic acid derivative that is reported to be a potent and efficacious analgesic agent in humans (Williams & Upton 1988). The pharmacokinetics of ketorolac have been studied in six standardbred trotters administered a single dose of 300 mg either i.v. or i.m. (Planborg et al 1994). Ketorolac had a small V_d (0.28 l/kg) and a plasma half-life of 6.7 h, which is longer than many other NSAIDs (Planborg et al 1994). No obvious side-effects were observed in this study, although it was not designed to evaluate the safety of ketorolac in horses.

In studies carried out in postoperative human patients, ketorolac provided analgesia equal to or superior to that provided by opiate agents (Grisneaux et al 1999, Sunshine et al 1993). Although its efficacy has not been evaluated in the horse, it has been used in clinical cases (Planborg et al 1994). Further studies are necessary, however, to determine the safety and efficacy of ketorolac in horses.

Eltenac

Eltenac is an acetic acid derivative that appears to be effective and relatively safe when used in horses (Prugner et al 1991). The pharmacokinetics of eltenac have been examined in several studies. It has a short plasma half-life of 1.7–3 h and a small V_d (approximately 0.2 l/kg) (Dyke et al 1998, Prugner et al 1991). There was no indication of accumulation in the plasma after 4 days of repeated i.v. administrations (0.5 mg/kg), unlike phenylbutazone (Dyke et al 1998).

The safety of eltenac in horses appears to be similar to other commonly used NSAIDs. In one study carried out in 24 horses, the four horses given eltenac at the recommended dose rate (0.5 mg/kg) i.v. once daily for 15 days either had no lesions or extremely mild erosions in the glandular mucosa of the stomach (Goodrich et al 1998). In the horses given higher doses of eltenac (1.5 and 2.5 mg/kg) i.v. daily for 15 days, there was a dose-related increase in signs of toxicity, such as gastric ulcers, and decreases in white blood cell counts and total serum protein concentrations, although these effects were not profound (Goodrich et al 1998).

Although not extensive, there is evidence that eltenac is an efficacious NSAID in horses when used at recommended doses (Table 14.1). In one study, eltenac (0.5 mg/kg) was as effective as flunixin meglumine (1.1 mg/kg) in relieving pain and inflammation in an experimentally induced carpitis model in horses (Hamm et al 1997). In addition, the effects of eltenac are long lasting with a dosing interval of once every 24 h recommended for most conditions (Dyke et al 1998). Together these findings suggest that eltenac may be an effective and useful NSAID in horses.

REFERENCES

Abebe W 2002 Herbal medication: potential for adverse interactions with analgesic drugs. Journal of Clinical Pharmacy and Therapeutics 27:391–401

Anfossi P, Villa R, Montesissa C et al 1997 Intramuscular bioavailability of ketoprofen lysine salt in horses. Veterinary Quarterly 19:65–68

Avouac B, Teule M 1988 Ketoprofen: the European experience. Journal of Clinical Pharmacology 28:S2–S7

Betley M, Sutherland S F, Gregoricka M J et al 1991 The analgesic effect of ketoprofen for use in treating equine colic as compared to flunixin meglumine. Equine Practice 13:11–16

Boothe D M 1995 The analgesic–antipyretic–anti-inflammatory drugs. In: Adams H R (ed) Veterinary pharmacology and therapeutics, 7th edn. Iowa State University Press, Ames, IA, pp. 432–449

Brune K, Menzel-Soglowek S, Zeilhofer H U 1992 Differential analgesic effects of aspirin-like drugs. Drugs 44(suppl 5):52–59

Cambridge H, Lees P, Hooke R E et al 1991 Antithrombotic actions of aspirin in the horse. Equine Veterinary Journal 23:123–127

Campbell W B, Halushka P V 1996 Lipid-derived autocoids: eicosanoids and platelet-activating factor. In: Hardman J G, Limbird L E, Molinoff P B et al (eds) Goodman and Gilman's the pharmacological basis of therapeutics, 9th edn. McGraw-Hill, New York, pp. 601–616

Chay S, Woods W E, Nugent T E et al 1982 The pharmacology of nonsteroidal anti-inflammatory drugs in the horse: flunixin meglumine (Banamine). Equine Practice 4:16–23

Collier H O 1971 Prostaglandins and aspirin. Nature 232:17–19

Collins L G, Tyler D E 1985 Experimentally induced phenylbutazone toxicosis in ponies: description of the syndrome and its prevention with synthetic prostaglandin E_2. American Journal of Veterinary Research 46:1605–1615

Corveleyn S, Deprez P, van der Weken G et al 1996 Bioavailability of ketoprofen in horses after rectal administration. Journal of Veterinary Pharmacology and Therapeutics 19:359–363

DiBona G F 1986 Prostaglandins and nonsteroidal anti-inflammatory drugs. Effects on renal hemodynamics. American Journal of Medicine 80:12–21

Dunn M J 1984 Clinical effects of prostaglandins in renal disease. Hospital Practice (Office Edition) 19:99–103, 109–113

Dunn M J, Simonson M, Davidson E W et al 1988 Nonsteroidal anti-inflammatory drugs and renal function. Journal of Clinical Pharmacology 28:524–529

Dyke T M, Sams R A, Thompson K G et al 1998 Pharmacokinetics of multiple-dose administration of eltenac in horses. American Journal of Veterinary Research 59:1447–1450

European Medicines Evaluation Agency 2003a European public assessment report, revision 3, 8 April 2003. Online: http://www.eudra.org/vetdocs/vets/Epar/quardisol50/quadrisol50.htm

European Medicines Evaluation Agency 2003b European public assessment report, revision 4, 8 April 2003. Online: http://www.eudra.org/vetdocs/vets/Epar/quadrisol100/quadrisol100.htm

Flower R J, Moncada S, Vane J R 1985 Analgesic, antipyretic and anti-inflammatory agents. In: Gilman A G, Goodman L S, Wall T W et al (eds) Goodman and Gilman's the pharmacological basis of therapeutics, 7th edn. Macmillan, New York, pp. 674–715

Foreman J H, Grubb T L, Inoue O J 1994 Comparison of the effects of fluxinin meglumine and ketoprofen on experimentally-induced lameness in the horse. In: Proceedings of the 40th American Association of Equine Practitioners Annual Convention, Vancouver BC, pp. 51–52

Forrester S D, Troy G C 1999 Renal effects of nonsteroidal anti-inflammatory drugs. Compendium on Continuing Education for the Practicing Veterinarian 21:910–919

Fry S W, Seeff L B 1995 Hepatotoxicity of analgesics and anti-inflammatory agents. Gastroenterology Clinics of North America 24:875–905

Galbraith L A, McKellar Q A 1996 Protein binding and in vitro serum thromboxane B_2 inhibition by flunixin meglumine and meclofenamic acid in dog, goat and horse blood. Research in Veterinary Science 61:78–81

Gerring E L, Lees P, Taylor J B 1981 Pharmacokinetics of phenylbutazone and its metabolites in the horse. Equine Veterinary Journal 13:152–157

Glaser K, Sung M L, O'Neill K et al 1995 Etodolac selectively inhibits human prostaglandin G/H synthase 2 (PGHS-2) versus human PGHS-1. European Journal of Pharmacology 281:107–111

Goodrich L R, Furr M O, Robertson J L et al 1998 A toxicity study of eltenac, a nonsteroidal anti-inflammatory drug, in horses. Journal of Veterinary Pharmacology and Therapeutics 21:24–33

Grisneaux E, Pibarot P, Dupuis J et al 1999 Comparison of ketoprofen and carprofen administered prior to orthopedic surgery for control of postoperative pain in dogs. Journal of the American Veterinary Medical Association 215:1105–1110

Gunson D E 1983 Renal papillary necrosis in horses. Journal of the American Veterinary Medical Association 182:263–266

Guth P H, Aures D, Paulsen G 1979 Topical aspirin plus HCl gastric lesions in the rat. Cytoprotective effect of prostaglandin, cimetidine and probanthine. Gastroenterology 76:88–93

Hamm D, Turchi P, Johnson J C et al 1997 Determination of an effective dose of eltenac and its comparison with that of flunixin meglumine in horses after experimentally induced carpitis. American Journal of Veterinary Research 58:298–302

Hardee M M, Moore J N, Hardee G E 1986 Effects of flunixin meglumine, phenylbutazone and a selective thromboxane synthetase inhibitor (UK-38,485) on thromboxane and prostacyclin production in healthy horses. Research in Veterinary Science 40:152–156

Hickford F H, Barr S C, Erb H N 2001 Effect of carprofen on hemostatic variables in dogs. American Journal of Veterinary Research 62:1642–1646

Higgins A J, Lees P, Sedgwick A D et al 1987 Use of a novel non-steroidal anti-inflammatory drug in the horse. Equine Veterinary Journal 19:60–66

Homedes J, Sabate D, Mayos I 1997 General and gastrointestinal tolerance of suxibuzone orally administered to horses, compared to phenylbutazone. Journal of Veterinary Pharmacology and Therapeutics 20:163–164

Insel P A 1996 Analgesic, antipyretic and anti-inflammatory agents and drugs employed in the treatment of gout. In: Hardman J G, Limbird L E, Molinoff P B et al (eds) Goodman and Gilman's the pharmacological basis of therapeutics, 9th edn. McGraw-Hill, New York, pp. 617–657

Jackman B R, Moore J N, Barton M H et al 1994 Comparison of the effects of ketoprofen and flunixin meglumine on the in vitro response of equine peripheral blood monocytes to bacterial endotoxin. Canadian Journal of Veterinary Research 58:138–143

Jensen R C, Fischer J H, Cwik M J 1990 Effect of age and training status on pharmacokinetics of flunixin meglumine in thoroughbreds. American Journal of Veterinary Research 51:591–594

Johansson I M, Kallings P, Hammarlund-Udenaes M 1991 Studies of meclofenamic acid and two metabolites in horses: pharmacokinetics and effects on exercise tolerance. Journal of Veterinary Pharmacology and Therapeutics 14:235–242

Jones E W, Hamm D 1978 Comparative efficacy of phenylbutazone and naproxen in induced equine myositis. Journal of Equine Medicine and Surgery 2:341–347

Kahn L H, Styrt B A 1997 Necrotizing soft tissue infections reported with nonsteroidal anti-inflammatory drugs. Annals of Pharmacotherapy 31:1034–1039

Karcher L F, Dill S G, Anderson W I et al 1990 Right dorsal colitis. Journal of Veterinary Internal Medicine 4:247–253

King J N, Gerring E L 1989 Antagonism of endotoxin-induced disruption of equine bowel motility by flunixin meglumine and phenylbutazone. Equine Veterinary Journal Supplement 7:38–42

Kopp K J, Moore J N, Byars T D et al 1985 Template bleeding time and thromboxane generation in the horse: Effects of three non-steroidal anti-inflammatory drugs. Equine Veterinary Journal 17:322–324

Landoni M F, Lees P 1995a Comparison of the anti-inflammatory action of flunixin meglumine and ketoprofen in horses applying PK/PD modeling. Equine Veterinary Journal 27:247–256

Landoni M F, Lees P 1995b Influence of formulation on the pharmacokinetics and bioavailability of racemic ketoprofen in horses. Journal of Veterinary Pharmacology and Therapeutics 18:446–450

Landoni M F, Foot R, Frean S et al 1996 Effects of flunixin, tolfenamic acid, $R(-)$ and $S(+)$ ketoprofen on the response of equine synoviocytes to lipopolysaccharide stimulation. Equine Veterinary Journal 28:468–475

Landuyt J, Delbeke F T, Debackere M 1993 The intramuscular bioavailability of a phenylbutazone preparation in the horse. Journal of Veterinary Pharmacology and Therapeutics 16:494–500

Lee S H, Soyoola E, Chanmugam P et al 1992 Selective expression of mitogen-inducible cyclooxygenase in macrophages stimulated with lipopolysaccharide. Journal of Biological Chemistry 267:25934–25938

Lees P, Higgins A J 1985 Clinical pharmacology and therapeutic uses of non-steroidal anti-inflammatory drugs in the horse. Equine Veterinary Journal 17:83–96

Lees P, Higgins A J 1986 Effects of a phenylbutazone paste in ponies: model of acute nonimmune inflammation. American Journal of Veterinary Research 47:2359–2363

Lees P, Maitho T E, Taylor J B O 1985 Pharmacokinetics of phenylbutazone in two age groups of ponies: a preliminary study. Veterinary Record 116:229–232

Lees P, Taylor J B O, Higgins A J et al 1986 Phenylbutazone and oxyphenbutazone distribution into tissue fluids in the horse. Journal of Veterinary Pharmacology and Therapeutics 9:204–212

Lees P, Ewins C P, Taylor J B O et al 1987a Serum thromboxane in the horse and its inhibition by aspirin, phenylbutazone and flunixin. British Veterinary Journal 143:462–476

Lees P, Taylor J B, Maitho T E et al 1987b Metabolism, excretion, pharmacokinetics and tissue residues of phenylbutazone in the horse. Cornell Veterinarian 77:192–211

Lees P, McKellar Q A, May S A et al 1994 Pharmacodynamics and pharmacokinetics of carprofen in the horse. Equine Veterinary Journal 26:203–208

Lees P, May S A, Hoeijmakers M et al 1999 A pharmacodynamic and pharmacokinetic study with vedaprofen in an equine model of acute nonimmune inflammation. Journal of Veterinary Pharmacology and Therapeutics 22:96–106

Lichtenberger L M, Wang Z M, Romero J J et al 1995 Non-steroidal anti-inflammatory drugs (NSAIDs) associate with zwitterionic phospholipids: insight into the mechanism and reversal of NSAID-induced gastrointestinal injury. Nature Medicine 1:154–158

MacAllister C G, Morgan S J, Borne A T et al 1993 Comparison of adverse effects of phenylbutazone, flunixin meglumine and ketoprofen in horse. Journal of the American Veterinary Association 202:71–77

MacKay R J, French T W, Nguyen H T et al 1983 Effects of large doses of phenylbutazone administration to horses. American Journal of Veterinary Research 44:774–780

MacPhail C M, Lappin M R, Meyer D J et al 1998 Hepatocellular toxicosis associated with administration of carprofen in 21 dogs. Journal of the American Veterinary Medical Association 212:1895–1901

Maitho T E, Lees P, Taylor J B 1986 Absorption and pharmacokinetics of phenylbutazone in Welsh Mountain ponies. Journal of Veterinary Pharmacology and Therapeutics 9:26–39

Mathews K A, Pettifer G, Foster R et al 2001 Safety and efficacy of preoperative administration of meloxicam, compared with that of ketoprofen and butorphanol in dogs undergoing abdominal surgery. American Journal of Veterinary Research 62:882–888

May S A, Lees P 1999 Nonsteroidal anti-inflammatory drugs In: MacIlwraith C W, Trotter G W (eds) Joint disease in the horse. Saunders, Philadelphia, PA, pp. 223–237

McCormack K 1994 The spinal actions of nonsteroidal anti-inflammatory drugs and the dissociation between their anti-inflammatory and analgesic effects. Drugs Supplement 5:28–45

McIlwraith C W 1996 Intra-articular and systemic medications for the treatment of equine joint disease. In: Proceedings of the 42nd American Association of Equine Practitioners Annual Convention, Denver, CO, pp. 101–125

McKellar Q A, Bogan J A, von Fellenberg R L et al 1991 Pharmacokinetic, biochemical and tolerance studies on carprofen in the horse. Equine Veterinary Journal 23:280–284

Meade E A, Smith W L, Dewitt D L 1993 Differential inhibition of prostaglandin endoperoxide synthase (cyclooxygenase) isozymes by aspirin and other non-steroidal anti-inflammatory drugs. Journal of Biological Chemistry 268:6610–6614

Mieszczak C, Winther K 1993 Lack of interaction of ketoprofen with warfarin. European Journal of Clinical Pharmacology 44:205–206

Mills P C, Ng J C, Auer D E 1996 The effect of inflammation on the disposition of phenylbutazone in thoroughbred horses. Journal of Veterinary Pharmacology and Therapeutics 19:475–481

Mitchell J A, Akarasereenont P, Thiemermann C et al 1993 Selectivity of nonsteroidal anti-inflammatory drugs as inhibitors of constitutive and inducible cyclooxygenase. Proceedings of the National Academy of Sciences of the USA 90:11693–11697

Moncada S, Flower R, Vane J 1985 Prostaglandins, prostacyclin, thromboxane A_2 and leukotrienes. In: Gilman A G, Goodman L S, Rall T W et al (eds) Goodman and Gilman's the pharmacological basis of therapeutics, 7th edn. Macmillan, New York, pp. 660–673

Moore J N, Hardee M M, Hardee G E 1986 Modulation of arachidonic acid metabolism in endotoxic horses: comparison of flunixin meglumine, phenylbutazone and a selective thromboxane synthetase inhibitor. American Journal of Veterinary Research 47:110–113

Moss M S, Haywood P E 1973 Persistence of phenylbutazone in horses producing acid urine. Veterinary Record 93:124–125

Murray M J 1985 Phenylbutazone toxicity in a horse. Compendium on Continuing Education for the Practicing Veterinarian 7:S389–S394

Owens J G, Kamerling S G, Barker S A 1995a Pharmacokinetics of ketoprofen in healthy horses and horses with acute synovitis. Journal of Veterinary Pharmacology and Therapeutics 18:187–195

Owens J G, Kamerling S G, Stanton S R et al 1995b Effects of ketoprofen and phenylbutazone on chronic hoof pain and lameness in the horse. Equine Veterinary Journal 27:296–300

Owens J G, Kamerling S G, Stanton S R et al 1996 Effects of pretreatment with ketoprofen and phenylbutazone on experimentally induces synovitis in horses. American Journal of Veterinary Research 57:866–874

Palmoski M J, Brandt K D 1983 Benoxaprofen stimulates proteoglycan synthesis in normal canine knee cartilage in vitro Arthritis and Rheumatism 26:771–774

Pasargiklian M, Bianco S 1986 Perspectives in the treatment of reversible airway obstruction. Respiration 50(suppl 2):131–136

Patrono C, Dunn M J 1987 The clinical significance of inhibition of renal prostaglandin synthesis. Kidney International 32:1–12

Planborg S, Bondesson U, Fredriksson E et al 1994 Pharmacokinetic properties of ketorolac in the horse. In: Proceedings of the 10th International Conference of Racing Analysts and Veterinarians, Stockholm, Sweden, pp. 359–363

Plumb D C 1999 Veterinary drug handbook, 3rd edn. Iowa State University Press, Ames, IA

Prugner W, Huber R, Luhmann R 1991 Eltenac, a new anti-inflammatory and analgesic drug for horses: clinical aspects. Journal of Veterinary Pharmacology and Therapeutics 14:193–199

Raekallio M, Taylor P M, Bennet R C 1997 Preliminary investigations of pain and analgesia assessment in horses administered phenylbutazone or placebo after arthroscopic surgery. Veterinary Surgery 26:150–155

Ramirez S, Seahorn T L, Williams J 1998 Renal medullary rim sign in 2 adult quarter horses. Canadian Veterinary Journal 39:647–649

Reimer M E, Johnston S A, Leib M S et al 1999 The gastroduodenal effects of buffered aspirin, carprofen and etodolac in healthy dogs. Journal of Veterinary Internal Medicine 13:427–477

Ricketts A P, Lundy K M, Seibel S B 1998 Evaluation of selective inhibition of canine cyclooxygenase 1 and 2 by carprofen and other nonsteroidal anti-inflammatory drugs. American Journal of Veterinary Research 59:1441–1446

Rogstad A, Yndestad M 1981 Analysis of xylazine in biological material by gas chromatography using packed and capillary columns. Journal of Chromatography 216:350–354

Sabate D, Homedes J, Mayos I 1997 Comparative study of the clinical efficacy of suxibuzone and phenylbutazone in the treatment of musculoskeletal inflammatory disorders in horses. Journal of Veterinary Pharmacology and Therapeutics 20:162–163

Sams R A, Gerken D F, Ashcraft S M 1995 Pharmacokinetics of ketoprofen after multiple i.v. doses to mares. Journal of Veterinary Pharmacology and Therapeutics 18:108–116

Schary W L, Lewis R J, Rowland M 1975 Warfarin–phenylbutazone interaction in man: a long term multiple dose study. Research Communications in Chemical Pathology and Pharmacology 10:663–672

Semrad S D, Sams R A, Harris O N et al 1993a Effects of concurrent administration of phenylbutazone and flunixin meglumine of pharmacokinetic variables and in vitro generation of thromboxane B_2 in mares. American Journal of Veterinary Research 54:1901–1905

Semrad S D, Sams R A, Ashcraft S M 1993b Pharmacokinetics of and serum thromboxane suppression by flunixin meglumine in healthy foals during the first month of life. American Journal of Veterinary Research 54:2083–2087

Sigurdsson G H, Youssef H 1994 Amelioration of respiratory and circulatory changes in established endotoxic shock by ketoprofen. Acta Anaesthesiologica Scandinavica 38:33–39

Snow D H, Baxter P, Whiting B 1981 The pharmacokinetics of meclofenamic acid in the horse. Journal of Veterinary Pharmacology and Therapeutics 4:147–156

Soma L R, Gallis D E, Davis W L et al 1983 Phenylbutazone kinetics and metabolic concentrations in the horse after five days of administration. American Journal of Veterinary Research 44:2104–2109

Soma L R, Behrend E N, Rudy J A et al 1988 Disposition and excretion of flunixin meglumine in horses. American Journal of Veterinary Research 49:1894–1898

Soraci A, Benoit E, Jaussaud P et al 1995 Enantioselective glucuronidation and subsequent biliary excretion of carprofen in horses. American Journal of Veterinary Research 56:358–361

Stadler I, Kapui Z, Ambrus J L 1994 Study on the mechanisms of action of sodium meclofenamic acid (meclomen) a "double inhibitor" of the arachidonic acid cascade. Journal of Medicine 25:371–382

Stillman M, Schlesinger P 1990 Nonsteroidal anti-inflammatory drugs nephrotoxicity. Archives of Internal Medicine 150:268–270

Strub K M, Aeppli L, Müller R K 1982 Pharmacological properties of carprofen. European Journal of Rheumatology and Inflammation 5:478–487

Sullivan M, Snow D H 1982 Factors affecting absorption of non-steroidal anti-inflammatory agents in the horse. Veterinary Record 110:554–558

Sunshine A, Olson N Z, Zighelboim I et al 1993 Ketoprofen, acetaminophen plus oxycodone and acetaminophen in the relief of postoperative pain. Clinical Pharmacology and Therapeutics 54:546–555

Taylor J B O, Walland A, Lees P et al 1983 Biochemical and haematological effects of a revised dosage schedule of phenylbutazone in horses. Veterinary Record 112:599–602

Templeton C B, Bottoms G D, Fessler J F et al 1987 Endotoxin-induced hemodynamic and prostaglandin changes in ponies: effects of flunixin meglumine, dexamethasone and prednisolone. Circulatory Shock 23:231–240

Tobin T 1979 Pharmacology review: the nonsteroidal anti-inflammatory drugs II. Equiproxen, meclofenamic acid, flunixin meglumine and others. Journal of Equine Medicine and Surgery 6:298–302

Tobin T, Blake J W, Valentine R W 1977 Drug interactions in the horse: effects of chloramphenicol, quinidine and oxyphenbutazone on phenylbutazone metabolism. American Journal of Veterinary Research 38:123–127

Tobin T, Chay S, Kamerling S et al 1986 Phenylbutazone in the horse: a review. Journal of Veterinary Pharmacology and Therapeutics 9:1–25

Toutain P L, Autefage A, Legrand C et al 1994 Plasma concentrations and therapeutic efficacy of phenylbutazone and flunixin meglumine in the horse: pharmacokinetic/pharmacodynamic modeling. Journal of Veterinary Pharmacology and Therapeutics 17:459–469

Trillo M, Soto G, De G 1984 Flunixin meglumine toxicity in a pony. Equine Practice 6:21–29

Vane J R, Botting R M 1995 New insights into the mode of action of anti-inflammatory drugs. Inflammation Research 44:1–10

Venturini C M, Isakson P, Needleman P 1998 Non-steroidal anti-inflammatory drug-induced renal failure: a brief review of the role of cyclooxygenase isoforms. Current Opinion in Nephrology and Hypertension 7:79–82

Welsh J C M, Lees P, Stodulski G et al 1992 Influence of feeding schedule on the absorption of orally administered flunixin meglumine in the horse. Equine Veterinary Journal Supplement 124:62–65

Whittem T, Firth E C, Hodge H et al 1996 Pharmacokinetic interactions between repeated dose phenylbutazone and gentamicin in the horse. Journal of Veterinary Pharmacology and Therapeutics 19:454–459

Wilcke J R, Crisman M V, Scarratt W K et al 1998 Pharmacokinetics of ketoprofen in healthy foals less than 24 hours old. American Journal of Veterinary Research 59:290–292

Williams R L, Upton R A 1988 The clinical pharmacology of ketoprofen. Journal of Clinical Pharmacology 28:S13–S22

Wood T W, Weckman T J, Henry P A et al 1990 Equine urine pH: normal population distributions and methods of acidification. Equine Veterinary Journal 22:118–121

Ziel R, Krupp P 1975 The significance of inhibition of prostaglandin synthesis in the selection of non-steroidal anti-inflammatory agents. International Journal of Clinical Pharmacology and Biopharmacy 12:186–191

CHAPTER CONTENTS

Introduction 267

Sedatives and tranquillizers 267
  α_2 adrenoceptor agonists 268
  Phenothiazines 271
  Benzodiazepines 273

Opioid analgesics 276

Intravenous anesthetic agents 282
  Dissociative anesthetics 282
  Barbiturates 286
  Propofol 288
  Guaifenesin 290

Inhalation anesthetic agents 290

Local anesthetic agents 297

References 301

15

Anesthetics, tranquillizers and opioid analgesics

Diane E. Mason

INTRODUCTION

Prior to using any therapeutic agent, it is important to have an understanding of the pharmacology of the drug. This is perhaps nowhere more important than when using anesthetics, tranquillizers and opioid analgesics in equine medicine. These classes of agent include drugs with very narrow margins of safety, requiring precise dosing and administration. There are also agents that can produce significant untoward effects, contraindicating their use in certain disease states. There are drugs whose pharmacokinetics dictates the circumstances under which they can be used. Knowledge of this is essential to make the appropriate choice of drugs. In the horse, anesthetics, tranquillizers and opioid analgesics are used primarily to allow completion of a procedure or treatment that otherwise would be difficult or impossible to perform. It is important that the right drug is chosen for the situation. Not only is the humane treatment and health safety of the horse at issue, but also the safety of all who are working with the horse is a critical concern. This chapter will review the drugs used most commonly in equine practice for providing sedation, tranquillization, anesthesia and analgesia in horses.

SEDATIVES AND TRANQUILLIZERS

Traditionally sedatives and tranquillizers are classified into groups according to their chemical structure, with all of the drugs in a group sharing a common mechanism of action. In human pharmacology, there is a distinction made between designating an agent as a sedative or a tranquillizer. This distinction is made based on the sites in the central nervous system (CNS) that the drug exerts its primary effect, for instance cortical versus subcortical activity. In horses, the site of activity is not always well established; we often extrapolate from the literature on studies in humans or laboratory animals. In addition, the pharmacological effects of many of these agents in the horse may differ substantially from the effects described in other species. Therefore, in equine pharmacology, such a specific distinction between the groups of drugs in this class is not made and all drugs in these groups are designated as sedative–tranquillizers.

α_2 ADRENOCEPTOR AGONISTS

Mechanism of action

The α_2 agonists produce their clinical effects by binding to α_2 adrenoceptors. Three subtypes have been identified: $\alpha_{2A/D}$, α_{2B} and α_{2C}; however, the presence and/or distribution of each of these subtypes has not yet been described in the horse (Guimaraes & Moura 2001, Saunders & Limbird 1999). The α_2 adrenoceptors are cell membrane receptors that are coupled to membrane-associated G proteins, which mediate their signaling to intracellular effector molecules such as cyclic adenosine monophosphate (cAMP) and the phosphoinositide system (Kamibayashi & Maze 2000). Depending on the cell type, stimulation of α_2 adrenoceptors may inhibit adenylate cyclase, inhibit the opening of voltage-gated calcium channels, activate potassium channels and activate phospholipase A_2, C and D or influence sodium/hydrogen ion exchange (Guimaraes & Moura 2001). Despite the fact that the precise effector molecules activated upon agonist binding seems to be specific to a receptor subtype, the α_2 agonist drugs available currently for clinical use are not selective for receptor subtype (Kamibayashi & Maze 2000, MacDonald & Scheinin 1995). Consequently, the pharmacological

effects of the α_2 agonists used commonly in horses are similar, and differences between drugs are primarily a function of duration of effect (England & Clarke 1996, England et al 1992). In addition to having α_2 agonist activity, many of these drugs also have affinity and efficacy at α_1 adrenoceptors. There are differences among the α_2 agonist drugs with respect to their α_2/α_1 adrenoceptor selectivity: reported values are 160:1 for xylazine, 260:1 for detomidine and 1620:1 for medetomidine (which has a very high level of α_2 selectivity) (Virtanen et al 1988). The extent to which the difference in selectivity of these drugs affects the pharmacological response in horses has not been established.

The α_2 adrenoceptors are present in the brain, spinal cord and in a number of other important tissues throughout the body. They can be located presynaptically at nerve terminals, where they play a role in feedback inhibition of release of the neurotransmitter norepinephrine. This is the primary role of α_2 adrenoceptors in the CNS. The α_2 adrenoceptors can also be located postsynaptically, where they respond to the neurotransmitter norepinephrine or to circulating catecholamines.

Pharmacological effects

The α_2 agonists produce a spectrum of pharmacological effects, some of which are attributable to central effects and others to their action on peripheral receptors in target tissues. Within the CNS, α_2 adrenoceptors mediate sedation, analgesia and decreased output from the sympathetic nervous system. The peripheral effects of α_2 agonists include vasoconstriction and impaired insulin release.

The pharmacological effects of α_2 agonists in the horse are well described. They are very good sedatives in the horse, producing a lower head carriage, decreased locomotor activity and decreased response to touch, sound or visual stimulation (England et al 1992, Harkins et al 1997). The degree of sedation is dose related for all α_2 agonists and ataxia is typical at higher doses. Medetomidine is reported to produce the greatest degree of ataxia and romifidine causes the least ataxia at similar levels of sedation when compared with xylazine or detomidine (Bryant et al 1991, England et al 1991).

The α_2 agonists are very good analgesics, with efficacy demonstrated for pain associated with tendon injury (Chambers et al 1993) and colic (Chambers et al 1993, Jochle 1989, Jochle et al 1989). They reduce the minimum alveolar concentration (MAC, p. 291) of inhalation anesthetics (Steffey et al 2000). The magnitude of MAC reduction is dose and time dependent, with xylazine (0.05–1.0 mg/kg) reducing the MAC of isoflurane from 24 to 34% (Steffey et al 2000). The α_2 agonists are effective agents for epidural anesthesia. Xylazine (0.15 mg/kg) administered into the epidural space significantly decreased the MAC of halothane (Doherty et al 1997a). Xylazine (0.15–0.25 mg/kg) diluted in 8–10 ml 0.9% sodium chloride produced perineal analgesia for more than 2.5 h with minimal systemic effects (Le Blanc et al 1988, Skarda & Muir 1996). Extradural administration of detomidine (60 µg/kg) in 8–10 ml 0.9% sodium chloride has also been reported to produce perineal analgesia, although the response to this dose was not consistent (Skarda 1991, Skarda & Muir 1992, Wittern et al 1998).

Xylazine, detomidine, medetomidine and romifidine are all associated with an initial period of arterial hypertension, which develops within seconds of intravenous (i.v.) administration (Bryant et al 1998, Gasthuys et al 1990, Sarazan et al 1989, Yamashita et al 2000a). Increased peripheral vascular resistance is evident (Yamashita et al 2000a). The hypertension is caused by a direct agonist effect on the peripheral postsynaptic α_2 and α_1 adrenoceptors that mediate vasoconstriction in vascular smooth muscle. Initial hypertension is followed within minutes by a hypotensive phase after both xylazine (1 mg/kg) and medetomidine (3.0–7.5 µg/kg). Hypertension is more prolonged when detomidine or higher doses of medetomidine (10 µg/kg) are administered (Yamashita et al 2000a). Hypertension caused by detomidine reached maximum at 20 µg/kg, with higher doses prolonging the hypertension without further increases in systemic blood pressure (Sarazan et al 1989). At the same time α_2 agonists produce a rapid and significant decrease in heart rate, often

accompanied by the development of second-degree atrioventricular block, which is a result of a vagal reflex response to hypertension (Gasthuys et al 1990, Sarazan et al 1989, Yamashita et al 2000a). The antimuscarinic agents atropine and glycopyrrolate will prevent the bradycardia produced by the α_2 agonists but potentiate arterial hypertension, which introduces the concern of increased ventricular work and increased myocardial oxygen consumption (Alibhai et al 1996, Gasthuys et al 1990). In addition, antimuscarinic agents are often avoided in horses because they decrease gastrointestinal motility (see Ch. 6). However, it has been shown that glycopyrrolate (2.5 µg/kg) prior to xylazine sedation did not significantly change the duration of bowel immobility compared with xylazine alone (Singh et al 1997). In addition, glycopyrrolate prevented bradycardia, increased cardiac output and potentiated hypertension but did not significantly alter left ventricular work (Singh et al 1997). The α_2 agonists reduce cardiac output by causing a marked decrease in heart rate, but they also have a negative inotropic effect, primarily as a result of decreased sympathetic output from the CNS (Sarazan et al 1989, Wagner et al 1991, Yamashita et al 2000a).

The α_2 agonists relax smooth muscle in the distal airways of horses. *In vitro* evidence suggests that this should temporarily improve pulmonary function in horses with chronic obstructive pulmonary disease (heaves) (Le Blanc et al 1993). Airway relaxation is a result of the presynaptic inhibition of acetylcholine release from cholinergic nerves in airways, which is mediated by stimulation of α_2 adrenoceptors (Le Blanc et al 1993). However, sedation with α_2 agonists can increase the total respiratory resistance and the work of breathing in normal horses through an increase in upper airway resistance (Tomasic et al 1997). Endoscopic evaluation indicates that xylazine induces significant relaxation of the pharyngeal soft tissue and increases the incidence of laryngeal asynchrony in horses. These are likely contributing factors to the increase in upper airway resistance produced by α_2 agonists (Valdez-Vasquez et al 1993). The α_2 agonists also reduce mucociliary clearance in the equine airway (Willoughby et al 1991).

The α_2 agonists slow gastrointestinal motility (see Ch. 6). Xylazine (0.5 mg/kg) slows duodenal motility, although the effect is mild and short lived (<30 min) (Merritt et al 1989a, 1998). Detomidine (12.5 μg/kg) produces a more significant suppression of duodenal motility that can be prolonged (at least 1 h) (Merritt et al 1998). Borborygmus is significantly reduced in horses for up to 3 h after detomidine administration (20 μg/kg i.v.) (Jones 1993).

The α_2 agonists are associated with hyperglycemia, hypoinsulinemia and increased micturition (through antagonism of antidiuretic hormone) in adult horses but not in foals (Robertson et al 1990). The α_2 agonist-induced hyperglycemia and hypoinsulinemia result from inhibition of insulin release from the pancreatic islet β cells.

In the horse, α_2 agonists are associated with a decrease in levels of catecholamines (Raekallio et al 1991). This is attributed to decreased sympathetic outflow from the CNS as well as decreased stress response owing to the sedative effects of these drugs (Raekallio et al 1991, 1992). Cortisol levels do not decrease following the administration of α_2 agonists even though the release of adrenocorticotropic hormone from the pituitary is depressed (Alexander & Irvine 2000, Raekallio et al 1991). However, plasma total cortisol levels may not be an accurate indicator of stress levels in the horse (Alexander & Irvine 1998).

The α_2 agonists can produce profuse sweating, cause mydriasis (Kamerling et al 1988) and decrease the hematocrit (Wood et al 1992) in horses. They also decrease rectal temperature and suppress shivering in foals (Robertson et al 1990).

The α_2 agonists increase intrauterine pressure in non-pregnant mares (Schatzmann et al 1994). The effects on the uterus of pregnant mares have not been established, although α_2 agonists are known to increase uterine motility in gravid goats (Perez et al 1994, Sakamoto et al 1996). They increase intrauterine pressure in ruminants by stimulating postsynaptic myometrial α_2 adrenoceptors, causing uterine smooth muscle contraction (Perez et al 1994, Taneike et al 1999). Isolated studies in pregnant mares have not been able to demonstrate an increased risk of abortion after the administration of α_2 agonists even in late gestation (Katila & Oijala 1988, Luukkanen et al 1997).

Physicochemical properties

The α_2 agonists are water soluble and are formulated in solution for parenteral use. Xylazine is available as an injectable solution of 20 mg/ml and 100 mg/ml concentrations, the latter being most frequently used for horses. Detomidine and romifidine are available in 10 mg/ml injectable solutions and medetomidine is available as a 1 mg/ml solution.

Bioavailability and route of administration

The bioavailability of xylazine after intramuscular (i.m.) injection is 40–48% (Garcia-Villar et al 1981). The α_2 agonists are effective when administered by i.v. or i.m. injection. Sublingual administration of romifidine (120 μg/kg) has been shown to be ineffective in producing a sedative effect (Freeman & England 1999). Detomidine is approximately 68% protein bound in equine blood (Singh et al 1987).

Onset, elimination, duration of effect

The onset of sedation after i.v. injection of any of the α_2 agonists is rapid and occurs within minutes. Peak plasma concentrations of xylazine occur 12–15 min after i.m. administration (Garcia-Villar et al 1981). The α_2 agonists undergo hepatic biotransformation with aliphatic hydroxylation followed by glucuronic acid conjugation (Salonen 1991, Salonen & Suolinna 1988). The metabolites are then cleared primarily by renal elimination. Animals with severely impaired liver function may exhibit prolonged effects owing to impaired metabolism of the α_2 agonist. Chloramphenicol, an inhibitor of oxidative metabolism in the liver, can interfere with the metabolism of α_2 agonists. There is a report of the successful use of yohimbine for the treatment of prolonged effects of xylazine in a horse treated with chloramphenicol (Grubb et al 1997). The elimination half-life of xylazine is reported to be 50–75 min after i.v. administration (Dyer et al 1987, Garcia-Villar et al 1981). The elimination half-life of detomidine is approximately 70 min (Salonen et al 1989). The elimination half-life of medetomidine is approximately 50 min after i.v. administration (Bettschart-Wolfensberger et al 1999).

Major uses in the horse

The major uses of the α_2 agonists in the horse are for sedation, as premedication prior to general anesthesia and for analgesia. The recommended dose rates are 0.2–1.1 mg/kg i.v. or up to 2.2 mg/kg i.m. for xylazine, 4–20 µg/kg i.v. or up to 40 µg/kg i.m. for detomidine and 40–100 µg/kg i.v. or up to 120 µg/kg i.m. for romifidine (Freeman & England 1999). Medetomidine is recommended for i.v. use at 5 µg/kg. At 10 µg/kg, medetomidine can cause significant ataxia. For sedation, medetomidine can be administered as a constant rate infusion to horses using a loading dose of 5 µg/kg followed by an i.v. infusion at 3.5 µg/h per kg (Bettschart-Wolfensberger et al 1999). Equipotent sedative doses for the major α_2 agonists are xylazine (1 mg/kg), detomidine (20 µg/kg), romifidine (80 µg/kg) and medetomidine (10 µg/kg) (Bryant et al 1991, England et al 1992). The duration of sedation does not necessarily correlate with the potency. Xylazine sedation lasts 10–15 min. The duration of detomidine sedation is variable, lasting approximately 60–120 min, depending on the dose. Romifidine produces sedation of longer duration than either xylazine or detomidine at equivalent doses (England et al 1992).

The effects of α_2 agonists can be reversed with the specific α_2 adrenoceptor antagonists yohimbine, tolazoline, atipamezole or idazoxan. Yohimbine is an α_2 antagonist with an α_2/α_1 adrenoceptor selectivity of 60:1. Tolazoline is less α_2 specific than yohimbine. Atipamezole has an α_2/α_1 specificity that is 200–300 times that of yohimbine. Atipamezole, at a dose rate of 60 µg/kg, effectively reverses medetomidine action (plasma levels of 1–1.5 ng/ml) (Bettschart-Wolfensberger et al 1999). Doses of 100–160 µg atipamezole have

been recommended to antagonize detomidine sedation (Ramseyer et al 1998).

PHENOTHIAZINES

The phenothiazines are members of a family of drugs classified variously as neuroleptics, tranquillizers or antipsychotic agents, based primarily on their use in treating psychiatric disorders in human medicine. Their activity differs somewhat from other members of the sedative–tranquillizer group in that they produce a general calming effect with decreased spontaneous motor activity, while retaining sensitivity to noise. There is little interference in coordinated motor responses except at very high doses, so animals remain arousable. Ataxia is not generally a feature of phenothiazine use in horses.

Mechanism of action

Phenothiazines act as antagonists of the neurotransmitter dopamine at subcortical excitatory dopamine D_2 receptors in the basal ganglia and limbic forebrain. The dopamine D_2 receptor is present in the nerve cell membrane and is coupled to a G protein that mediates signal transduction to intracellular adenylate cyclase. Dopamine is the endogenous neurotransmitter that binds to the D_2 receptor. The phenothiazines have structural similarity to catecholamines, such as dopamine and norepinephrine, allowing the phenothiazines to bind to catecholamine receptors and block the activity of these neurotransmitters. In addition to their antidopaminergic activity, the phenothiazines are also antagonists at α_1 adrenoceptors, histamine H_1 receptors, muscarinic cholinergic 2 receptors and 5-hydroxytryptamine (serotonin) (5-HT$_2$) receptors. The phenothiazines produce a number of prominent side effects because of this broad antagonist activity at various receptors.

Pharmacological effects

Phenothiazines produce a calming effect in horses. A horse will lower its head carriage and decrease random movements following acepromazine, promazine or chlorpromazine. They tend to stay reactive to noise and visual stimulation and are arousable with adequate stimulus; consequently, the phenothiazines are probably not a good choice for the tranquillization of an intractable or aggressive horse.

Phenothiazines do not produce analgesia but can potentiate the efficacy of other analgesic drugs, such as the opioids (p. 276). An exception to this is levomepromazine (methotrimeprazine), a phenothiazine used formerly in the horse in combination with the opioid etorphine (Petts & Pleuvry 1983). Phenothiazines lower the MAC of inhalation anesthetics. In one controlled study, acepromazine was shown to decrease the MAC of halothane by approximately 37% (Doherty et al 1997b).

The phenothiazines produce a number of effects in addition to their effects on the CNS. Acepromazine decreases the hematocrit. The reduction in the hematocrit can be seen at very low doses (0.002 mg/kg) and its magnitude is dose related and can be clinically significant (25–50% decrease from baseline) especially after i.v. administration (Ballard et al 1982, Hashem & Keller 1993). This effect results from antagonism of α_1 adrenoceptors in the splenic capsule, causing splenic dilatation and the sequestration of red blood cells (Parry & Anderson 1983).

The hemodynamic effects of the phenothiazines can be significant. Acepromazine is associated with decreased systolic, mean and diastolic blood pressures (Marroum et al 1994). The heart rate is usually unchanged after acepromazine administration. The fall in blood pressure is a result of decreased total peripheral resistance caused by antagonism of α_1 adrenoceptors in the vasculature. Despite a fall in blood pressure, administration of acepromazine (0.05 mg/kg) can be associated with improved cardiac output, as stroke volume increases with the decrease in peripheral resistance (Steffey et al 1985). This would not be the case in a horse that is volume depleted as a result of colic or blood loss and acepromazine is contraindicated in these cases because of the potential for the development of extreme hypotension and cardiovascular collapse. There can be significant individual variability in the degree of hypotension that results from the same dose of acepromazine (Parry et al 1982). It is unclear why this variability exists; however, the initial level of stress or excitement may be a contributing factor. This phenomenon has been referred to as "epinephrine reversal." Antagonism of the visceral vasoconstrictive α adrenergic effects of the catecholamines, combined with catecholamine-induced β adrenergic vasodilatation to skeletal muscle, can markedly potentiate the hypotensive effect of the phenothiazines in horses with high levels of circulating catecholamines.

Phenothiazines can produce penile prolapse in horses. The magnitude and duration of this effect is dose related. As little as 0.01 mg/kg acepromazine may cause protrusion of the penis and at very high doses (0.4 mg/kg) this effect can persist for up to 10 h (Ballard et al 1982). The potential for penile trauma, swelling and edema exists and there are reports of priapism continuing long after the termination of the effect of acepromazine. As a result, phenothiazines are not generally recommended for use in breeding stallions. Successful treatment of persistent penile prolapse may be possible with the long-acting anticholinergic benzatropine (Sharrock 1982).

Phenothiazines may decrease the seizure threshold in small animal patients and are contraindicated in dogs and cats with seizure disorders. Although in the horse, seizure disorders are rare (see Ch. 9) and the influence of these drugs on the seizure threshold is unknown, the phenothiazines should be avoided in horses with a history of seizures. Phenothiazines are also contraindicated in animals recently exposed to organophosphate insecticides because of the potential to enhance the toxicity to these drugs (Fernandez et al 1975). In addition, the concomitant administration of phenothiazines and procaine or procaine benzylpenicillin is not advised because of the potential to enhance the adverse effects of procaine (Chapman et al 1992).

Physicochemical properties

Acepromazine is a water-soluble agent that appears yellow in color in solution. It is available as a 10 mg/ml solution or as 10 mg or 25 mg tablets for oral administration. Promazine (50 mg/ml) is available in solution for injection.

Bioavailability and route of administration

Phenothiazines can be administered i.v., i.m. and orally to horses. The bioavailability of orally administered acepromazine is approximately 55% (Hashem & Keller 1993). Side-effects such as penile prolapse and decreased blood pressure are less significant after oral acepromazine (0.5 mg/kg) than following i.v. administration (0.1 mg/kg) but the sedative effects are comparable.

Onset, elimination, duration of effect

The phenothiazines have a long duration of effect compared with many of the other sedative–tranquillizers used in horses. The onset of effect is relatively slow after i.v. administration and the maximum clinical effect occurs 20–30 min after i.v. administration. Peak plasma drug levels occur 30 min after the i.m. injection of acepromazine (Chou et al 1998). Acepromazine has a biphasic concentration decay pattern after i.v. administration (Marroum et al 1994). The distribution half-life is 3–5 min (Ballard et al 1982, Marroum et al 1994) and the elimination half-life is 2–3 h. The terminal half-life of acepromazine after oral administration is approximately 6 h. Acepromazine is highly protein bound in the plasma (>99%) with a large apparent volume of distribution (V_d, 6.61/kg) (Ballard et al 1982).

The phenothiazines undergo hepatic biotransformation (Dewey et al 1981). The primary metabolites are glucuronide conjugates of the parent drug. Acepromazine and promazine both produce a number of metabolites that are detectable in the urine of the horse. Since the duration of effect often exceeds the detection of the phenothiazine in plasma, it is possible that some metabolites retain pharmacological activity (Marroum et al 1994). Phenothiazines should be used with caution in horses with impaired liver function because of the potential for marked prolongation of effect.

Major uses in the horse

Acepromazine is the phenothiazine used by far the most commonly in horses. It can be used alone to provide tranquillization for minor procedures. It is not useful for providing pain relief and is often combined with an opioid (p. 276) or α_2 agonist (p. 268). Acepromazine can be used as a preanesthetic agent prior to general anesthesia at the recommended dose rate of 0.03 mg/kg i.v., 20–30 min prior to a procedure. Lower doses may also be effective in a calm or geriatric animal. Acepromazine can be given orally (0.04–0.1 mg/kg) as tablets for long-term tranquillization, such as for transport.

Promazine has been used extensively for tranquillization of horses at dose rates of 0.4–1.0 mg/kg by injection and up to twice that dose orally. Chlorpromazine is rarely used in the horse because of a greater tendency to produce extrapyramidal side-effects. Propriopromazine is also no longer used in the horse due to a relatively high incidence of penile prolapse.

BENZODIAZEPINES

There are a number of pharmacological agents within the benzodiazepine group. However, there are only a few of these drugs that are currently used with any frequency in equine practice. The most commonly used benzodiazepine is diazepam. Zolazepam is used in combination with the dissociative anesthetic tiletamine (p. 248).

Midazolam, a more water-soluble benzodiazepine with higher bioavailability after i.m. administration, could potentially be used in horses. Midazolam has pharmacological and chemical structural properties closely similar to diazepam; however, its relatively greater lipid solubility results in a more rapid onset of action than diazepam. Midazolam is approximately three to four times more potent than diazepam, although the relative potencies differ among the benzodiazepines with respect to each of the pharmacological effects. According to metabolism and plasma clearance, midazolam is shorter acting than diazepam (Reeves 1984). Dose rates of 0.0045–0.01 mg/kg have been suggested for midazolam use in the horse (Muir & Hubbell 2000).

There may also be rare occasions when the benzodiazepine antagonist flumazenil could be used in horses (see Ch. 9).

Mechanism of action

Benzodiazepines all bind to a specific binding site on the gamma-aminobutyric acid (GABA) A chloride channel. The $GABA_A$ chloride channel is a multi-subunit protein complex that is found in the plasma membrane of nerve cells in various parts of the CNS. When the neurotransmitter GABA binds to the chloride channel, the channel opens, allowing the influx of chloride ions into the cell. This causes hyperpolarization of the nerve cell and diminishes its response to excitatory input. The $GABA_A$ chloride channel is considered the major inhibitory system to neurotransmission in the CNS.

Within the $GABA_A$ chloride channel is a binding site for benzodiazepines, referred to as the benzodiazepine receptor. Upon binding, a benzodiazepine drug will enhance the action of GABA on the chloride channel through an allosteric effect on the channel structure. The presence of a benzodiazepine potentiates the ability of GABA to open the channel (channel gating), increasing chloride ion conductance through the channel. The benzodiazepines alone exert no gating action; their presence on the benzodiazepine receptor will not initiate a chloride current in the absence of GABA. As with many agents that bind to a specific receptor, there are benzodiazepine compounds that are classified as full agonists, partial agonists and competitive antagonists.

Pharmacological effects

Benzodiazepine receptors are present in the cerebral cortex, thalamus, hippocampus, hypothalamus, cerebellar cortex and spinal cord. Each of the major pharmacological effects of benzodiazepines is attributable to the effect of the benzodiazepines on chloride channels at these sites in the CNS: sedation, muscle relaxation and an anticonvulsant effect. In humans, they are considered effective anxiolytics and they produce amnesia.

It is difficult to assess relief from anxiety and the effect on memory in horses, but one might assume a similar response.

Physicochemical properties

As a group, the benzodiazepines are lipid soluble and highly protein bound. Diazepam is 99%, midazolam is 95% and flumazenil is 50% bound to plasma albumin. Only unbound drug can cross the blood–brain barrier. An animal with hypoalbuminemia may have a higher sensitivity to a given dose of a benzodiazepine. The presence of another drug that competes for binding sites on albumin could increase the amount of unbound, active benzodiazepine, potentiating the clinical effect of a given dose of that agent. However, because of the rather mild effects and wide margin of safety, few clinically significant drug interactions are noted after i.v. administration of these drugs. Benzodiazepines are basic drugs with acidic dissociation constants (pK_a) that are much lower than normal blood pH, so they exist primarily in an unionized form in the circulation. Comparatively, diazepam is 99.9%, midazolam 94.1% and flumazenil 99.9% unionized in the circulation.

Bioavailability and route of administration

Although diazepam has a high bioavailability after oral administration (approaching 100%), it is administered in equine practice primarily by the i.v. route. Because of its low water solubility, diazepam is solubilized in propylene glycol for injection. The bioavailability of this formulation is poor after i.m. administration and diazepam is not recommended for i.m. use. When i.m. administration of a benzodiazepine is desired, the more water-soluble agent midazolam is recommended. In contrast to diazepam, midazolam has a poor oral bioavailability (42%) because of its high hepatic clearance and first-pass metabolism. Zolazepam, in combination with tiletamine, can also be administered i.m.

Onset, elimination, duration of effect

The onset of effect is rapid after i.v. administration of the benzodiazepines because of their lipid solubility and the high percentage of unionized drug in the circulation. Benzodiazepines also cross into the placental circulation very rapidly.

After i.v. administration, the primary factors influencing the termination of effect of the benzodiazepines are redistribution away from the CNS and uptake into other tissues, such as skeletal muscle. After an i.v. dose of diazepam or midazolam, redistribution results in diminished effects within 10–15 min. The competitive antagonist flumazenil also has a short duration of effect and, if used to reverse an overdose of a benzodiazepine, may need to be administered repeatedly or by infusion to prevent sedation recurring.

Benzodiazepines, like most lipid-soluble drugs, undergo biotransformation to more water-soluble glucuronide compounds, which are eventually eliminated in the urine. The primary metabolites of diazepam (N-desmethyldiazepam) and midazolam (α-hydroxymidazolam) are pharmacologically active, with similar potency to their parent compounds. These active metabolites are probably of little clinical significance after i.v. administration, because of their rapid elimination and the significance of redistribution in the termination of the CNS effect.

The influence of the active metabolites becomes more significant with repeated administration of the parent drug, as might occur for the control of seizures (see Ch. 9), or chronic oral administration for continued sedation of a neonatal foal. Foals less than 21 days of age have a lower total body clearance of diazepam than older foals and adult horses and, therefore, a greater tendency to develop effects caused by drug accumulation (Norman et al 1997).

Biotransformation of benzodiazepines occurs in the liver, where the drugs undergo phase I metabolism by the cytochrome P450 enzyme complex. Other drugs that may compete with benzodiazepines for liver microsomal enzymes and result in decreased metabolism of benzodiazepines are erythromycin, ketoconazole, verapamil and cimetidine. Geriatric horses or animals with concurrent liver disease may have impaired metabolism of benzodiazepines.

Major uses in the horse

Diazepam produces very mild sedation and muscle relaxation and ataxia in horses after i.v. administration (Muir et al 1982). The ataxia may be significant at doses >0.1 mg/kg and recumbency may result. Foals develop a greater degree of sedation following i.v. diazepam than mature horses.

There are reports that diazepam can produce paradoxical excitability immediately after i.v. administration to humans and small animals. Although this paradoxical effect is not well described in horses, diazepam should be administered with caution to mature horses when used as a sole agent. It can be used as the sole agent for sedation and restraint in young foals. Diazepam is recommended for i.v. use at doses of 0.02–0.1 mg/kg. Diazepam is primarily used in adult horses to provide muscle relaxation and for its anticonvulsant effect prior to anesthetic induction with ketamine. Diazepam (0.04 mg/kg) reduces the MAC of halothane by approximately 29% (Matthews et al 1990). Diazepam is considered the acute treatment of choice for status epilepticus in all species (see Ch. 9). Diazepam (0.02–0.04 mg/kg) is an appetite stimulant in horses, although its effect is of short duration (Brown et al 1976).

Midazolam is recommended for i.v. or i.m. use at doses of 0.01–0.05 mg/kg. Because of its increased cost, midazolam currently offers little advantage over diazepam in clinical use except when i.m. administration of a benzodiazepine is desired.

The benzodiazepine antagonist flumazenil is available for the complete reversal of benzodiazepine effects; however, because of the mild degree of effects, the relative safety of benzodiazepines and the potential to produce excitability, the reversal of benzodiazepines is rarely indicated. Flumazenil is contraindicated in head trauma because it may elevate intracranial pressure (ICP).

OPIOID ANALGESICS

Opioids interact specifically with opioid receptors that are present throughout the body but are of primary importance within the CNS. Opioid drugs are used widely in both human and veterinary medicine as adjuncts to anesthesia and post-operatively because of their efficacy as analgesics and their relative safety even in critically ill or compromised patients. However, there are significant species differences in the pharmacological response to opioid administration and their use in the horse has been limited by undesirable physiological and behavioral side-effects and equivocal or short duration of analgesic efficacy (Bennett & Steffey 2002).

The combination of opioids with other sedatives such as acepromazine (p. 271) and α_2 agonists (p. 268) provides very good quality standing restraint in the horse. Opioids are used as part of a balanced anesthesia techniques in horses to improve analgesic effects, although few opioids decrease the MAC of inhalation agents in the horse. Epidural administration of certain opioids has also been shown to be efficacious in providing analgesia in horses, while avoiding some of the more prominent behavioral side-effects that occur after systemic administration.

The behavioral response of horses to systemic opioid administration has resulted in the illicit use of opioid drugs in the racing and show horse industry and measures to detect opioid residues are part of postperformance drug testing in many venues (McDonald et al 1987, Lehner et al 2000). In addition, though not unique to this class of drugs, the significant abuse potential for opioids in people and government regulatory control means that excellent record keeping and security are fundamental to the use of opioids in clinical practice.

Mechanism of action

Three opioid receptor families have been identified: μ, κ and δ receptors (Carvey 1998). These receptors have been cloned, their nucleotide sequences delineated and a great deal is understood about their molecular pharmacology (Pasternak & Standifer 1996). All opioid receptors are complex protein structures located in the cell membrane with an extracellular amino-terminal segment and an intracellular carboxy-terminal segment sandwiching seven transmembrane domains. The opioid receptor protein is coupled to a G protein on the cytoplasmic side of the cell membrane that mediates the intracellular events which result from receptor activation by an agonist.

The binding of an agonist activates an opioid receptor, which results in primarily inhibitory effects within the cell. Opioid agonists inhibit adenylate cyclase, decreasing the production of cAMP, they activate inwardly rectifying potassium channels, increasing potassium conductance, hyperpolarizing the cell membrane and decreasing neuronal excitability. Opioid agonists also inhibit voltage-gated calcium channels, decreasing calcium influx into the cell, which inhibits neurotransmitter release (Carvey 1998). These intracellular events produce a variety of physiological responses to opioids, some inhibitory and some excitatory as a result of the widespread distribution of opioid receptors throughout the nervous system. Opioid receptors are located in many areas in the brain, in the spinal cord and in the myenteric plexus, and they have been identified in various other tissues, such as synovial membranes. The actions of opioid drugs were recognized long before an understanding of the opioid receptor system developed.

There are three families of endogenous opioid neuropeptides that interact with opioid receptors: enkephalins, endorphins and dynorphins (Carvey 1998). These neuropeptides have varying affinities for the three types of opioid receptors, though none binds exclusively to only one receptor type (Meunier et al 1995). Beta-endorphin shows equal activity at μ and δ opioid receptors with lesser affinity for κ receptors. Met-enkephalin and leu-enkephalin have high affinity for δ receptors, their affinity for μ receptors is one-tenth of that for δ receptors and they have negligible affinity for κ receptors. Dynorphins A and B have high affinity for κ receptors but also bind to μ and δ receptors (Corbett et al 1993).

The opioids used clinically also have differing affinities and efficacy at various opioid receptor types and this is the basis of the classification scheme used typically to describe opioids. Opioid drugs are classified either as agonists, agonist–antagonists or antagonists. Opioid agonists (or full agonists) cause opioid receptor activation and elicit the characteristic pharmacological response with full efficacy. Opioid agonist–antagonists are drugs that have an agonist or partial agonist activity (lower efficacy) at one or more types of opioid receptor and have the ability to antagonize the effect of a full agonist at one or more types of receptor. An opioid antagonist binds to opioid receptors and causes no pharmacological effect and may compete with the binding of other opioids (a competitive antagonist) (Branson et al 1995).

Pharmacological effects

Opioids are the "gold standard" for analgesia. Analgesia is mediated at both the supraspinal and spinal levels through the effects of opioids at all three receptor types. At the spinal level, opioids inhibit the release of the neurotransmitter substance P from primary afferent C fiber nerve terminals in the substantia gelatinosa of the dorsal horn of the spinal cord. This reduces the transmission of nociceptive signals to the spinothalamic tract, which would be carried to higher centers in the brain. Supraspinal analgesia is mediated at many sites in the brain including the periaqueductal gray matter, median raphe and locus ceruleus, where opioids acting on μ and κ receptors further inhibit ascending nociceptive signaling arriving via the spinothalamic tract. In addition, opioids activate both serotoninergic and norepinephrinergic (noradrenergic) descending inhibitory efferent fibers, which project to the spinal cord dorsal horn, to depress further pain signals at the level of the spinal cord. Descending inhibitory pathways are activated by opioid-induced, presynaptic inhibition of spontaneous GABA release from neurons that are inhibitory to descending norepinephrinergic (noradrenergic) and serotonergic pathways. Therefore, opioids disinhibit other inhibitory nerves resulting in pathway activation (Vaughan et al 1997).

Opioids are associated with behavioral changes that are quite variable across species. Dose-dependent euphoria and sedation are typical responses following opioid administration to dogs and primates (including humans). CNS excitation and dysphoria are more typical responses in cats, horses, pigs and ruminants (Branson et al 1995). CNS excitation may at first seem inconsistent with the neuroinhibitory nature of the opioid effect, but there is evidence to suggest that the excitatory effects of the opioids are indirect, caused by interactions with brain dopaminergic and norepinephrinergic (noradrenergic) pathways that control motor and behavioral responses. The excitement and increased locomotion seen in horses seem to be effectively diminished by the concomitant administration of the dopaminergic antagonist acepromazine (p. 271), or α_2 adrenoceptor agonists (p. 268), which depress norepinephrinergic (noradrenergic) transmission centrally (Clarke & Paton 1988, Combie et al 1981).

Opioids are potent respiratory depressants, causing a dose-dependent decrease in respiratory frequency, tidal volume and minute ventilation and increased arterial partial pressure of carbon dioxide (Pa_{CO_2}) (Carvey 1998). Opioids depress chemosensors in the brainstem, decreasing the ventilatory response to carbon dioxide. Opioids also depress rhythmicity in the dorsal respiratory group in the nucleus tractus solitarius, attenuating the respiratory cycle. Opioids, however, do not diminish hypoxic ventilatory drive. Significant elevations in Pa_{CO_2} can result in increased ICP after opioid administration.

The opioids are considered relatively safe from a cardiovascular standpoint. Myocardial depression is minimal. Changes in heart rate are species dependent and usually manifest as a mild decrease in heart rate; however, a significant increase in heart rate can be seen in horses, which is consistent with the central excitatory effect that often occurs. Opioids inhibit the baroreceptor reflex response to changes in blood pressure. Certain opioids may cause systemic vasodilatation, decreased peripheral vascular resistance and hypotension secondary to histamine release. Morphine and meperidine (pethidine) are the opioids most likely associated with this effect. This is typically seen after rapid i.v. administration, is dose dependent and does not result from mast cell degranulation but from displacement of histamine from the heparin–protein complex (Carvey 1998). Opioids are located in the myenteric plexus of the gastrointestinal tract and opioid administration has a significant effect on gastrointestinal motility (see Ch. 6). In the horse, gastrointestinal effects are variable depending on the segment of bowel and the opioid agent used. In general, opioids decrease the propulsive activity of the gastrointestinal tract by inhibiting peristalsis, while increasing tone in intestinal smooth muscle. Opioids also induce spastic tone in gastrointestinal sphincters.

Major uses of opioid agonists in the horse

The opioid agonists include morphine, meperidine, methadone, fentanyl, alfentanil, remifentanil and carfentanil.

Morphine

Morphine is the prototypical μ receptor agonist that produces CNS stimulation, increased locomotor activity, analgesia, cardiorespiratory stimulation and decreased gastrointestinal motility in the horse. It is most often used in combination with a sedative for standing chemical restraint (Geiser 1990) or as anesthetic premedication. Morphine is also used to provide epidural analgesia in horses. The recommended dose rate of morphine for standing restraint is 0.3–0.6 mg/kg i.v. in combination with acepromazine (0.05 mg/kg) or xylazine (0.5–1.0 mg/kg), detomidine (0.01–0.02 mg/kg) or romifidine (0.05–0.08 mg/kg).

Morphine (0.66 mg/kg i.m.) alone stimulates motor activity, characterized by muscle tremors and restlessness from 1 to 3 h after administration (Kalpravidh et al 1984). Morphine increases arterial blood pressure, heart rate and respiratory rate in ponies for up to 4 h (Kalpravidh et al 1984). The cardiopulmonary response to morphine (0.12–0.66 mg/kg) administered i.v. with xylazine (0.66 mg/kg) is characterized by quiet standing, decreased heart rate, cardiac output and respiratory rate and increased arterial blood pressure (Muir et al 1979). In the same study,

morphine significantly increased the threshold response to a thermal stimulus for 30 min and to visceral pain, in a cecal balloon model, at 30 and 60 min. Locomotor stimulation after morphine (2.4 mg/kg) is significant for up to 7 h postadministration. This locomotor response is reduced 75% by the narcotic antagonist naloxone (0.015 mg/kg) and is diminished by acepromazine for up to 6 h (Combie et al 1981).

Analgesia occurs after epidural administration of morphine (0.1 mg/kg) as measured by increased avoidance threshold to an electrical stimulus. The onset of analgesia was 5 h in the sacral and perineal region, 6 h in the lumbar region and 8 h in the thoracic region. The duration of effect was 6 h postonset in the sacral and perineal region, 5 h in the lumbar region and 3 h in the thoracic dermatomes (Natalini & Robinson 2000). Preoperative epidural administration of morphine (0.2 mg/kg) with detomidine (0.03 mg/kg) resulted in a significant decrease in lameness scores in an experimental model of tarsal synovitis; however, the horses were only observed for the first 6 h postoperatively so the effect may have been more attributable to the α_2 agonist than to the opioid (Sysel et al 1996). When the same combination was used in horses undergoing bilateral stifle arthroscopy, the investigators observed a significant decrease in lameness scores with a maximum effect at 1–2 h postrecovery (Goodrich et al 2002). Epidural morphine (0.1 mg/kg) significantly decreased the MAC of halothane in horses by approximately 15% for a stimulus applied to the pelvic but not the thoracic limbs (Doherty et al 1997c).

Morphine (0.5–1.0 mg/kg) inhibited jejunal and cecocolonic motility from 30 min to 3 h in ponies after i.v. administration. Overall resting muscle tone in the colon was increased (Roger et al 1985).

Morphine has very low bioavailability after oral administration because of significant first-pass metabolism. It is interesting to note, however, that the oral intake of as little as 1 g poppy seeds results in detectable urine levels of morphine for up to 24 h postingestion (Kollias-Baker & Sams 2002). Morphine (0.1 mg/kg) is detectable in blood for 48 h and in urine for 144 h after administration. The elimination half-life of morphine is 88 min in the horse. The degree of protein binding is 31% (Combie et al 1983).

Meperidine (pethidine)

Meperidine is a μ receptor agonist that is one-tenth as potent as morphine and has a shorter duration of effect. Its effects in the horse are similar to those described for morphine and it is used primarily as an anesthetic adjunct, or along with other sedatives for standing chemical restraint or anesthetic premedication. The recommended dose rate is 0.6–1.0 mg/kg i.v. in combination with either acepromazine (0.05 mg/kg) or xylazine (0.5–1.0 mg/kg).

Meperidine (1 mg/kg i.v.) given alone caused a significant increase in respiratory rate, heart rate and cardiac output for the first 30 min after administration and it increased mean arterial blood pressure significantly for at least 60 min (total duration of the observation period) (Muir & Robertson 1985). In a cecal balloon model, meperidine provided visceral analgesia for 36 min (Muir & Robertson 1985). Meperidine (1 mg/kg i.v.) also induced visual and auditory hyper-responsiveness, shivering, head shaking and restlessness for 5–10 min after i.v. administration to horses (Muir & Robertson 1985, Waterman & Amin 1992). Caudal epidural administration of meperidine (0.8 mg/kg) in horses induced superficial analgesia in the coccygeal and first sacral (S1) dermatomes with an onset at 12 min and duration lasting for 4–5 h. No sedative, ataxia, or hyperresponsiveness was evident after epidural administration (Skarda & Muir 2001). Meperidine reduced intestinal motility in the jejunem, but not at the pelvic flexure in horses (Sojka et al 1988). The elimination half-life of meperidine is 57 min in the horse (Waterman & Amin 1992). Total body clearance is relatively rapid (17.7 ml/kg/min).

Methadone (dolophine hydrochloride)

Methadone is a synthetic μ opioid receptor agonist that is three times as potent as morphine. It is unique in that it has significant bioavailability after oral administration. Methadone is typically used i.v. in the horse in combination with acepromazine to produce sedation that lasts for several hours. The recommended dose rate is 0.1 mg/kg i.v. in combination with either acepromazine (0.05 mg/kg), xylazine (0.5–1.0 mg/kg), detomidine (0.01 mg/kg) or romifidine (0.05–0.08 mg/kg). In some countries, the L-isomer (eutomer) of methadone (levomethadone), with the consequent dose rate reductions, is approved for use in horses.

Fentanyl, alfentanil and remifentanil

Fentanyl, alfentanil and remifentanil are all highly potent, short-duration, μ receptor agonists that have relatively limited clinical application in the horse but represent drugs with a high potential for abuse in performance horses. Fentanyl and alfentanil are phenylperadine derivatives that are highly lipid soluble, have a rapid onset of effect after i.v. administration and a short duration of action, the termination of effect being primarily a result of redistribution of drug from the brain to other tissues. Fentanyl is 150–250 times as potent and alfentanil is approximately 30–50 times as potent as morphine. Remifentanil is a new synthetic opioid that has potency roughly equivalent to fentanyl (p. 280). Remifentanil has a rapid onset of effect and a short half-life owing to rapid metabolism of the drug by non-specific tissue and plasma esterases (Lehner et al 2000). There are currently no published reports on the clinical use of remifentanil in horses. Administration of remifentanil (5 mg i.v.) induces increased locomotor responses in horses similar to that produced by other μ receptor agonists. The major metabolite of remifentanil is produced by ester hydrolysis and peak levels are found in the urine 1 h post-administration.

Alfentanil pharmacokinetics, analgesic efficacy and behavioral effects have been evaluated in the horse. Alfentanil (0.02–0.04 mg/kg i.v.) produces a significant increase in locomotor activity in horses (Pascoe et al 1991). Electroencephalography (EEG) after alfentanil administration (0.04 mg/kg) during halothane anesthesia in the horse shows a reduction in the frequency power spectrum similar to that seen in other species, suggesting that the excitatory response of horses does not originate from the cerebral cortex (Johnson & Taylor 1997). Alfentanil infusion did not significantly alter the MAC of halothane in the anesthetized horse (Pascoe et al 1993). Alfentanil infusion during halothane anesthesia resulted in a dose-dependent increase in blood pressure without a change in heart rate (Pascoe et al 1993). Epidural administration of alfentanil (0.02 mg/kg) did not result in a significant change in avoidance threshold to a noxious stimulus in horses (Natalini & Robinson 2000). The elimination half-life of alfentanil in the horse is 22 min with a clearance of 14 ml/min per kg (Pascoe et al 1991).

Fentanyl is a μ receptor agonist that significantly increases locomotor activity in horses (0.02 mg/kg). Addition of a specific κ receptor agonist (U50, 488H) to fentanyl enhanced the locomotory effect, with a more rapid onset and longer duration. This may indicate that locomotor activity is mediated by both μ and κ receptors or it may be the result of altered pharmacokinetics of fentanyl in the presence of the second drug (Mama et al 1993). Fentanyl (0.01–0.05 mg/kg i.v.) caused marked inhibition of propulsive activity in the equine colon with closure of the cecocolic sphincter that lasted for 60–120 min (Roger et al 1994).

Fentanyl (0.001 mg/kg i.v.) can be used with xylazine (0.44 mg/kg i.v.) for anesthetic premedication. Fentanyl is sometimes used as an anesthetic adjunct during inhalation anesthesia to improve analgesia. The pharmacokinetics of fentanyl make it ideal for administration by constant rate infusion and it can be administered intraoperatively at a rate of 0.001–0.004 mg/kg/h after a 0.001 mg/kg loading dose. To prevent excitement or locomotory stimulation in recovery, the infusion should be discontinued 30 min prior to recovery or the horse should be sedated with xylazine (0.1 mg/kg i.v.) prior to recovery.

Carfentanil

Carfentanil is the most potent opioid available commercially for use in veterinary medicine. It is a μ receptor agonist that is 10 000 times as potent

as morphine. Because of this potency, very small volumes of this agent are needed for injection, making it potentially ideal for immobilizing free-ranging equids (Shaw et al 1995). Carfentanil is never used as the sole agent for wildlife capture but is typically combined with an α2 agonist, such as xylazine. This helps to reduce the total dose of carfentanil needed for capture, improves the level of muscle relaxation and helps to reduce the excitatory response that may occur with carfentanil alone. Carfentanil (0.015–0.33 mg/kg i.m.) with xylazine (0.014–0.29 mg/kg i.m.) has been used to immobilize feral horses, Przewalski's horses and zebras. Immobilization after i.m. injection is rapid and occurs in 8–9 min (Shaw et al 1995). Domestic horses and ponies may not show a favorable response to this combination. Muscle fasciculations, paddling of the limbs while in recumbency, and sweating are prominent. Tachycardia and marked hypertension are characteristic of the hemodynamic response to carfentanil in the horse. Hyperthermia may occur. An unexpected death was reported in one of three horses immobilized with this combination, with pulmonary edema being found at postmortem examination.

Major uses of opioid agonist/antagonists

The opioid agonist–antagonists include butorphanol, pentazocine, and buprenorphine

Butorphanol

Butorphanol is the opioid agonist–antagonist that is most frequently used in the horse. It is a κ receptor agonist and can antagonize the effect of μ agonists at the μ opioid receptor (Sellon et al 2001). Butorphanol is used in combination with another sedative for standing chemical restraint and as part of premedication protocols for anesthesia. Recommended dose rates for butorphanol are 0.02–0.05 mg/kg i.v. in combination with acepromazine (0.05 mg/kg), xylazine (0.5–1.0 mg/kg) or detomidine (10–20 μg/kg).

The pharmacological response to butorphanol is well described in the horse. Administration of butorphanol (0.1–0.13 mg/kg i.v.) results in significant ataxia, decreased gastrointestinal motility and decreased defecation (Sellon et al 2001). Constant rate infusion of butorphanol (23.7 mg/kg/h) after an initial loading dose (0.018 mg/kg) induced no changes in behavior or gastrointestinal function. Butorphanol (0.22 mg/kg) produced very mild increases in heart rate and blood pressure, but this change was only significant for heart rate 60 min postadminstration (Kalpravidh et al 1984).

Butorphanol is used as an analgesic in horses. Butorphanol (0.1 mg/kg i.v.) increased the pain threshold in a rectal balloon model in mares (Skarda & Muir 2003). It had analgesic efficacy for 60 min in a cecal balloon model (Muir & Robertson 1985). Butorphanol (0.025 mg/kg i.v.) combined with detomidine (0.01 mg/kg) increased the nociceptive threshold for an electrical stimulus within 15 min of administration and prolonged the duration of analgesia by 15–75 min compared with detomidine alone (Schatzmann et al 2001). Butorphanol (0.05 mg/kg) either i.v. or epidurally did not reduce the MAC of halothane in horses (Doherty et al 1997b,c). Epidural butorphanol (0.08 mg/kg) did not increase the threshold for noxious stimulation in perineal, sacral or lumbar dermatomes (Natalini & Robinson 2000). In a multicenter trial examining the efficacy of a variety of analgesic drugs in horses with colic, butorphanol (0.1 mg/kg) was not considered clinically effective as an analgesic (Jochle et al 1989).

Butorphanol combined with xylazine decreased esophageal motility, including a reduction in spontaneous swallowing and peristaltic activity in the horse (Wooldridge et al 2002). Butorphanol combined with detomidine prolonged gastric emptying time (Sutton et al 2002). Combined with xylazine, it resulted in a significant reduction of duodenal motility for 1 h after treatment (Merritt et al 1998). Butorphanol alone did not adversely effect antroduodenal motility in the horse (Merritt et al 1989b). However, in combination with xylazine, it reduced cecal motility for 150 min and prolonged the depression of cecal mechanical activity induced by xylazine alone (Rutkowski et al 1991). During halothane anesthesia, i.v. administration of butorphanol (0.2 mg/kg) caused

hypotension and a secondary decrease in intestinal blood flow without increasing intestinal vascular resistance or compromising intestinal viability (Stick et al 1989). Butorphanol (0.04 mg/kg) decreased progressive cecocolic motility but only for 10 min (Rutkowski et al 1989).

Pentazocine

Pentazocine is an agonist–antagonist opioid with a potency one-third that of morphine. It is a benzomorphan derivative of ketazocine, a selective κ agonist. The binding affinity of pentazocine is not selective for κ opioid receptors but κ opioid effects predominate with use of this drug. As a κ agonist, pentazocine produces a lesser degree of respiratory depression than μ agonists. After i.v. administration of pentazocine, horses exhibited auditory hypersensitivity, incoordination and muscle tremors (Branson et al 1995). Pentazocine (0.33–1.1 mg/kg i.v.) has been recommended to provide analgesia for horses with colic; however, in cecal balloon models of equine colic, pentazocine either did not provide detectable analgesia or provided analgesia of less than 30 min duration (Muir et al 1978).

After i.m. administration of pentazocine, the peak plasma concentration is achieved at 30 min in the horse. Pentazocine has an elimination half-life of 97 min in ponies and 138 min in the horse (Davis & Sturm 1970). After i.v. administration, pentazocine has been shown to be 80% bound to plasma protein. The glucuronide metabolite of pentazocine is cleared in the urine and pentazocine metabolites can be detected in the urine for up to 5 days in the horse.

Buprenorphine

Buprenorphine is a partial agonist at μ receptors, with high binding affinity that provides a long duration of action. Buprenorphine (0.003–0.006 mg/kg i.v.) like other opioids can be combined with another sedative, such as xylazine (p. 268) or acepromazine (p. 271), but because of the long duration of effect of buprenorphine compared with other opioids, acepromazine

(0.04–0.05 mg/kg) or detomidine (10–20 µg/kg) are the best match. Buprenorphine (0.003 mg/kg i.v.) caused an increase in respiratory frequency and minute ventilation while decreasing tidal volume and pulmonary resistance; it produced no significant change in the partial pressure of oxygen (PaO_2) or $PaCO_2$ (Szoke et al 1998). Buprenorphine also caused increased heart rate and arterial blood pressure for at least 3 h (total observation time). Buprenorphine (0.003 mg/kg) is associated with a mild degree of CNS stimulation, characterized by pawing, chewing and muscle rigidity in the neck with a duration of less than 30 min (Szoke et al 1998). Buprenorphine does not have significant respiratory depressant effects in normal horses or in horses with chronic obstructive pulmonary disease.

Major uses of opioid antagonists

Naloxone

Naloxone is a pure opioid antagonist that has no known agonist activity. Naloxone can produce rapid reversal of the effects of other opioids within minutes of i.v. administration but it has a relatively short duration of action and renarcotization of horses may occur if the effect of naloxone dissipates before the opioid agonist drug is cleared sufficiently from the body (Shaw et al 1995). Naloxone (0.02–0.04 mg/kg) has been shown to be effective in preventing crib-biting (Dodman et al 1987; see Ch. 9). However, the duration of effect is short lived. Although naloxone has been used experimentally to improve hemodynamic function in hypovolemic shock in several species, it did not alleviate the hemodynamic or metabolic changes accompanying endotoxic shock in ponies (Moore et al 1983).

Naloxone has been investigated as a prokinetic agent for the gastrointestinal tract in horses (Ruckebusch & Roger 1988; see Ch. 6). Naloxone increased the frequency of defecation, softened feces and increased the intensity of borborygmus in normal horses (Aurich et al 1993). Naloxone decreased heart rate and respiratory frequency in these horses and was associated with behavioral changes, such as yawning and flehmen. In another study in normal horses, high doses of naloxone (0.75 mg/kg) caused rapid onset of diarrhea, restlessness, tachycardia, tachypnea and flank checking, signs similar to those seen in spasmodic colic (Kamerling et al 1990). Naloxone (0.05 mg/kg) caused an increase in propulsive contractile activity in the cecum and colon of horses that was as effective as cisapride and superior to that metoclopramide (Ruckebusch & Roger 1988).

INTRAVENOUS ANESTHETIC AGENTS

DISSOCIATIVE ANESTHETICS

Ketamine and tiletamine are the major dissociative anesthetic drugs used in veterinary medicine. They are commonly referred to as dissociative anesthetic agents because of their unique mechanism of producing anesthesia. In contrast to most anesthetics, which exert their action via a generalized depressant effect on the CNS, dissociative agents produce both excitatory and depressant effects on the CNS, as seen in EEG of anesthetized patients. Humans report feeling an "out of body" experience because of the dissociation of the cerebral cortex from the lower thalamic centers in the brain. Dissociative agents produce amnesia, analgesia and a cataleptic state. Seizure discharges can be seen on an EEG during dissociative anesthesia. In humans, dissociative anesthetics produce hallucinogenic, vivid dreaming; in animals, they can produce a state of dysphoria. As a result, dissociative anesthetics are rarely used alone and are always combined with a sedative/tranquillizer to improve the anesthetic effect. Ketamine is the drug used most commonly for anesthetic induction of the horse in both ambulatory and clinic practice. Tiletamine has properties very similar to ketamine. It is commercially available in a combination anesthetic product that consists of a 1:1 ratio of tiletamine with the benzodiazepine zolazepam (p. 273). Zolazepam is added to the dissociative tiletamine for its muscle relaxation and anticonvulsant effects.

Mechanism of action

Dissociative anesthetic agents produce their effects through action as a non-competitive N-methyl-D-aspartate (NMDA) receptor antagonist. The NMDA receptor is activated by the amino acid neurotransmitter glutamate, the primary excitatory neurotransmitter in the CNS. Ketamine binds at a site within the ion channel of the receptor, which is separate from the binding site of glutamate. Therefore, ketamine does not competitively inhibit the binding of glutamate to the NMDA receptor, rather it prevents the sodium and calcium ion conductance through the channel pore that normally results from channel activation by glutamate (Carvey 1998). Antagonism of the action of glutamate throughout the CNS produces a variety of effects both excitatory and inhibitory, as glutamate is instrumental in nerve signal processing at many levels in the brain and spinal cord.

Pharmacological effects

Ketamine

Ketamine produces a dose-dependent loss of consciousness, ultimately progressing to a trance-like rather than a sleep-like state, described as catalepsy. This loss of consciousness is usually associated with an increase in skeletal muscle tone. Ocular and pharyngeal reflexes remain intact and nystagmus is common. Because of its tendency to produce excitation, ketamine should not be used in horses without prior tranquillization. Most studies on the pharmacological effects of ketamine in the horse are undertaken in this context. Inadequate sedation in the horse prior to administration of ketamine may result in the failure of ketamine to induce general anesthesia (Trim et al 1987). Ketamine can cause an increase in ICP, cerebral blood flow and metabolic oxygen consumption. In goats, these changes can be attenuated if the $PaCO_2$ remains normal (Schwedler et al 1982). In other species, elevations of ICP can be attenuated by the concomitant administration of benzodiazepines or other CNS depressants (Artru 1990). It is not known to what extent ketamine might elevate ICP in the horse.

Xylazine decreases ICP in the horse, so the combination of xylazine and ketamine may not be associated with elevated ICP, as long as the $PaCO_2$ remains within the normal range (Moore & Trim 1992). Xylazine and ketamine anesthesia is associated with a decrease in intraocular pressure in the horse (Smith et al 1990, Trim et al 1985).

There is ample evidence that ketamine is an effective analgesic that acts at the level of both the spinal cord and the brain. In horses, epidural administration of ketamine provided perineal analgesia for up to 75 min (Gomez de Segura et al 1998). Epidural ketamine reduced the MAC of halothane for hind- but not forelimb procedures, indicating a localized effect in the spinal cord after epidural administration (Doherty et al 1997c). Constant rate i.v. infusions of ketamine caused a reduction in the MAC value for halothane in the horse when plasma ketamine concentrations exceeded 1 μg/ml (Muir & Sams 1992).

One of the potential advantages of dissociative agents over other types of anesthetic agent is the stimulatory effect on cardiovascular function. This results from indirect cardiac stimulation via centrally mediated sympathetic stimulation and inhibition of neuronal uptake of catecholamines at the sympathetic neuroeffector junction. In dogs, heart rate and blood pressure increase, as does cardiac output and myocardial oxygen consumption, while systemic vascular resistance remains unchanged (Folts et al 1975). Ketamine is never used as the sole anesthetic agent in the horse. The cardiovascular stimulation produced by ketamine is blunted by prior administration of α_2 agonists and concomitant use of inhalation agents. Ketamine-based total i.v. anesthetic (TIVA) techniques, such as guaifenesin and ketamine with an α_2 agonist given as constant rate infusion, provide superior hemodynamic stability in horses compared with maintenance of anesthesia using inhalation agents (Taylor et al 1995, 1998, Yamashita et al 2000b, Young et al 1993).

Ketamine is not a significant respiratory depressant and the ventilatory response to hypoxia is maintained. Ketamine has a bronchodilatory effect subsequent to sympathetic stimulation. Airway reflexes are well maintained after ketamine administration. However, since ketamine is not used as a sole anesthetic in horses, the respiratory depressant effects of the α_2 agonists and the addition of inhalation agents, after anesthetic induction with ketamine, typically result in hypercarbia in the anesthetized horse. Ketamine-based TIVA techniques do not result in as severe respiratory depression as anesthetic maintenance with an inhalation agent (Luna et al 1996, Marlin et al 2001).

Tiletamine

The pharmacological effects of tiletamine plus zolazepam are very similar to the effects produced by ketamine. When used as the sole anesthetic in the horse, tiletamine plus zolazepam can cause excitation and hyperresponsiveness. This combination is only used in the horse after adequate sedation. In general, it produces a dose-related loss of consciousness, characterized as a cataleptic state, and analgesia. Ocular and airway reflexes are well maintained. The combination induces mild cardiovascular stimulation secondary to centrally mediated sympathetic nervous system stimulation. There is minimal respiratory depression.

Physicochemical properties

Ketamine

Ketamine is a low-molecular-weight, highly lipid- and water-soluble molecule. As such, it can quickly cross the blood–brain barrier, producing a maximal effect in the CNS within 1 min of i.v. administration. Ketamine exists as a racemic mixture of the two optical isomers $S(+)$-ketamine and $R(-)$-ketamine. The majority of the hypnosis and analgesia produced by ketamine is contributed by the $S(+)$-isomer (Joo et al 2000, Muir & Hubbell 1988, Redig et al 1984). A purified $S(+)$-ketamine pharmaceutical product is not yet available commercially for veterinary use and the possible advantages of such a product in the horse have not been established. Ketamine is 45–60% bound to equine plasma proteins (Kaka et al 1979) meaning that the maximal effect of ketamine is unlikely to be altered substantially by hypoproteinemic states.

Tiletamine

Tiletamine is a highly lipid- and water-soluble compound, similar to ketamine. It has a higher potency than ketamine and a longer duration of effect after i.v. administration.

Bioavailability and route of administration

Ketamine

Ketamine is almost always administered i.v. in the horse. Ketamine has been administered i.m. in combination with medetomidine for field immobilization of feral horses (Matthews et al 1995). The pH of an aqueous solution of ketamine is 3.5. Because of its acidity, ketamine can cause pain upon i.m. injection, although it does not produce any lasting tissue damage when given by this route.

Tiletamine

Tiletamine in combination with zolazepam is almost always administered i.v. to horses. It has been used successfully to induce recumbency in horses after i.m. administration (Matthews 1993).

Onset, elimination, duration of effect

Ketamine

Ketamine produces a rapid onset of anesthesia when given i.v. with recumbency occurring within 1 min (Kaka et al 1979). After i.m. administration, a combination of medetomidine and ketamine produced recumbency in feral horses with a mean induction time of 11 min, although 3 out of the 14 horses were still standing, sedated but not manageable (Matthews et al 1995).

Ketamine has a short duration of effect after i.v. bolus administration. Ketamine induction after xylazine sedation generally provides 12–20 min duration of anesthesia (Muir et al 1977). The termination of the effects of ketamine in the CNS primarily results from redistribution of the drug from the brain to other tissues (Waterman et al

1987). Ketamine undergoes hepatic biotransformation in the horse. The primary metabolites are norketamine and dehydronorketamine (Delatour et al 1991, Sams & Pizzo 1987, Seay et al 1993). Up to 40% of ketamine can be excreted unchanged in the urine. Upon recovery from ketamine anesthesia, 40% of the ketamine dose still remains in the horse at levels insufficient to produce anesthesia (Kaka et al 1979). In the horse, the elimination half-life of ketamine is reported to be 42–65 min with a total body clearance of 23–26 ml/kg/min (Kaka et al 1979, Waterman et al 1987).

Tiletamine

After sedation, i.v. tiletamine plus zolazepam rapidly results in anesthetic induction, typically within 1 min (Muir et al 1999). Recumbency cannot always be achieved with tiletamine plus zolazepam after i.m. administration, but the onset of recumbency was reported to be 10 min on average (Matthews 1993). The duration of tiletamine plus zolazepam anesthesia after xylazine or detomidine sedation is in the range of 26–40 min (Cuvelliez et al 1995, Hubbell et al 1989, Muir et al 1999, Wan et al 1992). Tiletamine plus zolazepam provides a longer duration of anesthesia than ketamine in the horse, but the quality of recovery is not as good, with significantly more attempts made to achieve standing postanesthesia (Matthews et al 1991, Muir et al 2000).

Major uses in the horse

Ketamine

Ketamine is used as an i.v. anesthetic in the horse, always after adequate sedation. Ketamine can be used as an anesthetic induction agent, prior to intubation and maintenance with inhalation anesthesia. The typical dose used in the horse for induction of anesthesia is 2.2 mg/kg i.v. xylazine (1.1 mg/kg i.v.) followed by ketamine (2.2 mg/kg i.v.) is the most common anesthetic technique used for short procedures in horses in the field. Sedatives other than xylazine may be used prior to ketamine anesthetic induction, for example detomidine

(0.02 mg/kg) or romifidine (0.1 mg/kg). Total anesthetic time is short and anesthesia can be prolonged by administering one-third to one-half of the original dose of each drug again. To improve the degree of muscle relaxation during ketamine anesthesia, either diazepam (0.05–0.1 mg/kg), butorphanol (0.02–0.04 mg/kg; p. 280) or guaifenesin (50–100 mg/kg; p. 290) can be administered i.v. after sedation and immediately prior to injection of ketamine.

Ketamine can also be used in combination with other agents for maintenance of anesthesia. Xylazine plus ketamine anesthesia can be prolonged by the administration of a mixture of guaifenesin, ketamine and xylazine (G-K-X) by constant rate i.v. infusion. The G-K-X mixture typically consists of 50 mg/ml guaifenesin with 0.5 mg/ml xylazine and 1–2 mg/ml ketamine, although variations using 10% guaifenesin are also used (Greene et al 1986, Lin et al 1994, Young et al 1993). Anesthesia is prolonged by infusion of the G-K-X mixture at 2.75–4.5 ml/kg/h to effect. Anesthesia can also be induced with G-K-X at a dose of 1.1 ml/kg i.v. Detomidine or romifidine can be substituted for xylazine in the G-K-X regimen with satisfactory results. Recovery from ketamine-based anesthesia is considered to be good and superior in quality to recovery from inhalation anesthesia.

Tiletamine

Tiletamine plus zolazepam is primarily used for i.v. induction of anesthesia. Tiletamine plus zolazepam can be used for induction and intubation, with subsequent maintenance of anesthesia with an inhalation agent. The recommended i.v. dose of tiletamine in the tiletamine plus zolazepam combination is 1.1–1.65 mg/kg. After sedation with xylazine (1.1 mg/kg i.v.), detomidine (0.02 mg/kg i.v.) or romifidine (0.1 mg/kg i.v.), tiletamine plus zolazepam can be used to provide field anesthesia of intermediate duration. Tiletamine plus zolazepam can be used, in combination with xylazine and butorphanol or detomidine, as part of an i.m. combination protocol for the capture of feral horses (Matthews 1993).

BARBITURATES

Many barbituric acid derivatives have been formulated since the early 1920s. Only a few remain in regular clinical usage and only one, thiopental, is used with any regularity in equine anesthesia. Thiopental is classified as a thiobarbiturate because there is a sulfur atom on the second carbon of the barbituric acid ring. It is also classified as an ultrashort-acting barbiturate. The presence of the sulfur atom decreases the stability of the molecule and shortens the duration of anesthetic action (Branson & Booth 1995).

Mechanism of action

Barbiturates exert their anesthetic effects via interaction with $GABA_A$ chloride channels in the CNS. Barbiturates bind to a distinct site on the $GABA_A$ receptor called the barbiturate-binding site. They enhance the binding of GABA to its receptor and also increase the amount of time the chloride channel remains open for chloride ion influx (Carvey 1998). In contrast to the benzodiazepines (p. 273), barbiturates can increase $GABA_A$ channel chloride conductance in the absence of the neurotransmitter GABA. Barbiturate interaction with the $GABA_A$ receptor results in hyperpolarization of neurons and depression of neuronal activity.

Pharmacological effects

Barbiturates depress neuronal activity in the CNS. This is accompanied by decreased cerebral metabolic oxygen consumption and decreased cerebral blood flow, since the coupling of blood flow to brain metabolism is preserved with the barbiturates. It also results in a decrease in ICP. Barbiturates depress neuronal activity in the cerebral cortex, thalamus and motor centers. Barbiturates are effective anticonvulsants (see Ch. 9), reduce intraocular pressure, increase the threshold of spinal reflexes and provide excellent muscle relaxation. The barbiturates lack specific analgesic effects and are, therefore, not suitable as the sole anesthetic for invasive procedures.

Barbiturates cause significant centrally mediated respiratory depression and overdose or rapid i.v. administration may cause apnea. Barbiturates decrease the ventilatory response to carbon dioxide, abolishing the response at very deep planes of anesthesia (McDonell 1996). Both tidal volume and respiratory frequency decrease after barbiturate administration. Barbiturates also diminish the sensitivity of the hypoxic drive for ventilation.

Barbiturates are associated with dose-dependent cardiovascular depression. However, because of preservation of the baroreceptor reflex, the hemodynamic response to an induction dose of thiopental is mild. Heart rate generally increases to compensate for a brief fall in arterial blood pressure. As a result of this reflex response, blood pressure remains unchanged and cardiac output may increase slightly with the elevation in heart rate (Ilkiw et al 1991). Without the compensatory heart rate response, or if the change in heart rate is small, a decrease in systemic blood pressure and cardiac output would predominate.

Physicochemical properties of thiopental

Thiopental is a weak acid formulated as a sodium salt that is water soluble at alkaline pH. The pH of sodium thiopental is >10. The extreme alkalinity of thiopental solution can cause significant local tissue damage if the drug is administered into the perivascular region or by the intraarterial route. Following i.v. administration, thiopental dissociates and is present in both its ionized and unionized forms. The pK_a of thiopental is 7.6. At normal physiological pH (7.4), approximately 61% of the administered drug is in the unionized form, which is available to cross the blood–brain barrier and produce CNS effects. Systemic acidosis can increase the proportion of unionized thiopental, resulting in increased delivery of active drug to the brain.

Thiopental is highly lipid soluble in its unionized form and has a very rapid onset of effect after i.v. administration. It also binds to serum albumin and only the unbound drug is available to cross the blood–brain barrier. The extent of protein binding for thiopental is reported to be 65–85% in humans and 74% in dogs. Other drugs, such as non-steroidal anti-inflammatory drugs (NSAIDs) may compete with thiopental for protein binding sites when administered concurrently, increasing the proportion of active thiopental in the plasma; however, whether this would occur at clinically relevant levels of thiopental is questionable (Young et al 1994).

Thiopental is available commercially as a powder for reconstitution just prior to use. The shelf-life of reconstituted thiopental is limited. It is suggested that reconstituted thiopental be kept at room temperature no longer than 3 days before discarding. The solution should be examined before use for turbidity or signs of precipitation and discarded if either of these exists. Reconstituted thiopental can be kept refrigerated for a maximum of 7 days (Haws et al 1998). Because of its alkalinity, thiopental is not susceptible to bacterial contamination. Its limited shelf life is a function of the instability of the compound in solution and loss of efficacy over time. The alkalinity of thiopental makes it incompatible for mixing with certain other drugs. Thiopental can be mixed with guaifenesin or propofol but cannot be mixed with lidocaine. Any drug mixture should always be examined carefully for signs of precipitation. If precipitation occurs, the mixture should be discarded and the drugs administered separately.

Thiopental: bioavailability and route of administration

Thiopental is used only as an i.v. induction agent. Tissue damage, as a result of inadvertent extravascular use, can be significant. The higher the concentration of thiopental in solution, the more likely the tissue is to become necrotic and slough after perivascular administration. In horses, it is not unusual to use concentrations as high as 10% thiopental (100 mg/ml), compared with 2.5% thiopental, which is typically used in small animal practice. If thiopental is accidentally administered perivascularly, the recommendation is to infuse 0.9% sodium chloride into the site of injection to dilute the local concentration of thiopental and to inject 2% lidocaine to provide immediate analgesia.

Thiopental: onset, elimination, duration of effect

Thiopental rapidly induces general anesthesia with recumbency occurring 20–30 s after i.v. bolus administration. Induction with thiopental is not recommended without prior sedation because a brief excitement phase may occur. If no further anesthetic is administered, recovery from a single i.v. bolus of thiopental will take 10 to 30 min in horses. Redistribution of the thiopental from the brain to other body tissues is the primary mechanism for termination of the anesthetic effect. Thiopental undergoes hepatic biotransformation but total body elimination is a very slow process. The elimination half-life of thiopental is 147 min in horses and 222 min in ponies (Abass et al 1994). Total body clearance of thiopental in horses and ponies is 3.5 ml/min per kg. This very slow clearance means that repeated dosing of thiopental can significantly prolong recovery and the use of thiopental by constant rate infusion for maintenance anesthesia is not recommended unless the infusion time is very short (<30 min).

Major uses of thiopental in the horse

Thiopental is used for i.v. anesthetic induction in the horse, usually to precede intubation and maintenance with inhalation anesthetics. It is used at 5–10% in the horse, with the higher concentration allowing for a significant reduction of the volume of injection. Thiopental at these concentrations should only be injected i.v. via a preplaced i.v. catheter, preferably placed in a large vein, such as the jugular vein. Even with these precautions, evidence of jugular thrombophlebitis can be seen at 48 h after the routine administration of guaifenesin and 10% thiopental to horses (Dickson et al 1990).

Anesthetic induction with thiopental alone requires a dose of 10 to 15 mg/kg and this is not recommended. Thiopental induction typically occurs after sedation with an α_2 agonist or acepromazine with or without opioids. Guaifenesin can be used prior to thiopental at 50–100 mg/kg until significant ataxia is evident, followed by bolus administration of thiopental (5–6 mg/kg). Another technique for induction involves adding 5–6 mg/kg thiopental to 5% guaifenesin (1000 ml) or 10% guaifenesin (500 ml) and infusing the mixture until recumbency is achieved. This technique works well if the horse is well restrained but produces a slow, ataxic induction that may be unsuitable in open field conditions.

In the horse, induction with thiopental usually results in a brief increase in heart rate and a decrease in cardiac output but no significant change in arterial blood pressure. Arterial blood pressure is typically lower after thiopental induction than in ketamine-based anesthetic techniques (Bennett et al 1998, Muir et al 2000). However, when horses are placed on inhalation anesthetics for maintenance of anesthesia, the hemodynamic effects of the induction agents is short lived and the hypotension and reduced cardiac output typical of inhalation anesthesia predominates (Bennett et al 1998, Wagner et al 1996). Respiratory depression is significant with an accompanying increase in $PaCO_2$ and decrease in pH.

PROPOFOL

Propofol is a non-barbiturate, i.v. anesthetic that provides rapid-onset, short-duration anesthesia. It is widely used in human and small animal anesthesia. Propofol has not yet reached widespread use in equine anesthesia but a number of investigations into its clinical use have now been reported.

Mechanism of action

Propofol, like thiopental (p. 286) and the benzodiazepines (p. 273), potentiates the effect of GABA on the $GABA_A$ chloride channel. In addition, like thiopental and in contrast to benzodiazepines, propofol activates the $GABA_A$ receptor in the absence of GABA, mediating channel opening and the influx of chloride ions into the cell, thus suppressing neuronal transmission (Carvey 1998). The binding site for propofol appears to be separate from the barbiturate-, GABA- and benzodiazepin-binding sites on the membrane receptor and is putatively located on the β-subunit of the $GABA_A$ chloride channel (Krasowski et al 2001).

Pharmacological effects

Propofol induces rapid CNS depression through the potentiation of the GABA inhibitory system in the brain. Along with a generalized decrease in brain activity, there is a decrease in cerebral blood flow, cerebral perfusion pressure and ICP after propofol administration (Myburgh et al 2002, Trapani et al 2000). Propofol also has an anticonvulsant effect and has been effective for short-term control of refractory seizures in small animals (Heldmann et al 1999, Steffen & Grasmueck 2000). Propofol is not an effective analgesic and, therefore, is not suitable as the sole anesthetic for invasive surgical procedures. Intraocular pressure decreases or remains unchanged during propofol anesthesia (Batista et al 2000, Sator-Katzenschlager et al 2002). In dogs, propofol causes a transient decrease in arterial blood pressure as a result of vasodilatation and the absence of a baroreceptor-mediated reflex increase in heart rate (Bufalari et al 1998, Pagel et al 1998). In the horse, constant rate infusion of propofol is associated with arterial hypotension, although a combination infusion of propofol and ketamine has been shown to maintain cardiovascular parameters well (Flaherty et al 1997). Constant infusion of propofol also maintained arterial blood pressure better than inhalant anesthesia with isoflurane (Deryck et al 1996, Keegan & Greene 1993). Propofol has a direct negative inotropic effect in the dog heart (Pagel et al 1998). Propofol has been shown to enhance epinephrine-induced arrhythmias in halothane-anesthetized dogs (Kamibayashi et al 1991). Propofol is a respiratory depressant; postinduction apnea occurs more frequently in dogs after propofol administration than after thiopental (Murison, 2001). In horses anesthetized with propofol after α_2 agonist sedation, hypercarbia and decreases in PaO_2 are common and supplemental oxygen insufflation is recommended to prevent significant hypoxemia (Mama et al 1996, Bettschart-Wolfensberger et al 2001a).

Physicochemical properties

Propofol is an alkylphenol compound that is highly lipid soluble but water insoluble. Its lipid solubility allows rapid penetration of the blood–brain barrier after i.v. administration, with rapid onset of CNS effects. This physicochemical property also means that rapid redistribution of propofol from the brain to other body tissues plays a significant role in the termination of the anesthetic effect.

The commercially available veterinary preparations are emulsions of propofol in soybean oil, glycerol and egg lecithin. These formulations do not contain preservatives and provide a suitable substrate for bacterial growth, so aseptic technique is recommended when drawing the drug from the vial into a syringe and opened vials should be discarded within 24 h.

Propofol is highly bound to serum proteins (98%); consequently, hypoproteinemic states or the concomitant administration of drugs that compete for protein binding sites may increase the unbound fraction of propofol and increase the clinical effect (Mazoit & Samii 1999).

Onset, elimination, duration of effect

Because of propofol's high lipid solubility, the onset of anesthesia after i.v. administration of propofol is rapid, with recumbency occurring within 24 s (Matthews et al 1999). Excitement at induction or paddling limb movements upon recumbency occur occasionally despite adequate premedication with α_2 agonists (Mama et al 1995, 1996). Recovery from a single dose of propofol (2 mg/kg), after sedation with either xylazine or detomidine, was smooth and recovery times were 25 min with xylazine premedication at 0.5 mg/kg i.v. and 35 min with xylazine premedication at 1.0 mg/kg i.v. (Mama et al 1996). When detomidine was used for premedication, recovery to standing took 41 and 52 min after 0.015 and 0.030 mg/kg, respectively. In foals, the recovery time after xylazine (1.1 mg/kg), butorphanol (0.01 mg/kg) and propofol (2 mg/kg) averaged 12 min.

The pharmacokinetic parameters for propofol in the horse are derived from a study of propofol and ketamine constant rate infusion (Nolan et al 1996). In that study, propofol had an elimination half-life of 69 min in the horse, with a total body clearance of 33 ml/kg/min. The principal site of elimination of propofol is the liver; however, the clearance of propofol exceeds hepatic blood flow, suggesting an extrahepatic site of metabolism (Kuipers et al 1999). In dogs, propofol undergoes biotransformation to 4-hydroxypropofol by cytochrome P450 enzymes (Court et al 1999).

Major uses in the horse

Propofol is being examined for its potential as a routine i.v. induction agent in the horse, as well as a component of TIVA, as an alternative to maintenance of anesthesia with inhalant agents. Propofol has not been adopted for widespread use in equine anesthesia yet and cost plays a role currently.

Propofol is effective as an anesthetic induction agent in foals and has been used to maintain anesthesia during diagnostic procedures such as magnetic resonance imaging (Chaffin et al 1997). The recommended dose for propofol induction in the foal is 2 mg/kg i.v., given after xylazine (0.5 mg/kg) with or without butorphanol (0.01 mg/kg) as premedication. Constant rate infusion of propofol (0.26–0.47 mg/kg/min) can be used to maintain anesthesia in the foal for non-invasive procedures.

In adult horses, propofol induction is undesirable without prior sedation (Mama et al 1995). Even with an adequate level of sedation provided by an α_2 agonist, induction with propofol is not always smooth. The incorporation of guaifenesin in the induction protocol prior to administration of propofol markedly improves the quality of anesthetic induction (Aguiar et al 1993). Recoveries from propofol-based anesthesia are generally good. The dose rate recommended for anesthetic induction with propofol is 2 mg/kg i.v. after premedication with xylazine (0.5 mg/kg i.v.) or detomidine (0.015 mg/kg) followed by administration of guaifenesin (50–100 mg/kg i.v.) until muscle relaxation and ataxia are evident. Maintenance of anesthesia in adult horses with propofol infusion (0.2 mg/kg/min) is useful for relatively non-invasive procedures, although significant respiratory depression occurs and may be exacerbated by positioning in dorsal recumbency (Matthews et al 1999). Propofol has also been combined with medetomidine (0.0035 mg/kg/min) or ketamine (0.04 mg/kg/min) for anesthetic maintenance by constant infusion (Bettschart-Wolfensberger et al 2001b, Flaherty et al 1997).

GUAIFENESIN

The centrally acting muscle relaxant guaifenesin is discussed further in Chapter 8.

INHALATION ANESTHETIC AGENTS

Mechanism of action

Despite more than 100 years of medical use, the mechanism of action of inhalation anesthetics is not well understood. Early theories of mechanism were based on the fact that anesthetic potency was highly correlated to an inhalation agent's lipid solubility. Consequently, it was believed that inhalation agents dissolved in the lipid bilayer of the cell membrane, increasing membrane fluidity and non-specifically disrupting the normal function of membrane proteins such as ion channels (Ueda & Suzuki 1998). Increasing evidence now suggests that, rather than a non-specific cell membrane effect, there may in fact be relatively specific sites of action at cell and tissue level for

inhalation anesthetic agents (Ueda & Suzuki 1998). In certain sites in the brain, inhalation anesthetics alter neuronal firing selectively rather than globally (Angel 1993). Certain inhalation agents show stereoselectivity, which implies a specific protein binding site (Hall et al 1994). It is also possible to demonstrate inhalant anesthetic binding to ligand-gated ion channels and inhalant-induced increases in chloride conductance in channels such as the $GABA_A$ receptor complex (Franks & Lieb 1998). Whether these actions have relevance in producing general anesthesia in animals remains to be determined Inhalant agents also have actions on neural transmission. For example, nitrous oxide has been shown to activate inhibitory (GABA) pathways in the spinal cord (Hashimoto et al 2001).

Physicochemical properties

Inhalation anesthetic agents are small, highly lipophilic molecules that cross the alveolar–capillary membrane and the blood–brain barrier quite rapidly. The onset of anesthesia and drug elimination are markedly influenced by the physicochemical properties of each agent. With the exception of nitrous oxide, which is commercially available as a gas stored in cylinders at a pressure of 50 atmospheres, the inhalation agents are all volatile liquids that vaporize at room temperature. The degree of vaporization is a function of the vapor pressure of the agent, an index of drug volatility. All of the modern inhalation agents, halothane, isoflurane, sevoflurane and desflurane, are highly volatile (Table 15.1). At room temperature (20°C), these agents can vaporize to concentrations that are 15–30 times

Table 15.1 Properties of the inhalation anesthetic agents

Agent	Vapor pressure at 20°C (mmHg)	Maximum concentration at 20°C (%)	Blood:gas partition coefficient	Minimum alveolar concentration in the horse (%)	Percentage of agent recovered as metabolite (%)
Halothane	244	32	2.5	0.88	16–20
Isoflurane	240	31	1.4	1.31	0.2
Sevoflurane	160	21	0.7	2.31	3
Desflurane	664	87	0.4	7.6	0.02

their anesthetic dose, which could be rapidly lethal to an animal. Inhalation agent vaporization is also influenced by ambient temperature; as temperature rises a much higher concentration of the agent can be achieved. As a result of this volatility, agent-specific vaporizers, adjusted for the vapor pressure of the drug and able to compensate for temperature, are used to administer inhalation agents so that the delivery of anesthetic can be controlled more precisely. Desflurane has a very high vapor pressure and its boiling point is 22.8°C, which means that liquid desflurane will boil in a warm room (Eger 1994). As a result, clinical delivery of desflurane requires an even more specialized vaporizer than those used for other inhalation agents. Desflurane vaporizers have an electrically heated chamber that converts liquid anesthetic to gas and meters this vapor into the diluent fresh gas flow (Eger 1994). These vaporizers are much more expensive than conventional agent-specific vaporizers and are not yet in widespread use in veterinary medicine.

Inhalation agents are inhaled as gases; therefore, it is necessary to discuss their anesthetic activity in relation to partial pressure rather than just concentration. Partial pressure is sometimes described as the tendency for a gas to leave its current medium. Gas molecules move from one phase to another down a partial pressure gradient. The partial pressure of a gas is equal between the two phases at equilibrium. In the gaseous phase, the partial pressure of gas is its percentage concentration multiplied by the total atmospheric pressure. However, in either liquid or tissue phase, a particular partial pressure of gas may represent markedly different concentrations in the liquid or tissue, depending on the solubility of the gas in that phase. Blood:gas partition coefficients represent the ratio between the concentration of a gas in blood versus that in the alveoli at equilibrium (Eger 1974). It is an index of an inhalation agent's relative solubility in blood (Table 15.1). Higher blood:gas partition coefficients represent inhalation agents that are more soluble in blood. Intuitively, it might follow that an agent that is highly soluble in the blood would be taken up from the alveoli rapidly and result in a rapid onset of anesthesia; however, the opposite

is true. Inhalation anesthetics enter the blood and exist in solution as unbound drug in the aqueous phase, which is in equilibrium with drug bound to blood components, such as red blood cells and protein (Carvey 1998). Only the unbound drug in the aqueous phase is free to diffuse from the arterial blood into the brain. Agents with high blood:gas partition coefficients have a greater tendency to bind to blood components and more anesthetic must enter the blood in order for the partial pressure to rise to the point at which the drug will diffuse from the blood into the brain. Based on the blood:gas partition coefficients of these commonly used agents, the onset of anesthesia would be most rapid with desflurane, followed by sevoflurane, isoflurane then halothane.

Pharmacological effects

All of the volatile anesthetics are dose-dependent CNS depressants. They produce unconsciousness, muscle relaxation, analgesia, respiratory depression and cardiovascular depression to varying degrees depending on the particular agent. The depth of anesthesia varies directly with the partial pressure of the inhalation agent in the brain. Because of the significant degree of respiratory and cardiovascular depression, all of these drugs have a very narrow margin of safety, with therapeutic indices ranging from two to four (Carvey 1998). Therefore, inhalation agents are considered some of the most dangerous drugs used commonly in veterinary medicine.

The potency of inhalation agents can be compared using their respective MAC values. The MAC is the minimum alveolar concentration of an inhalation anesthetic (percentage concentration at sea level) that would prevent movement in response to a surgical incision in 50% of subjects. At equilibrium, the concentration of the inhalation agent in the pulmonary alveoli correlates well with the partial pressure of the anesthetic in the brain, while the inspired concentration of the anesthetic and the concentration of the anesthetic in the blood do not correlate well with brain partial pressure. In order to achieve surgical anesthesia for most subjects, one needs to achieve an alveolar concentration of 1.2–1.5 times the MAC for that agent (Table 15.1). MAC is a useful value for comparing anesthetic potency; in part because it is remarkably consistent among individuals of the same species. In addition, it is clinically applicable and altered by few patient characteristics, only extremes of age, body temperature, thyroid function and pregnancy.

Halothane

Halothane is the most potent of the inhalation agents used currently in horses. A great deal of information on the effects of general anesthesia in the horse has been obtained over the years from studies of halothane. Halothane causes significant dose-dependent depression of cardiovascular function (Steffey & Howland 1978a, 1980). Halothane anesthesia may decrease cardiac output by up to 50% of the value when awake (Gasthuys et al 1991, Mizuno et al 1994, Purchase 1966). The decreased cardiac output is accompanied by a decrease in stroke volume and arterial blood pressure without a significant change in total peripheral resistance (Raisis et al 2000). Although there is a significant depression of hemodynamics upon induction of halothane anesthesia, during prolonged periods of halothane anesthesia (>5 h) cardiovascular parameters (cardiac output and arterial blood pressure) gradually improve as a result of decreasing total peripheral resistance and increasing stroke volume (Steffey et al 1987b). Halothane is a potent myocardial depressant; administration of the inotropic agent dobutamine (1–5 μg/kg/min; see Ch. 12) or ephedrine (0.06 mg/kg) to horses can counteract this effect, resulting in improved stroke volume, cardiac output and mean arterial blood pressure (Gasthuys et al 1991, Grandy et al 1989). Halothane sensitizes the myocardium to catecholamine-induced arrhythmias, most notably premature ventricular extrasystoles (Purchase 1966). Some agents administered commonly in combination with inhalation anesthetic agents increase (e.g. xylazine, thiopental) or decrease (e.g. acepromazine, lidocaine) the arrhythmogenicity of halothane. Skeletal muscle,

liver and renal blood flow are reduced during halothane anesthesia as a result of the overall decrease in cardiac output.

Halothane causes dose-dependent respiratory depression in the horse (Whitehair et al 1993). Minute ventilation decreases during halothane anesthesia, mainly as a result of decreased tidal volume; however, at deeper planes of anesthesia, respiratory rate decreases as well. Respiratory effort ceases entirely at approximately 2.6 times the MAC of halothane in the absence of other depressant drugs (Steffey et al 1977). Elevations in $PaCO_2$ as a result of halothane anesthesia may diminish halothane-induced cardiovascular depression (Wagner et al 1990). However, the presence of hypercapnia lowers the arrhythmogenic dose of epinephrine (adrenaline) in the halothane-anesthetized horse (Gaynor et al 1993). An increased $PaCO_2$ during halothane anesthesia is associated with higher plasma levels of epinephrine (adrenaline) and norepinephrine (noradrenaline); and $PaCO_2$ augmentation of cardiovascular parameters is prevented by the prior administration of propranolol, suggesting that carbon dioxide acts as a sympathetic nervous system stimulant (Wagner et al 1990). Elevations in $PaCO_2$ during halothane anesthesia result in increased cerebrospinal fluid pressure (Cullen et al 1990). Halothane increases cerebral blood flow more than isoflurane, contraindicating the use of halothane in animals with elevated ICP.

Halothane provides skeletal muscle relaxation and potentiates the action of neuromuscular blocking agents. Halothane has been reported to trigger a malignant hyperthermia-like reaction in horses infrequently, often in association with the use of the depolarizing neuromuscular blocking agent succinylcholine (suxamethonium) (Hildebrand & Howitt 1983, Hildebrand et al 1990, Klein et al 1989, Manley et al 1983, Riedesel & Hildebrand 1985, Waldron-Mease et al 1981). The signs associated with the malignant hyperthermia-like reactions included hyperthermia, sweating, tachypnea, increased $PaCO_2$, hypertension and postanesthetic myopathy (see Ch. 8). However a positive halothane–caffeine contracture test, diagnostic of malignant hyperthermia in swine and humans, has been found only in a few of these horses, so the exact etiology of this syndrome in horses has not been determined.

Isoflurane

Like halothane, isoflurane causes dose-dependent depression of cardiovascular function during anesthesia. At 1.2 times the MAC, isoflurane lowers the systemic arterial pressure and stroke volume but does not significantly change heart rate or decrease cardiac output compared with the values in awake animals (Steffey et al 1987b). A significant reduction in cardiac output and systemic blood pressure is seen at 1.55 times the MAC with no change in heart rate compared with unanesthetized horses (Manohar et al 1987). Despite this cardiovascular depression, the cardiac index is higher in horses anesthetized with isoflurane than with halothane anesthesia (Raisis et al 2000, Whitehair et al 1996). Cardiac contractility is significantly better during isoflurane than during halothane anesthesia (Raisis et al 2000). Isoflurane is associated with better aortic flow indices and higher arterial and venous flow in the femoral arteries (Raisis et al 2000). Isoflurane anesthesia results in better oxygen delivery to tissues with a significantly lower oxygen extraction ratio than halothane (Branson et al 1992).

Isoflurane is a potent respiratory depressant, causing a dose-dependent decrease in respiratory rate and minute ventilation and an increase in $PaCO_2$ (Steffey et al 1987a). The respiratory depression produced by isoflurane is significantly greater in magnitude than that caused by halothane (Whitehair et al 1993).

Isoflurane has a lower blood:gas partition coefficient than halothane, so more rapid induction and recovery would be anticipated. A number of studies have tried to compare the speed and quality of recovery from isoflurane and halothane, with variable results. In clinical cases undergoing either halothane or isoflurane maintenance anesthesia, more rapid recovery from isoflurane was not evident but coordination at the time of recovery was judged to be significantly worse in horses anesthetized with isoflurane than with halothane (Bramlage et al 1993). Another study examined the recovery from halothane and isoflurane anesthesia

in equines undergoing surgery and non-surgical anesthetic events. No significant difference in the quality of recovery or the number of attempts to stand could be demonstrated. Early indicators of recovery, such as the time to first movement and to sternal recumbency, were shorter in the animals anesthetized with isoflurane than in those given halothane. However, the time to standing was significantly shorter only in the non-surgical cases anesthetized with isoflurane (Matthews et al 1992). A controlled study, in horses given no other drugs, compared the recovery from 1 h halothane anesthesia with recovery from 3 h of either halothane or isoflurane anesthesia (Whitehair et al 1993). This study did not reveal a significant difference in the standing time, quality of recovery or the number of attempts to stand. The authors reported large interindividual variation and preanesthetic temperament was the only factor that influenced the nature of recovery significantly (Whitehair et al 1993). An 8-year clinical study of the quality of recovery in 99 horses undergoing arthroscopy with either halothane or isoflurane as maintenance anesthesia indicated that recovery times were significantly shorter with isoflurane (Donaldson et al 2000). The scores for the quality of recovery were lower in isoflurane-anesthetized horses (Donaldson et al 2000). A better quality of recovery was highly correlated with a longer recovery time. Interestingly, on average, halothane-anesthetized horses were maintained under anesthesia at a higher multiple of MAC, were at a higher multiple of MAC at the end of surgery, had longer total MAC-hours of anesthesia and received intraoperative supplemental ketamine more often, all of which may have contributed to the longer recovery times (Donaldson et al 2000).

Sevoflurane

Sevoflurane is a relatively new inhalation anesthetic in veterinary medicine. It has a low solubility in the blood. With a blood:gas partition coefficient that is half that of isoflurane, sevoflurane should produce a more rapid induction, allow rapid change of anesthetic plane during surgery and result in a more rapid recovery in horses (Aida et al 1996). In one study in horses, mask induction followed by 2.5–3 h sevoflurane anesthesia resulted in an average time to standing of 8 min (Aida et al 1996). Recovery after 90 min of isoflurane or sevoflurane anesthesia (1.2 times the MAC) was characterized by a significant decrease in the time to standing for horses anesthetized with sevoflurane (13.9 min) compared with isoflurane (17.4 min) or sevoflurane-anesthetized horses given xylazine (0.1 mg/kg i.v.) prior to recovery (18.0 min) (Matthews et al 1998). Another study reported no significant difference in the recovery times between isoflurane and sevoflurane (1.5 times MAC for 90 min), while halothane was associated with statistically longer recovery times (Grosenbaugh & Muir 1998). Administration of xylazine to horses prior to recovery tended to equalize the recovery times for all three inhalation agents (Grosenbaugh & Muir 1998). The quality of recovery was consistently shown to be significantly better in sevoflurane-anesthetized horses than in either isoflurane- or halothane-anesthetized horses (Grosenbaugh & Muir 1998, Matthews et al 1998).

In the horse, the cardiovascular and respiratory effects of sevoflurane are equivalent to those of isoflurane (Aida et al 1996, Grosenbaugh & Muir 1998, Matthews et al 1998). Sevoflurane is associated with a decrease in cardiac output, blood pressure, contractility and systemic vascular resistance without a significant change in heart rate (Grosenbaugh & Muir 1998). The decreases in cardiac output and blood pressure are equivalent to those produced by isoflurane and significantly less than those produced by halothane (Grosenbaugh & Muir 1998). Sevoflurane decreases the respiratory rate and increases the $PaCO_2$ in a manner similar to isoflurane and is associated with significantly greater respiratory depression than halothane (Grosenbaugh & Muir 1998).

Desflurane

Desflurane has the lowest blood:gas partition coefficient of all of the modern inhalation anesthetic agents. Rapid onset of anesthesia and short recovery times are associated with its use in horses (Tendillo et al 1997). Mask induction with desflurane in unsedated horses (vaporizer setting 18%, 10 l/min oxygen flow rate) resulted in lateral recumbency in approximately 6 min; after approximately 98 min of anesthesia, the time to standing was 14 min on average, with the quality of recovery reported to be good to excellent in all of the horses (Tendillo et al 1997). The authors did not comment on the ease of desflurane mask induction in horses. However, desflurane is pungent and in humans is considered irritating at high inspired concentrations, producing coughing, breath holding and laryngospasm in some patients during mask induction (Smiley 1992).

In ponies, desflurane (MAC) caused a decrease in arterial blood pressure and systemic vascular resistance while heart rate and cardiac index were not changed significantly (Clarke et al 1996). Increasing the concentration of desflurane to 1.3 times MAC resulted in further depression of the arterial blood pressure and a significant decrease in the cardiac index, attributed to the onset of cardiac depression at higher concentrations (Clarke et al 1996). Desflurane also results in respiratory depression; there is a significant increase in $PaCO_2$ at MAC (Clarke et al 1996). In other species, the cardiopulmonary effects of desflurane are considered to be approximately equal to those of isoflurane, but a direct comparison of desflurane and other inhalation anesthetics has not yet been carried out in the horse.

Nitrous oxide

Nitrous oxide (laughing gas) has been used as an inhalant anesthetic since 1844 and is still widely used in human anesthesia because of its potent analgesic actions. Although it has many desirable properties, including rapid onset and recovery, limited cardiopulmonary depression and minimal toxicity, it is a weak anesthetic. Its lack of potency, its relatively high cost and its possible contribution to hypoxia and accumulation in gas-filled spaces limits its use in the horse.

Nitrous oxide is highly insoluble in lipids and has a very low anesthetic potency. The nitrous oxide MAC in the horse is nearly 205% (Steffey & Howland 1978b) compared with 100% in humans. In addition, the use of nitrous oxide requires a higher fresh gas flow rate than when using oxygen alone. Accordingly the total amount of the primary anesthetic that is vaporized is increased, further increasing the cost. Like desflurane, nitrous oxide has a very low solubility in blood (blood:gas solubility 0.47) and tissues resulting in a rapid induction and recovery. In fact, induction of unconsciousness using nitrous oxide alone is impossible in most animal species. This low solubility can, however, be exploited during anesthesia, where nitrous oxide enhances the uptake of other inhalation agents and is, therefore, used to facilitate the induction and rate of change in anesthetic depth: the *second gas effect*. In other words, the presence of nitrous oxide causes the other inhalation agent to reach a desirable blood concentration more rapidly than when used alone and induction of anesthesia is more rapid.

Nitrous oxide is particularly useful in conjunction with other inhalant agents since it has minimal effects on the respiratory and circulatory systems. Of all the inhalant agents, it produces the least respiratory depression and little myocardial depression, little reduction in cardiac output and little reduction in systemic vascular resistance. It does, however, stimulate the sympathetic nervous system, which may counteract some of the cardiovascular depression induced by other anesthetic agents administered concurrently. The addition of nitrous oxide to the anesthetic regimen for horses allows the concentration of other inhalation agents used to be reduced (e.g. by 25%; Steffey & Howland 1978b), thus reducing the degree of depression at a particular depth of anesthesia. However, more recently it was shown in horses that concentrations of nitrous oxide of greater than 25% had no effect on the amount of halothane required or on cardiovascular and respiratory parameters compared with halothane alone (Testa et al 1990).

Nitrous oxide is used in high concentrations because of its low potency; therefore, the inspired oxygen concentration is reduced proportionally. This makes nitrous oxide unsuitable for animals with pulmonary disease, which may require as much as 100% inspired oxygen to maintain acceptable blood oxygenation. The lowest concentration of oxygen in inspired air during inhalation anesthesia should be 33%.

Nitrous oxide is 20–30 times more soluble in blood or tissues than nitrogen. It diffuses rapidly into closed gas cavities within the body at a faster rate than nitrogen diffuses out, resulting in an increase in either volume or pressure. When nitrous oxide administration is stopped, its uptake is reversed and it moves from the blood to the alveoli. During the initial period after discontinuing nitrous oxide, the volume moving into the lung is large and dilutes the oxygen in the alveoli. If breathing room air (21% oxygen), this may result in hypoxia. To prevent this diffusion (dilutional) hypoxia occurring, 100% oxygen must be administered during the first 5–10 min after stopping nitrous oxide administration. Similarly, any air bubbles within the body will be greatly expanded from diffusion of nitrous oxide into them. This enhances hypoxia-related problems in animals with gastric or intestinal distension or pneumothorax. In fact, the use of nitrous oxide is contraindicated in animals with pneumothorax, pneumoperitoneum or intestinal obstruction with gaseous distension. Nitrous oxide has also been shown to increase the volume of naturally produced intestinal gas in normal, anesthetized ponies (Steffey et al 1979).

Route of administration and onset of effect

Inhalation anesthetic agents enter and leave the body via the lungs. Controlling the amount of an inhalation agent that reaches its site of action (the brain) is a function of regulating the partial pressure of the inhalation agent in the alveoli, which in turn regulates the partial pressure of the inhalation agent in the blood. The first step in this process is controlling the inspired concentration of the anesthetic agent that is delivered by an agent-specific vaporizer. With delivery of an adequate inspired concentration of anesthetic, the solubility of the inhalation agent in the blood is the most important determinant of the speed of onset of the anesthetic effect. In addition to this physicochemical property of the inhalation agent, physiological factors in the animal being anesthetized also influence the onset and elimination of these agents. The two physiological factors that influence the speed of induction are alveolar ventilation and cardiac output. Because onset and recovery from anesthesia mirror the change in the alveolar partial pressure of an inhalation anesthetic agent, ventilation is extremely important in determining the delivery or removal of an anesthetic to and from the alveoli. The rate of increase of alveolar partial pressure that results from ventilation is offset by the uptake of the agent from alveoli into the blood. Cardiac output determines the amount of blood moving through the pulmonary capillaries with time. Higher cardiac outputs result in greater pulmonary blood flow and, therefore, greater uptake of inhalation agent into the arterial blood. This slows the increase in alveolar partial pressure, which partially explains why inhalation anesthesia is more difficult to induce in an excited animal.

Elimination and duration of effect

The primary route of elimination for the inhalation anesthetics is through the lungs. Drug metabolism is insignificant for most modern inhalation agents with respect to the termination of their effects. Drug metabolism may, however, play a role in the potential toxicity of an inhalation agent. Inhalation agents can undergo metabolism by cytochrome P450 enzymes in hepatocytes. The extent of hepatic metabolism differs between the agents and is a function of both the relative lipid solubility of the drug and its inherent chemical stability (Table 15.1). Halothane undergoes the greatest degree of hepatic metabolism; in humans 20–25% of an inhaled dose of halothane is recovered as drug metabolites. Halothane has relatively high lipid solubility so there is greater uptake of the drug into the body and residual halothane diffuses slowly out of the tissues at the end of anesthesia. Although a large percentage of halothane is eliminated via the lungs, halothane remains in the body for a longer period of time than agents with a lower solubility and the liver, therefore, has more opportunity to biodegrade this drug. The biodegradation of halothane does not produce an appreciable amount of fluoride ion; chlorine, bromine and trifluoroacetic acid are released. The incidence of hepatitis is low in human patients exposed repeatedly to halothane anesthesia in a short period. The mechanism of hepatic damage is not completely understood but is attributed to a reactive intermediate metabolite, which may bind to cellular proteins or phospholipids eliciting an immune-mediated response against hepatocytes, resulting in hepatic necrosis (Pumford et al 1997). There are no reports of halothane-induced hepatic necrosis in horses. Three consecutive days of short-duration halothane anesthesia did not result in significant changes in liver enzymes or liver histopathology in horses (Stover et al 1988). Halothane anesthesia for 2 h did not impair liver function or biliary excretion during anesthesia (Engelking et al 1984). However, prolonged halothane anesthesia (>12 h) resulted in significantly increased serum bilirubin, aspartate aminotransferase, alkaline phosphatase and L-iditol dehydrogenase values for up to 9 days after anesthesia (Steffey et al 1993).

The fluoride ion is a potent inhibitor of renal metabolic processes and is the cause of the renal toxicity produced by the inhalation agent methoxyflurane. None of the inhalation agents used currently in equine practice are likely to produce direct nephrotoxicity via the inorganic fluoride ion. Isoflurane can be metabolized to produce fluoride ions, but the low blood solubility of isoflurane results in its rapid elimination via the lungs. Only approximately 0.2% of the isoflurane taken up during anesthesia undergoes biotransformation and no appreciable levels of fluoride ion accumulate in the renal tubules. Sevoflurane also has very low blood solubility but it is less biologically stable than isoflurane and undergoes a much greater degree of biotransformation, approximately 3%, with the fluoride ion released as a byproduct. Prolonged sevoflurane anesthesia in humans results in fluoride accumulation to levels that are generally thought to produce nephrotoxicity. However, no clinically significant changes in renal function have been correlated with these increased fluoride ion concentrations (Mazze et al 2000). In addition to the production of the fluoride ion, sevoflurane also decomposes in the carbon dioxide absorbent of a circle system to produce the nephrotoxic substance fluoromethyl-2,2-difluoro-1-(trifluoromethyl)vinyl ether (compound A). Compound A can accumulate to high concentrations in a circle system. The production of compound A during anesthesia is enhanced by high sevoflurane concentrations, when barium hydroxide is used instead of soda lime, when the absorbent is dry, when low fresh gas flows are used, at higher absorbent temperatures or with higher carbon dioxide production (Bito & Ikeda 1995). In dogs anesthetized with sevoflurane using an in-circle vaporizer, low oxygen flow rates have been shown to result in an increased accumulation of compound A in a circle system (Muir & Gadawski 1998). Despite the demonstration of significant accumulation of compound A, sevoflurane has not been shown to be a cause of significant renal dysfunction in humans (Obata et al 2000). Although little evidence of renal impairment exists under the usual clinical circumstances, it may be wise to avoid low oxygen flow rates ($<15\,ml/kg/min$) when using sevoflurane in horses with an underlying renal disorder or undergoing prolonged anesthesia. Desflurane has very low solubility and very high biological stability and is, therefore, resistant to degradation by the liver, with only 0.02% of an inhaled dose undergoing metabolism. Nitrous oxide has little or no effect on hepatic or renal function and is eliminated by exhalation. Minimal metabolism of nitrous oxide (0.004%) takes place by intestinal bacteria such as *Escherichia coli* (Drummond & Matthews 1994). Prolonged and repeated exposure to nitrous oxide has been reported to cause neurological disease and pernicious anemia (Stimpfel & Gershey 1991). Unnecessary exposure of personnel to gases from volatile anesthetics must be avoided by use of appropriate scavenger systems.

Major uses in the horse

In horses, the inhalation anesthetics are used solely for general anesthesia. They are almost always delivered using a precision vaporizer with oxygen as the carrier gas. Inhalation agents are then administered via a breathing circuit into the equine respiratory system typically using an endotracheal tube.

LOCAL ANESTHETIC AGENTS

Local anesthesia is used commonly in equine practice, often in combination with other agents such as opioid analgesics (p. 276) or α_2 agonists

(p. 268) (Stashak 1987). An understanding of the pharmacology of local anesthesia is important for selection of a local anesthetic for use in the equine (Day & Skarda 1991).

Mechanism of action

Local anesthetics prevent the voltage-dependent increase in sodium ion conductance and thus block the initiation and propagation of action potentials. This occurs via two mechanisms. Firstly, non-specific activity on the membrane surface causes the membrane to swell, physically preventing sodium ions getting through the membrane pores. Secondly, blockade of sodium channels occurs.

Pharmacological effects

Local anesthetics are used in the clinical situation to interrupt the nociceptive process at one or more points between the peripheral, high-threshold nociceptor and the cerebral cortex, by blocking transduction; by infiltration at the site of injury or incision; by preventing transmission in afferent myelinated A δ and unmyelinated C fibers; by blockade of peripheral nerves or nerve plexuses or by epidural injection.

Local anesthetics do not act selectively on pain fibers; following a nerve block, sensation is lost in the following order: pain, cold, warmth, touch and pressure. In fact, local anesthetics depress all excitable cells (e.g. cardiac muscle cells) and this, in part, explains some of their undesired effects.

Local tissue reactions, including inflammation and necrosis, can occur, particularly if local anesthetic formulations containing epinephrine (adrenaline) have been administered. Allergic reactions can also occur and are most commonly associated with the esters (e.g. procaine, see Ch. 2). Neurotoxicity is rare but may occur when 200 ml or more of a local anesthetic is administered by infiltration in a short period. It is more likely that a horse will become ataxic, which can lead to self-trauma, after nerve blockade in the limbs, and severe hindlimb ataxia can follow the caudal epidural administration of lidocaine to horses (Le Blanc et al 1988).

Systemic reactions often occur as a result of inadvertent intravascular injection or overdosage and systemic absorption. CNS toxicity is dose dependent and ranges from depression (sedation) to excitation, muscle twitching and convulsions. This most commonly occurs following administration in areas with large blood vessels (e.g. with epidural administration) and usually occurs before cardiovascular toxicity. High doses produce generalized CNS depression and an isoelectric electroencephalogram (EEG).

Cardiovascular reactions include bradycardia and/or conduction disturbances, myocardial depression and peripheral vasodilatation resulting in hypotension, as a result of direct effects on the myocardium and blood vessels. In extreme cases, cardiovascular collapse (cardiac arrest) may result from decreased ventricular contractility, decreased myocardial conduction and loss of peripheral vasomotor tone.

If undesired effects are noted in time, seizure activity can be treated with benzodiazepines or thiobarbiturates (see Ch. 9) and cardiovascular collapse can be treated symptomatically (volume expansion, adrenergic agonists, oxygen, sodium bicarbonate; see Ch. 12).

Physicochemical properties

Each local anesthetic molecule has three general areas: a lipophilic portion containing an aromatic ring, an intermediate chain and a hydrophilic amine functionality. The structure–activity relationships for local anesthetics can be described in terms of structural modifications to each of these three areas. Depending on the structure of the intermediate chain, local anesthetics are classified as either esters or amides.

Route of administration

Local anesthetics are effective when applied to mucous membranes or to the cornea (see Ch. 13) but, with the exception of EMLA cream (a mixture of 2.5% prilocaine and 2.5% lidocaine), are ineffective when applied to intact skin. Common administration techniques in the horse include perineural infiltration (nerve block), field block (ring block), direct infiltration, or intrasynovial anesthesia (Stashak 1987; see Ch. 7). The volume injected depends on the joint size (coffin joint 6 ml, stifle joint 50 ml), but in practice the smallest volume possible should be administered (Le Blanc 1992, Stashak 1987). Caudal epidural anesthesia is useful for procedures that require analgesia of the tail, perineal skin, anus, rectum, vulva and vagina (Le Blanc 1992). It is important that the horse is adequately restrained and that the site is properly and aseptically prepared.

Onset, elimination and duration of effect

The physicochemical properties of a local anesthetic agent determine the onset, potency and duration of action (Table 15.2). The acidic dissociation constant (pK_a) determines the rate of onset of action of a local anesthetic. Local anesthetics are weak bases with pK_a values in the range 7.7–9.0. This means that at physiological pH they are mostly ionized (positively charged, active). However, to reach their site of action on the inner side of the ion channel they need to be unionized. For the quaternary ammonium compounds, the sodium channel must be open for the block to take place, but the tertiary ammonium compounds (e.g. lidocaine) can block the channel when it is not open by diffusing through the membrane. An agent's lipid solubility (oil/water partition coefficient) determines its intrinsic potency since more lipid-soluble agents are better able to cross the nerve cell membrane. Local anesthetics with a higher degree of protein binding have a longer duration of action.

The activity of the local anesthetics is enhanced by increased extraneuronal pH and by coadministration of a vasoconstrictor (e.g. epinephrine (adrenaline)) or hyaluronidase. Sodium channel blockade is pH dependent, increasing when the pH is alkaline, and can be reduced in disease conditions associated with acid pH (e.g. inflammation). The addition of bicarbonate (e.g. to lidocaine) speeds up the onset and prolongs the duration of action. If bicarbonate is added to

Table 15.2 Features of some local anesthetic agents used in the horse

Agent	pK_a	Onset	Potency	Tissue penetration	Duration
Procaine	8.9	Moderate	Low	Slow	Short
Lidocaine (lignocaine)	7.8	Rapid: 4 min[a]	Intermediate	Rapid	Medium: 60–150 min[b]
Mepivacaine	7.7	Rapid: 5–10 min[c]	Intermediate	Rapid	Medium: 68–210 min[d]
Bupivacaine	8.16	Moderate	High	Moderate	Long
Ropivacaine	8.16	Moderate	High	Moderate	Long

[a] Grubb et al 1992
[b] Perineural infiltration around 60 min (Kristinsson et al 1996); caudal epidural 90–150 min (Fikes et al 1989, Grubb et al 1992, Le Blanc et al 1988)
[c] Skarda and Muir 1982, Skarda et al 1984
[d] Subarachnoidal around 68 min (Skarda & Muir 1982, Skarda et al 1984); caudal epidural 80.0 ± 11.5 min (Skarda et al 1984); infiltration around palmar and metacarpal nerves 210 min (Kamerling et al 1984)

a local anesthetic, these solutions should always be made up freshly and used within 30 min of preparation.

The ester-linked agents, such as procaine (see Ch. 2), are readily hydrolyzed in the blood by plasma cholinesterases and have half-lives measured in minutes; they are no longer widely used as local anesthetics. The amides (e.g. lidocaine, mepivacaine, bupivacaine and ropivacaine) undergo hepatic metabolism and have half-lives measured in hours. Local anesthetics and/or their metabolites can be readily detected in equine urine, in some cases for prolonged periods (Kamerling 1993). Although approved in the USA for use in horses in training by the American Association of Equine Practitioners (AAEP), local anesthetics (e.g. lidocaine, mepivacaine, bupivacaine) are also classified as a Class 2 foreign substance by the Association of Racing Commissioners International (ARCI) and their detection in urine samples can result in significant penalties (Dirikolu et al 2000, Harkins et al 1998, 1999a,b).

Major uses in the horse

Lidocaine (lignocaine)

Lidocaine (lignocaine) is an amide local anesthetic that is approved (2% solution, 20 mg/ml) for use in horses. This agent is also used widely in humans and is available as 1% and 2% solutions also in combination with epinephrine (adrenaline) at a concentration of 1 in 200 000.

Following abaxial sessamoid administration or perineural infiltration (forelimb) in horses, lidocaine was rapidly absorbed into the systemic circulation, with peak concentrations reached after 20–30 min (Harkins et al 1998, Kristinsson et al 1996). After hepatic metabolism, lidocaine is excreted in urine as 3-hydroxylidocaine glucuronide (Dirikolu et al 2000), with peak urine concentrations occurring around 60 min after injection. The terminal half-life of lidocaine, following perineural administration to horses, was 48 min (Kristinsson et al 1996). Lidocaine has a rapid onset and medium duration of action in horses (Table 15.2). For a prolonged duration of action (200 min) following caudal epidural injection, lidocaine can be administered in combination with the α_2 agonist xylazine (Grubb et al 1992; see p. 268).

Lidocaine is used in cardiovascular medicine for its antiarrhythmic properties (see Ch. 12). More recently, studies have looked at the i.v. administration of lidocaine to horses with colic (see Ch. 6). It appears that i.v. lidocaine (without epinephrine (adrenaline)) may have some desirable effects on jejunal distension and peritoneal fluid accumulation and is well-tolerated perioperatively in horses with colic (Brianceau et al 2002). In addition, i.v. lidocaine reduced the halothane MAC significantly (Doherty & Frazier 1998) in ponies.

Toxic effects of lidocaine may be seen in horses if it is administered as an i.v. loading dose of 1.5 mg/kg followed by constant i.v. infusion of 0.3 mg/kg/min (Meyer et al 2001). The mean

(±SD) concentrations of serum lidocaine at which the clinical signs of intoxication (skeletal muscle tremors) were observed was $3.24 \pm 0.74\,\mu g/ml$ (range $1.85–4.53\,\mu g/ml$) (Meyer et al 2001). Although, these concentrations induced significant changes in the electrocardiogram (ECG) (P wave duration, P–R interval, R–R interval and Q–T interval), these were within the published reference range and were not clinically significant (Meyer et al 2001). Consequently, it is considered that serum lidocaine concentrations lower than those required to produce toxicity do not induce significant cardiovascular changes in the conscious horse. Some authors report severe hindlimb ataxia following the caudal epidural administration of lidocaine to horses (Le Blanc et al 1988), which does not appear to be improved by use in combination with butorphanol (Csik-Salmon et al 1996); other authors report the ataxia to be mild and transient (Fikes et al 1989). Lidocaine is irritant when injected into joint spaces (White et al 1989).

In an abaxial sessamoid local anaesthetic model, the highest no-effect dose for the local anaesthetic effect of lidocaine was 4 mg (Harkins et al 1998). For caudal epidural anesthesia, dose rates of lidocaine alone of 0.25 (Csik-Salmon et al 1996) or 0.35 mg/kg (Fikes et al 1989) have been proposed (i.e. 6–10 ml of a 2% solution). A maximum of 200 ml should be used for field blocks. The dose rates quoted for i.v. administration of either a 1% or 2% solution of lidocaine (without epinephrine (adrenaline)) are for loading doses of 0.65–5 mg/kg followed by a constant i.v. infusion of 25–100 μg/kg/min (Brianceau et al 2002, Doherty & Frazier 1998).

Mepivacaine

Mepivacaine is a racemic, tertiary amide local anesthetic that is approved (2% solution) for use in horses. This agent is also used widely in humans and is available as 1% and 2% solutions also in combination with 1:200 000 epinephrine (adrenaline).

Although slightly less lipid soluble than lidocaine, mepivacaine diffuses readily out of joint spaces (Gough et al 2002a,b, Keegan et al 1996). It is absorbed rapidly into the systemic circulation, with peak plasma concentrations observed approximately 1 h after midsacral, subarachnoidal or sacral epidural administration (Skarda et al 1984). Mepivacaine is more highly bound to plasma proteins (77–80%) than lidocaine. It is excreted in urine both as parent compound and 3-hydroxymepivacine, with peak concentrations achieved within 2 h of subcutaneous (s.c.) administration (Harkins et al 1999a). Both mepivacaine and its main metabolite can be detected in horse urine for prolonged periods, at least 50 and 33 h, respectively. Mepivacaine has a rapid onset and a slightly longer duration of action than lidocaine in horses (Table 15.2).

Mepivacaine is irritant when injected into joint spaces (White et al 1989); however, it is reportedly less tissue irritating than lidocaine. Mepivacaine does not produce vasodilatation and epinephrine (adrenaline) is not required to prolong its effect. Although mepivacaine does not appear to influence local bone uptake of ^{99m}Tc-methylene diphosphonate (MDP) or nuclear medical bone images significantly (Gaughan et al 1990), it may affect the ultrasonographic appearance (such as mild hypoechoic swelling of the surrounding soft tissues and gas in the region of the injections) of equine palmar metacarpal structures requiring repeat examinations to be carried out 24 h later (Zekas & Forrest 2003).

The dosage of mepivacaine used commonly in the horse aims to achieve an estimated effective tissue concentration of 0.3 μg/mg (Keegan et al 1996) and ranges from 20 to 200 mg/animal depending on the site of administration. Smaller doses (approximately 30 mg, or 1.5 ml of 2% solution) are required for subarachnoid techniques (Skarda & Muir 1982, Skarda et al 1984), doses of 40–100 mg (2–5 ml) for field blocks, mid-range doses (80–90 mg or 4–4.5 ml of 2% solution) for epidural techniques (Skarda & Muir 1982, Skarda et al 1984), high doses (160 mg or 8 ml of a 2% solution) for distal interphalangeal joint injection (Keegan et al 1996) and doses of 40–200 mg for perineural injection.

Bupivacaine

Bupivacaine is a racemic aminoamide local anesthetic that is also now used widely in equine medicine. It has a longer duration of action than lidocaine and mepivacaine (Table 15.2). For this reason, nerve blocks should not be repeated within 4–6 h to avoid accumulation and hence toxicity. The (S)-isomer of bupivacaine has local anesthetic actions whilst the (R)-isomer is responsible for cardiotoxicity, because of prolonged sodium channel blockade (de Jong 1995). This has led recently to the introduction of ropivacaine, the (S)-isomer of bupivacaine, for local anesthesia. Bupivacaine is excreted in urine as 3-hydroxybupivacaine (Harkins et al 1999b) with peak urine concentrations reached approximately 2 h after intra-articular and 4 h after s.c. administration (Harkins et al 1999b). Urine pH, creatinine concentration and specific gravity appear to have no effect on the concentration of 3-hydroxybupivacaine recovered (Harkins et al 1999b). Bupivacaine does not appear to influence local bone uptake of ^{99m}Tc-MDP or nuclear medical bone images significantly (Gaughan et al 1990). Following abaxial sessamoid block with bupivacaine, the highest no-effect dose was about 0.25 mg/site (Harkins et al 1996). It is suggested that the maximal dose should not exceed 2 mg/kg. For perineural injection in horses, a dose rate of 1–2 ml/site of a 0.5% (5 mg/ml) solution has been proposed.

Ropivacaine

Ropivacaine is a potent local anesthetic that has been introduced recently in human medicine. Ropivacaine is the (S)-isomer of bupivacaine and retains the local anesthetic properties while having lower cardiotoxic potential than racemic bupivacaine (de Jong 1995). Ropivacaine has a high potential for abuse in horses; if administered in clinically effective doses to horses, it can be detected as 3-hydroxyropivacine glucuronide in equine urine (Harkins et al 2000). Based on an abaxial sessamoid block model, it has an estimated highest no-effect dose of about 0.4 mg/site (Harkins et al 2001).

REFERENCES

Abass B T, Weaver B M, Staddon G E et al 1994 Pharmacokinetics of thiopentone in the horse. Journal of Veterinary Pharmacology and Therapeutics 17:331–338

Aguiar A J A, Hussni C A, Luna S P L 1993 Propofol compared with propofol/guaiphenesin after detomidine premedication for equine surgery. Journal of Veterinary Anaesthesia 20:26–28

Aida H, Mizuno Y, Hobo S et al 1996 Cardiovascular and pulmonary effects of sevoflurane anesthesia in horses. Veterinary Surgery 25:164–170

Alexander S L, Irvine C H 1998 The effect of social stress on adrenal axis activity in horses: the importance of monitoring corticosteroid-binding globulin capacity. Journal of Endocrinology 157:425–432

Alexander S L, Irvine C H 2000 The effect of the α_2-adrenergic agonist clonidine on secretion patterns and rates of adrenocorticotropic hormone and its secretagogues in the horse. Journal of Neuroendocrinology 12:874–880

Alibhai H I, Clarke K W, Lee Y H et al 1996 Cardiopulmonary effects of combinations of medetomidine hydrochloride and atropine sulphate in dogs. Veterinary Record 138:11–13

Angel A 1993 Central neuronal pathways and the process of anaesthesia. British Journal of Anaesthesia 71:148–163

Artru A A 1990 Hypocapnia and diazepam reverse and midazolam or fentanyl attenuates ketamine induced increase of cerebral blood volume and/or cerebrospinal fluid pressure. In: Domino E F (ed) Status of ketamine in anesthesiology. NPP Books, Ann Arbor, MI, p. 119

Aurich C, Aurich J E, Klug E 1993 Naloxone affects gastrointestinal functions and behaviour in horses. Deutsche Tierarztliche Wochenschrift 100:314–315

Ballard S, Shults T, Kownacki A A et al 1982 The pharmacokinetics, pharmacological responses and behavioral effects of acepromazine in the horse. Journal of Veterinary Pharmacology and Therapeutics 5:21–31

Batista C M, Laus J L, Nunes N et al 2000 Evaluation of intraocular and partial CO_2 pressure in dogs anesthetized with propofol. Veterinary Ophthalmology 3:17–19

Bennett R C, Steffey E P 2002 Use of opioids for pain and anesthetic management in horses. Veterinary Clinics of North America Equine Practice 18:47–60

Bennett R C, Taylor P M, Brearley J C et al 1998 Comparison of detomidine/ketamine and guaiphenesin/thiopentone for induction of anaesthesia in horses maintained with halothane. Veterinary Record 142:541–545

Bettschart-Wolfensberger R, Clarke K W, Vainio O et al 1999 Pharmacokinetics of medetomidine in ponies and elaboration of a medetomidine infusion regime which provides a constant level of sedation. Research in Veterinary Science 67:41–46

Bettschart-Wolfensberger R, Freeman S L, Jaggin-Schmucker N et al 2001a Infusion of a combination of propofol and medetomidine for long-term anesthesia in ponies. American Journal of Veterinary Research 62:500–507

Bettschart-Wolfensberger R, Bowen M I, Freeman S L et al 2001b Cardiopulmonary effects of prolonged anesthesia via propofol–medetomidine infusion in ponies. American Journal of Veterinary Research 62:1428–1435

Bito H, Ikeda K 1995 Degradation products of sevoflurane during low-flow anaesthesia. British Journal of Anaesthesia 74:56–59

Bramlage D, Bednarski R, Muir W 1993 Recovery from halothane and isoflurane in the horse. Veterinary Surgery 22:546

Branson K, Benson C, Thurmon J et al 1992 Comparison of isoflurane and halothane in horses: hemodynamics, tissue oxygen delivery and extractions. Veterinary Surgery 21:80

Branson K R, Booth N H 1995 Injectable anesthetics. In: Adams H R (ed) Veterinary pharmacology and therapeutics. Iowa State University Press, Ames, IA, pp. 209–273

Branson K R, Gross M E, Booth N H 1995 Opioid agonists and antagonists. In: Adams H R (ed) Veterinary pharmacology and therapeutics. Iowa State University Press, Ames, IA, pp. 274–307

Brianceau P, Chevalier H, Karas A 2002 Intravenous lidocaine and small-intestinal size, abdominal fluid, and outcome after colic surgery in horses. Journal of Veterinary Internal Medicine 16:736–741

Brown R F, Houpt K A, Schryver H F 1976 Stimulation of food intake in horses by diazepam and promazine. Pharmacology, Biochemistry and Behavior 5:495–497

Bryant C E, England G C, Clarke K W 1991 Comparison of the sedative effects of medetomidine and xylazine in horses. Veterinary Record 129:421–423

Bryant C E, Thompson J, Clarke K W 1998 Characterisation of the cardiovascular pharmacology of medetomidine in the horse and sheep. Research in Veterinary Science 65:149–154

Bufalari A, Miller S M, Giannoni C et al 1998 The use of propofol as an induction agent for halothane and isoflurane anesthesia in dogs. Journal of the American Animal Hospital Association 34:84–91

Carvey P 1998 Drug action in the central nervous system. Oxford University Press, New York

Chaffin M K, Walker M A, McArthur N H et al 1997 Magnetic resonance imaging of the brain of normal neonatal foals. Veterinary Radiology and Ultrasound 38:102–111

Chambers J P, Livingston A, Waterman A E et al 1993 Analgesic effects of detomidine in thoroughbred horses with chronic tendon injury. Research in Veterinary Science 54:52–56

Chapman C, Courage P, Nielsen I et al 1992 The role of procaine in adverse reactions to procaine penicillin in horses. Australian Veterinary Journal 69:129–133

Chou C C, Chen C L, Asbury A C et al 1998 Development and use of an enzyme-linked immunosorbent assay to monitor serum and urine acepromazine concentrations in thoroughbreds and possible changes associated with exercise. American Journal of Veterinary Research 59:593–597

Clarke K W, Paton B S 1988 Combined use of detomidine with opiates in the horse. Equine Veterinary Journal 20:331–334

Clarke K W, Song D Y, Alibhai H I et al 1996 Cardiopulmonary effects of desflurane in ponies, after induction of anaesthesia with xylazine and ketamine. Veterinary Record 139:180–185

Combie J, Shults T, Nugent E C et al 1981 Pharmacology of narcotic analgesics in the horse: selective blockade of narcotic-induced locomotor activity. American Journal of Veterinary Research 42:716–721

Combie J D, Nugent T E, Tobin T 1983 Pharmacokinetics and protein binding of morphine in horses. American Journal of Veterinary Research 44:870–874

Corbett A D, Paterson S, Kosterlitz H 1993 Selectivity of ligands for opioid receptors. In: Herz A, Akil H, Simon E J (eds) Handbook of experimental pharmacology, vol. 104 Springer-Verlag, Berlin, pp. 645–679

Court M H, Hay-Kraus B L, Hill D W et al 1999 Propofol hydroxylation by dog liver microsomes: assay development and dog breed differences. Drug Metabolism and Disposition 27:1293–1299

Csik-Salmon J, Blais D, Vaillancourt D 1996 Use of a mix of lidocaine and butorphanol as a caudal epidural anesthesia in a mare. Canadian Journal of Veterinary Research 60:288–295

Cullen L K, Steffey E P, Bailey C S et al 1990 Effect of high $PaCO_2$ and time on cerebrospinal fluid and intraocular pressure in halothane-anesthetized horses. American Journal of Veterinary Research 51:300–304

Cuvelliez S, Rosseel G, Blais D et al 1995 Intravenous anesthesia in the horse: comparison of xylazine–ketamine and xylazine–tiletamine–zolazepam combinations. Canadian Veterinary Journal 36:613–618

Davis L E, Sturm B L 1970 Drug effects and plasma concentrations of pentazocine in domesticated animals. American Journal of Veterinary Research 31:1631–1635

Day T K, Skarda R T 1991 The pharmacology of local anesthetics. Veterinary Clinics of North America Equine Practice 7:489–500

de Jong R H 1995 Gaston Labat lecture. Ropivacaine: white knight or dark horse? Regional Anesthesia 20:474–481

Delatour P, Jaussaud P, Courtot D et al 1991 Enantioselective N-demethylation of ketamine in the horse. Journal of Veterinary Pharmacology and Therapeutics 142:209–212

Deryck Y L, Brimioulle S, Maggiorini M et al 1996 Systemic vascular effects of isoflurane versus propofol anesthesia in dogs. Anesthesia and Analgesia 83:958–964

Dewey E A, Maylin G A, Ebel J G et al 1981 The metabolism of promazine and acetylpromazine in the horse. Drug Metabolism and Disposition 9:30–36

Dickson L R, Badcoe L M, Burbidge H et al 1990 Jugular thrombophlebitis resulting from an anaesthetic induction technique in the horse. Equine Veterinary Journal 22:177–179

Dirikolu L, Lehner A F, Karpiesiuk W et al 2000 Identification of lidocaine and its metabolites in postadministration equine urine by ELISA and MS/MS. Journal of Veterinary Pharmacology and Therapeutics 23:215–222

Dodman N H, Shuster L, Court M H et al 1987 Investigation into the use of narcotic antagonists in the treatment of a stereotypic behavior pattern (crib-biting) in the horse. American Journal of Veterinary Research 48:311–319

Doherty T J, Frazier D L 1998 Effect of intravenous lidocaine on halothane minimum alveolar concentration in ponies. Equine Veterinary Journal 30:300–303

Doherty T J, Geiser D R, Rohrbach B W 1997a The effect of epidural xylazine on halothane minimum alveolar concentration in ponies. Journal of Veterinary Pharmacology and Therapeutics 20:246–248

Doherty T J, Geiser D R, Rohrbach B W 1997b Effect of acepromazine and butorphanol on halothane minimum alveolar concentration in ponies. Equine Veterinary Journal 29:374–376

Doherty T J, Geiser D R, Rohrbach B W 1997c Effect of high volume epidural morphine, ketamine and butorphanol on halothane minimum alveolar concentration in ponies. Equine Veterinary Journal 29:370–373

Donaldson L L, Dunlop G S, Holland M S et al 2000 The recovery of horses from inhalant anesthesia: a comparison of halothane and isoflurane. Veterinary Surgery 29:92–101

Drummond J, Matthews R 1994 Nitrous oxide inactivation of cobalamin-dependent methionine synthase from *Escherichia coli*: characterization of the damage to the enzyme and prosthetic group. Biochemistry 33:3742–3750

Dyer D C, Hsu W H, Lloyd W E 1987 Pharmacokinetics of xylazine in ponies: influence of yohimbine. Archives Internationales de Pharmacodynamie et de Therapie 289:5–10

Eger E 1974 Concentration and second gas effects In: Eger E (ed) Anesthetic uptake and action. Williams & Wilkins, Baltimore, MD, pp. 113–121

Eger E I 1994 New inhaled anesthetics. Anesthesiology 80:906–922

Engelking L R, Dodman N H, Hartman G et al 1984 Effects of halothane anesthesia on equine liver function. American Journal of Veterinary Research 45:607–615

England G C, Clarke K W 1996 α_2 adrenoceptor agonists in the horse: a review. British Veterinary Journal 152:641–657

England G C, Clarke K W, Goossens L 1991 The sedative effects of romifidine compared with detomidine and xylazine in the horse. Journal of Veterinary Anaesthesia 63–65(suppl.):25–31

England G C, Clarke K W, Goossens L 1992 A comparison of the sedative effects of three α_2-adrenoceptor agonists (romifidine, detomidine and xylazine) in the horse. Journal of Veterinary Pharmacology and Therapeutics 15:194–201

Fernandez G, Gomez M D, Castro J 1975 Cholinesterase inhibition by phenothiazine and nonphenothiazine antihistaminics: analysis of its postulated role in synergizing organophosphate toxicity. Toxicology and Applied Pharmacology 31:179–190

Fikes L W, Lin H C, Thurmon J C 1989 A preliminary comparison of lidocaine and xylazine as epidural analgesics in ponies. Veterinary Surgery 18:85–86

Flaherty D, Reid J, Welsh E et al 1997 A pharmacodynamic study of propofol or propofol and ketamine infusions in ponies undergoing surgery. Research in Veterinary Science 62:179–184

Folts J D, Alfonso S, Rowe G G 1975 Systemic and coronary hemodynamic effects of ketamine in intact anaesthetized and unanaesthetized dogs. British Journal of Anaesthesia 47:686–694

Franks N P, Lieb W R 1998 Which molecular targets are most relevant to general anaesthesia? Toxicology Letters 100–101:1–8

Freeman S L, England G C 1999 Comparison of sedative effects of romifidine following intravenous, intramuscular and sublingual administration to horses. American Journal of Veterinary Research 60:954–959

Garcia-Villar R, Toutain P L, Alvinerie M 1981 The pharmacokinetics of xylazine hydrochloride: an interspecific study. Journal of Veterinary Pharmacology and Therapeutics 4:87–92

Gasthuys F, de Moor A, Parmentier D 1990 Haemodynamic changes during sedation in ponies. Veterinary Research Communications 14:309–327

Gasthuys F, de Moor A, Parmentier D 1991 Influence of dopamine and dobutamine on the cardiovascular depression during a standard halothane anaesthesia in dorsally recumbent, ventilated ponies. Zentralblatt für Veterinarmedizin Reihe A 38:494–500

Gaughan E M, Wallace R J, Kallfelz F A 1990 Local anesthetics and nuclear medical bone images of the equine fore limb. Veterinary Surgery 19:131–135

Gaynor J S, Bednarski R M, Muir W W III 1993 Effect of hypercapnia on the arrhythmogenic dose of epinephrine in horses anesthetized with guaifenesin, thiamylal sodium and halothane. American Journal of Veterinary Research 54:315–321

Geiser D R 1990 Chemical restraint and analgesia in the horse. Veterinary Clinics of North America Equine Practice 6:495–451

Gomez de Segura I A, De Rossi R, Santos M et al 1998 Epidural injection of ketamine for perineal analgesia in the horse. Veterinary Surgery 27:384–391

Goodrich L R, Nixon A J, Fubini S L et al 2002 Epidural morphine and detomidine decreases postoperative hindlimb lameness in horses after bilateral stifle arthroscopy. Veterinary Surgery 31:232–239

Gough M R, Mayhew G, Munroe G A 2002a Diffusion of mepivacaine between adjacent synovial structures in the horse. Part 1: forelimb foot and carpus. Equine Veterinary Journal 34:80–84

Gough M R, Munroe G A, Mayhew G 2002b Diffusion of mepivacaine between adjacent synovial structures in the horse. Part 2: tarsus and stifle. Equine Veterinary Journal 34:85–90

Grandy J L, Hodgson D S, Dunlop C I 1989 Cardiopulmonary effects of ephedrine in halothane-anesthetized horses. Journal of Veterinary Pharmacology and Therapeutics 12:389–396

Greene S A, Thurmon J C, Tranquilli W J et al 1986 Cardiopulmonary effects of continuous intravenous infusion of guaifenesin, ketamine, and xylazine in ponies. American Journal of Veterinary Research 47:2364–2367

Grosenbaugh D A, Muir W W 1998 Cardiorespiratory effects of sevoflurane, isoflurane and halothane anesthesia in horses. American Journal of Veterinary Research 59:101–106

Grubb T L, Riebold T W, Huber M J 1992 Comparison of lidocaine, xylazine, and xylazine/lidocaine for caudal epidural analgesia in horses. Journal of the American Veterinary Medical Association 201:1187–1190

Grubb T L, Muir W W III, Bertone A L et al 1997 Use of yohimbine to reverse prolonged effects of xylazine hydrochloride in a horse being treated with chloramphenicol. Journal of the American Veterinary Medical Association 210:1771–1773

Guimaraes S, Moura D 2001 Vascular adrenoceptors: an update. Pharmacological Reviews 53:319–356

Hall A C, Lieb W R, Franks N P 1994 Stereoselective and non-stereoselective actions of isoflurane on the GABA$_A$ receptor. British Journal of Pharmacology 112:906–910

Harkins J D, Karpiesiuk W, Lehner A et al 2001 Ropivacaine in the horse: its pharmacological responses, urinary detection and mass spectral confirmation. Journal of Veterinary Pharmacology and Therapeutics 24:89–98

Harkins J D, Karpiesiuk W, Tobin T et al 2000 Identification of hydroxyropivacaine glucuronide in equine urine by ESI+/MS/MS. Canadian Journal of Veterinary Research 64:178–183

Harkins J D, Karpiesiuk W, Woods W E et al 1999a Mepivacaine: its pharmacological effects and their relationship to analytical findings in the horse. Journal of Veterinary Pharmacology and Therapeutics 22:107–121

Harkins J D, Lehner A, Karpiesiuk W et al 1999b Bupivacaine in the horse: relationship of local anaesthetic responses and urinary concentrations of 3-hydroxybupivacaine. Journal of Veterinary Pharmacology and Therapeutics 22:181–195

Harkins J D, Mundy G D, Stanley S 1996 Determination of highest no effect dose (HNED) for local anaesthetic responses to procaine, cocaine, bupivacaine and benzocaine. Equine Veterinary Journal 28:30–37

Harkins J D, Mundy G D, Woods W E et al 1998 Lidocaine in the horse: its pharmacological effects and their relationship to analytical findings. Journal of Veterinary Pharmacology and Therapeutics 21:462–476

Harkins J D, Queiroz-Neto A, Mundy G D 1997 Development and characterization of an equine behaviour chamber and the effects of amitraz and detomidine on spontaneous locomotor activity. Journal of Veterinary Pharmacology and Therapeutics 20:396–401

Hashem A, Keller H 1993 Disposition, bioavailability and clinical efficacy of orally administered acepromazine in the horse. Journal of Veterinary Pharmacology and Therapeutics 16:359–368

Hashimoto T, Maze M, Ohashi Y et al 2001 Nitrous oxide activates GABAergic neurons in the spinal cord in Fischer rats. Anesthesiology 95:463–469

Haws J L, Herman N, Clark Y et al 1998 The chemical stability and sterility of sodium thiopental after preparation. Anesthesia and Analgesia 86:208–213

Heldmann E, Holt D E, Brockman D J et al 1999 Use of propofol to manage seizure activity after surgical treatment of portosystemic shunts. Journal of Small Animal Practice 40:590–594

Hildebrand S V, Howitt G A 1983 Succinylcholine infusion associated with hyperthermia in ponies anesthetized with halothane. American Journal of Veterinary Research 44:2280–2284

Hildebrand S V, Arpin D, Cardinet G III 1990 Contracture test and histologic and histochemical analyses of muscle biopsy specimens from horses with exertional rhabdomyolysis. Journal of the American Veterinary Medical Association 196:1077–1083

Hubbell J A, Bednarski R M, Muir W W 1989 Xylazine and tiletamine–zolazepam anesthesia in horses. American Journal of Veterinary Research 50:737–742

Ilkiw J E, Haskins S C, Patz J D 1991 Cardiovascular and respiratory effects of thiopental administration in hypovolemic dogs. American Journal of Veterinary Research 52:576–580

Jochle W 1989 Field trial evaluation of detomidine as a sedative and analgesic in horses with colic. Equine Veterinary Journal Supplement 136:117–120

Jochle W, Moore J N, Brown J et al 1989 Comparison of detomidine butorphanol, flunixin meglumine and xylazine in clinical cases of equine colic. Equine Veterinary Journal Supplement 136:111–116

Johnson C B, Taylor P M 1997 Effects of alfentanil on the equine electroencephalogram during anaesthesia with halothane in oxygen. Research in Veterinary Science 62:159–163

Jones D 1993 Clinical effects of detomidine with or without atropine used for arthrocentesis in horses. Canadian Veterinary Journal 34:296–300

Joo G, Horvath G, Klimscha W et al 2000 The effects of ketamine and its enantiomers on the morphine- or dexmedetomidine-induced antinociception after intrathecal administration in rats. Anesthesiology 93:231–241

Kaka J S, Klavano P A, Hayton W L 1979 Pharmacokinetics of ketamine in the horse. American Journal of Veterinary Research 40:978–981

Kalpravidh M, Lumb W V, Wright M et al 1984 Effects of butorphanol, flunixin, levorphanol, morphine, and xylazine in ponies. American Journal of Veterinary Research 45:217–223

Kamerling S G 1993 Narcotics and local anesthetics. Veterinary Clinics of North America Equine Practice 9:605–620

Kamerling S G, Dequick D J, Weckman T J et al 1984 Differential effects of phenylbutazone and local anesthetics on nociception in the equine. European Journal of Pharmacology 107:35–41

Kamerling S G, Cravens W M, Bagwell C A 1988 Dose-related effects of detomidine on autonomic responses in the horse. Journal of Autonomic Pharmacology 8:241–249

Kamerling S G, Hamra J G, Bagwell C A 1990 Naloxone-induced abdominal distress in the horse. Equine Veterinary Journal 22:241–243

Kamibayashi T, Hayashi Y, Sumikawa K et al 1991 Enhancement by propofol of epinephrine-induced arrhythmias in dogs. Anesthesiology 75:1035–1040

Kamibayashi T, Maze M 2000 Clinical uses of α_2-adrenergic agonists. Anesthesiology 93:1345–1349

Katila T, Oijala M 1988 The effect of detomidine (Domosedan) on the maintenance of equine pregnancy and foetal development: ten cases. Equine Veterinary Journal 20:323–326

Keegan R D, Greene S A 1993 Cardiovascular effects of a continuous two-hour propofol infusion in dogs. Comparison with isoflurane anesthesia. Veterinary Surgery 22:537–543

Keegan K G, Wilson D A, Kreeger J M 1996 Local distribution of mepivacaine after distal interphalangeal joint injection in horses. American Journal of Veterinary Research 57:422–426

Klein L, Ailes N, Fackelman G E 1989 Postanesthetic equine myopathy suggestive of malignant hyperthermia. A case report. Veterinary Surgery 18:479–482

Kollias-Baker C, Sams R 2002 Detection of morphine in blood and urine samples from horses administered poppy seeds and morphine sulfate orally. Journal of Analytical Toxicology 26:81–86

Krasowski M D, Nishikawa K, Nikolaeva N et al 2001 Methionine 286 in transmembrane domain 3 of the GABA$_A$ receptor beta subunit controls a binding cavity for propofol and other alkylphenol general anesthetics. Neuropharmacology 41:952–964

Kristinsson J, Thordarson T H, Johannesson T 1996 Pharmacokinetics of lignocaine in Icelandic horses after infiltration anaesthesia. Veterinary Record 138:111–112

Kuipers J A, Boer F, Olieman W et al 1999 First-pass lung uptake and pulmonary clearance of propofol: assessment with a recirculatory indocyanine green pharmacokinetic model. Anesthesiology 91:1780–1787

Le Blanc P H 1992 Regional anesthesia In: Robinson N E (ed) Current therapy in equine medicine, 3rd edn. Saunders, Philadelphia, PA, pp. 25–28

Le Blanc P H, Caron J P, Patterson J S et al 1988 Epidural injection of xylazine for perineal analgesia in horses. Journal of the American Veterinary Medical Association 193:1405–1408

Le Blanc P H, Eberhart S W, Robinson N E 1993 In vitro effects of α_2-adrenergic receptor stimulation on cholinergic contractions of equine distal airways. American Journal of Veterinary Research 54:788–792

Lehner A F, Almeida P, Jacobs J et al 2000 Remifentanil in the horse: identification and detection of its major urinary metabolite. Journal of Analytical Toxicology 24:309–315

Lin H C, Wallace S S, Robbins R L et al 1994 A case report on the use of guaifenesin–ketamine–xylazine anesthesia for equine dystocia. Cornell Veterinarian 84:61–66

Luna S P, Taylor P M, Wheeler M J 1996 Cardiorespiratory, endocrine and metabolic changes in ponies undergoing intravenous or inhalation anaesthesia. Journal of Veterinary Pharmacology and Therapeutics 19:251–258

Luukkanen L, Katila T, Koskinen E 1997 Some effects of multiple administrations of detomidine during the last trimester of equine pregnancy. Equine Veterinary Journal 29:400–402

Mama K R, Pascoe P J, Steffey E P 1993 Evaluation of the interaction of mu and kappa opioid agonists on locomotor behavior in the horse. Canadian Journal of Veterinary Research 57:106–109

Mama K R, Steffey E P, Pascoe P J 1995 Evaluation of propofol as a general anesthetic for horses. Veterinary Surgery 24:188–194

Mama K R, Steffey E P, Pascoe P J 1996 Evaluation of propofol for general anesthesia in premedicated horses. American Journal of Veterinary Research 57:512–516

Manley S V, Kelly A B, Hodgson D 1983 Malignant hyperthermia-like reactions in three anesthetized horses. Journal of the American Veterinary Medical Association 183:85–89

Manohar M, Gustafson R, Nganwa D 1987 Skeletal muscle perfusion during prolonged 2.03% end-tidal isoflurane–O$_2$ anesthesia in isocapnic ponies. American Journal of Veterinary Research 48:946–951

Marlin D J, Young L E, McMurphy R et al 2001 Effect of two anaesthetic regimens on airway nitric oxide production in horses. British Journal of Anaesthesia 86:127–130

Marroum P J, Webb A I, Aeschbacher G et al 1994 Pharmacokinetics and pharmacodynamics of acepromazine in horses. American Journal of Veterinary Research 55:1428–1433

Matthews N S 1993 The use of tiletamine–zolazepam for "darting" feral horses. Journal of Equine Veterinary Science 13:264–267

Matthews N S, Dollar N S, Shawley R V 1990 Halothane-sparing effect of benzodiazepines in ponies. Cornell Veterinarian 80:259–265

Matthews N S, Hartsfield S M, Cornick J L et al 1991 A comparison of injectable anesthetic combinations in horses. Veterinary Surgery 20:268–273

Matthews N S, Hartsfield S M, Hague B et al 1999 Detomidine–propofol anesthesia for abdominal surgery in horses. Veterinary Surgery 28:196–201

Matthews N S, Hartsfield S M, Mercer D et al 1998 Recovery from sevoflurane anesthesia in horses: comparison to isoflurane and effect of postmedication with xylazine. Veterinary Surgery 27:480–485

Matthews N S, Miller S M, Hartsfield S M et al 1992 Comparison of recoveries from halothane vs isoflurane anesthesia in horses. Journal of the American Veterinary Medical Association 201:559–563

Matthews N S, Petrini K R, Wolff P L 1995 Anesthesia of Przewalski's horses with medetomidine/ketamine and antagonism with atipamezole. Journal of Zoo and Wildlife Medicine 26:231–236

Mazoit J X, Samii K 1999 Binding of propofol to blood components: implications for pharmacokinetics and for pharmacodynamics. British Journal of Clinical Pharmacology 47:35–42

Mazze R I, Callan C M, Galvez S T et al 2000 The effects of sevoflurane on serum creatinine and blood urea nitrogen concentrations: a retrospective, twenty-two-center, comparative evaluation of renal function in adult surgical patients. Anesthesia and Analgesia 90:683–688

McDonald J, Gall R, Wiedenbach P et al 1987 Immunoassay detection of drugs in horses. I. Particle concentration fluoroimmunoassay detection of fentanyl and its congeners. Research Communications in Chemical Pathology and Pharmacology 57:389–407

MacDonald E, Scheinin M 1995 Distribution and pharmacology of α2-adrenoceptors in the central nervous system. Journal of Physiology and Pharmacology 46:241–258

McDonell W 1996 Respiratory system. In: Thurmon J C, Tranquilli W J, Benson G J (eds) Lumb & Jones veterinary anesthesia. Williams & Wilkins, Baltimore, MD, pp. 115–147

Merritt A M, Burrow J A, Hartless C S 1998 Effect of xylazine, detomidine and a combination of xylazine and butorphanol on equine duodenal motility. American Journal of Veterinary Research 59:619–623

Merritt A M, Campbell-Thompson M L, Lowrey S 1989a Effect of xylazine treatment on equine proximal gastrointestinal tract myoelectrical activity. American Journal of Veterinary Research 50:945–949

Merritt A M, Campbell-Thompson M L, Lowrey S 1989b Effect of butorphanol on equine antroduodenal motility. Equine Veterinary Journal Supplement 7:21–23

Meunier J C, Mollereau C, Toll L et al 1995 Isolation and structure of the endogenous agonist of opioid receptor-like ORL1 receptor. Nature 377:535–535

Meyer G A, Lin H C, Hanson R R et al 2001 Effects of intravenous lidocaine overdose on cardiac electrical activity and blood pressure in the horse. Equine Veterinary Journal 33:434–437

Mizuno Y, Aida H, Hara H et al 1994 Cardiovascular effects of intermittent positive pressure ventilation in the anesthetized horse. Journal of Veterinary Medical Science 56:39–44

Moore A B, Roesel O F, Fessler J F et al 1983 Effects of naloxone on endotoxin-induced changes in ponies. American Journal of Veterinary Research 44:103–109

Moore R M, Trim C M 1992 Effect of xylazine on cerebrospinal fluid pressure in conscious horses. American Journal of Veterinary Research 53:1558–1561

Muir W W III, Gadawski J 1998 Cardiorespiratory effects of low-flow and closed circuit inhalation anesthesia, using sevoflurane delivered with an in-circuit vaporizer and concentrations of compound A. American Journal of Veterinary Research 59:603–608

Muir W W III, Gadawski J E, Grosenbaugh D A 1999 Cardiorespiratory effects of a tiletamine/zolazepam–ketamine–detomidine combination in horses. American Journal of Veterinary Research 60:770–774

Muir W W, Hubbell J A 1988 Cardiopulmonary and anesthetic effects of ketamine and its enantiomers in dogs. American Journal of Veterinary Research 49:530–534

Muir W W, Hubbell J A E 2000 Drugs used for preanaesthetic medication In: Muir W W, Hubbell J A E, Skarda R T et al (eds) Handbook of veterinary anaesthesia, 3rd edn. Mosby, St Louis, MO, p. 20

Muir W W III, Lerche P, Robertson J T et al 2000 Comparison of four drug combinations for total intravenous anesthesia of horses undergoing surgical removal of an abdominal testis. Journal of the American Veterinary Medical Association 217: 869–873

Muir W W, Robertson J T 1985 Visceral analgesia: effects of xylazine, butorphanol, meperidine, and pentazocine in horses. American Journal of Veterinary Research 46:2081–2084

Muir W W III, Sams R 1992 Effects of ketamine infusion on halothane minimal alveolar concentration in horses. American Journal of Veterinary Research 53:1802–1806

Muir W W, Sams R A, Huffman R H et al 1982 Pharmacodynamic and pharmacokinetic properties of diazepam in horses. American Journal of Veterinary Research 43:1756–1762

Muir W W, Skarda R T, Milne D W 1977 Evaluation of xylazine and ketamine hydrochloride for anesthesia in horses. American Journal of Veterinary Research 38:195–201

Muir W W, Skarda R T, Sheehan W C 1978 Cardiopulmonary effects of narcotic agonists and a partial agonist in horses. American Journal of Veterinary Research 39:1632–1635

Muir W W, Skarda R T, Sheehan W C 1979 Hemodynamic and respiratory effects of xylazine–morphine sulfate in horses. American Journal of Veterinary Research 40:1417–1420

Murison P J 2001 Effect of propofol at two injection rates or thiopentone on post-intubation apnoea in the dog. Journal of Small Animal Practice 42:71–74

Myburgh J A, Upton R N, Ludbrook G L et al 2002 Cerebrovascular carbon dioxide reactivity in sheep:

effect of propofol or isoflurane. Anaesthesia and Intensive Care 30:413–421

Natalini C C, Robinson E P 2000 Evaluation of the analgesic effects of epidurally administered morphine, alfentanil, butorphanol, tramadol, and U50488H in horses. American Journal of Veterinary Research 61:1579–1586

Nolan A, Reid J, Welsh E et al 1996 Simultaneous infusions of propofol and ketamine in ponies premedicated with detomidine: a pharmacokinetic study. Research in Veterinary Science 60:262–266

Norman W M, Court M H, Greenblatt D J 1997 Age-related changes in the pharmacokinetic disposition of diazepam in foals. American Journal of Veterinary Research 58:878–880

Obata R, Bito H, Ohmura M et al 2000 The effects of prolonged low-flow sevoflurane anesthesia on renal and hepatic function. Anesthesia and Analgesia 91:1262–1268

Pagel P S, Hettrick D A, Kersten J R et al 1998 Cardiovascular effects of propofol in dogs with dilated cardiomyopathy. Anesthesiology 88:180–189

Parry B W, Anderson G A 1983 Influence of acepromazine maleate on the equine haematocrit. Journal of Veterinary Pharmacology and Therapeutics 6:121–126

Parry B W, Anderson G A, Gay C C 1982 Hypotension in the horse induced by acepromazine maleate. Australian Veterinary Journal 59:148–152

Pascoe P J, Black W D, Claxton J M et al 1991 The pharmacokinetics and locomotor activity of alfentanil in the horse. Journal of Veterinary Pharmacology and Therapeutics 14:317–325

Pascoe P J, Steffey E P, Black W D et al 1993 Evaluation of the effect of alfentanil on the minimum alveolar concentration of halothane in horses. American Journal of Veterinary Research 54:1327–1332

Pasternak G W, Standifer K M 1996 Mapping of opioid receptors using antisense oligodeoxynucleotides: correlating their molecular biology and pharmacology. Trends in Pharmacological Sciences 16:344–350

Perez R, Cox J F, Arrue R 1994 Probable post-synaptic α_2 adrenergic mediated effect of xylazine on goat uterine motility. Journal of Veterinary Pharmacology and Therapeutics 17:59–63

Petts H V, Pleuvry B J 1983 Interactions of morphine and methotrimeprazine in mouse and man with respect to analgesia, respiration and sedation. British Journal of Anaesthesia 55:437–441

Pumford N R, Halmes N C, Hinson J A 1997 Covalent binding of xenobiotics to specific proteins in the liver. Drug Metabolism Reviews 29:39–57

Purchase I F 1966 Cardiac arrhythmias occur during halothane anaesthesia in cats. British Journal of Anaesthesia 38:13–22

Raekallio M, Vainio O, Scheinin M 1991 Detomidine reduces the plasma catecholamine but not cortisol concentrations in horses. Zentralblatt für Veterinarmedizin Reihe A 38:153–156

Raekallio M, Leino A, Vainio O et al 1992 Sympatho-adrenal activity and the clinical sedative effect of detomidine in horses. Equine Veterinary Journal Supplement 11:66–68

Raisis A L, Young L E, Blissitt K J et al 2000 A comparison of the haemodynamic effects of isoflurane and halothane anaesthesia in horses. Equine Veterinary Journal 32:318–326

Ramseyer B, Schmucker N, Schatzmann U et al 1998 Antagonism of detomidine sedation with atipamezole. Journal of Veterinary Anaesthesia 25:47–51

Redig P T, Larson A A, Duke G E 1984 Response of great horned owls given the optical isomers of ketamine. American Journal of Veterinary Research 45:125–127

Reeves J G 1984 Benzodiazepines In: Prys-Roberts C, Hug C G (eds) Pharmacokinetics of anaesthesia. Blackwell, Boston, MA, p. 157

Riedesel D H, Hildebrand S V 1985 Unusual response following use of succinylcholine in a horse anesthetized with halothane. Journal of the American Veterinary Medical Association 187:507–508

Robertson S A, Carter S W, Donovan M et al 1990 Effects of intravenous xylazine hydrochloride on blood glucose, plasma insulin and rectal temperature in neonatal foals. Equine Veterinary Journal 22:43–47

Roger T, Bardon T, Ruckebush Y 1994 Comparative effects of mu and kappa opiate agonists on the cecocolic motility in the pony. Canadian Journal of Veterinary Research 58:163–166

Roger T, Bardon T, Ruckebusch Y 1985 Colonic motor responses in the pony: relevance of colonic stimulation by opiate antagonists. American Journal of Veterinary Research 46:31–35

Ruckebusch Y, Roger T 1988 Prokinetic effects of cisapride, naloxone and parasympathetic stimulation at the equine ileo-caeco-colonic junction. Journal of Veterinary Pharmacology and Therapeutics 11:322–329

Rutkowski J A, Ross M W, Cullen K 1989 Effects of xylazine and/or butorphanol or neostigmine on myoelectric activity of the cecum and right ventral colon in female ponies. American Journal of Veterinary Research 50:1096–1101

Rutkowski J A, Eades S C, Moore J N 1991 Effects of xylazine butorphanol on cecal arterial blood flow, cecal mechanical activity, and systemic hemodynamics in horses. American Journal of Veterinary Research 52:1153–1158

Sakamoto H, Misumi K, Nakama M et al 1996 The effects of xylazine on intrauterine pressure, uterine blood flow, maternal and fetal cardiovascular and pulmonary function in pregnant goats. Journal of Veterinary Medical Science 58:211–217

Salonen J S 1991 Tissue-specificity of hydroxylation and N-methylation of arylalkylimidazoles. Pharmacology and Toxicology 69:1–4

Salonen J S, Suolinna E M 1988 Metabolism of detomidine in the rat. I. Comparison of ^{3}H-labelled metabolites formed in vitro and in vivo. European Journal of Drug Metabolism and Pharmacokinetics 13:53–58

Salonen J S, Vaha-Vahe T, Vainio O et al 1989 Single-dose pharmacokinetics of detomidine in the horse and cow. Journal of Veterinary Pharmacology and Therapeutics 12:65–72

Sams R, Pizzo P 1987 Detection and identification of ketamine and its metabolites in horse urine. Journal of Analytical Toxicology 11:58–62

Sarazan R D, Starke W A, Krause G F et al 1989 Cardiovascular effects of detomidine, a new α_2-adrenoceptor agonist, in the conscious pony. Journal of Veterinary Pharmacology and Therapeutics 12:378–388

Sator-Katzenschlager S, Deusch E, Dolezal S et al 2002 Sevoflurane and propofol decrease intraocular pressure equally during non-ophthalmic surgery and recovery. British Journal of Anaesthesia 89:764–766

Saunders C, Limbird L E 1999 Localization and trafficking of α_2-adrenergic receptor subtypes in cells and tissues. Pharmacology and Therapeutics 84:193–205

Schatzmann U, Jossfck H, Stauffer J L et al 1994 Effects of α_2-agonists on intrauterine pressure and sedation in horses: comparison between detomidine, romifidine and xylazine. Zentralblatt für Veterinarmedizin Reihe A 41:523–529

Schatzmann U, Armbruster S, Stucki F et al 2001 Analgesic effect of butorphanol and levomethadone in detomidine sedated horses. Journal of Veterinary Medicine A: Physiology, Pathology, Clinical Medicine 48:337–342

Schwedler M, Miletich D J, Albrecht R F 1982 Cerebral blood flow and metabolism following ketamine administration. Canadian Anaesthetists' Society Journal 29:222–226

Seay S S, Aucoin D P, Tyczkowska K L 1993 Rapid high-performance liquid chromatographic method for the determination of ketamine and its metabolite dehydronorketamine in equine serum. Journal of Chromatography 620:281–287

Sellon D C, Monroe V L, Roberts M C et al 2001 Pharmacokinetics and adverse effects of butorphanol administered by single intravenous injection or continuous intravenous infusion in horses. American Journal of Veterinary Research 62:183–189

Sharrock A G 1982 Reversal of drug-induced priapism in a gelding by medication. Australian Veterinary Journal 58:39–40

Shaw M L, Carpenter J W, Leith D E 1995 Complications with the use of carfentanil citrate and xylazine hydrochloride to immobilize domestic horses. Journal of the American Veterinary Medical Association 206:833–836

Singh A K, Mishra U, Ashraf M et al 1987 Analysis of detomidine in horse blood, plasma and urine samples utilizing a sensitive gas chromatography-mass spectrometry method. Journal of Chromatography 404:223–232

Singh S, Young S S, McDonell W N et al 1997 Modification of cardiopulmonary and intestinal motility effects of xylazine with glycopyrrolate in horses. Canadian Journal of Veterinary Research 61:99–107

Skarda R T 1991 Antagonists effects of atipamezole on epidurally administered detomidine-induced sedation, analgesia and cardiopulmonary depression in horses. Journal of Veterinary Anaesthesia 4(suppl):79–81

Skarda R T, Muir W W 1982 Segmental thoracolumbar spinal (subarachnoid) analgesia in conscious horses. American Journal of Veterinary Research 43:2121–2128

Skarda R T, Muir W W 1992 Physiologic responses after caudal epidural administration of detomidine in horses and xylazine in cattle In: Short C E, Poznack A (eds) Animal pain. Churchill Livingstone, London, pp. 292–302

Skarda R T, Muir W W 1996 Comparison of antinociceptive, cardiovascular and respiratory effects, head ptosis and position of pelvic limbs in mares after caudal epidural administration of xylazine and detomidine hydrochloride solution. American Journal of Veterinary Research 57:1338–1345

Skarda R T, Muir W W III 2001 Analgesic, hemodynamic, and respiratory effects induced by caudal epidural administration of meperidine hydrochloride in mares. American Journal of Veterinary Research 62:1001–1007

Skarda R T, Muir W W III 2003 Comparison of electroacupuncture and butorphanol on respiratory and cardiovascular effects and rectal pain threshold after controlled rectal distention in mares. American Journal of Veterinary Research 64:137–144

Skarda R T, Muir W W, Ibrahim A I 1984 Plasma mepivacaine concentrations after caudal epidural and subarachnoid injection in the horse: comparative study. American Journal of Veterinary Research 45:1967–1971

Smiley R M 1992 An overview of induction and emergence characteristics of desflurane in pediatric, adult and geriatric patients. Anesthesia and Analgesia 75:S38–S46

Smith P J, Gum G G, Whitley R D et al 1990 Tonometric and tonographic studies in the normal pony eye. Equine Veterinary Journal Supplement 10:36–38

Sojka J E, Adams S B, Lamar C H et al 1988 Effect of butorphanol, pentazocine, meperidine, or metoclopramide on intestinal motility in female ponies. American Journal of Veterinary Research 49:527–529

Stashak T S 1987 Diagnosis of lameness. In: Stashak T S (ed) Adams' lameness in horses, 4th edn. Lea and Febiger, Philadelphia, PA, pp. 134–151

Steffen F, Grasmueck S 2000 Propofol for treatment of refractory seizures in dogs and a cat with intracranial disorders. Journal of Small Animal Practice 41:496–499

Steffey E P, Dunlop C I, Farver T B et al 1987a Cardiovascular and respiratory measurements in awake and isoflurane-anesthetized horses. American Journal of Veterinary Research 48:7–12

Steffey E P, Giri S N, Dunlop C I et al 1993 Biochemical and haematological changes following prolonged halothane anaesthesia in horses. Research in Veterinary Science 55:338–345

Steffey E P, Howland D Jr 1978a Cardiovascular effects of halothane in the horse. American Journal of Veterinary Research 39:611–615

Steffey E P, Howland D Jr 1978b Potency of halothane-N20 in the horse. American Journal of Veterinary Research 39:1141–1146

Steffey E P, Howland D Jr 1980 Comparison of circulatory and respiratory effects of isoflurane and halothane anesthesia in horses. American Journal of Veterinary Research 41:821–825

Steffey E P, Howland D Jr, Giri S et al 1977 Enflurane, halothane and isoflurane potency in horses. American Journal of Veterinary Research 38:1037–1039

Steffey E P, Johnson B H, Eger E I II et al 1979 Nitrous oxide: effect on accumulation rate and uptake of bowel gases. Anesthesia and Analgesia 58:405–408

Steffey E P, Kelly A B, Farver T B et al 1985 Cardiovascular and respiratory effects of acetylpromazine and xylazine on halothane-anesthetized horses. Journal of Veterinary Pharmacology and Therapeutics 8:290–302

Steffey E P, Kelly A B, Woliner M J 1987b Time-related responses of spontaneously breathing, laterally recumbent horses to prolonged anesthesia with halothane. American Journal of Veterinary Research 48:952–957

Steffey E P, Pascoe P J, Woliner M J et al 2000 Effects of xylazine hydrochloride during isoflurane-induced anesthesia in horses. American Journal of Veterinary Research 61:1225–1231

Stick J A, Loeffler B S, Arden W A et al 1989 Effects of butorphanol tartrate on arterial pressure, jejunal blood flow, vascular resistance, O_2 extraction, and O_2 uptake in halothane-anesthetized ponies. American Journal of Veterinary Research 50:1202–1206

Stimpfel T M, Gershey E L 1991 Selecting anesthetic agents for human safety and animal recovery surgery. Federation of American Societies for Experimental Biology Journal 5:2099–2104

Stover S M, Steffey E P, Dybdal N O et al 1988 Hematologic and serum biochemical alterations associated with multiple halothane anesthesia exposures and minor surgical trauma in horses. American Journal of Veterinary Research 49:236–241

Sutton D G, Preston T, Christley R M et al 2002 The effects of xylazine, detomidine, acepromazine and butorphanol on equine solid phase gastric emptying rate. Equine Veterinary Journal 34:486–492

Sysel A M, Pleasant R S, Jacobson J D et al 1996 Efficacy of an epidural combination of morphine and detomidine in alleviating experimentally induced hindlimb lameness in horses. Veterinary Surgery 25:511–518

Szoke M O, Blais D, Cuvelliez S G et al 1998 Effects of buprenorphine on cardiovascular and pulmonary function in clinically normal horses and horses with chronic obstructive pulmonary disease. American Journal of Veterinary Research 59:1287–1291

Taneike T, Kitazawa T, Funakura H et al 1999 Smooth muscle layer-specific variations in the autonomic innervation of bovine myometrium. General Pharmacology 32:91–100

Taylor P M, Kirby J J, Shrimpton D J et al 1998 Cardiovascular effects of surgical castration during anaesthesia maintained with halothane or infusion of detomidine, ketamine and guaifenesin in ponies. Equine Veterinary Journal 30:304–309

Taylor P M, Luna S P, Sear J W et al 1995 Total intravenous anaesthesia in ponies using detomidine, ketamine and guaiphenesin: pharmacokinetics, cardiopulmonary and endocrine effects. Research in Veterinary Science 59:17–23

Tendillo F J, Mascias A, Santos M et al 1997 Anesthetic potency of desflurane in the horse: determination of the minimum alveolar concentration. Veterinary Surgery 26:354–357

Testa M, Raffe M R, Robinson E P 1990 Evaluation of 25%, 50%, and 67% nitrous oxide with halothane–oxygen for general anesthesia in horses. Veterinary Surgery 19:308–312

Tomasic M, Mann L S, Soma L R 1997 Effects of sedation, anesthesia and endotracheal intubation on respiratory mechanics in adult horses. American Journal of Veterinary Research 58:641–646

Trapani G, Altomare C, Liso G et al 2000 Propofol in anesthesia. Mechanism of action, structure–activity relationships, and drug delivery. Current Medicinal Chemistry 7:249–271

Trim C M, Adams J G, Hovda L R 1987 Failure of ketamine to induce anesthesia in two horses. Journal of the American Veterinary Medical Association 190:201–202

Trim C M, Colbern G T, Martin C L 1985 Effect of xylazine and ketamine on intraocular pressure in horses. Veterinary Record 117:442–443

Ueda I, Suzuki A 1998 Is there a specific receptor for anesthetics? Contrary effects of alcohols and fatty acids on phase transition and bioluminescence of firefly luciferase. Biophysical Journal 75:1052–1057

Valdez-Vasquez M, Aguilera-Tejero E, Mayer-Valor R 1993 Effect of xylazine during endoscopic evaluation of functional upper respiratory disorders in horses. Journal of Equine Veterinary Science 13:84–86

Vaughan C W, Ingram S L, Connor M A et al 1997 How opioids inhibit GABA-mediated neurotransmission. Nature 390:611–614

Virtanen R, Savola J M, Saano V et al 1988 Characterization of the selectivity, specificity and potency of medetomidine as an α_2-adrenoceptor agonist. European Journal of Pharmacology 150:9–14

Wagner A E, Bednarski R M, Muir W W III 1990 Hemodynamic effects of carbon dioxide during intermittent positive-pressure ventilation in horses. American Journal of Veterinary Research 51:1922–1929

Wagner A E, Dunlop C I, Wertz E M et al 1996 Evaluation of five common induction protocols by comparison of hemodynamic responses to surgical manipulation in halothane-anesthetized horses. Journal of the American Veterinary Medical Association 208:252–257

Wagner A E, Muir W W, Hinchcliff K W 1991 Cardiovascular effects of xylazine and detomidine in horses. American Journal of Veterinary Research 52:651–657

Waldron-Mease E, Klein L V, Rosenberg H et al 1981 Malignant hyperthermia in a halothane-anesthetized horse. Journal of the American Veterinary Medical Association 179:896–898

Wan P Y, Trim C M, Mueller P O 1992 Xylazine–ketamine and detomidine–tiletamine–zolazepam anesthesia in horses. Veterinary Surgery 21:312–318

Waterman A E, Amin A 1992 The influence of surgery and anaesthesia on the pharmacokinetics of pethidine in the horse. Equine Veterinary Journal Supplement 11:56–58

Waterman A E, Robertson S A, Lane J G 1987 Pharmacokinetics of intravenously administered ketamine in the horse. Research in Veterinary Science 42:162–166

White K K, Hodgson D R, Hancock D et al 1989 Changes in equine carpal joint synovial fluid in response to the injection of two local anesthetic agents. Cornell Veterinarian 79:25–38

Whitehair K J, Steffey E P, Willits N H et al 1993 Recovery of horses from inhalation anesthesia. American Journal of Veterinary Research 54:1693–1702

Whitehair K J, Steffey E P, Woliner M J et al 1996 Effects of inhalation anesthetic agents on response of horses to 3 hours of hypoxemia. American Journal of Veterinary Research 57:351–360

Willoughby R A, Ecker G L, McKee S L et al 1991 Use of scintigraphy for the determination of mucociliary clearance rates in normal, sedated, diseased and exercised horses. Canadian Journal of Veterinary Research 55:315–320

Wittern C, Hendrickson D A, Trumble T et al 1998 Complications associated with administration of detomidine into the caudal epidural space in a horse. Journal of the American Veterinary Medical Association 213:516–518

Wood T, Stanley S, Woods W E et al 1992 Evaluation of threshold doses of drug action in the horse using hematocrit values as an indicator. Research Communications in Chemical Pathology and Pharmacology 75:231–241

Wooldridge A A, Eades S C, Hosgood G L et al 2002 Effects of treatment with oxytocin, xylazine butorphanol, guaifenesin, acepromazine, and detomidine on esophageal manometric pressure in conscious horses. American Journal of Veterinary Research 63:1738–1444

Yamashita K, Satoh M, Umikawa A et al 2000b Combination of continuous intravenous infusion using a mixture of guaifenesin–ketamine–medetomidine and sevoflurane anesthesia in horses. Journal of Veterinary Medical Science 62:229–235

Yamashita K, Tsubakishita S, Futaok S et al 2000a Cardiovascular effects of medetomidine, detomidine and xylazine in horses. Journal of Veterinary Medical Science 62:1025–1032

Young L E, Bartram D H, Diamond M J et al 1993 Clinical evaluation of an infusion of xylazine, guaifenesin and ketamine for maintenance of anaesthesia in horses. Equine Veterinary Journal 25:115–119

Young D B, Ewing P J, Burrows G E et al 1994 Effects of phenylbutazone on thiamylal disposition and anaesthesia in ponies. Journal of Veterinary Pharmacology and Therapeutics 17:389–393

Zekas L J, Forrest L J 2003 Effect of perineural anesthesia on the ultrasonographic appearance of equine palmar metacarpal structures. Veterinary Radiology and Ultrasound 44:59–64

CHAPTER CONTENTS

Introduction   311

Inhalant bronchodilator therapy   313

Anti-inflammatory therapy   318

Antimicrobial therapy   322

References   324

16

Inhalation therapy for the respiratory system

Bonnie R. Rush

INTRODUCTION

Inhalation therapy has become increasingly popular for treatment of lower respiratory tract disease in horses. This route of administration reduces the total therapeutic dose, minimizes the exposure of other body systems to the drug and allows direct delivery of the drug to the lower respiratory tract. Delivery systems for the administration of aerosolized drugs to horses are being rapidly developed. The most important components of an aerosol administration system for horses are efficient pulmonary drug delivery and easy administration. To date, inhalation therapy for horses has focused predominately on the administration of bronchodilating agents and corticosteroid preparations for the treatment of recurrent airway obstruction (heaves). Aerosolized antimicrobial agents are under investigation for treatment of bacterial infection of the lower respiratory tract in horses.

Pulmonary deposition of an aerosol preparation is determined primarily by its size. Aerosols with a mass median aerodynamic diameter of 1–5 μm produce the best therapeutic results and are the target particle size for inhalation therapy. These small particles penetrate deep within the respiratory tract to ensure drug deposition in peripheral airways. The cross-sectional area (cm^2) of the lung increases dramatically at the level of the respiratory zone; therefore, the velocity of gas flow during inspiration rapidly decreases at this level. Moderate-sized particles (5–10 μm) frequently settle out by sedimentation in larger more central airways because the velocity of gas falls rapidly in the region of the terminal bronchioles.

Large aerosolized particles ($>10\,\mu m$) deposit in the upper respiratory tract via inertial impaction. The majority (90%) of particles below the target size ($<0.5\,\mu m$) are inhaled and exhaled freely and rarely impact within the respiratory tract. To avoid triggering bronchospasm, aerosolized solutions should be isotonic with a neutral pH and should not contain chemical irritants such as benzalkonium, ethylenediamine tetraacetic acid (EDTA), chlorbutol, edetic acid or metabisulfite (Duvivier et al 1999b).

Several devices have been designed for convenient administration of aerosolized drugs to horses with recurrent airway obstruction. The Equine AeroMask (Canadian Monaghan, Ontario, Canada) is a mask system designed to administer aerosolized drugs via metered-dose inhalant (MDI) devices or a nebulization solution (Tesarowski et al 1994). Drug is actuated or nebulized into a spacer device with a one-way inspiratory valve. To facilitate drug delivery, the mask must fit snugly around the muzzle, to ensure adequate negative inspiratory pressure. This system allows the clinician to administer any drug available for human asthma therapy to a horse with heaves. Drug delivery to the lower respiratory tract using the Equine AeroMask with a MDI is approximately 6% of actuated drug. Pulmonary drug delivery in humans using MDI devices is approximately 10–15%, with 85–90% of the drug deposited in the caudal pharynx (Barnes et al 1998). A novel hand-held device, the Equine Aerosol Drug Delivery System (3M Animal Care Products, St Paul, MN, USA) has been designed for administration of aerosolized drugs to horses (Derksen et al 1996, 1999). The device fits snugly into the left nostril of the horse. The operator actuates a puff at the onset of inhalation, denoted by a flow indicator within the device. This device delivers approximately 23% of actuated drug to the lower respiratory tract and the mean particle size generated using this system is $2.3 \pm 2.0\,\mu m$ (Geor & Johnson 1993). Ventilation imaging using radiolabeled aerosol confirmed that drug is deposited in all pulmonary fields with minimal deposition in the nasal cavity, oral pharynx or trachea. Currently, the Equine Aerosol Drug Deliver System is not available commercially.

Chlorofluorocarbon (CFC) propellant has been an essential component of MDI drug delivery systems. Since CFCs were recognized to have a depleting effect on the ozone layer in 1985, propellants containing CFCs are being phased out of most applications and newly developed inhalant products are formulated with CFC-free, ozone-friendly solution propellants. Hydrofluoroalkane-134a (HFA) is an inert, non-toxic replacement propellant for CFCs. It is eliminated from the body by ventilation, without evidence of accumulation or metabolism. HFA formulations are in solution, rather than in suspension; therefore, shaking is not necessary between actuations allowing immediate administration of drug with each breath. The efficacy of the HFA formulation of some drugs (e.g. salbutamol, fenoterol, ipratropium) is equivalent to the CFC preparations. However, the HFA formulation of beclometasone produces a greater total mass of fine drug particles, which improves pulmonary drug deposition and reduces the required daily dose by 50% in humans (Seale & Harrison 1998). With some devices, there is a 10-fold improvement in pulmonary drug delivery using an HFA formulation over a CFC formulation. Less medication is deposited in the pharynx using HFA propellants, which reduces the incidence of local side-effects.

Ultrasonic nebulizers, jet nebulizers and dry powder inhalants are ozone-friendly delivery systems that are used as alternatives to CFC propellant inhalers (Duvivier et al 1999b). Ultrasonic nebulizers produce aerosol particles using vibrations of a quartz crystal and jet nebulizers operate by the Venturi effect (dry air compressor) to fragment therapeutic solutions into aerosol particles. Ultrasonic nebulizers are silent, but they are fragile and expensive. Ultrasonic nebulization (Ultra-Neb, DeVilbiss, Somerset, PA, USA) delivers approximately 5% of the drug to the pulmonary system, and high-pressure jet nebulization (Hudson RCI, Temecula, CA, USA) using a delivery system developed for horses (Agritronix, Meux, Belgium) delivers approximately 7% of the drug to the pulmonary system (Votion et al 1997). Jet nebulizers are readily accessible, inexpensive and easy to use. Gas flow rates of 6–8 l/min are required to generate a suitable particle diameter

($<5\,\mu m$) for pulmonary delivery. The primary disadvantage is the noise generated by this type of system.

Deposition of radiolabeled drug into the peripheral pulmonary fields using jet nebulization is superior to ultrasonic nebulization. Pulmonary contamination with environmental bacteria and fungi may occur using these aerosolization systems; consequently, rigorous disinfection of the equipment is required. Aerosol therapy via ultrasonic and jet nebulization takes approximately 20 min. Dry powder inhalant devices offer several advantages over nebulization systems. Drug can be administered rapidly with minimal risk of environmental contamination and no requirement for electricity (Duvivier et al 1997). The dry powder inhalation device is breath actuated, which eliminates the need for the operator to synchronize administration with inhalation. The device punctures gelatin capsules containing powdered drug, releasing it into a chamber for inhalation by the patient. The mask used with this system must fit snugly around the muzzle to create adequate inspiratory pressures to ensure sufficient inhalant emptying rates (Duvivier et al 1997).

INHALANT BRONCHODILATOR THERAPY

The major classes of bronchodilating agent administered via inhalation include short-acting β_2 adrenoceptor agonists (β_2 agonists: albuterol, pirbuterol, fenoterol), long-acting β_2 agonists (salmeterol, formoterol) and anticholinergic agents (ipratropium bromide). Table 16.1 outlines the recommended dosages of aerosolized bronchodilators for horses.

Short-acting β_2 agonists

Sympathetic innervation of the respiratory tract is relatively sparse and is primarily associated with the regulation of mucosal blood flow. However, non-innervated β_2 adrenoceptors are widespread throughout the equine pulmonary system and are present on respiratory smooth muscle, epithelium and submucosal glands (Robinson et al 1996). Circulating (endogenous) epinephrine or β adrenergic drugs can activate non-innervated, β_2 adrenoceptors. Stimulation of these receptors induces relaxation of bronchial smooth muscle, via G_s protein activation, to increase intracellular cyclic adenosine monophosphate cAMP, resulting in decreased intracellular calcium ion concentrations. Non-selective β agonists are not used for bronchodilatation in clinical practice because of the adverse effects associated with β_1 adrenoceptor stimulation (tachycardia, sweating and excitement).

Albuterol sulfate (360–900 μg) and pirbuterol acetate (600 μg) are potent, short-acting β_2 adrenergic agents that rapidly produce bronchodilatation

Table 16.1 Aerosolized bronchodilator therapy in horses

Bronchodilator	Mechanism	Dose	Onset (min)	Duration (h)	Device
Albuterol sulfate	β_2 agonist: short acting	360 μg	5	1–3	Equine Aerosol Delivery Device (Derksen et al 1999, Page & Morley 1999)
Pirbuterol acetate	β_2 agonist: short acting	600 μg 1–2 μg/kg	5	1–4	Equine Aerosol Delivery Device (Derksen et al 1996)
Fenoterol	β_2 agonist: short acting	2–4 μg/kg	ND	4–6	MDI and Equine AeroMask (Tesarowski et al 1994)
Salmeterol	β_2 agonist: long acting	210 μg	ND	12	MDI and Equine AeroMask (Hoffman 1997)
Ipratropium bromide	Anticholinergic	90–180 μg	ND	4–6	MDI and Equine AeroMask (Hoffman 1997)
		2–3 μg/kg	<60	4–6	Ultrasonic nebulizer (Duvivier et al 1999a,b)
		4 μg/kg	15	>1	Dry powder inhaler (Duvivier et al 1997)

MDI, metered dose inhalant; ND, not determined

(5 min) in horses (Derksen et al 1992, 1996, 1999). The duration of effective bronchodilatation is approximately 1–3 h. Albuterol and pirbuterol improve parameters of pulmonary function by approximately 70% in horses during an episode of airway obstruction. Residual pulmonary dysfunction after bronchodilatory therapy is attributed to the obstruction of small airways by inflammatory exudate and mucosal edema. Aerosolized short-acting β_2 agonist bronchodilators produce minimal systemic effects and are safe for use in horses. Systemic administration of these agents requires 10 times the dose to achieve the same level of bronchodilatation and is associated with sweating, trembling, muscle tremors and excitement.

Rapid-onset, short-acting β_2 adrenergic agents are primarily indicated for 'rescue therapy' in horses suffering from dyspnea at rest. These agents allow the clinician to determine the reversibility of airway obstruction in individual horses with chronic disease. In addition, this type of β_2 agonist should be administered prior to administration of surface-active corticosteroid preparations and antimicrobial agents to improve the pulmonary distribution of these agents (Rush et al 1999a). It has been suggested that the administration of albuterol prior to exercise may improve the performance of horses with mild-to-moderate airway obstruction, although there are no objective data to support this recommendation. There are conflicting data relating to the effect of albuterol sulfate on exercise performance in normal horses. For most parameters, albuterol sulfate administered prior to exercise does not improve athletic performance; however, one investigation identified a small but significant, increase in run time and peak oxygen consumption ($\dot{V}O_2$ peak) in fit thoroughbred horses (Bailey et al 1999). In human asthmatics, the ability of β_2 agonists to improve athletic performance is dependent on the type of respiratory disease. Administration of albuterol prior to exercise consistently protects against exercise-induced bronchoconstriction in human athletes. However, β_2 agonists do not improve exercise performance in humans with chronic obstructive pulmonary disease. In general, chronic obstructive pulmonary disease is less responsive to bronchodilatory therapy and it appears that bronchodilatation stimulated by exercise appears to overshadow the effects of β_2 agonists in these patients.

In humans, the half-life of aerosolized albuterol sulfate is approximately 4 h. The kidney is the primary site of elimination with the majority of the drug excreted as sulfide and glucuronide metabolites (61%) and the remainder (39%) excreted unchanged. The absorption of albuterol from the gastrointestinal tract is poor (20% bioavailability); the primary site of absorption into the systemic circulation is the pulmonary system. There are currently no data available on the pharmacokinetics of albuterol in horses.

Most albuterol sulfate preparations contain an equimolar, racemic mixture of the (R)- and (S)-stereoisomers (Page & Morley 1999). (R)-albuterol has bronchodilator and bronchoprotective activity. (S)-Albuterol does not activate β_2 adrenoceptors and does not modify the activation of these receptors by (R)-albuterol. (S)-Albuterol is metabolized more slowly than (R)-albuterol and is retained preferentially in the airways. Until recently, (S)-albuterol was considered biologically inert; however, it has been shown to intensify allergic bronchospasm and eosinophilic activation in laboratory animals and appears to have the potential to induce paradoxical reactions in some asthmatic patients. In horses, (S)-albuterol does not have bronchodilatory activity and stimulates acetylcholine release via prejunctional β_2 adrenoceptor stimulation (Zhang et al 1998). Levalbuterol (homochiral (R)-albuterol) has been marketed recently and reportedly dramatically reduces the incidence of the side-effects associated with racemic albuterol in some patients.

Long-acting β_2 agonists

Salmeterol is a long-acting β_2 agonist that is a chemical analog of albuterol. The receptor-binding site of salmeterol is structurally similar to that of albuterol; however, salmeterol has an elongated (aliphatic) side chain thought to bind to a membrane exosite proximal to the region of the β_2 adrenoceptor protein (Linden et al 1996). Exosite binding allows salmeterol to contact the β_2 adrenoceptor repeatedly while the drug remains anchored adjacent to the receptor site, producing an extended duration of action. In addition, salmeterol has a higher lipophilicity, β_2 affinity, β_2 selectivity and potency (10-fold) than albuterol. Lipophilicity may be the most important determinant regarding duration of action, by influencing the amount of drug entering the cell membrane in the vicinity of the β_2 adrenoceptor. The $\beta_2:\beta_1$ activity ratio of salmeterol is 50 000:1 compared with 650:1 for albuterol; isoproterenol (isoprenaline) is the standard (1:1) for the β adrenoceptor activity ratio. Enhanced β_2 adrenoceptor selectivity provides a greater margin of safety by reducing the frequency of β_1 effects (nervousness, tachycardia and sweating) at therapeutic doses. In humans, twice daily administration of salmeterol provides superior control of bronchoconstriction compared with regular (four times a day) or as needed administration of albuterol. In addition to bronchodilatory activity, salmeterol appears to have some anti-inflammatory properties, such as inhibition of leukotriene and histamine release from mast cells and the reduction of eosinophil activity. Salmeterol (210 µg via Equine AeroMask) provides relief of the clinical signs of airway obstruction for 8 to 12 h in heaves-affected horses. Salmeterol has been recommended for maintenance therapy and pre-exercise administration to horses with mild-to-moderate airway obstruction (Hoffman 1997).

There is growing concern in human medicine that the overuse of the β_2 agonists for asthma is associated with increased morbidity and even mortality (Sears 1995). Regular use of β_2 agonists as monotherapy is associated with deterioration in asthma control, increased non-specific and allergen-induced airway responsiveness, increased eosinophilic pulmonary infiltration and progressive deterioration of lung function. Poor control of asthma symptoms triggers a vicious cycle of intensifying need for symptomatic relief and more frequent administration of β_2 agonists. This β_2 tolerance (loss of bronchodilator response) and deterioration in pulmonary function appears to occur through downregulation or desensitization of β_2 adrenoceptors. This downregulation may

occur via receptor phosphorylation, internalization or destruction. Deterioration in pulmonary function, increased airway responsiveness and failure to respond to β_2 adrenoceptor stimulation has been documented in asthmatic human patients after 3 weeks of regular (four times a day) administration of albuterol as monotherapy. Preliminary studies in horses with recurrent airway obstruction indicate that tolerance to bronchodilatator therapy may occur within 5 days of regular administration of albuterol sulfate. Given that the β_2 agonists have little or no anti-inflammatory activity, it is difficult to justify their use as monotherapy for a disease characterized by airway inflammation. Despite the National Asthma Education and Prevention Program issuing guidelines for asthma management in 1991, approximately 25–35% of asthmatic patients are still treated inappropriately with β_2 agonists as monotherapy, thereby failing to provide anti-inflammatory therapy (Emerman et al 1996).

Paradoxical bronchoconstriction can occur immediately after administration of aerosolized β_2 agonists in a small percentage of human patients (Finnerty & Howard 1993). This phenomenon can occur with long-term administration of any β_2 agonists but is most commonly documented in patients using albuterol sulfate followed by salmeterol. Paradoxical bronchoconstriction does not appear to be an effect of the propellant/vehicle and, in most instances, it is not a β_2 agonist class effect (i.e. patients developing paradoxical bronchoconstriction with albuterol will not necessarily demonstrate the response with an alternative β_2 agonist). Early reports of paradoxical bronchoconstriction suggested that the phenomenon resulted from increased airway deposition of noxious inhalant particles and induction of airway reactivity. This theory has been disproven. The most likely explanation involves stimulation of β_2 adrenoceptors on presynaptic cholinergic nerve endings, resulting in acetylcholine release. In the case of albuterol, the (S)-enantiomer stimulates acetylcholine release from cholinergic nerves via the presynaptic β_2 adrenoceptor (contributing to bronchospasm) and has proinflammatory activity. The mechanism of paradoxical bronchoconstriction with administration of other β_2 agonists is likely to involve cholinergic stimulation via presynaptic β_2 adrenoceptor in conjunction with dysfunctional presynaptic muscarinic autoreceptors (inhibitory to acetylcholine release). Although paradoxical bronchoconstriction has not been reported in horses at this time, clinicians should be aware of this response and consider administering levalbuterol or an alternative β_2 agonist to those cases.

Anticholinergic agents

The parasympathetic division is the dominant portion of the pulmonary autonomic nervous system in all mammals. Airway smooth muscle is richly supplied with muscarinic receptors and stimulation of M_3 receptors results in smooth muscle contraction and bronchoconstriction. Cholinergic stimulation is the primary mechanism of bronchospasm in horses with recurrent airway obstruction (Robinson et al 1996). Parasympathetic innervation can be demonstrated throughout the tracheobronchial tree of the horse but smooth muscle contraction evoked by stimulation of cholinergic nerves is more pronounced in the trachea than in the smaller bronchi. It is expected that parasympathetic blockade with a muscarinic antagonist will have the greatest effect in large, central airways.

Atropine

Atropine is the classic anticholinergic bronchodilator. It antagonizes acetylcholine, resulting in reduced intracellular cyclic guanosine monophosphate (cGMP) and smooth muscle relaxation. In horses, the therapeutic index of atropine is narrow and the duration of action is short (0.5–2.0 h). Adverse systemic effects associated with parenteral atropine administration include mydriasis, ileus, dry mucous membranes, blurred vision, excitement and tachycardia. Atropine is not suitable for routine administration to horses with recurrent airway obstruction.

Ipratropium bromide

Ipratropium bromide is a synthetic, anticholinergic compound that produces bronchodilatation,

inhibits cough and protects against bronchoconstrictive stimuli. Like atropine, ipratropium bromide is a non-selective (M_1, M_2, M_3) muscarinic antagonist: bronchodilatation results from blockade of the M_3 receptor. Because of its quaternary ammonium structure, ipratropium is absorbed poorly from the respiratory system (6%) or gastrointestinal tract (2%). Therefore, ipratropium has minimal systemic adverse effects and does not inhibit gastrointestinal motility. In addition, ipratropium does not cause drying of respiratory secretions and does not inhibit mucociliary clearance. In humans, paradoxical bronchoconstriction was observed with previous formulations of ipratropium bromide; however, reformulation of the nebulization solution without the preservatives EDTA and benzalkonium chloride has eliminated this response (Rafferty et al 1998).

Ipratropium bromide can be administered to horses via ultrasonic nebulizer (2 to 3 µg/kg), dry powder inhaler (200 µg/100 kg; 2400 µg/horse) or MDI via the Equine AeroMask (180–360 µg/500 kg horse) (Duvivier et al 1999a, Hoffman 1997, Robinson et al 1993). The onset of bronchodilatation in heaves-affected horses is approximately 15–30 min and the effect lasts approximately 4–6 h. Administration of ipratropium (and atropine) produces a more significant improvement in pulmonary resistance than in dynamic compliance. Dynamic compliance provides a reflection of peripheral airway function whereas pulmonary resistance is more easily influenced by larger, more central airways. This finding is consistent with the greater bronchodilatory effect of ipratropium in larger, more central airways. Administration of ipratropium prior to exercise in horses with recurrent airway obstruction does not improve exercise performance. Failure of ipratropium under these circumstances may result from the bronchodilatation normally associated with the sympathetic drive of exercise (Duvivier et al 1999a).

The combination of albuterol sulfate and ipratropium bromide is available commercially in a metered-dose inhaler device for humans. In human patients with chronic obstructive pulmonary disease, this anticholinergic β_2 agonist combination provides more complete bronchodilatation than either drug alone. The β_2 agonist predominately relaxes small (peripheral) airway smooth muscle whereas the anticholinergic drug has a greater effect on the relaxation of larger (more central) airways. Short-acting β_2 agonists provide rapid relief from bronchoconstriction whereas the response to ipratropium is delayed. In contrast, the relief provided by ipratropium will last longer (4–6 h) than the bronchodilatory activity of albuterol. Reversibility of airway obstruction using β_2 agonists does not predict the anticholinergic response in human asthmatics and visa versa. Therefore, combination anticholinergic/β_2 agonist therapy provides broad-spectrum relief of bronchoconstriction for a heterogeneous population of human patients.

Oxitropium and tiotropium bromides

Oxitropium and tiotropium bromides are quaternary scopolamine (hyoscine) derivatives; these anticholinergic agents have a prolonged duration of effect (>12 h) in human patients. Oxitropium is 10 times more potent than atropine and its bioavailability from the respiratory (12%) and gastrointestinal tract (0.48%) is poor in humans (Ensing et al 1989). Like ipratropium, tiotropium is a non-selective muscarinic antagonist; however, it dissociates slowly from muscarinic M_3 (and M_1) receptors. Slow dissociation from M_3 receptors results in the prolonged (12–24 h) duration of activity of tiotropium (Barnes 2000). Tiotropium is approximately 10-fold more potent than ipratropium. These newer-generation anticholinergic agents may prove attractive for treatment of recurrent airway obstruction in horses if their duration of action is similar to that in humans.

Combination therapy

Regular administration of bronchodilating agents as monotherapy to control the clinical signs of airway obstruction is inappropriate (Sears 1995). Although these agents provide symptomatic relief of the clinical signs of airway obstruction,

they do not alter the underlying inflammatory process. In human patients, tolerance to symptomatic bronchodilator therapy and deterioration in pulmonary function develops rapidly and may be associated with serious consequences (Varner & Busse 1996). Preliminary data in horses indicate that tolerance to β_2 agonists may occur within 1 week of commencing regular administration (Bayly et al 2000).

Combination therapy using aerosolized bronchodilators and corticosteroids is the most appropriate therapeutic approach for horses with recurrent airway obstruction. Bronchodilators provide immediate relief of bronchoconstriction, whereas corticosteroids reduce the underlying inflammation over a period of days to weeks. The pulmonary distribution of aerosolized preparations is poor in horses with severe airway obstruction; however, aerosolized β_2 agonists remain effective regardless of the severity of disease. Precedent short-acting, aerosolized bronchodilator therapy, such as albuterol sulfate, is recommended to improve the pulmonary distribution of surface-active corticosteroid preparations. Aerosolized corticosteroids do not improve the clinical signs of airway obstruction for several days; therefore, bronchodilators provide first-line (rescue) therapy for emergency treatment of acute, severe airway obstruction. In human asthmatics, corticosteroid therapy prevents and/or reverts tolerance to β_2 adrenergic drugs by preventing the downregulation of β_2 adrenoceptors and inducing the formation of new β_2 adrenoceptors on pulmonary cells. In human patients with poor asthma control despite appropriate maintenance corticosteroid therapy, optimal control of the clinical signs is obtained by the addition of a bronchodilator rather than by increasing the dose of corticosteroid. Increasing the dose of corticosteroid does not provide an equivalent improvement in the therapeutic efficacy in human asthmatics or heaves-affected horses and is typically not effective in stabilizing the clinical signs in human patients with severe disease. Dose-dependent therapeutic effects of inhaled steroids are not typically observed beyond the recommended dosage range; however, the risk of adverse side-effects is dose dependent.

ANTI-INFLAMMATORY THERAPY

In asthmatic human patients, the therapeutic emphasis has shifted away from symptomatic bronchodilator therapy and focused on daily anti-inflammatory therapy to prevent episodes of airway obstruction (Barnes et al 1998). It is now recognized that inflammation is the underlying component in all cases of bronchoconstriction and daily anti-inflammatory therapy often eliminates the need for symptomatic bronchodilator therapy. Corticosteroids are the only drug class that demonstrates sustained modification of the disease course in asthmatic human patients. Recent investigations indicate that early intervention is an important prognostic determinant and long-term, low-dose administration is associated with progressive improvement in pulmonary function and a reduction in non-specific and allergen-induce airway responsiveness (Barnes et al 1998).

Corticosteroids

Glucocorticoid receptors are located in the cytoplasm of target cells and are distributed widely throughout the pulmonary system. Immunocytochemical localization studies indicate that the greatest density of glucocorticoid receptor expression is in airway epithelial cells and bronchial vascular endothelial cells (Barnes et al 1998). Corticosteroids produce their effects on responsive cells by activating the glucocorticoid receptor, which directly or indirectly regulates the transcription of target genes. The number of genes per cell directly regulated by corticosteroids ranges from 10 to 100 and numerous genes are regulated indirectly through the interaction with other transcription factors. Corticosteroids suppress inflammation by decreasing the transcription of proinflammatory genes and increasing the transcription of anti-inflammatory genes, such as inhibitory protein κB (IκB), secretory leukocyte protease inhibitor and interleukin (IL) 10. IκB inhibits the activity of nuclear factor κB (NFκB), which appears to play a pivotal role in the inflammatory process in heaves (Bureau et al 2000). Transcription factor NFκB is highly activated in

bronchoalveolar lavage cells of heaves-affected horses during an episode of airway obstruction (Bureau et al 2000). Further, there is a strong correlation between NFκB activity and pulmonary dysfunction and inflammation (percent neutrophils) in horses with heaves. NFκB is activated by stimuli that lead to the exacerbation of airway obstruction and it induces the expression of multiple proinflammatory genes that are abnormally expressed in the airways of heaves-affected horses (intercellular adhesion molecule 1 (ICAM-1), IL-8). Corticosteroids increase the expression of IκB, which binds to NFκB within the cytoplasm, preventing the activation of proinflammatory genes. Secretory leukocyte protease inhibitor is the predominant antiprotease in conducting airways and appears to be pivotal to reducing airway inflammation in humans. IL-10 has anti-inflammatory activity via the suppression of transcription of many proinflammatory cytokines and chemokines. Corticosteroid administration has been shown to increase IL-10 production by pulmonary macrophages in asthmatic humans (Barnes et al 1998). In many tissues, corticosteroid administration increases the synthesis of lipocortin 1 (an inhibitor of phospholipase A_2), a primary anti-inflammatory protein. However, lipocortin 1 expression is not increased in pulmonary tissue in response to aerosolized corticosteroid administration and appears to play no role in reduction of pulmonary inflammation in asthmatic human patients.

Horses appear to be more sensitive to the adrenosuppressive effects of aerosolized corticosteroids than human patients. Documentation of systemic absorption (adrenal suppression) of inhaled beclometasone and fluticasone raises concerns that other systemic glucocorticoid effects may occur following aerosol administration of corticosteroids. The administration of adrenosuppressive doses ($>1600\,\mu g/day$) of beclometasone dipropionate to asthmatic human patients does not produce the other systemic side-effects of glucocorticoid administration, including a round face (Cushingoid facies), polyuria, polydipsia, hyperglycemia, obesity, altered carbohydrate metabolism, osteoporosis, abortion, posterior subcapsular cataract and aseptic necrosis of the femoral head (Barnes et al 1998). Adrenal suppression is the most sensitive indicator of the systemic absorption of inhaled corticosteroids and does not necessarily correlate with other systemic effects of the glucocorticoids. No cases of clinical adrenal insufficiency or adrenal exhaustion have been reported in asthmatic human patients treated for years at a time with inhaled corticosteroids. Clinical signs of iatrogenic Cushing's syndrome, such as laminitis, secondary bacterial infection, polyuria and polydipsia, have not been observed in horses given beclometasone or fluticasone. Adrenal responsiveness to exogenous adrenocorticotropic hormone (ACTH) is maintained in horses during treatment with aerosolized corticosteroids (Rush et al 1998c, Viel 1999). However, clinicians should administer inhaled corticosteroids judiciously and prescribe the lowest effective dose for a relatively short period.

The timing of corticosteroid administration has been pinpointed to interact with the diurnal rhythm of the hypothalamic–pituitary–adrenal axis in humans (Meibohm et al 1997). Dose timing has a pivotal effect on the safety profile and consequently the risk–benefit ratio of inhaled corticosteroids. In humans, maximum adrenal suppression occurs with the administration of aerosolized corticosteroids in the early morning hours, whereas endogenous cortisol production is least disrupted by administration in the afternoon. The circadian pattern results from the

temporal arrangement of the systemic drug activity in relation to endogenous cortisol release. In humans, adrenal suppression is maximized when systemic drug concentrations are high at the time of the maximum endogenous cortisol release (3 a.m.) and minimized if high systemic drug activity is synchronized with the minimum endogenous cortisol release (in the late evening). Therefore, in humans, the longer the terminal elimination half-life of a drug, the earlier in the afternoon it should be administered. The safety and efficacy of once daily administration (afternoon/evening) of aerosolized corticosteroids in horses has not been evaluated.

There are three aerosolized corticosteroid preparations available in MDI formulation for administration to horses via the Equine AeroMask: beclometasone dipropionate, fluticasone propionate and flunisolide (Table 16.2). In terms of the relative potency, fluticasone is more potent than beclometasone, which is more potent than flunisolide, which is equipotent to triamcinolone. Using dexamethasone as the standard (1.0), the relative glucocorticoid receptor affinity of the common corticosteroids is flunisolide 1.9, triamcinolone 2.0, beclometasone (active metabolite) 13.5 and fluticasone propionate 22.0 (Barnes et al 1998). The pulmonary residence time of the aerosolized corticosteroids is determined by the lipophilicity of each drug. Flunisolide has intermediate water solubility (10 mg/ml), similar to

Table 16.2 Aerosolized anti-inflammatory therapy

Drug	Drug class	Dose	Frequency	Device	Comments
Beclometasone	Corticosteroid	500 μg	b.i.d.	Equine Aerosol Delivery Device	Minimum adrenal suppression
Beclometasone	Corticosteroid	3750 μg	b.i.d.	MDI and Equine AeroMask	
Fluticasone	Corticosteroid	2000 μg	b.i.d.	MDI and Equine AeroMask	Minimum-to-moderate adrenal suppression
Sodium cromoglicate	Mast cell stabilizer	80 mg	Once daily	Jet nebulizer	Maintenance therapy, prophylaxis for heaves
Sodium cromoglicate	Mast cell stabilizer	200 mg	b.i.d.	Jet nebulizer	Inflammatory airway disease (mast cells > 2%)
Nedocromil sodium	Mast cell stabilizer	40 mg	q.i.d.	MDI and Equine AeroMask	Inflammatory airway disease (mast cells > 2%)

b.i.d., twice daily; q.i.d., four times a day; MDI, metered-dose inhalant triamcinolone; however, beclometasone (active metabolite) and fluticasone are more lipophilic (water solubility 0.1 mg/ml), resulting in more prolonged tissue retention. The therapeutic index is defined as the ratio between beneficial clinical effects and adverse effects. Drugs with a higher therapeutic index have a more favorable risk–benefit ratio. In general, the therapeutic index of the aerosolized corticosteroids is fluticasone > beclometasone > flunisolide > triamcinolone.

Beclometasone dipropionate

Beclometasone dipropionate is the most widely dispensed inhaled anti-inflammatory agent for asthmatic human patients. Inhaled beclometasone dipropionate reduces inflammatory cell populations in bronchoalveolar lavage fluid, controls clinical signs of airway obstruction and improves parameters of pulmonary function in human asthmatics. Consequently, aerosolized beclometasone dipropionate is the first line of therapy for moderate-to-severe allergic airway disease in human patients. Aerosolized beclometasone does not cause adrenal suppression in asthmatic human patients at therapeutic dosages (800–1600 μg/day) and initiation of beclometasone therapy as a replacement for systemic corticosteroid administration permits recovery of the hypothalamic–pituitary–adrenal axis (Barnes et al 1998).

Beclometasone (500–1500 μg twice daily via the Equine Aerosol Drug Delivery System) has been shown to reduce pulmonary inflammation (Rush et al 1998a), improve parameters of pulmonary function (Rush et al 1998b) and improve ventilation imaging of horses with recurrent airway obstruction. There was no immediate (15 min) therapeutic effect; however, the clinical signs and pulmonary function began to improve within 24 h of administration (Rush et al 1999b). Administration of beclometasone dipropionate (3750 μg twice daily using the Equine AeroMask) improved parameters of pulmonary function and arterial oxygen tension during a 2-week treatment period; however, parameters returned to pretreatment values 7 days after the discontinuation of drug treatment (Ammann et al 1998).

Neutrophilia (50–90%) in bronchoalveolar lavage fluid is the most consistent cytological abnormality in heaves-affected horses and is significantly reduced after beclometasone administration. Although pulmonary neutrophilic inflammation responds favorably to inhaled beclometasone, pulmonary neutrophil counts rebound to pretreatment values within 7 days after the discontinuation of drug treatment (Rush et al 1998b). The clinical signs of airway obstruction return 3 to 4 days after the discontinuation of beclometasone treatment and most pulmonary function abnormalities return to pretreatment values within 7 days after withdrawal of the drug. Short-term administration of inhaled beclometasone without minimizing environmental allergen exposure is not expected to provide prolonged anti-inflammatory benefit to horses with recurrent airway obstruction.

Endogenous cortisol production is suppressed by approximately 35 to 50% of baseline values within 24 h of administration of high-dose beclometasone (>1000 μg twice daily) to horses (Rush et al 1999c). After a 7-day treatment period, serum cortisol concentrations fall to 10–20% of baseline values. However, serum cortisol concentrations recover approximately 2 days after the discontinuation of drug treatment and adrenal responsiveness to exogenous ACTH administration is not affected by treatment for 7 days (Rush et al 1998c). Considering the known safety of long-term administration (years) of inhaled beclometasone to human patients at relatively low doses (800 μg twice daily) (Barnes et al 1998), marked suppression of endogenous cortisol production within 1 day of treatment commencing in horses was an unexpected finding. The threshold for adrenal suppression in normal and heaves-affected horses is approximately 500 μg beclometasone twice daily (Rush et al 1999c). The therapeutic efficacy of this minimally adrenosuppressive dose of beclometasone is equivalent to the efficacy of doses in excess of 1000 μg twice daily (Rush et al 1998b).

Beclometasone dipropionate is a synthetic, chlorinated, diester corticosteroid. The majority (>75%) of parent drug is hydrolyzed rapidly (within 5 min) in the lung to the more active metabolite beclometasone 17-monopropionate, which has a relative binding affinity that is 30 times greater than that of the parent drug. A smaller proportion of beclometasone dipropionate (approximately 7%) is hydrolyzed to the alternative metabolites beclometasone 21-monopropionate and beclometasone. The former is relatively inactive with 50 times less intrinsic activity than the parent drug, whereas the latter has approximately twice the activity of the parent drug. After oral administration (as a result of pharyngeal drug deposition), the majority of beclometasone dipropionate is converted to beclometasone 17-monopropionate in the small intestine, and the bioavailability is approximately 20%. The half-life of the active metabolite, beclometasone 17-monopropionate is approximately 2 h (children) to 6.5 h (adults), whereas the half-life of parent drug is approximately 6 min. First-pass metabolism of these two forms are approximately 79%.

In humans, the pulmonary drug deposition of HFA–beclometasone is superior to CFC–beclometasone and is improved by 10-fold in some studies (Sears 1995). Equivalent improvements in asthma control are seen with half of the daily dose of HFA–beclometasone compared with CFC–beclometasone. The greater systemic availability of HFA–beclometasone does not increase adrenal suppression; the adrenal effects and acute local tolerability are comparable to that of the CFC formulation at the same dose. Equivalent efficacy at a lower dose and equivalent safety at the same dose indicate a more favorable risk–benefit ratio for HFA–beclometasone. Comparative studies of HFA– and CFC–beclometasone have not been performed in horses. In theory, the enhanced drug delivery and efficacy of HFA–beclometasone may explain, in part, why relatively low doses of beclometasone are therapeutically effective in heaves-affected horses, compared with standard therapeutic doses in asthmatic humans.

Fluticasone propionate

Fluticasone propionate is an androstane, carbothioate corticosteroid. Of the available aerosolized corticosteroid preparations commercially, fluticasone propionate is the most potent, most lipophilic and most expensive. It has the longest pulmonary residence time because of its high lipophilicity. Fluticasone is not metabolized by the lung and is absorbed into systemic circulation unchanged. Oral bioavailability of fluticasone is negligible (<2%). Fluticasone undergoes extensive first-pass hepatic metabolism (99%) to inactive metabolites. As a result, it has a low bioavailability following oral administration and the least potential for adrenal suppression. The terminal half-life of fluticasone propionate after inhalation therapy is approximately 6 h.

In asthmatic human patients, fluticasone propionate improves asthma symptoms and parameters, improves pulmonary function and reduces pulmonary inflammation and airway reactivity (Barnes et al 1998). Regular fluticasone reduces or eliminates the need for rescue β_2 agonist therapy and produces progressive improvement in airway reactivity and pulmonary function. In clinical studies, equivalent efficacy is demonstrated with one-quarter of the dose of fluticasone compared with flunisolide and budesonide, and equivalent efficacy is demonstrated with one-half of the dose of fluticasone compared with beclometasone. Adrenal function is less affected by fluticasone propionate at therapeutic doses than with beclometasone, flunisolide or budesonide. Although all aerosolized corticosteroids are considered safe, fluticasone has the least potential for adverse systemic effects and has the most favorable therapeutic index.

In heaves-affected horses, fluticasone propionate (2000 μg twice daily by Equine AeroMask) has been shown to reduce pulmonary neutrophilia, improve parameters of pulmonary function and reduce responsiveness to histamine challenge during an episode of airway obstruction (Viel 1999). In normal horses, fluticasone propionate reduces serum cortisol concentrations by 40% after 1 day of therapy and by 65% after 7 days. Serum cortisol concentrations return to pretreatment values within 1–2 days after the discontinuation of drug treatment.

Flunisolide

Flunisolide is the least potent of the synthetic, topically active corticosteroids (Chaplin et al

1980) and, because it is the least lipophilic of the agents, it has the shortest pulmonary residence time. Flunisolide is similar to triamcinolone in terms of potency, lipophilicity and clinical efficacy. Much higher dosages are required to achieve therapeutic effects similar to those with fluticasone or beclometasone. Equivalent therapeutic effects can be achieved in asthmatic human patients with equipotent doses; however, adverse effects (adrenal suppression) occur more frequently with flunisolide. The primary advantage of flunisolide is its cost. Flunisolide has a relatively high oral bioavailability (21%) and is extensively absorbed as unchanged drug from the respiratory tract. The terminal half-life of flunisolide after inhalation therapy is approximately 1.7 h. Flunisolide undergoes rapid, extensive hepatic first-pass metabolism to relatively inactive compounds (6β-hydroxyl metabolite and conjugates). Despite its limitations, the therapeutic index of flunisolide is superior to corticosteroids administered systemically. In fact, initiation of flunisolide therapy as a replacement for oral prednisone allows recovery of the hypothalamic–pituitary–adrenal axis and superior control in human patients with steroid-dependent asthma. The safety and efficacy of aerosolized flunisolide has not been evaluated in heaves-affected horses.

Mast cell stabilizers (cromones)

Sodium cromoglicate and nedocromil sodium inhibit the degranulation of mast cells. Their structure is dissimilar and their mechanism of action unclear. Mast cell-stabilizing drugs have a delayed onset of action and are indicated for the prophylaxis of airway obstruction. They are ineffective for rescue therapy and are not recommended for the stabilization of clinical signs during an acute episode of airway obstruction. In clinical studies in human asthmatics, aerosolized corticosteroids provide superior improvements in pulmonary function and pulmonary inflammation compared with aerosolized cromones. In fact, mast cell stabilizers do not have any significant effect on inflammatory markers in bronchial biopsies of patients with asthma. Nonetheless, the addition of nedocromil sodium to high-dose

corticosteroid therapy improves asthma control in select patients (Barnes et al 1998).

Mast cell-stabilizing agents provide some benefit as maintenance therapy for heaves-affected horses during periods of remission (Table 16.2). The administration of disodium cromoglicate (80 mg via nebulization) 20–30 min prior to allergen challenge delays the induction of the clinical signs of airway obstruction (Thomson & McPherson 1981). Administration of 80 mg for 4 consecutive days (once daily) delayed the induction of airway obstruction for approximately 3 weeks. Another study demonstrated a minimal benefit with doses up to 500 mg daily for 2 days prior to allergen exposure (Soma et al 1987). It is important to recognize that mast cells do not appear to play a significant role in the pathophysiology of recurrent airway obstruction in horses and these drugs should not be considered an alternative to corticosteroid therapy in horses with heaves.

Mast cell stabilizers are indicated for the treatment of inflammatory airway disease in some horses. Inflammatory airway disease is observed in young horses; the clinical syndrome is characterized by poor exercise performance, chronic cough and the presence of exudate in the tracheobronchial tree. A subset of horses with inflammatory airway disease will have metachromatic inflammation in bronchoalveolar lavage, with mast cells constituting 2–5% of the total cell count. This form of chronic lower airway inflammation probably represents a local pulmonary hypersensitivity reaction. There is controversy as to whether this form of inflammatory airway disease represents an early form of recurrent airway obstruction. Nebulization of sodium cromoglicate (200 mg) will improve the clinical signs of respiratory disease and will stabilize mast cell histamine release (Hare et al 1994).

ANTIMICROBIAL THERAPY

Antimicrobial agents have been inhaled in human medicine for decades; however, this practice has always been controversial. There are relatively few accepted indications for this mode of administration. The chronic administration of tobramycin is effective in the maintenance of patients with cystic fibrosis; inhaled pentamidine is indicated for prophylaxis against *Pneumocystis carinii* infection in patients with human immunodeficiency virus infection and inhaled ribavirin (tribararin) is used to treat respiratory syncytial virus infection in children (O'Riordan & Faris 1999). The therapeutic efficacy of aerosolized antimicrobial agents for the treatment of bacterial alveolar and bronchial infections in humans is inconclusive, which may result from inconsistencies in the nebulization device, antimicrobial dose and the duration of therapy. The beta-lactams (penicillin, carbenicillin and cefaloradine), polymixins (polymixin B and colistin sulfate) and aminoglycosides (gentamicin, amikacin and tobramicin) have been administered safely via inhalation to human patients.

The advantages of aerosol therapy with an antimicrobial agent include direct delivery of the drug to the site of infection, rapid onset of action and reduced systemic drug concentrations (toxicity and cost). Aerosol administration results in high concentrations of antimicrobial agent on the mucosal surface of the lower respiratory tract. The efficacy of antimicrobial agents in the treatment of pulmonary bacterial infections is more closely associated with the antimicrobial concentration (time above minimal inhibitory concentration (MIC) for concentration-independent agents) within the respiratory tract than with antimicrobial concentrations in serum (McKenzie & Murray 2000).

In calves, nebulization of ceftiofur sodium (1 mg/kg) is superior to intramuscular (i.m.) administration (1 mg/kg) for the treatment of *Pasteurella haemolytica* pneumonia (Sustronck et al 1995). Aerosolized ceftiofur reduces mortality and clinical and hematological parameters return to normal significantly faster than in calves receiving ceftiofur i.m.

Aminoglycosides are ideal candidates for aerosol administration. This group exhibits concentration-dependent bacterial killing and induces long postantibiotic effects against susceptible organisms (see Ch. 2). In other words, the efficacy of the aminoglycosides is directly related to peak drug concentrations and the postantibiotic effect allows for less-frequent drug administration. In adult horses, aerosol administration of gentamicin sulfate (20 ml of 50 mg/ml) produced significantly higher drug concentrations in mucosal secretions than intravenous (i.v.) administration (6.6 mg/kg) for 8 h after administration (McKenzie & Murray 1998). Maximal gentamicin concentrations in bronchial lavage are approximately 12 times greater after aerosol administration than after i.v. administration.

The magnitude and duration of drug concentrations above MIC in respiratory secretions after aerosol administration indicate that inhalation therapy may be a suitable option for some bacterial infections of the lower respiratory tract. Pretreatment with a short-acting, aerosolized bronchodilator, such as albuterol sulfate, may improve the pulmonary distribution of aerosolized antimicrobial drugs.

The formulation of an antimicrobial nebulization solution can alter the characteristics of the aerosol and the response to drug administration. High solute concentrations decrease aerosol production and particle size (McKenzie & Murray 2000). Regardless of the drug, the concentration of the antimicrobial agent in the solution for nebulization should be 100 mg/ml or less in 0.23–0.45% saline. Antimicrobial concentrations >100 mg/ml decrease the efficiency of aerosol generation, thus prolonging the time required for drug administration.

There are several disadvantages to aerosol administration of antimicrobial agents, such as drug administration time (15–20 min), potential for pulmonary contamination with environmental pathogens and poor drug delivery to unventilated regions of lung. Inhalation therapy is ineffective in individuals with significant consolidation or interstitial involvement and should not be used as monotherapy. Some aerosol solutions will induce bronchoconstriction owing to irritation caused by the drug, drug carrier, tonicity or pH. In addition, topical administration of antibiotics to surfaces containing large numbers of diverse bacteria may select antibiotic resistant strains of bacteria. There are two potential mechanisms for the development of resistance with aerosol antimicrobial therapy: emergence of resistant organisms of the primary species or overgrowth of a genus intrinsically resistant to the agent administered. Both of these mechanisms have been observed in human patients receiving prophylactic aerosolized antimicrobial therapy to prevent nosocomial infection (Smith & Ramsey 1995).

Aerosol administration of antimicrobial drugs is technically feasible in horses and the available devices can readily deliver clinically relevant dosages to the lower respiratory tract. Controlled, prospective studies must be performed to determine appropriate indications in horses, including the need for concurrent systemic antimicrobial therapy, ideal drug concentrations and dosages and the susceptibility of specific respiratory pathogens.

Advances in the equipment for the administration of aerosol medication to horses have facilitated the widespread use of inhalation therapy in equine medicine. Newer aerosolization devices ease administration and make pulmonary drug delivery efficient. Aerosol therapy is likely to become the mainstay of treatment for horses with heaves and may prove beneficial in the treatment of infectious respiratory disease in horses.

REFERENCES

Ammann V, Vrins A, Lavoie J 1998 Effects of inhaled beclomethasone dipropionate on respiratory function in horses with chronic obstructive pulmonary disease (COPD). Equine Veterinary Journal 30:152–157

Bailey J, Colahan P, Kubilis P et al 1999 Effect of inhaled beta$_2$ adrenoceptor agonist, albuterol sulphate, on performance of horses. Equine Veterinary Journal Supplement 30:575–580

Barnes P 2000 The pharmacological properties of tiotropium. Chest 117(suppl 2):3–6

Barnes P, Pedersen S, Busse W 1998 Efficacy and safety of inhaled corticosteroids. American Journal of Respiratory and Critical Care Medicine 157:1–53

Bayly W M, Mitten L, Hines M et al 2000 Repeated doses of aerosolized albuterol sulfate in equidae with recurrent airway obstruction. In: Proceedings of the 18th Symposium of the Comparative Respiratory Society, Melbourne, Australia, p. A48

Bureau F, Bonizzi G, Kirschvink N et al 2000 Correction between Nuclear factor κB activity in bronchial brushing samples and lung dysfunction in an animal model of asthma. American Journal of Respiratory and Critical Care Medicine 161:1314–1321

Chaplin M, Rooks W, Swenson E et al 1980 Flunisolide metabolism and dynamics of a metabolite. Clinical Pharmacology and Therapeutics 27:402–413

Derksen F, Robinson N, Berney C 1992 Aerosol pirbuterol: bronchodilator activity and side-effects in ponies with recurrent airway obstruction (heaves). Equine Veterinary Journal 24:107–112

Derksen F, Olszewski M, Robinson N 1996 Use of a hand-held, metered-dose aerosol delivery device to administer pirbuterol acetate to horses with heaves. Equine Veterinary Journal 28:306–310

Derksen F, Olszewski M, Robinson N 1999 Aerosolized albuterol sulfate used as a bronchodilator in horses with recurrent airway obstruction. American Journal of Veterinary Research 60:689–693

Duvivier D, Votion D, Vandenput S et al 1997 Technical validation of a facemask adapted for dry powder inhalation in the equine species. Equine Veterinary Journal 29:471–476

Duvivier D, Bayly W, Votion D et al 1999a Effects of inhaled dry powder ipratropium bromide on recovery from exercise of horses with COPD. Equine Veterinary Journal 31:20–24

Duvivier D, Votion D, Roberts C et al 1999b Inhalation therapy of equine respiratory disorders. Equine Veterinary Education 11:124–130

Emerman C, Cydulka R, Skobeloff E 1996 Survey of asthma practice among emergency physicians. Chest 109:708–712

Ensing K, de Zeeuw R A, in't Hout W G et al 1989 Application of a radioreceptor assay in the pharmacokinetic study of oxitropium bromide in healthy volunteers after single iv, oral and inhalation doses. European Journal of Clinical Pharmacology 37:507–512

Finnerty J, Howard P 1993 Paradoxal bronchoconstriction with nebulized albuterol but not with terbutaline. American Review of Respiratory Disease 148:513

Geor R, Johnson G 1993 Deposition of radiolabeled aerosols within the equine respiratory tract. In: Proceedings of the 12th Veterinary Respiratory Symposium of the Comparative Respiratory Society, Kennett Square, PA, 1993

Hare J, Viel L, O'Byrne P 1994 Effect of sodium cromoglycate on light racehorses with elevated metachromatic cell numbers on bronchoalveolar lavage. Journal of Veterinary Pharmacology and Therapeutics 17:237–242

Hoffman A 1997 Inhaled medications and bronchodilator use in the horse. Veterinary Clinics of North America Equine Practice 13:519–530

Linden A, Rabe K, Lofdahl C-G 1996 Pharmacological basis for duration of effect: formoterol and salmeterol versus short-acting beta$_2$ adrenoceptor agonists. Lung 174:1–22

McKenzie H, Murray J 1998 Time/concentration relationships of gentamicin in serum and bronchial lavage fluid of horses administered gentamicin intravenously and by aerosol. In: Proceedings of the World Equine Airway Symposium, Guelph, Ontario, p. 29

McKenzie H C III, Murray M J 2000 Concentrations of gentamicin in serum and bronchial lavage fluid after intravenous and aerosol administration of gentamicin to horses. American Journal of Veterinary Research 61:1185–1190

Meibohm B, Hochhaus G, Rohatoagi S et al 1997 Dependency of cortisol suppression on the administration time of inhaled corticosteroids. Journal of Clinical Pharmacology 37:704–710

O'Riordan T, Faris M 1999 Inhaled antimicrobial therapy. Respiratory Care Clinics of North America 5:617–631

Page C, Morley J 1999 Contrasting properties of albuterol stereoisomers. Journal of Allergy and Clinical Immunology 104:31–41

Rafferty P, Beasley R, Holgate S T 1998 Comparison of the efficacy of preservative free ipratropium bromide and Atrovent nebuliser solution. Thorax 43:446–450

Robinson N, Derksen F, Berney C et al 1993 The airway response of horses with recurrent airway obstruction (heaves) to aerosol administration of ipratropium bromide. Equine Veterinary Journal 25:299–303

Robinson N, Derksen F, Olszewski M 1996 The pathogenesis of chronic obstructive pulmonary disease of horses. British Veterinary Journal 152:283–306

Rush B, Flaminio M, Matson C et al 1998a Cytologic evaluation of bronchoalveolar lavage fluid in horses with recurrent airway obstruction after aerosol and parenteral administration of beclomethasone dipropionate and dexamethasone, respectively. American Journal of Veterinary Research 59:1033–1038

Rush B, Raub E, Rhoads W et al 1998b Pulmonary function in horses with recurrent airway obstruction after aerosol and parenteral administration of beclomethasone dipropionate and dexamethasone, respectively. American Journal of Veterinary Research 59:1039–1043

Rush B R, Worster A A, Flaminio M J et al 1998c Alteration in adrenocortical function in horses with recurrent airway obstruction after aerosol and parenteral administration of beclomethasone dipropionate and dexamethasone, respectively. American Journal of Veterinary Research 59:1044–1047

Rush B, Hoskinson J, Davis E et al 1999a Pulmonary distribution of radioaerosol in horses with heaves after inhalation of single-dose albuterol sulfate. American Journal of Veterinary Research 60:764–769

Rush B, Raub E, Hakala J et al 1999b Incremental doses of aerosolized beclomethasone in horses with recurrent airway obstruction. In: Proceedings of the 17th Symposium of the Comparative Respiratory Society, Harrison Hot Springs, BC, p. 95

Rush B, Trevino I, Matson C 1999c Serum cortisol concentration in response to incremental doses of inhaled beclomethasone dipropionate. Equine Veterinary Journal 31:258–261

Seale J, Harrison L 1998 Effect of changing the fine particle mass of inhaled beclomethasone dipropionate on intrapulmonary deposition and pharmacokinetics. Respiratory Medicine 92:9–15

Sears M R 1995 Is the routine use of beta-adrenergic agonists appropriate in asthma treatment? American Journal of Respiratory and Critical Care Medicine 151:599–601

Smith A, Ramsey B 1995 Aerosol administration of antibiotics. Respiration 62(suppl 1):19–24

Soma L, Beech J, Gerber N 1987 Effects of cromolyn in horses with chronic obstructive pulmonary disease. Veterinary Research Communications 11:339–344

Sustronck B, Deprez P, Muylle E 1995 Evaluation of nebulization of sodium ceftiofur in the treatment of experimental *Pasteurella haemolytica* bronchopneumonia in calves. Research in Veterinary Science 59:267–271

Tesarowski D, Viel L, McOnell W 1994 The rapid and effective administration of a beta$_2$-agonist to horses with heaves using a compact inhalation device and metered-dose inhalers. Canadian Veterinary Journal 35:170–173

Thomson J, McPherson E 1981 Prophylactic effects of sodium cromoglycate on chronic obstructive pulmonary disease in the horse. Equine Veterinary Journal 13:243–251

Varner A, Busse W 1996 Are you undertreating inflammation in asthma? Journal of Respiratory Disease 17:656–668

Viel L 1999 Therapeutic efficacy of inhaled fluticasone propionate in horses with chronic obstructive pulmonary disease. In: Proceedings of the 45th American Association of Equine Practitioners Annual Convention, Albuquerque, NM, pp. 306–307

Votion D, Ghafir Y, Munsters K et al 1997 Aerosol deposition in equine lungs following ultrasonic nebulisation versus jet aerosol delivery system. Equine Veterinary Journal 29:388–393

Zhang X, Zhu F, Olszewski M et al 1998 Effects of enantiomers of beta2-agonists on ACh release and smooth muscle contraction in the trachea. American Journal of Physiology 274:32–38

CHAPTER CONTENTS

Principles of fluid therapy   327

Types of fluid   330
  Crystalloids   330
  Colloids   336

Blood and blood substitutes   343
  Whole blood   343
  Blood substitutes   344

Parenteral nutrition   344

Fluid therapy delivery   346
  Delivery systems   346
  Therapy plan: infusion rates and volumes   348

Correction of acid–base and electrolyte
disturbances   351

Complications of fluid therapy   357
  Thrombophlebitis   357
  Overhydration   357

Beyond fluid therapy   358

References   358

17

Fluid therapy

Kevin T. T. Corley

PRINCIPLES OF FLUID THERAPY

The main goal of fluid therapy is to increase cardiac output by increasing and then maintaining cardiac preload (Starling's law of the heart). This, in turn, increases oxygen delivery to the tissues. By selecting fluids with the appropriate electrolyte content, it is also possible to correct electrolyte and acid–base disturbances.

Formulating a fluid therapy plan

Fluid therapy should be based on an assessment of the horse's clinical status, an estimation of the severity of ongoing losses and available laboratory information. The plan should consist of selecting a type of fluid, a rate of administration and an appropriate delivery system. A fluid therapy plan will usually involve three phases. A resuscitation phase for treatment of hypovolemia, a rehydration phase for treatment of dehydration and a maintenance phase to provide ongoing fluid requirements. It should include a schedule of monitoring the effects of the fluid therapy, enabling adjustment as necessary. It is important to consider the practicality of administering fluids in the prevailing environmental conditions (e.g. fluids may freeze in cold weather). In horses destined for referral, the negative impact of any delay associated with fluid administration should be weighed against the perceived benefit of treatment, particularly when only small volumes can be administered.

The most important part of successful fluid therapy is to adjust the plan according to the response. Failure to do so will, at best, result in the client wasting money on unnecessary fluids. In the "worst case" scenario, this failure can cause severe iatrogenic electrolyte imbalances or severe hypovolemia, which may lead to the death of the animal.

Identifying patients requiring fluid therapy

Conditions that result in the loss of large volumes of body fluids, such as high-volume diarrhea and gastric reflux, obviously require aggressive fluid therapy. However, many other horses may require fluid therapy because of prolonged mild-to-moderate fluid losses or prolonged reduced fluid intake. In neonatal foals, reduced fluid intake can rapidly result in hypovolemia and severe dehydration. This section addresses the identification of these horses and foals.

Clinical signs

The clinical signs of hypovolemia and dehydration in the adult horse are listed in Table 17.1. Hypovolemia is defined as insufficient circulating blood volume, whereas dehydration is defined as loss of water from the tissues. It is important to distinguish between these conditions because hypovolemia requires immediate treatment but dehydration is optimally addressed over a period of 12–24 h. However, in most clinical scenarios, hypovolemia and dehydration occur concurrently.

Traditionally, clinical signs have been used to estimate percentage dehydration and formulate a fluid plan for replacement of the fluid deficit. Recent evidence from small animal medicine suggests that this method is unreliable (Hansen & DeFrancesco 2002). In the horse, at best, clinical signs may give an approximate guide to the severity of dehydration (Table 17.2). It should be noted that some signs associated with marked and severe dehydration are actually signs of hypovolemia. Horses that are considered to be moderately dehydrated probably require at least 50 ml/kg of crystalloid fluids to replace fluid deficits. In a 500 kg horse, this would represent 25 liters. The degree of dehydration is at best an approximation and should not be relied on to predict fluid requirements accurately. For this reason, the response to fluid therapy should always be monitored.

None of the clinical signs listed in Table 17.2 should be examined in isolation. It is important

Table 17.1 Clinical signs of hypovolemia and dehydration in the horse

	Signs
Hypovolemia	Tachycardia
	Cold extremities
	Tachypnea
	Decreased pulse pressure
	Reduced jugular fill
Dehydration	Prolonged skin tent
	Tacky mucous membranes
	Sunken eyes

Table 17.2 Clinical signs associated with different degrees of dehydration in the horse[a]

Degree of dehydration	Skin tent (s)	Mucous membranes	Capillary refill time	Heart rate (beats/min)[b]	Other signs
Moderate	1–3	Moist or slightly tacky	Normal (<2 s)	Normal	Decreased urine output
Marked	3–5	Tacky	Variable; often 2–3 s	40–60	Decreased arterial blood pressure
Severe	5 or more	Dry	Variable; often >4 s	≥60	Reduced jugular fill; barely detectable periph-eral pulse; sunken eyes

[a]Note that not all signs are consistently present in all horses
[b]Pain may also increase heart rate
Adapted with permission from Corley K T T 2002 Fluid therapy for horses with gastrointestinal diseases. In: Smith B P (ed) Large animal internal medicine, 3rd edn. Mosby, St Louis, MO, pp. 682–694

to make a judgement of the fluid status based on the whole animal. For example, in horses with colic, tachycardia may be caused by hypovolemia or by pain. To determine the source of the tachycardia, the accompanying clinical signs and the response to analgesics or fluid loading should be assessed.

In mature horses, tachycardia in hypovolemia is a physiological response to maintain cardiac output in the face of a falling stroke volume. Unfortunately, this physiological response appears not to occur in many critically ill neonatal foals. This means that hypovolemia can be more difficult to recognize in foals and that, because of poor compensation, it is associated with far higher morbidity and mortality. Other clinical signs of hypovolemia are also inconsistently present in neonatal foals. The clinical signs of dehydration are similar in the foal and the mature horse. However, the skin tent may be shorter in foals, because of increased elasticity of the skin.

Laboratory signs of hypovolemia

The laboratory tests used most commonly to assess hypovolemia are packed cell volume (PCV) and plasma total solids. Unfortunately, these tests are neither sensitive nor specific (Hansen & DeFrancesco 2002). The PCV may be increased substantially by splenic contraction, making small increases very hard to interpret. A PCV of >50% usually represents hypovolemia. The plasma total solids (protein measured by refractometer) or total protein concentration (measured by a chemistry analyzer) also increases with hypovolemia. How-ever significant protein loss can occur in disease (particularly colitis), resulting in a low or normal protein concentration despite hypovolemia. Further, hypergammaglobulinemia (e.g. in cyathostomiosis) can increase the plasma total protein concentration without the presence of hypovolemia. The PCV and plasma total solids are most useful when greatly increased or when used serially to monitor the response to fluid therapy.

Urine specific gravity is useful for monitoring the response to fluid therapy. Urine specific gravity can be measured easily in the field using a refractometer. High urine specific gravity (>1.040) indicates possible hypovolemia and normal renal concentration of urine. Isothenuria (1.010) indicates possible renal damage or a recent high fluid load. Rising or continually high specific gravity in the face of fluid therapy may indicate that insufficient fluid is being delivered to the horse. In the neonatal foal with normal renal function, urine specific gravity may increase early in fluid deprivation, before changes in other indicators such as heart rate, PCV, central venous pressure (CVP) and arterial blood pressure.

Plasma or serum creatinine concentrations are useful in the assessment of renal perfusion in the absence of renal dysfunction. High normal creatinine concentrations (1.5–1.8 mg/dl (130–160 μmol/l)) can be associated with subclinical hypovolemia and should be evaluated in the light of the history and clinical signs. Creatinine concentrations up to 3.5 mg/dl (310 μmol/l) are common in moderate-to-severe hypovolemia and concentrations as high as 5.0 mg/dl (450 μmol/l) are possible with prolonged hypovolemia. Even in severe hypovolemia, the creatinine concentration will not increase by much more than 2.3 mg/dl (200 μmol/l) per day (Tennant et al 1981). If the creatinine concentration is higher than would be suggested by the clinical signs and other laboratory parameters and if it does not decrease appropriately with fluid therapy, renal dysfunction should be suspected.

In the non-exercising horse, increased blood lactate concentrations are sufficient evidence of a metabolic disturbance to initiate fluid therapy. They are an indication of poor tissue perfusion or increased circulating epinephrine (adrenaline) concentrations (James et al 1999). Hypovolemia and endotoxemia are common causes of increased lactate concentrations in the horse. Endotoxemia increases tissue lactate production both through circulatory changes, which reduce blood flow to the tissues and inappropriate anaerobic metabolism (Fink 1997). Whereas lactate is a good indicator of the need to start fluid therapy, continued high lactate concentrations should be assessed in the context of cardiovascular parameters, such as pulse rate, urine output and blood pressure, because decreases in plasma lactate concentration can lag behind improved cardiovascular status (James et al 1999). High blood lactate concentrations have been associated with decreased survival in equine colic (Furr et al 1995). Lactate can be measured in the field using hand-held blood gas analyzers (i-STAT, Heska). The expected lactate concentration can also be calculated by means of equations based on electrolyte and acid–base measurements (Constable et al 1998, Corley & Marr 1998, Whitehair et al 1995). An increased circulating lactate concentration should be suspected when there is metabolic acidosis (decreased pH, negative base excess) in the absence of hyperchloremia or hyponatremia (Corley & Marr 1998).

Fluid requirements

Measurement of CVP and "fluid challenge" can be used to assess fluid requirements. Cardiac filling pressures, and the changes in these pressures in response to fluid therapy, are the most accurate method of determining fluid requirements in the hospitalized animal. It is relatively easy to measure CVP in the horse. In adult horses, sterile polyethylene tubing (PE190, outside diameter 1.70 mm, at least 1.5 m in length) can be passed through a 12 gauge jugular catheter into the thoracic vena cava or right atrium. In neonatal foals, the tip of a catheter 20 cm in length placed halfway down the jugular vein is usually intrathoracic and CVP can be measured directly from the catheter. The tubing or catheter is connected to a pressure transducer or manometer at the level of the sternal manubrium (Hall & Nigam 1975). The normal CVP of the adult horse is 5–14 mmHg (Hall & Nigam 1975). In foals less than 14 days old, the normal CVP is 2–9 mmHg (Thomas et al 1987). In horses with normal cardiac function, a high CVP indicates fluid overloading while a low CVP indicates insufficient circulating volume.

The change in CVP in response to a fluid challenge (bolus of fluid) (Webb 1997) is perhaps more accurate but this awaits formal evaluation in the horse. The fluid challenge method of monitoring fluid therapy may prove particularly useful in acute renal failure or pulmonary edema. In horses without pulmonary edema, a fluid challenge without measuring CVP can also be useful in the assessment of the fluid status of the horse. In horses with tachycardia, hypotension or oliguria, the purpose of the fluid challenge is to determine whether further fluids alone may reverse the abnormality or if another intervention is required. If there is no improvement after a 10 ml/kg bolus of crystalloids or a 2–3 ml/kg bolus of colloids, it is unlikely that fluid alone will be successful. The author uses this form of fluid challenge routinely in hypotensive individuals prior to starting a dobutamine infusion, as this drug may cause significant tachycardia in patients resuscitated with insufficient fluid (Hollenberg et al 1999).

TYPES OF FLUID

CRYSTALLOIDS

Crystalloid solutions consist of electrolytes in water. Crystalloid solutions may be isotonic, hypertonic or hypotonic. Isotonic solutions have approximately the same osmolality as plasma and, therefore, may be given rapidly in large volumes into peripheral veins. Hypertonic solutions act to draw water into the extracellular fluid (ECF) from the intracellular fluid and represent a method of rapidly restoring circulating volume at the expense of tissue hydration. Hypotonic solutions are usually only used to correct plasma hypertonicity. Because true hypotonic solutions (e.g. sterile water) cause erythrolysis (Krumbhaar 1914), they can only be given slowly via a central vein (Worthley 1986). For this reason, isotonic solutions containing a metabolizable substrate, such as dextrose, and no electrolytes are usually used.

Crystalloid fluids rapidly pass from the circulation to the interstitial fluid. This means that their resuscitation effect may be short lived and they can cause edema. Only 30% of isotonic fluids and 10% of hypotonic fluids remain in the circulation after 30 min (Spalding & Goodwin 1999). The increase in interstitial fluid may actually decrease tissue oxygen uptake in normal animals by increasing the diffusion distance between capillaries and cells (Gow et al 1998). However, crystalloids remain the cheapest and, in many circumstances, the best fluids for administration to the horse. All fluid therapy plans involve crystalloid fluids and these are frequently the only fluids administered.

Homemade or "Carboy" fluids, while considerably cheaper than fluids available commercially, have been associated with producing clinical signs of endotoxemia in normal horses (Denkhaus & van Amstel 1986) and a seven-fold increase in the risk of thrombophlebitis (Traub-Dargatz & Dargatz 1994) and, therefore, cannot be recommended.

Polyionic crystalloid solutions

Table 17.3 outlines the features of polyionic crystalloid solutions. For most situations in the field, commercial isotonic polyionic crystalloid solutions are the safest fluids with which to resuscitate hypovolemic horses (Table 17.3). They increase plasma volume without directly causing profound electrolyte disturbances because they contain

approximately the same electrolyte concentrations as plasma. Therefore, balanced polyionic fluids are always a good choice when laboratory information is not available immediately. It also follows that polyionic crystalloid solutions are often not sufficient to correct electrolyte imbalances.

Two classes of polyionic fluid are available, those for resuscitation and those for maintenance. Maintenance fluids (Normosol-M), Plasma-lyte M, Plasmalyte-56, contain higher potassium (15–30 mEq/l (15–30 mmol/l)) and lower sodium (40–60 mEq/l (40–60 mmol/l)) and chloride (40–60 mEq/l (40–60 mmol/l)) concentrations than resuscitation fluids (Normosol-R), Plasma-lyte 148, Isolec, lactated Ringer's solution. Currently, maintenance fluids are not available commercially in volumes of greater than 1 liter, which has led to the practice of adding potassium chloride (at 10–20 mEq/l) to resuscitation formulas so that they can be used as maintenance fluids in equine medicine. Commercial maintenance fluids should be considered as a treatment option in equine neonates.

The different alkalization agents ("bicarbonate substitutes") used in resuscitation fluids are clinically relevant. The alkalization agent in plasma is bicarbonate. Bicarbonate-containing fluids are unstable when stored and may produce profound metabolic alkalosis. Therefore Hartmann, an American pediatrician, replaced bicarbonate with lactate to make lactated Ringer's solution (also called Hartmann's solution). Lactate is metabolized in the liver but this process is slow enough to avoid the rapid changes in plasma pH seen with bicarbonate. Sodium bicarbonate and sodium lactate both increase the strong ion difference, resulting in a metabolic alkalosis. The cation (sodium) remains in the ECF while the anion (bicarbonate or lactate) is metabolized (Kellum 1999). It is the speed of metabolism of the anion and the renal excretion of sodium that determines the ultimate alkalization. It may seem counterintuitive to administer lactate-containing fluids to a horse with lactic acidosis resulting from poor tissue perfusion; however, clinical trials in human patients with hemorrhagic shock have shown that lactate-containing fluids do not exacerbate

Table 17.3 Polyionic crystalloid solutions

Features	Details
Resuscitation formulas	Sodium, potassium and chloride approximate plasma concentration Different alkalinizing agents used: lactate, acetate and/or gluconate Minor electrolytes (calcium/magnesium) differ between solutions
Maintenance formulas	Sodium, chloride lower than plasma concentration Potassium greater than plasma concentration Some solutions contain sugar, such as dextrose
Indications	Acute resuscitation (resuscitation fluids) Maintenance (resuscitation or maintenance fluids) Lactic acidosis (resuscitation fluids)
Possible indications	Hyperkalemia (resuscitation fluids)
Use with caution in	Pulmonary edema, generalized edema, hypoproteinemia, hypokalemia (resuscitation fluids), hyperkalemia (maintenance fluids), liver disease (lactate-containing fluids)

the lactic acidosis of hypoperfusion (Didwania et al 1997, Lowery et al 1971). It appears that the liver's capacity for metabolizing lactate in shock is not overwhelmed but instead the delivery of lactate to the liver by the circulation is impaired. Restoring the circulating volume, even with fluids containing moderate amounts of lactate, is sufficient to allow the liver to clear the circulating lactate (Lupo et al 1990). Although this is true for hemorrhagic shock, uptake of lactate by the liver may be impaired in severe septicemia (Chrusch et al 2000). In endotoxic and septic horses with these conditions, and those with liver disease, lactated Ringer's solution should be used with caution. Alternative alkalization agents to lactate are found in some commercial polyionic fluids (e.g. acetate and gluconate in Normosol-R). The muscles primarily metabolize acetate, and a variety of tissues throughout the body metabolize gluconate. Lactated Ringer's solution contains calcium whereas Normosol-R contains magnesium. Calcium solutions should not be mixed with whole blood; blood and its products should be stored with a compound that chelates calcium ions. Similarly, calcium solutions should not be mixed with sodium bicarbonate as they react to produce calcium carbonate. Clearly, calcium solutions are contraindicated in hypercalcemia. Fluids containing magnesium can, therefore, be used in more clinical situations than those containing calcium.

Isotonic sodium chloride (saline) solution

Isotonic (0.9%) sodium chloride is used commonly as an intraoperative intravenous (i.v.) replacement fluid in species other than the horse. Isotonic sodium chloride has a higher ratio of chloride to sodium than plasma and, therefore, reduces the strong ion difference and causes mild hyperchloremic acidosis in normal ponies (Gossett et al 1990a). This limits its utility as a resuscitation fluid in the horse, as most horses requiring fluid resuscitation already have acidosis. Isotonic sodium chloride should not be used for resuscitation unless indicated by measured electrolyte abnormalities. A possible exception is in foals with ruptured bladders, which are highly likely to be hypochloremic, hyponatremic and hyperkalemic.

Sodium chloride solution has been advocated in hyperkalemia, in order to avoid the potassium-containing polyionic fluids (Table 17.4). However this does not apply to the horse; in the absence of clinical signs of hyperkalemia and with the exception of horses with hyperkalemic periodic paralysis or with a ruptured bladder, the hyperkalemia is likely to reflect acidosis and polyionic fluids are probably appropriate.

Hypertonic sodium chloride (saline) solution

Hypertonic saline (2–4 ml/kg of 7–7.5% sodium chloride) has been advocated as a method of quickly restoring circulating volume in shock (Table 17.5). Its use results in an increase in the ECF of four to five times the infused volume for at least 60 min after it is infused (Onarheim 1995). Hypertonic saline draws fluid into the ECF from the intracellular fluid, principally from muscle and liver cells (Onarheim 1995) without providing significant fluid replacement. Administration of hypertonic saline should always be followed (within 2.5 h of administration: the point in experimental studies when cardiac output begins to

Table 17.4 Use of isotonic 0.9% sodium chloride

	Conditions
Indications	Hypochloremia, hyponatremia with hypochloremia
Possible indications	Hyperkalemia, acute resuscitation
Use with caution in	Acidosis, hyperchloremia, edema

Table 17.5 Uses of hypertonic sodium chloride solution 7.0–7.5% saline

	Conditions
Indications	Resuscitation in controlled hemorrhage, endotoxemia without dehydration
Possible indications	Following resuscitation to reduce endothelial swelling, head injury
Use with caution in	Dehydration, uncontrolled hemorrhage, hypernatremia or hyperchloremia, neonates

fall below baseline (Bertone et al 1990)) by the administration of large volumes of isotonic polyionic crystalloids. The volume of crystalloid fluids given should be based on the severity of clinical signs of hypovolemia and dehydration but should be in excess of five times the volume of hypertonic saline infused. As well as increasing ECF volume, hypertonic saline reduces the capillary endothelial swelling that may occur as part of the systemic inflammatory response syndrome and, therefore, improves tissue microcirculation and oxygen delivery (Mazzoni et al 1990). Furthermore, in experimental hemorrhagic shock, hypertonic saline reduced neutrophil activation resulting in reduced lung injury (Angle et al 1998).

Administration of hypertonic saline solution at 5 ml/kg immediately after experimental endotoxin infusion to horses attenuated the cardiovascular derangements associated with endotoxemia more effectively than an equivalent volume of isotonic saline (Bertone et al 1990). Despite positive experimental evidence for the use of hypertonic saline in endotoxemia, it should be used with caution during resuscitation in horses with significant dehydration. Cardiovascular improvements following the administration of hypertonic saline in 3–8% dehydrated rats were significantly reduced (Krausz et al 1993) and resuscitation of 8–10% dehydrated rats with hypertonic saline resulted in greater renal dysfunction and decreased survival compared with rats treated with lactated Ringer's solution (Malcolm et al 1993). Given the beneficial effects of hypertonic saline in experimental endotoxemia and sepsis, it may have a role after initial fluid resuscitation. However, this has not been evaluated clinically in horses with endotoxemia.

Because of the risks associated with rapid changes in plasma osmolality (Adrogue & Madias 2000a), 7% saline should probably not be administered to neonatal foals. The author has used 1.8% saline in foals with ruptured bladders (which are hyponatremic and hypochloremic) with apparently good clinical results.

The combination of dextran 70 (a colloid) with hypertonic saline resulted in acceptable resuscitation in experimental dehydration in calf and swine models (Constable et al 1996, McKirnan et al 1994). However, in the horse, the administration of a highly concentrated formula of hypertonic saline–dextran 70 resulted in clinically apparent intravascular hemolysis and hemoglobinuria (Moon et al 1991). Whether less-concentrated formulas are suitable for the horse remains to be investigated. The combination of an alternative colloid, hetastarch (10 ml/kg), and hypertonic saline (4 ml/kg) may be an appropriate solution for the resuscitation of horses that are both hypovolemic and dehydrated. Clinical experience suggests that hypertonic–saline–hetastarch is particularly useful in horses with marked hypovolemia and hypoproteinemia, such as those with severe colitis, but this has not been formally evaluated in experimental studies or clinical cases.

New research in human patients suggests a role for moderately hypertonic saline solutions (1.6–3%) in children with head injuries (Khanna et al 2000, Peterson et al 2000, Simma et al 1998). Whether this might also be useful in head injury or hypoxic ischemic encephalopathy in neonatal foals remains to be evaluated.

Dextrose solutions

Dextrose (5% dextrose (170 kcal/l) (D5W) is used to replace a deficit of pure water (without accompanying electrolyte deficits) and is effectively hypotonic because the dextrose is rapidly metabolized to carbon dioxide and water. It is indicated where fluid loss exceeds electrolyte loss, which can occur in horses with strangulating intestinal lesions (Table 17.6) (Brownlow & Hutchins 1982). Hypernatremia and hyperchloremia are also relatively common in neonatal foals, where

Table 17.6 Uses of dextrose solutions

	Conditions
Indications	Hypernatremia with hyperchloremia
Possible indications	Hypoglycemia
Use with caution in	Hyperglycemia, neurological disorders, hyponatremia or hypochloremia, when blood or urine glucose cannot be measured

resuscitation formulas are used as maintenance fluids. The volume of distribution of D5W is likely to be larger than that of a balanced electrolyte solution, which could result in a diminished ability to maintain the circulating volume. Horses receiving D5W should be monitored carefully because rapid administration can lead to hyperglycemia. If the plasma glucose concentration exceeds the renal threshold (approximately 180 mg/dl (10 mmol/l)), osmotic diuresis will result, which can reduce the benefit of the fluid administration. In species other than the horse (humans and dogs), high concentrations of glucose have been shown to be detrimental in both acute renal and acute cerebral injury (Li et al 1995, Moursi et al 1987). D5W should not be considered a form of parenteral nutrition. In order to provide 11.5 Mcal/day, the caloric requirement of a 500 kg horse standing in a stall (Ralston 1990), it would be necessary to administer 67.6 l/day, which would produce serious electrolyte abnormalities. Although the glucose in D5W may be helpful in the initial stages of resuscitation in foals, it is best to use 50% dextrose solution (or total parenteral nutrition (TPN) solutions) for nutritional support in addition to appropriate crystalloid solutions to meet fluid and electrolyte requirements.

An alternative is a solution of 2.5% dextrose and 0.45% sodium chloride (85 Kcal/L), which, once the dextrose has been metabolized, has an effective osmolality one-half of that of plasma. It is retained better in the circulation (20% after 30 min compared with 10% for D5W) (Spalding & Goodwin 1999) and can be used in the treatment of moderate plasma hypertonicity or when plasma glucose concentration is a concern. It should be noted that a rapid reduction in plasma tonicity has been associated with the development of cerebral edema, resulting in coma, seizures and death in other species (Adrogue & Madias 2000a). This has not been documented in the horse.

Sodium bicarbonate

Sodium bicarbonate (8.4%, 5% and 1.25% (isotonic)) has been advocated for the correction of metabolic acidosis in horses (Table 17.7) (Divers 1998, Johnson 1995). However, the cause of the

Table 17.7   Uses of sodium bicarbonate

	Conditions
Indications	Hyponatremia without hypochloremia, hyperchloremia without hypernatremia
Possible indications	Hyperkalemia
Use with caution in	Lactic acidosis, respiratory dysfunction, uncompensated metabolic alkalosis, hypocalcemia, hypokalemia, hypercapnia

acidosis needs to be considered carefully prior to starting treatment. Sodium bicarbonate may be beneficial in acidosis caused by hyponatremia or hyperchloremia (Corley & Marr 1998). However, in lactic acidosis, which is far more common in the horse, treatment with sodium bicarbonate is highly controversial.

It is the author's opinion that there are no grounds for using sodium bicarbonate to treat lactic acidosis, irrespective of the arterial (or venous) pH. This contradicts previous recommendations that it should be used when the pH decreases below 7.1 (Divers 1998) or 7.22 (Johnson 1995). The treatment of lactic acidosis with sodium bicarbonate is based on four suppositions: low blood pH is directly harmful, sodium bicarbonate is able to increase blood pH when infused i.v., raising the blood pH with sodium bicarbonate improves patient status and any adverse effects of sodium bicarbonate are outweighed by its benefits (Forsythe & Schmidt 2000). These suppositions are not supported by the data available currently in horses, humans and experimental animals.

Metabolic acidosis is reported to result in reduced cardiac contractility, constriction of the peripheral vasculature, inhibition of glycolysis, a decrease in oxygen uptake by hemoglobin in the lungs and central nervous system (CNS) depression (Cohen & Woods 1996, Smale et al 1994). The reduction in cardiac contractility clearly occurs with acidosis in isolated perfused rat and rabbit heart muscle preparations (Poole-Wilson & Langer 1975) but does not occur or is slight in whole animal models (Cooper et al 1993, Downing 1965). The lactate itself, rather than the pH, caused decreased contractility in a frog heart muscle model of lactic acidosis (Yatani et al 1981). Glycolysis is inhibited at low intracellular pH (Halperin et al 1969). However, the intracellular environment is protected from extracellular changes in pH. Lowering extracellular pH from 7.4 to 6.9 was not associated with any change in the pH gradient across the mitochondrial membrane in isolated rat hepatocytes, and an extracellular pH of 6.6 was not associated with any deleterious effects to the cells (Bonventre & Cheung 1985). Decreasing pH causes a shift to the right in the hemoglobin-oxygen dissociation curve (Smale et al 1994). Although this leads to decreased oxygen uptake in the lungs, it also results in increased oxygen liberation from hemoglobin in the tissues and the net effect may actually be an increase in tissue oxygen uptake. There is little compelling evidence that a low pH is directly harmful. Indeed, transient acidosis may actually be beneficial as it is associated with delayed cell death in anoxia (Bonventre & Cheung 1985) and decreased infarction size after myocardial ischemia (Kitakaze et al 1997).

In normal horses, the administration of sodium bicarbonate results in an increase in plasma pH (Pedrick et al 1998, Rumbaugh et al 1981), fulfilling the second supposition. Unfortunately, this is not true for the cerebrospinal fluid (CSF). In one study, i.v. administration of sodium bicarbonate to normal horses resulted in a mild decrease in CSF pH, which was still statistically significant 2 h after the infusion was complete (Pedrick et al 1998). The blood–brain barrier is not permeable to sodium and i.v. sodium bicarbonate administration does not change the CSF sodium concentration (Pedrick et al 1998) or the CSF strong ion gap. Consequently, i.v. sodium bicarbonate does not produce alkalization of the CSF. The bicarbonate ion from sodium bicarbonate combines with a hydrogen ion to produce carbon dioxide and water (Corley & Marr 1998). Carbon dioxide diffuses across the blood–brain barrier (Pedrick et al 1998) where it recombines with water and forms carbonic acid, resulting in a fall in CSF pH. Sodium bicarbonate may also cause a decrease in intracellular pH. The cell membrane is more permeable to carbon dioxide than to sodium and intracellular pH falls in response to extracellular sodium bicarbonate in the brain in normal humans (Nakashima

et al 1996) and in isolated lymphocytes (Bjerneroth et al 1994) and myocardial cells (Li et al 1997). The observed increase in plasma pH in normal horses may only be short-lived in clinical situations. In ponies treated with a low dose of endotoxin, the plasma pH was increased for less than 30 min after sodium bicarbonate administration (Gossett et al 1990b), whereas in normal horses the plasma pH was increased for at least 3 h (Pedrick et al 1998).

Many uncontrolled studies can be found in the literature demonstrating improved hemodynamics following the administration of sodium bicarbonate (Fanconi et al 1993, Vukmir et al 1995). However, this effect is almost certainly a result of increased cardiac preload, since no benefit was documented in studies where an equivalent sodium load was given as a control (Benjamin et al 1994, Graf et al 1985). This is true for human patients with a plasma pH below 7.2 (Cooper et al 1993); consequently specific recommendations to only give sodium bicarbonate below a certain pH threshold (Divers 1998, Johnson 1995) are hard to justify. No other clinical benefits of sodium bicarbonate administration have been documented. In diarrheic calves, there was no difference in clinical score between the sodium bicarbonate group and the saline controls at the end of infusion, despite a statistically different increase in plasma pH (Kasari & Naylor 1985). Some authors argue for the use of sodium bicarbonate in lactic acidosis based on the finding that acidosis results in decreased hepatic uptake of lactate (Lloyd et al 1973). The theory is that lactate cannot be cleared until pH is corrected and that low pH results in a vicious circle of increasing lactic acidosis. However, other authors have demonstrated that low pH does not inhibit hepatic lactate metabolism (Sestoft et al 1982, Sestoft & Marshall 1986). Furthermore, it has been demonstrated that increased extracellular carbon dioxide tension, a feature of bicarbonate administration, does inhibit hepatic lactate metabolism (Baron et al 1978).

It might be acceptable to administer sodium bicarbonate to improve plasma pH based on anecdotal evidence, if it caused no harmful effects. Unfortunately this is not the case. The production of carbon dioxide and accompanying respiratory acidosis causes a more profound depression in myocardial contractility than metabolic acidosis (Poole-Wilson & Langer 1975). Therefore, sodium bicarbonate is totally contraindicated in acidotic horses with normal or increased plasma carbon dioxide tensions, as they have not adequately compensated for the current acidosis and cannot be expected to eliminate the increased carbon dioxide load efficiently. Other potentially harmful effects of sodium bicarbonate include increasing plasma lactate concentration, hypernatremia, hypokalemia and hyperosmolality (Gossett et al 1990b).

Several alkalization agents have been developed as possible alternatives to sodium bicarbonate. These include carbicarb (a mixture of sodium carbonate and sodium bicarbonate) and trishydroxymethylaminomethane (also called THAM or tromethamine). These agents theoretically produce a lesser increase in plasma carbon dioxide tension and, therefore, less CSF and intracellular acidosis. However, this does not appear to be the case for tromethamine, which resulted in a decrease in CSF pH similar to sodium bicarbonate in healthy horses (Pedrick et al 1998).

In conclusion, the administration of sodium bicarbonate increases plasma pH but has the opposite effect in the CSF and intracellular fluid, which may be extremely detrimental to the acidotic patient. It may further increase the plasma lactate and sodium concentrations and may decrease the ionized calcium concentration. It corrects one laboratory value (pH) without addressing the underlying pathophysiology (poor tissue perfusion), by imposing a hypernatremic alkalosis on an already deranged metabolic balance.

Oral crystalloid therapy

It is possible to treat moderately dehydrated horses effectively with oral replacement solutions (ORSs) (McGinness et al 1996). Oral fluids do not need to be sterile and can be made up on the farm; they are, therefore, considerably cheaper and easier to transport than i.v. fluids. It is apparently not necessary to add glucose to oral fluids for horses (Sosa León et al 1995) but, if feasible, electrolytes should be added. Isotonic or hypotonic fluids should be administered (Sosa León et al 1995). A possible isotonic solution consists of 4.9 g/l table salt and 4.9 g/l lite salt (Morton Salt, Chicago, Illinois, USA) to produce final concentrations of 123 mmol/l sodium, 34 mmol/l potassium and 157 mmol/l chloride (Sosa León et al 1995). If using sodium chloride alone, no more than 9 g (approximately half a tablespoon) should be added per liter. A measured quantity of these fluids should be given via a nasogastric tube. The amount administered at any one time should not exceed 8–10 liters for a 500 kg horse, with at least 20 min allowed to elapse between each administration. Before each dose, the stomach should be refluxed and the administration delayed if more than 2 liters of fluid are recovered. Some horses will show signs of abdominal pain when large doses of oral fluids, especially if the fluids are cold, are administered.

Oral fluids can be a successful alternative or adjunct to i.v. fluids in many mildly dehydrated horses with large colon impactions (Lopes et al 1999). Unfortunately, oral fluids are insufficient for moderately to severely dehydrated horses: rapid administration of a glucose- and glycine-containing electrolyte solution (8 l/30 min) resulted in incomplete fluid absorption in horses with castor oil-induced diarrhea (Ecke et al 1998). The ORSs available commercially may not be ideal for fluid replacement in horses (Ecke et al 1998). Further research is necessary to refine oral fluid therapy for horses.

The administration of plain water is of minimal benefit to restore plasma volume in horses exercised in hot and humid conditions (Marlin et al 1998). However, the administration of an ORS or an electrolyte paste together with the provision of fresh drinking water may be sufficient to supplement water and electrolytes following vigorous or prolonged exercise in dehydrated horses with only mild hypovolemia (Marlin et al 1998, Sosa León et al 1998).

COLLOIDS

Colloids are solutions containing large sugar or protein molecules in addition to the water and electrolytes found in crystalloid solutions. All colloids, except albumin, contain a mixture of large and small protein or sugar molecules. The larger molecules allow colloid solutions to persist longer in the circulation than crystalloid solutions. The smaller molecules exert osmotic pressure to draw fluid into the circulation in a similar way to hypertonic saline. Solutions with a large number of smaller molecules allow a rapid increase in the circulating volume, greater than the actual volume infused.

The use of colloids has recently been advocated for the resuscitation of hypovolemic horses and for the treatment of severe hypoproteinemia (McFarlane 1999). Colloids have two advantages over crystalloids that makes them attractive for fluid therapy. Firstly, because of their persistence in the circulation, a three to six times lower volume of a colloid solution is required to produce the same resuscitative effect as a crystalloid solution (Rackow et al 1987). This is particularly useful in acute resuscitation of severely dehydrated horses or in the field where large amounts of crystalloids may be difficult to transport. Secondly, the administration of colloids can increase colloidal oncotic pressure, in contrast to the administration of large volumes of crystalloids, which decreases the colloidal oncotic pressure (Jones et al 1997, 2001).

Colloidal oncotic pressure refers to the osmotic pressure exerted by the molecules that do not freely pass from the vascular into the interstitial space. The oncotic pressure holds water in the circulation and draws fluid back into the circulation at the end of the capillary beds (Starling 1896). The number of particles in a solution determines its osmotic pressure. Therefore, solutions containing smaller molecules can exert a higher osmotic pressure since saturated solutions will contain more molecules per unit volume. However, small molecules diffuse more easily out of the vascular space. Therefore, the net oncotic pressure exerted by a solution is a balance between the osmotic pressure exerted by that solution and the rate of diffusion of that solution out of the vascular bed. In normal plasma, most of the oncotic pressure gradient (approximately 80%) is produced by albumin. Globulins contribute the remainder of the oncotic pressure, with fibrinogen exerting little effect (<0.01% of the total) (Roberts & Bratton 1998). The normal plasma colloid oncotic pressure of plasma is less in neonatal foals (17–21 mmHg) than in mature thoroughbred horses (20–22 mmHg) (Runk et al 2000).

As discussed briefly above, the molecular weight of a colloid solution is the most important factor in determining its pharmacology. All currently available synthetic colloids are polydisperse (made up of a mixture of molecules of differing molecular weights). Albumin is a monodisperse solution, as all molecules have a molecular mass of 69 kDa. The weight-average molecular weight refers to the average size of molecule in a polydisperse solution. As a rule, the higher the average molecular weight, the longer the colloid will persist in the circulation. The chemical nature of the colloid also influences the persistence in the circulation but generally to a lesser degree. The number of molecules in the solution determines the osmotic pressure, which can be considerably greater than plasma (e.g. 342 mmHg for urea-linked gelatin). Colloids with a smaller average molecular weight exert a higher osmotic pressure and expand the plasma volume more rapidly, by drawing fluid from the interstitial space into the vasculature and thus increasing the circulating volume in excess of the amount of fluid infused. However, colloids with smaller molecular weights are cleared faster from the circulation and may leak more readily into the interstitium.

Leakage of proteins into the interstitium is important in edema formation, a common feature in critically ill horses, particularly those with colitis. Edema impairs delivery of oxygen to the tissues, as it both compresses capillary beds and increases the diffusion distance between the capillaries and the cells. Therefore, edema may contribute significantly to morbidity and mortality. Endotoxin (Mills et al 1995) and ischemia–reperfusion injury (Dabareiner et al 1995, Henninger et al 1992) induce capillary damage, which allows plasma albumin to leak out into the interstitium. This not only reduces the oncotic pressure within the vasculature but also allows the extravasated albumin to exert an osmotic pressure that holds fluid in the interstitial space. Large colloid molecules do not leak as readily, allowing their oncotic pressure to draw fluid back into the vasculature. Larger colloid molecules may also plug the gaps in the capillary endothelium (Zikria et al 1989a,b). Even in conditions of severe capillary leak, very large molecules are not able to escape the vasculature unless the integrity of the capillary endothelium is totally destroyed (Conhaim et al 1999).

All of the colloid solutions available currently are removed from the circulation by the reticuloendothelial system, resulting in colloid-containing vacuoles, which may persist for years (Sirtl et al 1999, Thompson et al 1970). The presence of these vacuoles does not appear to interfere with the function of the reticuloendothelial system (Lenz et al 1986).

Hydroxyethyl starches

Hydroxyethyl starches are modified polymers of amylopectin. Several different hydroxyethyl starch preparations are marketed around the world. Hetastarch is available as a 6% solution in isotonic saline or a 6% solution in lactated electrolyte solution. Pentastarch is available as a 6% or 10% solution in isotonic saline. Indications for the use of hydroxyethyl starches are given in Table 17.8. They all consist of a polydisperse solution of starch molecules in which hydroxyethyl groups have been substituted for a number of the glucose subunits. The solutions differ in the number of glucose units substituted and the weight-average molecular weight. The greater the number of glucose molecules substituted, the longer the half-life of the solution *in vivo*. The degree of substitution is usually given as a proportion of substituted residues, which results in a number between 0 and 1, with higher numbers representing greater substitution and hence a longer half-life. The average molecular weight is also important, with lower molecular weight solutions having a greater oncotic pressure but a shorter persistence in the circulation.

Hydroxyethyl starches are eliminated by renal excretion, extravasation and uptake by the reticuloendothelial system and, for a very small percentage (<1%) of molecules, by biliary excretion (Lenz et al 2000, Thompson et al 1970). Larger molecules are cleaved by serum α amylase prior to elimination. Uptake by the reticuloendothelial system can result in the presence of phagocytic cells containing starch granules in the liver, spleen, skin, small intestine, striated muscle and lymph nodes (Sirtl et al 1999, Thompson et al 1970). These deposits are dose dependent and decrease with time but may persist for up to 4.5 years following the infusion of hydroxyethyl starch in humans (Sirtl et al 1999).

Hetastarch

Hetastarch is the only hydroxyethyl starch marketed for resuscitation in the USA. It is available as a 6% solution in isotonic saline or in an isotonic lactated electrolyte solution. Hetastarch is a polydisperse solution with a wide range of molecular sizes (10–3000 kDa), a high average molecular mass (450 kDa) and a high degree of substitution (0.75). Hetastarch exerts an osmotic pressure of approximately 31 mmHg in solution (Nearman & Herman 1991) and, at a dose of 10 ml/kg, increases the plasma colloidal oncotic pressure of normal ponies from 24 to 27 mmHg (Jones et al 1997). In normal dogs, hetastarch expands the plasma by 140% of the volume infused (Thompson et al 1970). The effects on plasma volume in the normal horse are likely to be similar but have not been investigated. Hetastarch is slowly degraded in the circulation and, therefore, has a long half-life. In normal ponies, the increase in colloidal oncotic pressure after a dose of 10 ml/kg lasts longer than 120 h (Jones et al 1997). However, in hypoproteinemic horses and foals, the clinical effects appear to be shorter, typically lasting 24–36 h (Jones et al 2001).

In normal ponies, hetastarch is safe, but high doses (20 ml/kg) decrease circulating von Willebrand factor, factor VIII coagulant activity and activated partial thromboplastin time and prolong bleeding times (Jones et al 1997). Although a dose of 10 ml/kg hetastarch did not affect hemostasis in normal ponies (Jones et al 1997), endotoxemia may produce coagulation derangements that might render endotoxic horses susceptible to

Table 17.8 Uses of hydroxyethyl starches

	Conditions
Indications	Hypoproteinemia, capillary leak syndrome
Possible indications	Acute fluid resuscitation
Use with caution in	Clotting disorders, renal failure

clinically important changes in the clotting profile at this or lower doses. A recent study from human medicine suggests administration of hydroxyethyl starches is associated with a higher incidence of renal failure than the administration of gelatins (Schortgen et al 2001). However, the hydroxyethyl starch and gelatin groups were not equivalent at study entry, the amount of fluid administered differed between the groups and the definition of acute renal failure was questionable in this study. Therefore, further work is required to establish any link between hydroxyethyl starch administration and renal failure.

Hetastarch may decrease vascular permeability following ischemia–reperfusion injury (Zikria et al 1989a,b), which makes it a theoretically attractive solution for administration to horses prior to the surgical correction of strangulating intestinal lesions. This effect on reperfusion injury is not simply a function of high molecular weight; a similar effect could not be demonstrated for a dextran solution with an average molecular mass of 250 kDa (Moore et al 1996). There is evidence that hetastarch reduces neutrophil chemotaxis through the endothelium in vitro (Hofbauer et al 1999). Thus, there is a potential for hetastarch to reduce neutrophil-mediated damage in ischemia–reperfusion, endotoxemia and other inflammatory tissue insults. However, this effect has not yet been demonstrated in vivo.

The rapid increase in circulating volume seen following the administration of hypertonic saline and the increase in oncotic pressure and more prolonged effects of hetastarch may make this combination appropriate for the resuscitation of severely dehydrated horses, especially those with severe colitis. Although hetastarch (up to 10 ml/kg) and hypertonic saline (2–4 ml/kg) have been combined with apparent success in a number of clinical cases, this combination has not been evaluated critically. If used, this combination should be followed up with crystalloid fluids.

Other hydroxyethyl starches

In Europe, several hydroxyethyl starch preparations are available commercially. Pentastarch, one of the more commonly used preparations, has been tested in horses (Hermann et al 1990, Meister et al 1992) and is approved for use in horses in Switzerland. It is available as a 6% or 10% solution in isotonic sodium chloride. Pentastarch has a smaller average molecular mass than hetastarch (200 kDa) and is, therefore, expected to produce a greater initial increase in the plasma volume. The initial increase in plasma volume in human patients is reported as 145% of the volume infused for the 10% solution and 100% of the volume infused for the 6% solution (HAES-steril, Fresenius AG, Bad Homburg, Germany). The degree of substitution (0.5) is less than in hetastarch, which is expected to lead to faster degradation by serum amylases.

In human medicine, starches with smaller average molecular weights have less profound effects on hemostasis (Treib et al 1999). This may also be the case in horses, although only one dose has been tested. In healthy horses, a 8 ml/kg dose of a 10% pentastarch solution resulted in a slight decrease in the thrombin time 12 h after administration, which returned to normal after 24 h. No effect on prothrombin time or partial thromboplastin time was documented (Meister et al 1992). In healthy horses, the initial phase half-life of pentastarch is 5.6 h and the terminal phase half-life is 122 h. However, the effects on PCV, plasma total solids and plasma viscosity appear to last only 12–24 h (Meister et al 1992). In equine clinical cases, the half-life may be as short as 2 h (Hermann et al 1990). Pentastarch, although available in the USA, is only approved for leukapheresis in human medicine.

A new hydroxyethyl starch has been developed to avoid the large-molecular-weight molecules that are thought to be mainly responsible for the effects on coagulation factors and the low-molecular-weight molecules, which are eliminated rapidly. This preparation, pentafraction, has an average molecular mass of 280 kDa with a range of 100–500 kDa. Initial results with this starch in experimental animals are promising (Webb et al 1992).

Dextrans

Dextrans are polysaccharides composed of linear glucose residues. They are produced from a polysaccharide synthesized by the bacteria *Leuconostoc mesenteroides* grown on sucrose media. Dextrans of different molecular weights are produced by acid hydrolysis of the parent molecule. Two dextran solutions are available commercially in the USA, dextran 40 (10% solution in isotonic saline) and dextran 70 (6% solution in isotonic saline). Both of these solutions are polydisperse. The number refers to the weight-average molecular mass: 40 and 70 kDa, respectively. Dextran molecules less than 50–55 kDa are excreted in the urine (Thompson et al 1970). Larger molecules are extravasated and taken up by the reticuloendothelial system or excreted through the gastrointestinal system (Nearman & Herman 1991).

In human patients, the peak plasma volume expansion after infusion of dextran 40 is 210% of the volume infused: the plasma expansion is approximately 140% of the volume infused at 1 h after infusion (Shoemaker 1976). In dogs, the peak effect of dextran 70 is a 140% plasma expansion: the expansion effect of dextran 70 is approximately 100% of the volume infused at 1 h after infusion (Thompson et al 1970). Within 12 h, 60% of the dextran 40 and 35% of the dextran 70 has been cleared from the vascular space (Nearman & Herman 1991). The increase in plasma volume in dogs is only 1.1% of the volume infused by 24 h after dextran 70 injection (Thompson et al 1970).

In humans, dextran administration is associated with a decrease in factor VIII activity, decreased fibrin clot formation and dilutional coagulopathy (Roberts & Bratton 1998). Dextran 70 inhibits equine platelet aggregation *in vitro* (Heath et al 1998) but other effects on hemostasis have not been investigated. Dextran 70 has been used for its presumed antithrombotic properties in horses with a clinical diagnosis of verminous aneurysm (Table 17.9) (Greatorex 1977). Dextran 70, when combined with hypertonic saline, resulted in a transient, severe intravascular hemolysis and hemoglobinuria in horses (Moon et al 1991). Dextran 40 was reported to cause acute renal failure in 4.7% of human patients (Biesenbach et al 1997). It is not known whether this is a risk in the horse.

Gelatins

Gelatins are produced by chemical modification of bovine collagen. Despite their bovine origin, the risk of transmission of bovine spongiform encephalopathy (BSE) by these products is apparently negligible (Peano et al 2000). Two types of gelatin are marketed in Europe, though neither is currently available in the USA. Urea-linked gelatin is marketed as a polydisperse solution (3.5% in polyionic electrolyte solution) with a weight-average molecular mass of 35 kDa and succinylated gelatin is marketed as a polydisperse solution (4% in polyionic electrolyte solution) with a weight-average molecular mass of 30 kDa. Because of their relatively small molecular size, gelatins have high osmotic pressure (342 mmHg) but are eliminated rapidly by the kidneys. The small size of the molecules in gelatin solutions also means that more of this colloid is extravasated than other colloids, leading to greater edema formation (Table 17.10) (Allison et al 1999, Holbeck & Grande 2000). The high osmotic pressure means that it is relatively easy to cause fluid overload in normal horses with gelatin. An average dose of 48 ml/kg caused significant fluid overload and pulmonary edema in normal ponies undergoing anesthesia (Taylor 1998). In human patients, allergic reactions are reported to both gelatin preparations, with urea-linked gelatins having the higher incidence at 0.146% (Ring & Messmer 1977). There is no evidence that urea-linked gelatin causes allergic reactions in horses (Taylor 1998).

Table 17.9 Uses of dextrans

	Conditions
Indications	Verminous aneurysm, deep vein thrombosis
Possible indications	Acute fluid resuscitation
Use with caution in	Combination with hypertonic saline, renal failure, clotting disorders

Table 17.10 Uses of gelatins

	Conditions
Indications	Unclear
Possible indications	Acute fluid resuscitation
Use with caution in	Edema, renal failure

Albumin

Hypoalbuminemia is common in horses with colitis and other protein-losing enteropathies, may occur following hemorrhage and burns and may be seen, rarely, in certain nephropathies. In none of these is albumin the ideal colloid for restoring plasma oncotic pressure. When there is protein loss through the gastrointestinal system or kidney, exogenous albumin will be lost at an equal rate to the endogenous albumin it is being used to replace. In burns, the endogenous albumin is extravasated and it can be expected that a proportion of the exogenous albumin administered will also be extravasated, adding to the tissue edema. This is also the case in endotoxin or capillary damage induced by ischemia–reperfusion, in which albumin leaks out of the vascular space into the tissues. In each of these cases, a larger colloid, such as a hydroxyethyl starch, should be used. If the hemorrhage is severe enough to result in clinically relevant hypoalbuminemia, whole blood or plasma represent better replacement fluids than albumin solutions (Table 17.11).

Albumin solutions are manufactured from pooled plasma. They can contain other plasma constituents, such as heme compounds, prekallikrein, endotoxins, bradykinin and bilirubin, in sufficient concentrations to cause clinical effects (Pulimood & Park 2000). Some batches of human albumin have been shown to induce the expression of adhesion molecules on endothelial cells *in vitro* (Nohe et al 1999), which could result in activation of the immune system *in vivo*. Despite appropriate precautions during the manufacturing process, there is always a theoretical chance of transmission of disease with any biological product.

An equine 5% albumin solution in isotonic saline has recently become available in the USA but, at the time of writing, no studies detailing its use have been published. A meta-analysis of clinical trials of albumin use in human critical care found an excess mortality of 6% in the albumin group (Cochrane Injuries Group Albumin Reviewers 1998). The methodology of this meta-analysis has been questioned repeatedly (Allison & Lobo 2000, Webb 1999) and a more recent meta-analysis using different criteria to select studies for inclusion found no effect of albumin on mortality (Wilkes & Navickis 2001). Neither meta-analysis demonstrated a beneficial effect of albumin on mortality, which suggests that the expense of this treatment might not be justified. Even albumin proponents do not recommend its use for either acute fluid replacement or the treatment of hypoalbuminemia (Allison & Lobo 2000). Albumin solutions have not been tested formally in horses and, because of the potential problems outlined above, should not be used until evaluated in controlled clinical trials.

Plasma

Plasma has been used extensively in horses with colitis and in neonatal foals for the passive transfer of immunity (Table 17.12). Plasma may either be purchased commercially or collected from donors and can be used fresh or stored frozen. Commercial plasma may be from donors who are hyperimmunized with certain equine pathogens and thus will contain antibodies to these pathogens. Hyperimmunized plasma may be preferable for the passive transfer of immunity

Table 17.11 Uses of albumin

	Conditions
Indications	Unclear
Possible indications	Maintenance fluid therapy, acute fluid resuscitation, edema
Use with caution in	Burn patients, edema

Table 17.12 Uses of plasma

	Conditions
Indications	Transfer of passive immunity, clotting disorders
Possible indications	Systemic inflammatory response syndrome, hypoproteinemia, if hydroxyethyl starch unavailable
Use with caution in	Horses previously transfused

but its utility in preventing specific diseases (e.g. *Rhodococcus equi* pneumonia) or in the specific treatment of diseases (e.g. anti-5 antibodies for endotoxemia) remains controversial (Becu et al 1997, Hurley & Begg 1995, Morris et al 1986, Spier et al 1989).

The ideal plasma donor is a young, healthy gelding with a known, complete history that has never been administered a blood product. For blood collection from the donor, a catheter is placed in the jugular vein with the tip pointing towards the head of the animal. Using a 10 or 12 gauge catheter speeds up collection. A collection bag containing anticoagulant (100 ml acid citrate dextrose for each 900 ml whole blood collected (Collatos 1997)) is connected to the catheter and the jugular vein occluded beneath the catheter until the bag is full. Centrifugation or plasmapheresis is the most effective methods of separating the plasma from the cells. It is possible to get reasonable separation of the plasma and cells by sedimentation. The bag should be placed with the administration set uppermost in an ice bucket. There is reasonable separation after 2 h but the bag should ideally be left for 12 h, if the circumstances allow (Durham 1996). However, if the plasma is being collected for replacement of clotting factors, no more than 6 h should elapse between collection and administration or freezing, since factors V and VIII are not stable beyond 6 h (Cotter 1991). These clotting factors are also depleted if plasma is stored frozen for longer than 1 year. Albumin, globulin and factors II, VII, IX and X are stable for at least 1 year (Cotter 1991).

Although classically prescribed for hypoalbuminemia, the utility of plasma for replacing protein is unclear. Approximately 80% of the colloidal oncotic pressure of plasma is provided by albumin and, therefore, many of the reservations expressed about albumin apply to plasma. At least 6 to 8 liters are required to treat clinically significant hypoproteinemia in adult horses (Collatos 1997) and even so the effects may be short lived. Plasma administration does not have the advantage of the larger-molecular-weight colloids of potentially drawing fluid back into the circulation in damaged capillaries, but it may prevent a low plasma oncotic pressure leading to generalized edema. Plasma may have a role in replacing antithrombin III, protein C and other cofactors that are depleted during the systemic inflammatory response syndrome. When used for this purpose, fresh plasma is preferable because plasma that has been frozen for longer than 1 year may no longer contain high concentrations of these proteins.

Clinical use of colloids

Although hetastarch and dextran 70 have been used clinically in horses (Greatorex 1977, McFarlane 1999), it remains to be seen whether either offers any advantage in terms of clinical outcome when compared with crystalloids. Furthermore, some of the theoretical benefits of colloids over crystalloids have not been observed in some experimental models and clinical trials. For example, increased extravascular lung water was found in an endotoxic pig model (Baum et al 1990) but not a septic rat model (Rackow et al 1989) when crystalloid and hetastarch resuscitation were compared. In preterm hypotensive human infants, treatment with 5% albumin resulted in significantly greater fluid retention than treatment with isotonic saline and the two treatments were equivalent in other respects (So et al 1997).

Recent meta-analyses of randomized trials of colloid administration to human critical care patients demonstrated no advantage of colloids over crystalloids and concluded that colloids increased mortality when used in some clinical syndromes (Choi et al 1999, Schierhout & Roberts 1998). When trauma patients were studied as a subpopulation, a 12.3% difference in mortality rate was identified in favor of crystalloid therapy. Conversely, analysis of pooled data from non-trauma patients identified a 7.8% difference in mortality rate in favor of colloid treatment (Velanovich 1989). The majority of clinical trials in these meta-analyses compared albumin with crystalloid solutions and thus these results should not discourage the use of hydroxyethyl starches in horses.

One precaution when using colloids is that the plasma total solids or total protein concentration is no longer a useful guide to plasma oncotic pressure (Bumpus et al 1998).

BLOOD AND BLOOD SUBSTITUTES

WHOLE BLOOD

Used judiciously, blood transfusion is a potentially life-saving treatment. It should be considered in all horses with a PCV of <18% (hemoglobin concentration less than 6 g/dl) and is imperative in horses with a PCV of less than 12% (Table 17.13). Blood transfusion is not necessary in mild anemia (PCV > 24%); human patients with mild anemia who received blood transfusion therapy have a worse outcome (Hébert et al 1999). Clinical situations in which blood transfusion are frequently indicated include neonatal isoerythrolysis, nasal passage or sinus surgery, trauma with large volume blood loss, hemolytic anemia and significant internal hemorrhage. In septic shock, blood transfusion has been suggested as a method of increasing oxygen delivery to the tissues by increasing the oxygen-carrying capacity of the blood. However, in septic human patients, blood transfusion was associated with an increase in oxygen delivery but not in oxygen uptake (Lorente et al 1993), suggesting that the increased supply of oxygen is not available to the tissues. This is supported by work in experimental animals that suggests that tissue oxygen uptake is superior at a PCV of 20% or 30% than at a PCV of 40%, despite the higher oxygen delivery at the higher PCV (Creteur et al 2001). The most likely explanation for this is that the increasing PCV increases blood viscosity (Stone et al 1968) causing blood sludging and reduced flow through the capillaries. This may be especially important in shock, where

blood viscosity may be increased independently from the PCV (Andrews et al 1990).

Blood transfusion recipients are usually cross-matched with potential donors prior to blood collection. However, the reliability of these tests in the horse is questionable (Durham 1996, Kallfelz et al 1978). It may be appropriate to select donors negative for the major antigens (Aa and Qa) so that cross-matching is not necessary (Durham 1996). Several laboratories offer blood-typing for horses. For neonatal isoerythrolysis, washed red cells from the dam are the transfusion of choice. Washing removes the plasma, which contains antierythrocyte antibodies. The red cells are washed by repeatedly separating the cells from the plasma and then resuspending them in isotonic saline. Ideally, the separation of the cells from the plasma or saline should be done with a centrifuge or plasmapheresis machine, but it is acceptable to allow the cells to settle, remove the plasma and then resuspend them. Three washes are usually adequate.

In all cases, the recipient should be monitored very closely for signs of a transfusion reaction during the infusion of the initial 50 ml of blood. Signs of transfusion reactions include pyrexia, tachycardia, tachypnea, sweating, icterus, lying down, frequent defecation, proteinuria and hemoglobinuria (Hata & Sonoda 1974). None of these signs are invariably present but pyrexia and sweating are frequently the most prominent signs. In one study of normal horses given repeated incompatible transfusions, icterus and proteinuria were the only clinical signs that lasted for longer than 24 h and transfusion reactions did not occur before the sixth incompatible transfusion (Hata & Sonoda 1974). In another study, one horse died, apparently of an anaphylactoid reaction, during the second transfusion (Kallfelz et al 1978). Disease transmission is possible with blood transfusion and is a particular concern in areas where equine infectious anemia is endemic (Issel et al 1982). All donor animals should be tested regularly for this disease.

Whole blood from donor animals should be collected into bags containing acid-citrate dextrose to give a 9:1 dilution, as described above for plasma. If possible, the blood should be used immediately but erythrocytes may remain viable in a refrigerator for as long as 3–4 weeks (Durham 1996).

Table 17.13 Uses of whole blood

	Conditions
Indications	Neonatal isoerythrolysis, large volume blood loss, packed cell volume (PCV) < 12%
Possible indications	PCV < 18%
Use with caution in	Horses with history of previous transfusion, uncontrolled hemorrhage, septicemia

The amount of blood needed for transfusion can be calculated using the following equation:

Amount of blood (in ml)

$$= \frac{\text{Bodyweight (kg)} \times (\text{Desired PCV} - \text{Current PCV}) \times Z}{\text{PCV of Donor}}$$

where Z is blood volume of the recipient per kg (i.e. 80 ml/kg for adult horses; 150 ml/kg for 2-day-old foals).

Studies of the length of survival of transfused erythrocytes in recipient horses have produced variable results. In adult horses, the half-life of ^{59}Fe-labeled donor erythrocytes was 4 days in three out of six horses and less than 24 h in the other three recipients (Kallfelz et al 1978). This methodology does not permit autologous transfusions as a control. In foals aged 2–5 days the mean half-life of ^{50}Cr-labeled donor erythrocytes was 5.5 days compared with 11.7 days for autologous erythrocytes (Smith et al 1992).

BLOOD SUBSTITUTES

Stroma-free hemoglobin preparations have been developed in response to the need for safe, infection-free, sustainable sources of blood in human medicine and to eliminate the need for cross-matching (Table 17.14). Unfortunately, unmodified free hemoglobin has too high an affinity for oxygen, is rapidly eliminated by the kidneys, causes a substantial increase in oncotic pressure and may cause renal injury. For this reason, research has focused on modified polymers of hemoglobin. At the time of writing four products are under development: polymerized bovine hemoglobin (13 g/dl in modified lactate Ringer's solution), diaspirin-linked human hemoglobin, recombinant engineered cross-linked hemoglobin and pyridoxylated polymerized human hemoglobin (Fromm 2000). Of these, polymerized bovine hemoglobin has already been registered in the USA and Europe for use in dogs, where the recommended dose is 10–30 ml/kg. Successful use of this product has been reported in a foal with neonatal isoerythrolysis (Perkins & Divers 2001) and an early version of the product was used with apparent success in an anemic miniature horse (Maxson et al 1993); in both cases, a compatible blood donor could not be found. Although not clinically significant in this case, the anemic mare showed increased pulmonary and systemic pressure, reported side-effects in humans (Fromm 2000), following infusion of the hemoglobin product (Maxson et al 1993). More concerning is that one out of six ponies experienced an anaphylactic reaction in an experimental trial of ponies with normovolemic anemia (Belgrave et al 2002).

These products are an exciting development, which may have a particular application in equine medicine because of the difficulty of reliable cross-matching for blood transfusion. However, the products available currently may not be the most optimal for use in the horse.

PARENTERAL NUTRITION

In the horse, any therapeutic plan should include a nutritional plan. In most horses, this will consist of an enteral diet based on the horse's normal diet. Enteral nutrition is always the first choice. In some horses with conditions of the oral cavity or esophagus, enteral nutrition may be supplied via a nasogastric tube or a tube inserted via an esophagostomy. Clinical experience suggests that hay-, pellet- and corn oil-based diets are preferable to commercial liquid enteral diets designed for humans, which appear to be associated with a high incidence of severe colitis and laminitis in horses.

In some horses, enteral nutrition is contraindicated or not practical. This includes adult horses with gastric reflux, ileus, intrathoracic esophageal obstruction or impaired digestive capacity (such

Table 17.14 Uses of blood substitutes

	Conditions
Indications	Not licensed for use in horses, transfusion where no compatible donor available
Possible indications	Any situation where transfusion is indicated
Use with caution in	Hypertension, uncontrolled hemorrhage, oliguria or anuria

as in severe colitis) in which the interruption to enteral feeding is predicted to last at least 3–5 days (Spurlock & Ward 1991). Gastrointestinal compromise and ileus are common in neonatal foals with sepsis or hypoxic ischemic encephalopathy, and parenteral nutrition should be considered if enteral nutrition is likely to be interrupted for more than 24 h (Table 17.15) (Spurlock & Ward 1991). In foals with severe hypoxic ischemic encephalopathy, enteral feeding, particularly with mare's milk substitutes, may increase the risk of necrotizing enterocolitis (Bosse et al 1993, Cudd & Pauly 1987, Martinez-Tallo et al 1997). Withholding enteral feeding in unweaned foals with severe diarrhea reduces the osmotic load in the intestine and can decrease the quantity of diarrhea. Typically, enteral nutrition is withheld for 48 to 72 h and nutritional support is supplied with partial or total parenteral nutrition (TPN) during this period.

TPN solutions commonly consist of dextrose, amino acids, lipids and a vitamin/mineral mix. The estimated energy and protein requirements of a normal adult horse standing in a stall can be calculated (Ralston 1990):

Energy requirement (Mcal/day)
$= 0.975 + [0.021 \times$ body weight (kg)]

Protein requirement (digestible protein in g/day)
$= 18 \times$ Energy requirement (in Mcal/day)

It is thought that both of these requirements are increased in disease (e.g. by an estimated 25–50% in sepsis; Ralston 1990). Therefore, the daily energy requirement of a hospitalized adult horse is approximately 30 kcal/kg and normal neonatal foals require 55–65 kcal/kg daily for maintenance and up to 150 kcal/kg daily for growth and normal

activity (Koterba 1990). In the intensive care unit, TPN is usually aimed at basal maintenance (approximately 70–80 kcal/kg daily in septic foals) because higher rates of administration may result in severe hyperglycemia.

The formulation of TPN solutions is described elsewhere (Spurlock & Ward 1991). It is important to mix the dextrose and amino acids prior to adding the lipids, since the pH of the amino acid solution can crack the lipid emulsion (Spurlock & Ward 1991). In some patients, such as those with pre-existing hyperlipemia or developing hyperlipemia in response to initial TPN, the solution may be formulated without lipids. In critically ill human patients, the inclusion or exclusion of lipids has no effect on mortality or morbidity (Heyland et al 1998). Formulating TPN without lipids significantly reduces the cost.

A convenient formula including lipids that can be used in many horses, but which is not suitable for all cases, is given in Table 17.16. This solution provides 72% of the non-nitrogen calories as dextrose, 28% as lipid and 131 non-nitrogen calories per gram of nitrogen. For foals, this solution delivers 80 kcal/kg daily if given at 3.76 ml/kg/h. For adult horses, this same formula provides 30 kcal/kg daily when given at 1.41 ml/kg/h.

The administration bag, and ideally the administration set and lines, should be covered to prevent exposure to daylight. This is unnecessary in totally artificially lit barns (Allwood 2000). TPN should be started at 50% of the target rate. After 4 h, the blood glucose concentration should be measured and the rate of administration increased to 75% of the target rate if the blood glucose concentration is <150 mg/dl (8.3 mmol/l). After a further 4 h and a further blood glucose

Table 17.15 Use of parenteral nutrition

	Conditions
Indications	When enteral nutrition is contraindicated and when interruption to feeding expected to last 3–5 days in adults or 24 h in neonates
Possible indications	To supplement low-volume enteral nutrition
Use with caution in	Hyperglycemia, hyperlipemia

Table 17.16 Total parenteral nutrition formula for horses[a]

Component	Volume (ml)
Dextrose 50% solution	1500
Lipids 20% solution	500
Amino acids 8.5% solution	2000
Vitamin/mineral mix	5

[a] Approximately four such bags per day for an adult horse

concentration determination, the rate of administration may be increased to the final target rate. There are two options if the blood glucose concentration increases to >150 mg/dl (8.3 mmol/l). Firstly, the rate of infusion can be reduced and then increased more slowly to allow more time for the animal to adapt to the high glucose load. Secondly, if the first strategy is unsuccessful, an insulin infusion may be started (titrated to the blood glucose concentration from an initial rate of 0.5–1 U/kg/h). If an insulin infusion is used, the blood glucose concentration should be monitored closely and maintained between 80 mg/dl (4.4 mmol/l) and 110 mg/dl (6.1 mmol/l) by adjusting the insulin infusion rate. Recent evidence from critically ill human patients demonstrated greatly improved survival if the blood glucose concentration is maintained within this narrow range (80–110 mg/dl (4.4–6.1 mmol/l)) than if patients are maintained at 80–200 mg/dl (4.4–11.1 mmol/l) (van den Berghe et al 2001). Although similar studies have not been yet carried out in the horse, it is likely that tight control of glucose will also be beneficial in critically ill equids.

During TPN, the serum should also be monitored for lipemia. If there is gross lipemia, the TPN can be formulated with a lower lipid concentration or without lipids. Lipemia may also respond to an insulin infusion. It is also important to monitor plasma electrolytes serially as hypokalemia and hypomagnesemia are common complications (Spurlock & Ward 1991).

When discontinuing TPN, it is advisable to decrease the rate of administration over several hours. TPN does not affect appetite in human children (Reifen et al 1999) and clinical experience suggests that this is also the case in foals. Therefore, if clinically indicated, it is possible to make the transition from TPN to nursing in foals. Although lactase production is reduced, compared with enteral nutrition, in neonatal pigs fed by parenteral nutrition (Park et al 1999), this is a function of a decrease in weight of the jejunum rather than a decrease in lactase synthesis per unit weight (Dudley et al 1998). Therefore, it is probably unnecessary to provide exogenous lactase during the transition from parenteral nutrition to enteral nutrition in neonatal foals.

Although there is much anecdotal evidence that TPN (as opposed to no nutrition) may be beneficial in hospitalized horses, this has not been proven (Lopes & White 2002). The administration of TPN increases the risk of sepsis and thrombophlebitis in hospitalized human patients (Ioannides-Demos et al 1995). This may result, at least in part, from decreased intracellular killing by neutrophils (Okada et al 2000) and increased plasma thrombin–antithrombin III concentrations, which result in increased plasma coagulability (van der Poll et al 1998).

FLUID THERAPY DELIVERY

DELIVERY SYSTEMS

During the early period of resuscitation of moderately to severely hypovolemic horses, it is important to use both a large-gauge catheter and a wide-bore sterile delivery system to allow rapid delivery of fluids. A 10 or 12 gauge catheter is recommended by the author for severely hypovolemic adult horses, a 12 or 14 gauge catheter for moderately hypovolemic horses, and 16 gauge catheters for neonatal foals and moderately hypovolemic weanlings and miniature horses. During TPN, double-lumen catheters can provide a dedicated line for the TPN and avoid the need to interrupt the TPN when administering incompatible drugs.

To place a catheter, the hair should be clipped over the vein and the area should be prepared aseptically, ideally with a chlorhexidine scrub solution (Mimoz et al 1996). The catheter should be handled and placed wearing sterile gloves. In young and fractious horses, a bleb of local anesthetic placed subcutaneously at the catheter site makes catheterization easier. The aseptic scrub should be repeated after the local anesthetic is deposited. A small stab incision through the skin can be helpful when using local anesthetic or if 10 gauge or Seldinger ("over the wire") catheters are used. For fluid therapy, the catheter should be directed towards the heart. After placement, the catheter should be flushed with heparinized saline

(5 U/ml) and fixed either with instant bonding glue (for short-term use), staples or sutures.

In the horse, the easiest vein to catheterize is the external jugular vein. The cephalic and the lateral thoracic veins may also be catheterized. These veins carry less-serious consequences if they become occluded by thrombophlebitis; however, the maximum fluid rate attainable in these smaller veins (approximately 5 l/h in adult horses) is less than that attainable in the jugular vein. Furthermore, infectious thrombophlebitis may be serious at any site. If one jugular vein is thrombosed or occluded, it is inadvisable to catheterize the contralateral jugular vein and risk bilateral jugular thrombosis, which can result in life-threatening swelling of the head. Both the cephalic and the lateral thoracic vein can be technically difficult to catheterize. Good sedation or restraint is required to catheterize the cephalic vein because horses have a tendency to move during catheter placement. The cephalic and saphenous veins are relatively easily catheterized in neonatal foals. The lateral thoracic vein can be hard to identify and has a flat profile, which can make it difficult to pass a catheter into the lumen. The vein can be identified by ultrasonography and is probably best catheterized using the Seldinger technique (Seldinger 1953). In the cephalic, saphenous and lateral thoracic veins, valves can impede the passing of a catheter stylet or wire.

A variety of fluid administration sets are available commercially. Sets that include large-bore tubing and a coil are suitable for most situations in adult horses and are recommended. Coils can also be helpful in neonatal foals, but wide-bore tubing is unnecessary. The flow rate can be estimated by counting the number of drops per 10 s in the drip chamber (Table 17.17) or can be set by using an electronic infusion pump. In all situations, a record should be kept of the time the infusion was started and the infusion rate to ensure that the desired volume is being delivered in the appropriate time.

The frequency of replacement of catheters and administration sets depends on the local environmental conditions and the catheter material. Catheters made from polytetrafluoroethylene (Teflon) are associated with an increased incidence of thrombophlebitis and have a tendency to crack

Table 17.17 Flow rates for various administration sets

Bag size (l)	Flow time (h)	Flow rate (l/h)	Drop rate in drip chamber (drops/10 s)					
			STAT set[a]	Straight set, single spike[b]	Coil set, single spike[c]	Six spike set[d]	10 solution set[e]	Mini (60) set[e]
5	1	5	150	–	–	–	138	–
5	1.5	3.33	100	–	–	–	92	–
5	2	2.5	75	–	–	–	69	–
5	3	1.66	50	32	–	–	46	–
5	4	1.25	38	23	25	–	35	–
5	5	1	30	21	24	29	28	–
1	1	1	30	21	24	29	28	167
1	1.5	0.75	–	15	17	21	21	125
1	2	0.5	–	11	11	13	14	83
1	3	0.33	–	9	8	12	9	55
1	4	0.25	–	7	7	11	7	42
1	5	0.2	–	6	5	10	–	33
1	6	0.16	–	4	4	5	–	28

[a] Stat Large Animal IV Set, International WIN, Kennett Square, PA, USA
[b] V-LACT-24-200-S-C-EC1, Cook Veterinary Products, Spencer, IN, USA
[c] V-LACT-24-450-S-C-EC2, Cook Veterinary Products, Spencer, IN, USA
[d] V-LACT-14-60-6S-C-EA3, Cook Veterinary Products, Spencer, IN, USA
[e] Baxter Healthcare Corp., Deerfield, IL, USA
Adapted with permission from Corley K T T 2002 Fluid therapy for horses with gastrointestinal diseases. In: Smith B P (ed) Large animal internal medicine, 3rd edn. Mosby, St Louis, MO, pp. 682–694

and kink (Spurlock et al 1990). These catheters should not be left in place for longer than 72 h. In contrast, soft catheters made from polyurethane or silicone rubber can often be left in place safely for at least 14 days (Spurlock et al 1990) or as long as 6 weeks when monitored properly. These catheters should only be replaced when there is a suspected problem. It is unclear how frequently administration sets should be replaced when used in a horse stall. The current US Centers for Disease Control and Prevention recommendations for human hospitals is not to replace administration sets more frequently than every 72 h, except when used to administer blood- or lipid-containing parenteral nutrition, in which case they should be changed every 24 h (O'Grady et al 2002).

Indwelling cecal catheters have been proposed for fluid therapy in horses to avoid the expense of sterile fluids. Although it is possible to deliver fluid by this technique, the high rate of serious complications precludes the use of cecal catheters (Mealey et al 1995). Repeated administration of oral fluids can be delivered through an indwelling nasogastric tube. The tube should be plugged with a syringe barrel between administrations to prevent excessive air influx. Continuous enteral fluid therapy can be provided with an enteral feeding tube (18 French, 100 inch nasogastric feeding tube, MILA International Inc., Florence, KY, USA) connected to a coiled administration set designed for i.v. fluid therapy (Lopes et al 2002).

THERAPY PLAN: INFUSION RATES AND VOLUMES

The fluid therapy plan should be divided into three stages: initial resuscitation, rehydration and maintenance. The focus of resuscitation is the rapid reversal of hypovolemia. Rehydration aims to replace fluid losses. The maintenance phase aims to prevent the occurrence of further fluid deficits. In severely hypovolemic horses, a transition phase, in which fluid rates are higher than those calculated for the rehydration phase, may be necessary after initial resuscitation. The need for this should be assessed based on the clinical and laboratory responses to the initial resuscitation. Although plasma electrolyte imbalances may

influence the choice of fluid during initial resuscitation, their correction usually takes place during the rehydration phase (Table 17.18).

Resuscitation phase

The resuscitation phase aims to restore circulating volume. There are two ways to think about the treatment of hypovolemia, both of which result in similar treatment patterns. Hypovolemic horses typically require 20–80 ml/kg of crystalloid fluids acutely.

The "shock dose" concept is borrowed from small animal medicine. The shock dose for adult horses and neonatal foals is 50–80 ml/kg crystalloid fluids. Depending on the perceived degree of hypovolemia, one-quarter to one-half of the shock dose is given as rapidly as possible (in less than 20 min) and the horse is reassessed. If the horse requires further fluid, another quarter of the shock dose is given and again the horse is reassessed. The final quarter of the shock dose is only given to severely hypovolemic horses.

The incremental "fluid bolus" concept is borrowed from human medicine. It is actually a much more practical method for the resuscitation of neonatal foals. The caveat is that it assumes that all patients have a similar body weight and, for this reason, it has not been adopted in small animal medicine. The bolus method is simply to give a bolus of 10 liters of crystalloids to an adult horse or 1 liter to neonatal foals (i.e. approximately 20 ml/kg) and reassess. The bolus should be given over 15–20 min. Up to three further boluses may be given, reassessing the horse after each. Most obviously hypovolemic animals require at least two boluses. In adult horses where their body weight is obviously different from 500 kg and neonatal foals that are not approximately 50 kg, the method needs to be adjusted so that the bolus delivers approximately 2 ml/kg. In pony foals and very premature thoroughbred foals, boluses of 500 ml are usually appropriate. In large draftbreed foals, the first bolus should be 2 liters.

It is important to include all fluids being administered in the calculation of fluid rates and volumes. This is especially true in neonatal foals, which often receive dextrose solutions, plasma and

Table 17.18 Fluids of choice for specific metabolic disturbances

Metabolic disturbance[a]	Recommended fluid	Dose[b]
Lactic acidosis	Polyionic crystalloids (Normosol-R, lactated Ringer's solution)	Up to 60 ml/h per kg
	Hetastarch	Up to 10 ml/h per kg
Hyponatremia		Sodium should be corrected at no faster than 1 mEq/l per h
With hypochloremia	Sodium chloride	
Without hypochloremia	Sodium bicarbonate	
Hypernatremia	5% dextrose or 2.5% dextrose/0.45% sodium chloride	To lower sodium no faster than 0.5 mEq/l per h
Hypochloremia	Sodium chloride	0.9% or 7.5%, to effect
Hyperchloremia		
With hypernatremia	5% dextrose	To lower sodium no faster than 0.5 mEq/l per h
Without hypernatremia	Sodium bicarbonate	5%, slowly, to effect
Hypokalemia	Potassium chloride	0.2–0.5 mEq/h per kg, never to exceed 1 mEq/h per kg
Hyperkalemia		
With clinical signs or >7 mEq/l	Calcium gluconate	1 ml/kg i.v.
	Sodium bicarbonate	Over 10 min
	50% dextrose solution	1–2 mEq/l i.v. over 15 min
Without clinical signs	Polyionic crystalloid fluids	2 ml/kg i.v. over 5 min
Hypocalcemia	Calcium gluconate	Typically requires 100–300 ml of 23% solution
Hypercalcemia	Non-calcium-containing polyionic fluids	
	Magnesium sulfate	4–16 mg/kg as an initial dose
Hypomagnesemia	Magnesium sulfate i.v.	4–16 mg/kg as an initial dose
	Magnesium oxide orally	8–32 mg/kg as an initial dose
Hypermagnesemia	Calcium gluconate	250–500 ml of 23% solution
Hypoalbuminemia	Fresh or fresh frozen equine plasma	To effect
	Hetastarch	Not to exceed 10 ml/kg

[a]Always take into account all disturbances present before commencing treatment
[b]1 Eq sodium = 1 mole
Adapted with permission from Corley K T T 2002 Fluid therapy for horses with gastrointestinal diseases. In: Smith B P (ed) Large animal internal medicine, 3rd edn. Mosby, St Louis, MO, pp. 682–694

dimethyl sulfoxide solutions early in the course of treatment. The exception to the recommendation for high initial fluid rates is uncontrolled hemorrhage, for which more conservative fluid volumes should be used until the hemorrhage is stopped (Burris et al 1999, Soucy et al 1999). If colloid solutions are used for initial resuscitation, 1 liter should be used to replace each 3–6 liters of crystalloid (Rackow et al 1987). The amount of hetastarch infused should probably not exceed 10 ml/kg (Jones et al 1997). For mildly hypovolemic adult horses with no significant ongoing

losses, oral fluid therapy alone may be used in the initial resuscitation phase (Lopes 2002). Up to 16 ml/kg (8 liters for a 500 kg horse) may be administered every 30 min (Ecke et al 1998), until the estimated fluid loss has been replaced.

In adult horses, the high end of the i.v. resuscitation rate (10 liters in 15 min for a 500 kg horse) may be difficult to achieve. In adult horses with severe hypovolemia, both jugular veins may be catheterized with large-bore catheters (10–12 gauge), allowing approximately 35 l/h to be administered by gravity if a wide-bore administration set (e.g. arthroscopy tubing) is used. One of the jugular catheters should be removed immediately after the initial resuscitation phase to reduce the risk of bilateral jugular vein thrombosis. An infusion pump may also be used to achieve high rates of fluid delivery, but the high pressures may cause damage to the intima of the vein and increase the risk of thrombosis. In neonatal foals, a 16 gauge catheter will allow flow rates of up to 58 ml/kg/h for a 50 kg foal and 48 ml/kg/h for a 60 kg foal. In larger foals and for higher flow rates, a larger-bore catheter should be used.

The rates of fluid administration recommended above are different from those published previously, which proposed the replacement of initial deficits over a 24 h period (Waterman 1977) or at a maximum fluid rate of 10 ml/kg/h (Seahorn & Cornick-Seahorn 1994). It was thought that these slow fluid rates were necessary to allow time for the fluid to diffuse into the extravascular space (Rose 1981, Seahorn & Cornick-Seahorn 1994). However, it has been shown that this diffusion takes place very rapidly. At the end of a 30 min infusion of lactated Ringer's solution, 67% has already diffused into the extravascular space (Vaupshas & Levy 1990). Another frequently expressed concern is the possibility of pulmo-nary edema with fluid resuscitation at high rates (Spurlock & Furr 1990). No increase in pulmonary edema has been demonstrated in septic humans or experimental pigs at higher fluid rates, despite increased pulmonary arterial occlusion pressure (Yu et al 1997, Zadrobilek et al 1989). Furthermore, there is good evidence from human medicine that high initial fluid rates are associated with better clinical outcomes (Holliday et al 1999). In septic children, fluid rates in excess of 40 ml/kg in the first hour after hospital admission are strongly associated with improved survival (Carcillo et al 1991, Thomas & Carcillo 1998). No studies of optimum fluid rates have been published for the horse, nor have high fluid rates been evaluated critically. Hypovolemic neonatal foals have been resuscitated routinely in the author's hospital with 40 ml/kg crystalloid fluids, with no evidence of any adverse effects and no clinical or radiographic evidence of pulmonary edema. It is this author's impression that aggressively resuscitated foals

remain hypotensive and recumbent for a shorter time and are able to tolerate enteral feeding earlier than foals in which the initial fluid therapy is more conservative. Clearly, controlled studies are required to substantiate or repudiate this impression. Maximum safe fluid rates are also unknown for the horse. The recommendations above are based on the experience in the author's hospital and on work in humans and calves (Kasari & Naylor 1985, Thomas & Carcillo 1998).

Rehydration phase

The rehydration phase aims to replace extravascular fluid losses. Crystalloid fluids are a logical choice for rehydration as they readily diffuse into the interstitial fluid from the vasculature (Spalding & Goodwin 1999, Vaupshas & Levy 1990). Rehydration should take place over the first 12–24 h of therapy. The amount given should be based on the clinical estimate of the degree of dehydration and the response to fluid therapy.

Typically, horses with obvious clinical signs of dehydration will require 50–100 ml/kg (25–50 liters for a 500 kg horse) of fluid to replace their deficits. Following treatment of hypovolemia, a fluid plan should be made for the first 24 h that includes fluids for rehydration, maintenance and ongoing losses. Clinical signs are not an accurate way of estimating fluid requirements (Hansen & DeFrancesco 2002) and so frequent monitoring is required to ensure that adequate fluids are being delivered. When fluid losses have been replaced adequately, the urine specific gravity should be <1.020, except in horses with renal failure. Ensuring adequate fluid therapy in horses with renal failure is difficult and is probably best achieved by measurement of the response of CVP to fluid therapy, as described above, but this is probably only practical in hospitals.

Maintenance phase

The goal of the maintenance phase of fluid therapy is to supply the basal fluid requirement of the horse ("maintenance" rate) and replace ongoing fluid losses. The mean daily water intake (including the water content of feed) of normal resting adult horses is 57–64 ml/kg at ambient temperatures of 41–77°F (5–25°C) (Groenendyk et al 1988, Tasker 1967). Although this may not strictly represent the minimal fluid requirements, it is a useful guideline for the "maintenance rate" (2.5 ml/kg/h) in adult horses. For example, a 500 kg horse requires approximately 30 l/day for maintenance, in addition to any fluids to replace ongoing losses. The maintenance requirement of neonatal foals is significantly higher and is usually taken to be 4–5 ml/kg/h (Spurlock & Furr 1990). Although the fluid intake of nursing foals considerably exceeds this figure (Martin et al 1992, Oftedal et al 1983), clinical experience suggests that these rates are appropriate for maintenance in foals receiving no enteral fluids. It should be emphasized that it is important to take into account the fluid component of all infusions when calculating fluid rates, to avoid inadvertent volume overload in neonatal foals receiving a number of i.v. infusions.

Significant ongoing fluid losses occur in horses with diarrhea, continued nasogastric reflux, polyuric renal failure and profuse sweating. Fluid loss may be as high as 200 ml/kg per day in those with diarrhea (100 l/day for a 500 kg horse) (Rose 1981). A horse with severe diarrhea might require approximately 260 ml/kg daily (approximately 5.5 l/h) of crystalloid fluids to provide basal requirements and replace ongoing losses. Horses with less-frequent or less-watery diarrhea require less fluid. The rate should be estimated based on the volume and consistency of the diarrhea. The adequacy of the rate should then be reassessed frequently based on both clinical signs and laboratory data. In horses with significant nasogastric reflux, the amount of reflux should be measured and replaced directly with i.v. fluids, in addition to the maintenance requirements. Again the results of the fluid therapy should be monitored frequently. With large urinary fluid losses, such as in polyuric renal failure, the amount of urine should be measured or estimated and replaced. In horses with low feed intake or fecal output, serial body weight measurements can be a useful way to monitor fluid losses, replacement and retention. Body weight measurements are most useful in neonatal foals, where the changes in gastrointestinal contents contribute less to weight fluctuations.

CORRECTION OF ACID–BASE AND ELECTROLYTE DISTURBANCES

The volume to be infused and rate of delivery are only part of the therapeutic plan for fluid therapy, albeit the most important in acute resuscitation. The electrolyte and acid–base status of the horse should also be considered and fluids chosen to help to correct physiological imbalances. Unfortunately, it is not possible to predict electrolyte and acid–base disturbances accurately based on clinical signs. Seemingly similar clinical presentations may have a quite different pathophysiology (Brownlow & Hutchins 1982, Svendsen et al 1979). The recent availability of relatively inexpensive, portable blood gas and electrolyte measuring equipment (Grosenbaugh et al 1998) has made determining the acid–base status possible in ambulatory equine practice and allows the field veterinarian to monitor and treat these disturbances. As stated earlier, in the absence of specific laboratory information, fluid therapy should probably be limited to isotonic polyionic crystalloid fluids, possibly with the addition of 10–20 mEq/l potassium chloride in the maintenance phase.

When laboratory information is available within 4–6 h, fluid therapy can be tailored to the individual horse, allowing correction of specific physiological abnormalities. Although calculations of whole body electrolyte or base deficits are possible (Carlson 1999), their relevance to managing the clinical case with ongoing losses and renal responses to changes in plasma electrolyte concentrations is unclear (Holliday 1996). A safer, more physiologically relevant approach is to monitor the clinical and laboratory responses to therapy frequently and to adjust the treatment accordingly, rather than to rely on a calculated electrolyte dose to restore normal plasma concentrations.

Acid–base disturbances

The most common acid–base disturbance in horses is metabolic acidosis, caused by lactic acidosis (e.g. hypovolemia, endotoxemia, strenuous exercise), hyponatremia (e.g. colitis, peritonitis, ruptured bladder, intestinal torsion, high-volume pleural drainage) or hyperchloremia (e.g. renal tubular acidosis). Metabolic alkalosis, caused by hypochloremia (high-volume gastric reflux, furosemide (frusemide) administration, rhabdomyolysis) or hypoalbuminemia (e.g. severe enterocolitis, glomerulonephritis, excessive fluid therapy), respiratory alkalosis (e.g. hyperventilation in response to pain) and respiratory acidosis (pneumonia, hypoventilation in response to extreme abdominal distension, central depression, botulism) can also occur (Corley & Marr 1998). The predominant clinical signs in horses with acid–base disturbances are likely to result from the disease, rather than from the direct effects of a change in plasma pH.

The treatment of acid–base disturbances should be directed at the underlying cause and the specific plasma constituent imbalance. It is possible to determine the relative contributions of sodium, chloride, unidentified anions (principally lactate in horses) and protein to the metabolic component of acid–base disturbances by the use of equations based on the calculated base excess (Corley & Marr 1998, Whitehair et al 1995). However, decisions on treatment can often be based on the absolute values of these blood constituents and it is only in complex disturbances, with changes in multiple plasma constituents, that the equations are usually necessary.

Lactate

As discussed, increased blood or plasma lactate concentrations are usually caused by poor tissue perfusion in gastrointestinal diseases but may also result from acute renal failure, hepatic failure and anaerobic metabolism during endotoxemia. The clinical signs related to the disease causing the lactic acidosis are likely to overshadow the direct effects of the lactemia, such as decreased myocardial contractility (Yatani et al 1981).

Although lactate can be measured directly, its plasma concentration can be accurately predicted by the anion gap in horses with normal plasma protein concentrations (Constable et al 1998). The anion gap is calculated from the plasma concentrations of sodium plus potassium minus the concentrations of chloride plus bicarbonate. The normal range is 7–15 mEq/l (Constable et al 1998). At low and high protein concentrations, equations should be used based on base excess (Corley & Marr 1998, Whitehair et al 1995) or the simplified strong ion gap (Constable et al 1998).

$$\frac{2.24 \times \text{Total protein (g/dl)}}{(1 + 10^{6.65-\text{pH}})} - \text{Anion gap}$$

Any of these calculations can be performed easily using a pocket calculator.

Lactic acidosis should be treated with large volumes of polyionic crystalloid solutions. As discussed above, the use of sodium bicarbonate in lactic acidosis is highly controversial and not recommended (Forsythe & Schmidt 2000).

Sodium

Low plasma sodium concentrations are most commonly seen in acute colitis. Hyponatremia is usually accompanied by hypochloremia because of the increased loss of electrolytes relative to water (Brownlow & Hutchins 1982). Other conditions associated with hyponatremia are those that result in the sequestration of sodium in a third space (e.g. bladder rupture, peritonitis, pleural effusion, intestinal torsion or volvulus) and sodium-wasting disorders (e.g. polyuric renal failure, esophageal obstruction leading to loss of saliva). Hyponatremia has also been reported in rhabdomyolysis in neonatal foals caused by selenium deficiency (Perkins et al 1998). Severe hyperglycemia can also contribute to hyponatremia. The plasma sodium concentration decreases by approximately 1.7 mmol/l for each increase of 100 mg/dl (5.6 mmol/l) in plasma glucose concentration (Adrogue & Madias 2000b). Clinical signs of hyponatremia include neurological disturbances, such as a reduced or absent menace response, intention tremor and hypermetric gait (Lakritz et al 1992); however, severe clinical signs do not usually occur until the sodium concentration is <110 mEq/l (Schaer 1999). Hyponatremia can also contribute to a metabolic acidosis (Corley & Marr 1998).

The fluid choice for hyponatremia depends on whether there is concurrent hypochloremia. Sodium chloride is the best choice, if the plasma chloride concentration is also low. If the chloride concentration is normal or increased, then sodium bicarbonate should be used. If the horse is not clinically dehydrated (Malcolm et al 1993) and the hyponatremia is severe, then hypertonic solutions may be indicated (7–7.5% sodium chloride and 5–8.4% sodium bicarbonate, respectively). In other species, the rapid correction of sodium deficits has been shown to cause demyelination of the pontine and extra pontine neurons, resulting in severe neurological dysfunction (Adrogue & Madias 2000b). It has not been established whether this is a risk or not in the horse and, therefore, it is necessary to follow the guidelines for sodium restoration in other species. These guidelines state that sodium should be corrected at a rate of 1 mEq/l per h in acute hyponatremia and at less than 0.5 mEq/l per h in chronic hyponatremia, in neither case to exceed 8 mEq/l during the first 24 h (Schaer 1999).

Hypernatremia is rare in horses (Brownlow & Hutchins 1982). It is usually a result of water loss in excess of electrolytes and is accompanied by hyperchloremia. Iatrogenic hypernatremia may occur in horses in which resuscitation formulas are used for maintenance and is not an uncommon sequela in neonates. To correct hypernatremia, low sodium fluids such as 5% dextrose or 2.5% dextrose and 0.45% sodium chloride should be given. Again, in other species, it is recommended that hypernatremia not be corrected too rapidly: sodium should be lowered by 0.5 mEq/l per h, not to exceed 12 mEq/l in the first 24 h (Schaer 1999).

Clinical signs associated with hypo- and hypernatremia result from changes in the plasma osmolality. Sodium is the major cation in plasma, and sodium and glucose concentrations are the main determinants of plasma osmolality (Brownlow & Hutchins 1982). Changes in plasma osmolality can lead to CNS edema or dehydration (Rose 1994), because the CSF equilibrates slowly with the plasma but will change rapidly if osmotic gradients are high.

Chloride

Hypochloremia is common in gastrointestinal disease (Svendsen et al 1979), because of the loss of gastric hydrochloric acid in high volume reflux from the stomach (in proximal enteritis and grass sickness) and the secretion and/or lack of absorption of chloride in severe colitis. It may also occur in exhausted horse syndrome, chronic compensated respiratory acidosis and following furosemide (frusemide) administration. Hypochloremia in the absence of hyponatremia results in a metabolic alkalosis (Corley & Marr 1998). The alkalosis associated with hypochloremia may also result in increased cellular uptake of potassium, leading to hypokalemia (Schaer 1999).

Treatment of hypochloremia can usually be achieved with i.v. 0.9% sodium chloride, which contains more chloride relative to sodium than plasma. In horses with high-volume gastric reflux, administration of i.v. histamine H_2 receptor antagonists (e.g. cimetidine at 6.6 mg/kg i.v. four times a day) reduces gastric hydrochloric acid secretion and may, therefore, reduce chloride loss. In humans, i.v. hydrochloric acid has been used to treat severe hypochloremia (Kwun et al 1983) but carries substantial risks for the patient (Rothe & Schimek 1986).

Hyperchloremia is rare in horses but may occur in renal tubular acidosis (Ziemer et al 1987, Trotter et al 1986) and severe colitis. In the absence of hypernatremia, hyperchloremia results in a metabolic acidosis (Corley & Marr 1998). It should be treated with 5% dextrose if accompanied by hypernatremia and with sodium bicarbonate if severe and accompanied by a low or normal plasma sodium concentration (Schaer 1999).

Potassium

Hypokalemia is seen commonly in horses following major surgery, as a result of enhanced mineralocorticoid and glucocorticoid release and following the infusion of large amounts of sodium-containing fluids, which increase distal tubular flow and renal potassium loss (Rose 1994). Hypokalemia can also occur in colitis, following heavy sweating and in metabolic alkalosis.

In patients with colic, the most relevant clinical sign of hypokalemia is reduced intestinal motility (Gennari 1998, Schaer 1999). However, the association between hypokalemia and ileus in the horse remains undetermined. Other clinical signs include muscle weakness, lethargy and inability to concentrate urine (Schaer 1999). Cardiac conduction abnormalities are rare except in severe hypokalemia and in pre-existing cardiac dysfunction (Gennari 1998). The effect of potassium on acid–base status is small and need not be considered clinically (Corley & Marr 1998).

Potassium is primarily an intracellular ion and, consequently, decreases in whole-body potassium may not be detected by plasma measurements (Muylle et al 1984). Although erythrocyte potassium content has been used to estimate whole-body potassium (Muylle et al 1984), its accuracy has not been validated. Moreover, the extracellular potassium concentration (reflected in the plasma) is critical for neuromuscular transmission and is, therefore, more relevant to clinical signs than whole-body potassium stores (Rose 1994). The intervention level for treatment of hypokalemia has not been established. In postoperative colic and proximal enteritis, where the prevention of ileus is a primary goal, it may be prudent to supplement if the plasma potassium concentration falls to <3.5 mEq/l. In other situations, especially those being fed enterally, it may not be necessary to treat if the plasma potassium concentration is >3.0 mEq/l.

Hypokalemia is treated with i.v. potassium chloride solution. The rate of administration is more important than the amount. Normally the rate should not exceed 0.5 mEq/kg/h and should never exceed 1 mEq/kg/h (Schaer 1999). The addition of 40 mEq/l potassium chloride to crystalloid fluids is safe at infusion rates of up to 10 ml/kg/h (5 l/h for a 500 kg horse). This amount is usually only required in severe hypokalemia (<2.7 mEq/l) and smaller disturbances can often be treated successfully with 20 mEq/l. If hypokalemia does not respond to potassium chloride administration, magnesium should be supplemented (Hamill-Ruth & McGory 1996).

Hyperkalemia may occur in acidosis, colitis, ruptured bladder and renal failure and in horses with hyperkalemic periodic paralysis. Artifactual hyperkalemia may be seen in blood samples stored for longer than 2 h before separation of the plasma, as a result of leaching of potassium from the erythrocytes. The clinical signs of hyperkalemia result from the disruption of neuromuscular transmission and are, therefore, similar to those of hypokalemia. In the absence of clinical signs, polyionic fluids should be administered. Possible treatments for symptomatic or severe (>7 mEq/l) hyperkalemia include calcium gluconate (1 ml/kg i.v. over 10 min), sodium bicarbonate (1–2 mEq/l i.v. over 15 min) and 50% dextrose solution (2 ml/kg i.v. over 5 min) (Schaer 1999).

Calcium

Low plasma ionized calcium concentrations are common in surgical colic (Dart et al 1992) and colitis. Hypocalcemia may also occur following vigorous or prolonged exercise, especially in hot and humid conditions (Taylor 1996). Possible causes of hypocalcemia include lactic acidosis (Cooper et al 1992), endotoxin-induced changes in calcium homeostasis (Todd & Mollitt 1995), loss of calcium in sweat (Taylor 1996) and functional disturbances of the small intestine (the main site of calcium absorption in the horse (Schryver et al 1970)). Clinical signs of hypocalcemia reported in the horse include synchronous diaphragmatic flutter, tetany, muscle spasm and seizures (Beyer et al 1997). In horses following surgery for colic, decreasing ionized calcium concentrations have been correlated with a number of electrocardiographic changes: increased heart rate, increased Q–T interval corrected for heart rate, decreased P–R interval and decreased Q–R–S interval (Garcia-Lopez et al 2001). Experimentally induced hypocalcaemia (<3.52 mg/dl (<0.83 mmol/l)) produced cardiac arrhythmias in four out of seven ponies, which were fatal in two (Glazier et al 1979). Hypocalcemia may be associated with postoperative ileus in the horse (Dart et al 1992) but this has not been investigated.

Approximately 50% of the total calcium in plasma is either bound to albumin or complexed to small ligands. The remaining ionized fraction is the biologically active form. Whenever possible, the plasma ionized calcium concentration should be measured rather than the total concentration. If total plasma calcium measurements are used to guide therapy, the calcium concentration should be corrected for changes in albumin concentration. The level at which intervention is required in the treatment of hypocalcemia is not known. Administration of calcium exacerbates endotoxemia in rodent models (Malcolm et al 1989, Zaloga et al 1992). While the relevance of these observations to the horse has not been determined, aggressive supplementation of calcium in endotoxemic horses may be inadvisable. However, the plasma ionized calcium concentration is directly related to myocardial contractility (Lang et al 1988) and, therefore, close attention to the ionized calcium concentration is warranted. Even in endotoxic horses, calcium should probably be supplemented if the ionized calcium concentration is <3.6 mg/dl (0.9 mmol/l).

Hypocalcemia is usually treated with 23% calcium gluconate solution administered i.v. A volume of 100–300 ml is typically required (Dart et al 1992) but the amount will depend on the ongoing losses and the ionized calcium concentration should be checked frequently during therapy. Calcium solutions are irritating to the veins and should be diluted in crystalloid fluids prior to administration. Calcium solutions should not be mixed with sodium bicarbonate or whole blood. Following calcium supplementation, the plasma calcium concentration should be checked after 4–8 h because ongoing losses and redistribution into cells may result in further hypocalcemia. Hypocalcemia can be a sequel to magnesium deficiency and, therefore, magnesium should be supplemented in horses with refractory hypocalcemia.

Hypercalcemia occurs in horses with chronic renal failure and in a few neoplastic conditions. The clinical signs are usually those of the underlying pathophysiology but soft tissue calcification may occur. In experimental ponies, hypercalcemia induced ventricular fibrillation or cardiac arrest at ionized calcium concentrations of 18.2–40 mg/dl (4.55–10.0 mmol/l) (Glazier et al 1979). Treatment for severe hypercalcemia (ionized

calcium concentration of >9 mg/dl (2.25 mmol/l)) should include non-calcium-containing i.v. fluids (sodium chloride or Normosol-R) and i.v. magnesium sulfate (see treatment of hypomagnesemia below).

Ionized calcium concentrations of <3.6 mg/dl (0.9 mmol/l) or >9 mg/dl (2.25 mmol/l) are rarely seen in clinical patients (Garcia-Lopez et al 2001).

Magnesium

In a recent study, 54% of horses with gastrointestinal disease had low plasma ionized magnesium concentrations (Garcia-Lopez et al 2001). Causes of hypomagnesemia include decreased intake, gastrointestinal losses (e.g. prolonged nasogastric reflux, malabsorption), alterations in distribution (e.g. endotoxemia, TPN), renal losses (e.g. prolonged administration of lactated Ringer's solution or other magnesium-free fluids, hypophosphatemia, acidemia, renal tubular acidosis; Olerich & Rude 1994, Salem et al 1991) and excessive sweating (Taylor 1996). In the horse, severe hypomagnesemia can result in ventricular arrhythmias and also muscle tremors, ataxia, seizures and calcification of elastic tissue (Harrington 1974). Other clinical manifestations of hypomagnesemia reported in humans include supraventricular tachycardia, atrial fibrillation, thrombosis, anemia, decreased muscle strength, increased nephrotoxicity of aminoglycoside drugs, increased pulmonary vascular resistance and sudden death (Gunther 1992, Landon & Young 1993, Salem et al 1991, Tso & Barish 1992). Hypomagnesemia can also result in hypokalemia that is refractory to potassium supplementation (Hamill-Ruth & McGory 1996).

ECF contains approximately 1% of the total body magnesium and, consequently, the serum magnesium concentration may not reflect the total body magnesium status (Olerich & Rude 1994), making the diagnosis of hypomagnesemia difficult. Fortunately it is safe to administer moderate amounts of magnesium, irrespective of the magnesium status of the horse, provided that the horse has normal renal function. Magnesium sulfate (at 2 mg/kg/min i.v., not to exceed 50 mg/kg) is recommended for the treatment of ventricular arrhythmias associated with hypo-magnesemia (Bonagura & Reef 1998). Higher doses should be avoided because they cause significant muscle weakness: 140 mg/kg i.v. magnesium sulfate can induce recumbency in normal horses (Bowen et al 1970). For the treatment of hypomagnesemia in the absence of cardiac signs, 2–8 mg/kg magnesium sulfate can be used as an initial dose in horses with normal renal function. Supplementation with oral magnesium–lactate–citrate or magnesium oxide is possible but oral magnesium sulfate should be avoided because of its laxative effects.

In one study, 11% of horses with gastrointestinal disease were identified as clinically hypermagnesemic but associated clinical signs were not reported (Costa et al 1999). Severe clinical signs have been reported following nasogastric administration of magnesium sulfate to two horses. The dose given was between 1600 and 2000 mg/kg. Both horses recovered 1 to 6 h after the onset of clinical signs, which included flaccid paralysis with recumbency, tachycardia, tachypnea and non-detectable peripheral pulses. The horses were treated i.v. with 250 ml 23% calcium gluconate solution, repeated after 1 h, and polyionic i.v. fluids to promote diuresis (Henninger & Horst 1997).

Phosphorus

Hypophosphatemia has been reported in horses with strangulating intestinal lesions, intestinal ileus (Svendsen et al 1979) and as a sequel to renal dysfunction (Tennant et al 1981). Hypophosphatemia has also been reported in humans during prolonged administration of lactate-containing fluids (Walton 1979), in metabolic or respiratory alkalosis, during repeated gastric magnesium sulfate administration (because magnesium binds phosphate to form an insoluble complex) and after prolonged administration of non-lipid-containing parenteral nutrition solutions (Bugg & Jones 1998). Reduced intestinal phosphate absorption, apparently without hypophosphatemia, is a reported sequel to large colon resection (Bertone et al 1989). Hypophosphatemia is also a feature of "refeeding syndrome" (Fisher et al 2000), which may have relevance to care of malnourished

"rescue" horses. The clinical signs of hypophosphatemia reported in small animals and humans include hemolysis, skeletal muscle weakness and rhabdomyolysis, leukocyte dysfunction, ventricular arrhythmias and reduced cardiac output (Bugg & Jones 1998, Macintire 1997).

The clinical manifestations and treatment of hypophosphatemia in the horse have not been reported and in humans there is no good evidence for commencing treatment in the absence of clinical signs (Bugg & Jones 1998). Treatment options reported in small animals include i.v. (0.01–0.03 mmol/h per kg) and oral (0.5–2 mmol/kg daily) potassium phosphate or sodium potassium phosphate (Macintire 1997). The author has used this dose rate of phosphate in mature horses, with apparent clinical success. The potential effects of potassium phosphate on the plasma potassium concentration must be considered before commencing treatment. Glucose 1-phosphate (Bollaert et al 1995) and sodium phosphate administration i.v. have also been reported in humans. The safety of these treatments has not been evaluated in the horse.

Hyperphosphatemia occurs without specific clinical signs in horses with strangulating intestinal lesions (Arden & Stick 1988) and severe colitis (Svendsen et al 1979). The clinical findings reported in small animals include diarrhea, hypocalcemia, hypernatremia and an increased propensity to metastatic soft-tissue calcification. The treatment recommended in small animals includes i.v. fluids to correct any acidosis and promote renal phosphorus excretion and dextrose-containing fluids to promote translocation of phosphorus into cells (Macintire 1997).

It appears that increased plasma phosphate concentrations are not directly toxic (Sutters et al 1996). Hypocalcemia and metastatic soft-tissue calcification caused by hyperphosphatemia result from the calcium/phosphate product exceeding that required for precipitation of calcium phosphate in the tissues (Macintire 1997, Sutters et al 1996).

Albumin

Hypoalbuminemia is common in horses with moderate-to-severe compromise of the colon. It may also occur as a result of parasitism, renal failure and overaggressive fluid therapy. Advanced hepatic failure may also lead to hypoalbuminemia but it is exceedingly rare to reach this stage of disease in horses. Clinical signs of hypoalbuminemia are peripheral edema (owing to reduced plasma oncotic pressure) and tissue and organ edema, leading to reduced oxygen uptake by cells (increased perfusion distance) and, in severe cases, organ failure. Albumin is a weak acid and severe hypoalbuminemia may contribute to a metabolic alkalosis or mask a concurrent metabolic acidosis (Corley & Marr 1998). A decrease in albumin concentration of 1 g/dl results in an increase in the base excess of 3.7 mEq/l (Whitehair et al 1995).

Hypoalbuminemia should be treated when acute or if there are clinical signs. Although it is advisable to treat all horses with a plasma total solids concentration of <4.0 g/dl, a few horses with chronic hypoproteinemia can have plasma total solids concentrations of 3.5–4.0 g/dl with no apparent clinical signs. The treatment options for hypoalbuminemia include hetastarch and fresh or fresh frozen equine plasma.

COMPLICATIONS OF FLUID THERAPY

THROMBOPHLEBITIS

Thrombophlebitis is a common complication of i.v. fluid therapy (Traub-Dargatz & Dargatz 1994). A thrombus may cause mechanical blockage of venous drainage, resulting in local edema, and may be a nidus for infection. Edematous occlusion of the nasal passages can result from bilateral jugular vein thrombosis and can be fatal. It is, therefore, advisable not to catheterize the contralateral jugular vein if one jugular vein shows signs of thrombosis. Bacterial endocarditis, particularly of the tricuspid valve, can occur as a sequel to septic thrombosis.

Thrombophlebitis can be identified by heat, swelling or the presence of any exudate around the catheter insertion site or a palpable thrombus ("corded" feel) in the catheterized vein. Catheterized veins should be examined at least daily.

Ultrasonography of a catheterized vein can help to identify thrombus formation. It is prudent to continue to check the vein for 2–3 days after catheter removal because thrombophlebitis may develop or become apparent in this period.

Topical nitroglycerin (glycerol trinitrate) ointment has been shown to be an effective treatment for thrombophlebitis in humans (Berrazueta et al 1993). Local application of hot packs and topical dimethyl sulfoxide ointment are also used for treatment in the horse. Catheters should be removed aseptically from thrombosed veins and bacterial culture (preferably by the roll-plate technique (Maki et al 1977)) and in vitro susceptibility testing carried out. A fine needle aspirate of the thrombus can also be submitted for bacterial culture. Fluid-filled pockets within the thrombus can often be identified by ultrasound (Gardner et al 1991) and should be aspirated following surgical preparation of the overlying skin. Empirical antimicrobial treatment should include an agent with a broad spectrum of activity including streptococci and staphylococci (Gardner et al 1991) and good tissue penetration, such as doxycycline.

The risk factors for thrombophlebitis include administration of "Carboy" fluids (Traub-Dargatz & Dargatz 1994), the presence of diarrhea (Traub-Dargatz & Dargatz 1994) or endotoxemia (Morris 1989), polytetrafluoroethylene (Teflon) catheter material and a long duration of catheterization (Spurlock et al 1990). Several other risk factors for thrombophlebitis have been identified in humans but not studied in horses. These include inexperienced personnel placing the catheter (Armstrong et al 1986), administration of TPN (Ioannides-Demos et al 1995) and large-bore catheters (Swanson & Aldrete 1989).

OVERHYDRATION

Clinical signs of overhydration are rare in horses with normal cardiac and renal function. The most important clinical sign of overhydration is pulmonary edema, manifested by dyspnea and a pink-white foamy nasal discharge. Treatment for overhydration should include i.v. furosemide (frusemide) (0.5–1 mg/kg) and a reduction in the rate of fluid administration. Intranasal oxygen supplementation is indicated where there is significant hypoxemia (based on arterial blood gas analysis). Further fluid therapy in these horses should be monitored carefully, ideally using CVP measurements.

BEYOND FLUID THERAPY

Some horses and foals will not respond to initial resuscitation fluid therapy. These animals have continued tachycardia, lactic acidosis, oliguria and hypo- or hypertension despite appropriate fluid therapy. A proportion of these patients will respond to inotropes, pressors and/or vasodilators. Before initiating treatment with vasoactive drugs, it is important to establish that the abnormality detected is a function of the cardiovascular system (for example tachycardia may be caused by pain and lactic acidosis may be caused by liver disease) and to reassess the adequacy of ongoing fluid therapy. The most expedient method of confirming that no further improvement can be expected with fluid therapy is to assess the response to a bolus of fluid (fluid challenge). If no response is seen to the fluid challenge, vasoactive agents such as dobutamine, norepinephrine (noradrenaline), vasopressin or nitroprusside should be considered (see Ch. 12).

REFERENCES

Adrogue H J, Madias N E 2000a Hypernatremia. New England Journal of Medicine 342:1493–1499

Adrogue H J, Madias N E 2000b Hyponatremia. New England Journal of Medicine 342:1581–1589

Allison K P, Gosling P, Jones S et al 1999 Randomized trial of hydroxyethyl starch versus gelatin for trauma resuscitation. Journal of Trauma 47:1114–1121

Allison S P, Lobo D N 2000 Debate: albumin administration should not be avoided. Critical Care 4:147–150

Allwood M C 2000 Light protection during parenteral nutrition infusion: is it really necessary? Nutrition 16:234–235

Andrews F M, Hamlin R L, Stalnaker P S 1990 Blood viscosity in horses with colic. Journal of Veterinary Internal Medicine 4:183–186

Angle N, Hoyt D B, Coimbra R et al 1998 Hypertonic saline resuscitation diminishes lung injury by suppressing neutrophil activation after hemorrhagic shock. Shock 9:164–170

Arden W A, Stick J A 1988 Serum and peritoneal fluid phosphate concentrations as predictors of major intestinal injury associated with equine colic. Journal of the American Veterinary Medical Association 193:927–931

Armstrong C W, Mayhall C G, Miller K B et al 1986 Prospective study of catheter replacement and other risk factors for infection of hyperalimentation catheters. Journal of Infectious Disease 154:808–816

Baron P G, Iles R A, Cohen R D 1978 Effect of varying PCO_2 on intracellular pH and lactate consumption in the isolated perfused rat liver. Clinical Science and Molecular Medicine 55:175–181

Baum T D, Wang H, Rothschild H R et al 1990 Mesenteric oxygen metabolism, ileal mucosal hydrogen ion concentration, and tissue edema after crystalloid or colloid resuscitation in porcine endotoxic shock: comparison of Ringer's lactate and 6% hetastarch. Circulatory Shock 30:385–397

Becu T, Polledo G, Gaskin J M 1997 Immunoprophylaxis of *Rhodococcus equi* pneumonia in foals. Veterinary Microbiology 56:193–204

Belgrave R L, Hines M T, Keegan R D et al 2002 Effects of a polymerized ultrapurified bovine hemoglobin blood substitute administered to ponies with normovolemic anemia. Journal of Veterinary Internal Medicine 16:396–403

Benjamin E, Oropello J M, Abalos A M et al 1994 Effects of acid–base correction on hemodynamics, oxygen dynamics, and resuscitability in severe canine haemorrhagic shock. Critical Care Medicine 22:1616–1623

Berrazueta J R, Poveda J J, Ochoteco J et al 1993 The anti-inflammatory and analgesic action of transdermal glyceryltrinitrate in the treatment of infusion-related thrombophlebitis. Postgraduate Medical Journal 69:37–40

Bertone J J, Gossett K A, Shoemaker K E et al 1990 Effect of hypertonic vs. isotonic saline solution on responses to sublethal *Escherichia coli* endotoxemia in horses. American Journal of Veterinary Research 51:999–1007

Bertone A L, van Soest P J, Stashak T S 1989 Digestion, fecal, and blood variables associated with extensive large colon resection in the horse. American Journal of Veterinary Research 50:253–258

Beyer M J, Freestone J F, Reimer J M et al 1997 Idiopathic hypocalcemia in foals. Journal of Veterinary Internal Medicine 11:356–360

Biesenbach G, Kaiser W, Zazgornik J 1997 Incidence of acute oligoanuric renal failure in dextran 40 treated patients with acute ischemic stroke stage III or IV. Renal Failure 19:69–75

Bjerneroth G, Sammeli O, Li Y-C et al 1994 Effects of alkaline buffers on cytoplasmic pH in lymphocytes. Critical Care Medicine 22:1550–1556

Bollaert P E, Levy B, Nace L et al 1995 Hemodynamic and metabolic effects of rapid correction of hypophosphatemia in patients with septic shock. Chest 107:1698–1701

Bonagura J D, Reef V B 1998 Cardiovascular diseases. In: Reed S M, Bayly W M (eds) Equine internal medicine. Saunders, Philadelphia, PA, pp. 290–370

Bonventre J V, Cheung J Y 1985 Effects of metabolic acidosis on viability of cells exposed to anoxia. American Journal of Physiology 249:C149–C159

Bosse U, Abel H T, Bannert N et al 1993 Necrotizing enterocolitis in the newborn infant. Pathogenetic risk factors in a 3 year analysis. Monatsschrift Kinderheilkrankheid 141:602–606

Bowen J M, Blackmon D M, Heavner J E 1970 Effect of magnesium ions on neuromuscular transmission in the horse, steer, and dog. Journal of the American Veterinary Medical Association 157:164–173

Brownlow M A, Hutchins D R 1982 The concept of osmolality: its use in the evaluation of dehydration in the horse. Equine Veterinary Journal 14:106–110

Bugg N C, Jones J A 1998 Hypophosphataemia. Pathophysiology, effects and management on the intensive care unit. Anaesthesia 53:895–902

Bumpus S E, Haskins S C, Kass P H 1998 Effect of synthetic colloids on refractometric readings of total solids. Journal of Veterinary Emergency and Critical Care 8:21–26

Burris D, Rhee P, Kaufmann C et al 1999 Controlled resuscitation for uncontrolled hemorrhagic shock. Journal of Trauma 46:216–223

Carcillo J A, Davis A L, Zaritsky A 1991 Role of early fluid resuscitation in pediatric septic shock. Journal of the American Medical Association 266:1242–1245

Carlson G P 1999 Quantative estimation of fluid and electrolyte deficits. In: Proceedings of the Bluegrass Equine Medical and Critical Care Symposium, Lexington, KY 1999 pp.

Choi P T, Yip G, Quinonez L G et al 1999 Crystalloids vs. colloids in fluid resuscitation: a systematic review. Critical Care Medicine 27:200–210

Chrusch C, Bands C, Bose D et al 2000 Impaired hepatic extraction and increased splanchnic production contribute to lactic acidosis in canine sepsis. American Journal of Respiratory and Critical Care Medicine 161:517–526

Cochrane Injuries Group Albumin Reviewers 1998 Human albumin administration in critically ill patients: systematic review of randomised controlled trials. British Medical Journal 317:235–240

Cohen R D, Woods H F 1996 Disturbances of acid–base homeostasis. In: Weatherall D J, Ledingham J G G, Warrell D A (eds) Oxford textbook of medicine, 3rd edn. Oxford University Press, Oxford, pp. 1533–1544

Collatos C 1997 Blood and blood component therapy. In: Robinson N E (ed) Current therapy in equine medicine, 4th edn. Saunders, Philadelphia, PA, pp. 290–292

Conhaim R L, Watson K E, Potenza B M et al 1999 Pulmonary capillary sieving of hetastarch is not altered by LPS-induced sepsis. Journal of Trauma 46: 800–810

Constable P D, Gohar H M, Morin D E et al 1996 Use of hypertonic saline–dextran solution to resuscitate hypovolemic calves with diarrhea. American Journal of Veterinary Research 57:97–104

Constable P D, Hinchcliff K W, Muir W W 1998 Comparison of anion gap and strong ion gap as predictors of unmeasured strong ion concentration in plasma and serum from horses. American Journal of Veterinary Research 59:881–887

Cooper D J, Herbertson M J, Werner H A et al 1993 Bicarbonate does not increase left ventricular contractility during L-lactic acidemia in pigs. American Review of Respiratory Disease 148:317–322

Cooper D J, Walley K R, Dodek P M et al 1992 Plasma ionized calcium and blood lactate concentrations are inversely associated in human lactic acidosis. Intensive Care Medicine 18:286–289

Corley K T T 2002 Fluid therapy for horses with gastrointestinal diseases. In: Smith B P (ed) Large animal internal medicine, 3rd edn. Mosby, St Louis, MO, pp. 682–694

Corley K T T, Marr C M 1998 Pathophysiology, assessment and treatment of acid–base disturbances in the horse. Equine Veterinary Education 10:255–265

Costa L R R, Eades S E, Tulley R T et al 1999 Plasma magnesium concentrations in horses with gastrointestinal tract disease. Journal of Veterinary Internal Medicine 13:274

Cotter S M 1991 Clinical transfusion medicine. Advances in Veterinary Science and Comparative Medicine 36:187–223

Creteur J, Sun Q, Abid O et al 2001 Normovolemic hemodilution improves oxygen extraction capabilities in endotoxic shock. Journal of Applied Physiology 91:1701–1707

Cudd A, Pauly T H 1987 Necrotizing enterocolitis in two equine neonates. Compendium on Continuing Education for the Practicing Veterinarian 9:88–92

Dabareiner R M, Snyder J R, White N A et al 1995 Microvascular permeability and endothelial cell morphology associated with low-flow ischemia/reperfusion injury in the equine jejunum. American Journal of Veterinary Research 56:639–648

Dart A J, Snyder J R, Spier S J et al 1992 Ionized calcium concentration in horses with surgically managed gastrointestinal disease: 147 cases (1988–1990). Journal of the American Veterinary Medical Association 201:1244–1248

Denkhaus M, van Amstel S 1986 Adverse effects following intravenous fluid therapy in the horse using non-commercial fluids: preliminary findings. Journal of the South African Veterinary Association 57:105–107

Didwania A, Miller J, Kassel D et al 1997 Effect of intravenous lactated Ringer's solution infusion on the circulating lactate concentration: Part 3. Results of a prospective, randomized, double-blind, placebo-controlled trial. Critical Care Medicine 25:1851–1854

Divers T J 1998 Diarrheal diseases: adults. In: Orsini J A, Divers T J (eds) Manual of equine emergencies. Saunders, Philadelphia, PA, pp. 217–225

Downing S E, Talner N S, Gardner T H 1965 Cardiovascular responses to metabolic acidosis. American Journal of Physiology 208:237–242

Dudley M A, Wykes L J, Dudley A W J et al 1998 Parenteral nutrition selectively decreases protein synthesis in the small intestine. American Journal of Physiology 274:G131–G137

Durham A E 1996 Blood and plasma transfusion in the horse. Equine Veterinary Education 8:8–12

Ecke P, Hodgson D R, Rose R J 1998 Induced diarrhoea in horses. Part 2: Response to administration of an oral rehydration solution. Veterinary Journal 155:161–170

Fanconi S, Burger R, Ghelfi D et al 1993 Hemodynamic effects of sodium bicarbonate in critically ill neonates. Intensive Care Medicine 19:65–69

Fink M 1997 Cytopathic hypoxia in sepsis. Acta Anaesthesiologic Scandinavica Supplementum 110:87–95

Fisher M, Simpser E, Schneider M 2000 Hypophosphatemia secondary to oral refeeding in anorexia nervosa. International Journal of Eating Disorders 28: 181–187

Forsythe S M, Schmidt G A 2000 Sodium bicarbonate for the treatment of lactic acidosis. Chest 117:260–267

Fromm R E 2000 Blood substitutes. Critical Care Medicine 28:2150–2151

Furr M O, Lessard P, White N A 1995 Development of a colic severity score for predicting the outcome of equine colic. Veterinary Surgery 24:97–101

Garcia-Lopez J M, Provost P J, Rush J E et al 2001 Prevalence and prognostic importance of hypomagnesemia and hypocalcemia in horses that have colic surgery. American Journal of Veterinary Research 62:7–12

Gardner S Y, Reef V B, Spencer P A 1991 Ultrasonographic evaluation of horses with thrombophlebitis of the jugular vein: 46 cases (1985–1988). Journal of the American Veterinary Medical Association 199:370–373

Gennari F J 1998 Hypokalemia. New England Journal of Medicine 339:451–458

Glazier D B, Littledike E T, Evans R D 1979 Electrocardiographic changes in induced hypocalcemia and hypercalcemia in horses. Journal of Equine Medicine & Surgery 3:489–494

Gossett K A, French D D, Cleghorn B et al 1990a Effect of acute acidemia on blood biochemical variables in healthy ponies. American Journal of Veterinary Research 51:1375–1379

Gossett K A, French D D, Cleghorn B et al 1990b Blood biochemical response to sodium bicarbonate infusion during sublethal endotoxemia in ponies. American Journal of Veterinary Research 51:1370–1374

Gow K W, Phang P T, Tebbutt-Speirs S M et al 1998 Effect of crystalloid administration on oxygen extraction in endotoxemic pigs. Journal of Applied Physiology 85:1667–1675

Graf H, Leach W, Arieff A I 1985 Evidence for a detrimental effect of bicarbonate therapy in hypoxic lactic acidosis. Science 227:754–756

Greatorex J C 1977 Diagnosis and treatment of verminous aneurysm formation in the horse. Veterinary Record 101:184–187

Groenendyk S, English P B, Abetz I 1988 External balance of water and electrolytes in the horse. Equine Veterinary Journal 20:189–193

Grosenbaugh D A, Gadawski J E, Muir W W 1998 Evaluation of a portable clinical analyzer in a veterinary hospital setting. Journal of the American Veterinary Medical Association 213:691–694

Gunther T 1992 Biochemical bases of the therapeutic actions of magnesium. Magnesium Bulletin 13:46–52

Hall L W, Nigam J M 1975 Measurement of central venous pressure in horses. Veterinary Record 97:66–69

Halperin M L, Connors H P, Relman A S et al 1969 Factors that control the effect of pH on glycolysis in leukocytes. Journal of Biological Chemistry 244:384–390

Hamill-Ruth R J, McGory R 1996 Magnesium repletion and its effect on potassium homeostasis in critically ill adults: results of a double-blind, randomized, controlled trial. Critical Care Medicine 24:38–45

Hansen B, DeFrancesco T 2002 Relationship between hydration estimate and body weight change after fluid therapy in critically ill dogs and cats. Journal of Veterinary Emergency and Critical Care 2:235–243

Harrington D D 1974 Pathological features of magnesium deficiency in young horses fed purified rations. American Journal of Veterinary Research 35:503–513

Hata R, Sonoda M 1974 Clinical and hematological observations on repeated experimental blood transfusions in horses. Experimental Report of the Equine Health Laboratory 11:133–151

Heath M F, Evans R J, Hayes L J 1998 Dextran-70 inhibits equine platelet aggregation induced by PAF but not by other agonists. Equine Veterinary Journal 30:408–411

Hébert P C, Wells G, Blajchman M A et al 1999 A multicenter, randomized, controlled clinical trial of transfusion requirements in critical care. New England Journal of Medicine 340:409–417

Henninger R W, Horst J 1997 Magnesium toxicosis in two horses. Journal of the American Veterinary Medical Association 211:82–85

Henninger D D, Snyder J R, Pascoe J R et al 1992 Microvascular permeability changes in ischemia/reperfusion injury in the ascending colon of horses. Journal of the American Veterinary Medical Association 201:1191–1196

Hermann M, Bretscher R, Thiébaud G et al 1990 Preliminary experiences with the treatment of shock in horses with a plasma expander from a starch base. Schweizer Archiv für Tierheilkunde 132:5–12

Heyland D K, MacDonald S, Keefe L et al 1998 Total parenteral nutrition in the critically ill patient: a meta-analysis. Journal of the American Medical Association 280:2013–2019

Hofbauer R, Moser D, Hornykewycz S et al 1999 Hydroxyethyl starch reduces the chemotaxis of white cells through endothelial cell monolayers. Transfusion 39:289–294

Holbeck S, Grande P-O 2000 Effects on capillary fluid permeability and fluid exchange of albumin, dextran, gelatin, and hydroxyethyl starch in cat skeletal muscle. Critical Care Medicine 28:1089–1095

Hollenberg S M, Ahrens T S, Astiz M E 1999 Practice parameters for hemodynamic support of sepsis in adult patients in sepsis. Critical Care Medicine 27:639–660

Holliday M 1996 The evolution of therapy for dehydration: should deficit therapy still be taught? Pediatrics 98:171–177

Holliday M A, Friedman A L, Wassner S J 1999 Extracellular fluid restoration in dehydration: a critique of rapid versus slow. Pediatric Nephrology 13:292–297

Hurley J R, Begg A P 1995 Failure of hyperimmune plasma to prevent pneumonia caused by Rhodococcus equi in foals. Australian Veterinary Journal 72:418–420

Ioannides-Demos L L, Liolios L, Topliss D J et al 1995 A prospective audit of total parenteral nutrition at a major teaching hospital. Medical Journal of Australia 163:233–237

Issel C J, Adams W V J, Meek L et al 1982 Transmission of equine infectious anemia virus from horses without clinical signs of disease. Journal of the American Veterinary Medical Association 180:272–275

James J H, Luchette F A, McCarter F D et al 1999 Lactate is an unreliable indicator of tissue hypoxia in injury or sepsis. Lancet 354:505–508

Johnson P J 1995 Electrolyte and acid–base disturbances in the horse. Veterinary Clinics of North America Equine Practice 11:491–514

Jones P A, Bain F T, Byars T D et al 2001 Effect of hydroxyethyl starch infusion on colloid oncotic pressure in hypoproteinemic horses. Journal of the American Veterinary Medical Association 218:1130–1135

Jones P A, Tomasic M, Gentry P A 1997 Oncotic, hemodilutional, and hemostatic effects of isotonic saline and hydroxyethyl starch solutions in clinically normal ponies. American Journal of Veterinary Research 58:541–548

Kallfelz F A, Whitlock R H, Schultz R D 1978 Survival of ^{59}Fe-labeled erythrocytes in cross-transfused equine blood. American Journal of Veterinary Research 39:617–620

Kasari T R, Naylor J M 1985 Clinical evaluation of sodium bicarbonate, sodium L-lactate, and sodium acetate for the treatment of acidosis in diarrheic calves. Journal of the American Veterinary Medical Association 187:392–397

Kellum J A 1999 Diagnosis and treatment of acid–base disturbances. In: Grenvik A, Ayres S M, Holbrook P R et al (eds) Textbook of critical care, 4th edn. Saunders, Philadelphia, PA, pp. 839–853

Khanna S, Davis D, Peterson B et al 2000 Use of hypertonic saline in the treatment of severe refractory posttraumatic intracranial hypertension in pediatric traumatic brain injury. Critical Care Medicine 28:1144–1151

Kitakaze M, Takashima S, Funaya H et al 1997 Temporary acidosis during reperfusion limits myocardial infarct size in dogs. American Journal of Physiology 272:H2071–H2078

Koterba A M 1990 Nutritional support: enteral feeding. In: Koterba A M, Drummond W H, Kosch P C (eds) Equine clinical neonatology. Lea & Febiger, Philadelphia, PA, pp. 728–746

Krausz M M, Ravid A, Izhar U et al 1993 The effect of heat load and dehydration on hypertonic saline solution treatment of controlled hemorrhagic shock. Surgery, Gynecology and Obstetrics 177:583–592

Krumbhaar E B 1914 Hemolysis due to intravenous injection of distilled water. Journal of the American Medical Association 62:992–993

Kwun K B, Boucherit T, Wong J et al 1983 Treatment of metabolic alkalosis with intravenous infusion of concentrated hydrochloric acid. American Journal of Surgery 146:328–330

Lakritz J, Madigan J, Carlson G P 1992 Hypovolemic hyponatremia and signs of neurological disease associated with diarrhea in a foal. Journal of the American Veterinary Medical Association 200:1114–1116

Landon R A, Young E A 1993 Role of magnesium in regulation of lung function. Journal of the American Dietetic Association 93:674–677

Lang R M, Fellner S K, Neumann A et al 1988 Left ventricular contractility varies directly with blood ionized calcium. Annals of Internal Medicine 108:524–529

Lenz G, Hempel V, Junger H et al 1986 Effect of hydroxyethyl starch, oxypolygelatin and human albumin on the phagocytic function of the reticuloendothelial system in healthy subjects. Anaesthesist 35:423–428

Lenz K, Schimetta W, Polz W et al 2000 Intestinal elimination of hydroxyethyl starch? Intensive Care Medicine 26:733–739

Li P A, Shamloo M, Katsura K et al 1995 Critical values for plasma glucose in aggravating ischaemic brain damage: correlation to extracellular pH. Neurobiology of Disease 2:97–108

Li Y-C, Wiklund L, Bjerneroth G 1997 Influence of alkaline buffers on cytoplasmic pH in myocardial cells exposed to hypoxia. Resuscitation 34:71–77

Lloyd M H, Iles R A, Simpson B R et al 1973 The effect of simulated metabolic acidosis on intracellular pH and lactate metabolism in the isolated perfused rat liver. Clinical Science and Molecular Medicine 45:543–549

Lopes M A F 2002 Physiological aspects, indications and contraindications of enteral fluid therapy. Equine Veterinary Education 14:257–262

Lopes M A F, Moura G S, Filho J D 1999 Treatment of large colon impaction with enteral fluid therapy. In: Proceedings of the 45th American Association of Equine Practitioners Annual Convention, Albuquerque NM, pp. 99–102

Lopes M A, Walker B L, White N A et al 2002 Treatments to promote colonic hydration: enteral fluid therapy versus intravenous fluid therapy and magnesium sulphate. Equine Veterinary Journal 34:505–509

Lopes M A, White N A 2002 Parenteral nutrition for horses with gastrointestinal disease: a retrospective study of 79 cases. Equine Veterinary Journal 34:250–257

Lorente J A, Landin L, De Pablo R et al 1993 Effects of blood transfusion on oxygen transport variables in severe sepsis. Critical Care Medicine 21:1312–1318

Lowery B D, Cloutier C T, Carey L C 1971 Electrolyte solutions in resuscitation in human hemorrhagic shock. Surgery, Gynecology and Obstetrics 133:273–284

Lupo M A, Cefalu W T, Pardridge W M 1990 Kinetics of lactate transport into rat liver in vivo. Metabolism 39:374–377

Macintire D K 1997 Disorders of potassium, phosphorus, and magnesium in critical illness. Compendium on Continuing Education for the Practicing Veterinarian 19:41–48

Maki D G, Weise C E, Sarafin H W 1977 A semiquantitative culture method for identifying intravenous-catheter-related infection. New England Journal of Medicine 296:1305–1309

Malcolm D S, Friedland M, Moore T et al 1993 Hypertonic saline resuscitation detrimentally affects renal function and survival in dehydrated rats. Circulatory Shock 40:69–74

Malcolm D S, Zaloga G P, Holaday J W 1989 Calcium administration increases the mortality of endotoxic shock in rats. Critical Care Medicine 17:900–903

Marlin D J, Scott C M, Mills P C et al 1998 Rehydration following exercise: effects of administration of water versus an isotonic oral rehydration solution (ORS). Veterinary Journal 156:41–49

Martin R G, McMeniman N P, Dowsett K F 1992 Milk and water intakes of foals sucking grazing mares. Equine Veterinary Journal 24:295–299

Martinez-Tallo E, Claure N, Bancalari E 1997 Necrotizing enterocolitis in full-term or near-term infants: risk factors. Biology of the Neonate 71:292–298

Maxson A D, Giger U, Sweeney C R et al 1993 Use of a bovine hemoglobin preparation in the treatment of cyclic ovarian hemorrhage in a miniature horse. Journal of the American Veterinary Medical Association 203:1308–1311

Mazzoni M C, Borgström P, Intaglietta M et al 1990 Capillary narrowing in hemorrhagic shock is rectified by hyperosmotic saline-dextran reinfusion. Circulatory Shock 31:407–418

McFarlane D 1999 Hetastarch: a synthetic colloid with potential in equine patients. Compendium on Continuing Education for the Practicing Veterinarian 21: 867–877

McGinness S G, Mansmann R A, Breuhaus B A 1996 Nasogastric electrolyte replacement in horses.

Compendium on Continuing Education for the Practicing Veterinarian 18:942–951

McKirnan M D, Williams R L, Limjoco U et al 1994 Hypertonic saline/dextran versus lactated Ringer's treatment for hemorrhage in dehydrated swine. Circulatory Shock 44:238–246

Mealey R H, Carter G K, Roussel A J et al 1995 Indwelling cecal catheters for fluid administration in ponies. Journal of Veterinary Internal Medicine 9:347–352

Meister D, Hermann M, Mathis G A 1992 Kinetics of hydroxyethyl starch in horses. Schweizer Archiv für Tierheilkunde 134:329–339

Mills P C, Ng J C, Seawright A A et al 1995 Kinetics, dose response, tachyphylaxis and cross-tachyphylaxis of vascular leakage induced by endotoxin, zymosan-activated plasma and platelet-activating factor in the horse. Journal of Veterinary Pharmacology and Therapeutics 18:204–209

Mimoz O, Pieroni L, Lawrence C et al 1996 Prospective, randomized trial of two antiseptic solutions for prevention of central venous or arterial catheter colonization and infection in intensive care unit patients. Critical Care Medicine 24:1818–1823

Moon P F, Snyder J R, Haskins S C et al 1991 Effects of a highly concentrated hypertonic saline–dextran volume expander on cardiopulmonary function in anesthetized normovolemic horses. American Journal of Veterinary Research 52:1611–1618

Moore R M, Bertone A L, Muir W W 1996 Effect of high-molecular weight dextran macromolecules on low-flow ischemia and reperfusion of the large colon in horses. American Journal of Veterinary Research 57:1067–1073

Morris D D 1989 Thrombophlebitis in horses: The contribution of hemostatic dysfunction to pathogenesis. Compendium on Continuing Education for the Practicing Veterinarian 11:1386–1394

Morris D D, Whitlock R H, Corbeil L B 1986 Endotoxemia in horses: protection provided by antiserum to core lipopolysaccharide. American Journal of Veterinary Research 47:544–550

Moursi M, Rising C L, Zelenock G B et al 1987 Dextrose administration exacerbates acute renal ischemic damage in anesthetized dogs. Archives of Surgery 122:790–794

Muylle E, Nuytten J, Van den Hende C et al 1984 Determination of red blood cell potassium content in horses with diarrhoea: a practical approach for therapy. Equine Veterinary Journal 16:450–452

Nakashima K, Yamashita T, Kashiwagi S et al 1996 The effect of sodium bicarbonate on CBF and intracellular pH in man: stable Xe-CT and ^{31}P-MRS. Acta Neurologica Scandinavica Supplementum 166:96–98

Nearman H S, Herman M L 1991 Toxic effects of colloids in the intensive care unit. Critical Care Clinics 7:713–723

Nohe B, Dieterich H-J, Eichner M et al 1999 Certain batches of albumin solutions influence the expression of endothelial cell adhesion molecules. Intensive Care Medicine 25:1381–1385

Oftedal O T, Hintz H F, Schryver H F 1983 Lactation in the horse: milk composition and intake by foals. Journal of Nutrition 113:2096–2106

O'Grady N P, Alexander M, Dellinger E P et al 2002 Guidelines for the prevention of intravascular catheter-related infections. Pediatrics 110:e51

Okada Y, Klein N J, van Saene H K F et al 2000 Bactericidal activity against coagulase-negative staphylococci is impaired in infants receiving long-term parenteral nutrition. Annals of Surgery 231:276–281

Olerich M A, Rude R K 1994 Should we supplement magnesium in critically ill patients? New Horizons 2:186–192

Onarheim H 1995 Fluid shifts following 7% hypertonic saline (2400 mosmol/l) infusion. Shock 3:350–354

Park Y K, Monaco M H, Donovan S M 1999 Enteral insulin-like growth factor-I augments intestinal disaccharidase activity in piglets receiving total parenteral nutrition. Journal of Pediatric Gastroenterology and Nutrition 29:198–206

Peano S, Reiner G, Carbonatto M et al 2000 Determination of the clearance factor for transmissible spongiform encephalopathy agents during the manufacturing process of polygeline. Intensive Care Medicine 26:608–612

Pedrick T P, Moon P F, Ludders J W et al 1998 The effects of equivalent doses of tromethamine or sodium bicarbonate in healthy horses. Veterinary Surgery 27:284–291

Perkins G A, Divers T J 2001 Polymerized hemoglobin therapy in a foal with neonatal isoerythrolysis. Journal of Veterinary Emergency and Critical Care 11:141–146

Perkins G, Valberg S J, Madigan J M et al 1998 Electrolyte disturbances in foals with severe rhabdomyolysis. Journal of Veterinary Internal Medicine 12:173–177

Peterson B, Khanna S, Fisher B et al 2000 Prolonged hypernatremia controls elevated intracranial pressure in head-injured pediatric patients. Critical Care Medicine 28:1136–1143

Poole-Wilson P A, Langer G A 1975 Effect of pH on ionic exchange and function in rat and rabbit myocardium. American Journal of Physiology 229:570–581

Pulimood T B, Park G R 2000 Debate: albumin administration should be avoided in the critically ill. Critical Care 4:151–155

Rackow E C, Astiz M E, Schumer W et al 1989 Lung and muscle water after crystalloid and colloid infusion in septic rats: effect on oxygen delivery and metabolism. Journal of Laboratory and Clinical Medicine 113:184–189

Rackow E C, Weil M H, Macneil A R et al 1987 Effects of crystalloid and colloid fluids on extravascular lung water in hypoproteinemic dogs. Journal of Applied Physiology 62:2421–2425

Ralston S L 1990 Clinical nutrition of adult horses. Veterinary Clinics of North America Equine Practice 6:339–354

Reifen R, Khoshoo V, Dinari G 1999 Effect of parenteral nutrition on oral intake. Journal of Pediatric Endocrinology and Metabolism 12:203–205

Ring J, Messmer K 1977 Incidence and severity of anaphylactoid reactions to colloid volume substitutes. Lancet i:466–469

Roberts J S, Bratton S L 1998 Colloid volume expanders. Problems, pitfalls and possibilities. Drugs 55:621–630

Rose B D 1994 Introduction to disorders of potassium balance. In: Rose B D (ed) Clinical physiology of acid–base and electrolyte disorders, 4th edn. McGraw Hill, New York, pp. 763–775

Rose R J 1981 A physiological approach to fluid and electrolyte therapy in the horse. Equine Veterinary Journal 13:7–14

Rothe K F, Schimek F 1986 Necrotic skin lesion following therapy of severe metabolic alkalosis. A case report. Acta Anaesthesiologica Belgica 37:137–139

Rumbaugh G E, Carlson G P, Harrold D 1981 Clinicopathologic effects of rapid infusion of 5% sodium bicarbonate in 5% dextrose in the horse. Journal of the American Veterinary Medical Association 178:267–271

Runk D T, Madigan J E, Rahal C J et al 2000 Measurement of plasma colloid osmotic pressure in normal thoroughbred neonatal foals. Journal of Veterinary Internal Medicine 14:475–478

Salem M, Munoz R, Chernow B 1991 Hypomagnesemia in critical illness. A common and clinically important problem. Critical Care Clinics 7:225–252

Schaer M 1999 Disorders of serum potassium, sodium, magnesium and chloride. Journal of Veterinary Emergency and Critical Care 9:209–217

Schierhout G, Roberts I 1998 Fluid resuscitation with colloid or crystalloid solutions in critically ill patients: a systematic review of randomised trials. British Medical Journal 316:961–964

Schortgen F, Lacherade J C, Bruneel F et al 2001 Effects of hydroxyethylstarch and gelatin on renal function in severe sepsis: a multicentre randomised study. Lancet 357:911–916

Schryver H F, Craig P H, Hintz H F et al 1970 The site of calcium absorption in the horse. Journal of Nutrition 100:1127–1131

Seahorn T L, Cornick-Seahorn J 1994 Fluid therapy. Veterinary Clinics of North America Equine Practice 10:517–525

Seldinger S I 1953 Catheter replacement of the needle in percutaneous arteriography. Acta Radiologica 39:368–376

Sestoft L, Bartels P D, Folke M 1982 Pathophysiology of metabolic acidosis: effect of low pH on the hepatic uptake of lactate, pyruvate and alanine. Clinical Physiology 2:51–58

Sestoft L, Marshall M O 1986 Hepatic lactate uptake is enhanced by low pH at low lactate concentrations in perfused rat liver. Clinical Science 70:19–22

Shoemaker W C 1976 Comparison of the relative effectiveness of whole blood transfusions and various types of fluid therapy in resuscitation. Critical Care Medicine 4:71–78

Simma B, Burger R, Falk M et al 1998 A prospective, randomized, and controlled study of fluid management in children with severe head injury: lactated Ringer's solution versus hypertonic saline. Critical Care Medicine 26:1265–1270

Sirtl C, Laubenthal H, Zumtobel V et al 1999 Tissue deposits of hydroxyethyl starch (HES): dose-dependent and time-related. British Journal of Anaesthesia 82:510–515

Smale K, Anderson L S, Butler P J 1994 An algorithm to describe the oxygen equilibrium curve for the thoroughbred racehorse. Equine Veterinary Journal 26:500–502

Smith J E, Dever M, Smith J et al 1992 Post-transfusion survival of [50]Cr-labeled erythrocytes in neonatal foals. Journal of Veterinary Internal Medicine 6:183–185

So K W, Fok T F, Ng P C et al 1997 Randomised controlled trial of colloid or crystalloid in hypotensive preterm infants. Archive of Diseases in Childhood 76:F43–F46

Sosa León L A, Davie A J, Hodgson D R et al 1995 The effects of tonicity, glucose concentration and temperature of an oral rehydration solution on its absorption and elimination. Equine Veterinary Journal Supplement 20:140–146

Sosa León L A, Hodgson D R, Carlson G P et al 1998 Effects of concentrated electrolytes administered via a paste on fluid, electrolyte, and acid base balance in horses. American Journal of Veterinary Research 59:898–903

Soucy D M, Rudé M, Hsia W C et al 1999 The effects of varying fluid volume and rate of resuscitation during uncontrolled hemorrhage. Journal of Trauma 46:209–215

Spalding H K, Goodwin S R 1999 Fluid and electrolyte disorders in the critically ill. Seminars in Anesthesia, Perioperative Medicine and Pain 18:15–26

Spier S J, Lavoie J P, Cullor J S et al 1989 Protection against clinical endotoxemia in horses by using plasma containing antibody to an Rc mutant E. coli (J5). Circulatory Shock 28:235–248

Spurlock S L, Furr M 1990 Fluid therapy. In: Koterba A M, Drummond W H, Kosch P C (eds) Equine clinical neonatology. Lea & Febiger, Philadelphia, PA, pp. 671–700

Spurlock S L, Spurlock G H, Parker G 1990 Long-term jugular vein catheterization in horses. Journal of the American Veterinary Medical Association 196:425–430

Spurlock S L, Ward M V 1991 Parenteral nutrition in equine patients: principles and theory. Compendium on Continuing Education for the Practicing Veterinarian 13:461–490

Starling E H 1896 On the absorption of fluids from the connective tissue spaces. Journal of Physiology 19:312–326

Stone H O, Thompson H K J, Schmidt-Nielsen K 1968 Influence of erythrocytes on blood viscosity. American Journal of Physiology 214:913–918

Sutters M, Gaboury C L, Bennett W M 1996 Severe hyperphosphatemia and hypocalcemia: a dilemma inpatient management. Journal of the American Society of Nephrology 7:2056–2061

Svendsen C K, Hjortkjaer R K, Hesselholt M 1979 Colic in the horse. A clinical and clinical chemical study of 42 cases. Nordisk Veterinaermedicin 31(Suppl):1–32

Swanson J T, Aldrete J A 1989 Thrombophlebitis after intravenous infusion. Factors affecting its incidence. Rocky Mountain Medical Journal 66:48–51

Tasker J B 1967 Fluid and electrolyte studies in the horse III. Intake and output of water, sodium and potassium in normal horses. Cornell Veterinarian 57:649–657

Taylor P 1996 Heat stroke, exhaustion and synchronous diaphragmatic flutter (SDF). In: Dyson S (ed) A guide to the management of emergencies at equine competitions. Equine Veterinary Journal (A British Equine Veterinary Association Manual), Newmarket, UK, pp. 102–113

Taylor PM 1998 Endocrine and metabolic responses to plasma volume expansion during halothane anesthesia in ponies. Journal of Veterinary Pharmacology and Therapeutics 21:485–490

Tennant B, Lowe JE, Tasker JB 1981 Hypercalcemia and hypophosphatemia in ponies following bilateral nephrectomy. Proceedings of the Society for Experimental Biology and Medicine 167:365–368

Thomas N J, Carcillo J A 1998 Hypovolemic shock in pediatric patients. New Horizons 6:120–129

Thomas W P, Madigan J E, Backus K Q et al 1987 Systemic and pulmonary haemodynamics in normal neonatal foals. Journal of Reproduction and Fertility Supplement 35:623–628

Thompson W L, Fukushima T, Rutherford R B et al 1970 Intravascular persistence, tissue storage, and excretion of hydroxyethyl starch. Surgery, Gynecology and Obstetrics 131:965–972

Todd J C, Mollitt D L 1995 Effect of sepsis on erythrocyte intracellular calcium homeostasis. Critical Care Medicine 23:459–465

Traub-Dargatz J L, Dargatz D A 1994 A retrospective study of vein thrombosis in horses treated with intravenous fluids in a veterinary teaching hospital. Journal of Veterinary Internal Medicine 8:264–266

Treib J, Baron J F, Grauer M T et al 1999 An international view of hydroxyethyl starches. Intensive Care Medicine 25:258–268

Trotter G W, Miller D, Parks A et al 1986 Type II renal tubular acidosis in a mare. Journal of the American Veterinary Medical Association 188:1050–1051

Tso E L, Barish R A 1992 Magnesium: clinical considerations. Journal of Emergency Medicine 10:735–745

van den Berghe G, Wouters P, Weekers F et al 2001 Intensive insulin therapy in critically ill patients. New England Journal of Medicine 345:1359–1367

van der Poll T, Levi M, Braxton C C 1998 Parenteral nutrition facilitates activation of coagulation but not of fibrinolysis during human endotoxemia. Journal of Infectious Diseases 177:793–795

Vaupshas H J, Levy M 1990 Distribution of saline following acute volume loading: postural effects. Clinical and Investigative Medicine 13:165–177

Velanovich V 1989 Crystalloid versus colloid fluid resuscitation: a meta-analysis of mortality. Surgery 105:65–71

Vukmir R B, Bircher N G, Radovsky A et al 1995 Sodium bicarbonate may improve outcome in dogs with brief or prolonged cardiac arrest. Critical Care Medicine 23:515–522

Walton R J 1979 Effect of intravenous sodium lactate on renal tubular reabsorption of phosphate in man. Clinical Science 57:125–127

Waterman A 1977 A review of the diagnosis and treatment of fluid and electrolyte disorders in the horse. Equine Veterinary Journal 9:43–48

Webb A R 1997 Fluid management in intensive care: avoiding hypovolaemia. British Journal of Intensive Care 7:59–64

Webb A R 1999 Crystalloid or colloid for resuscitation. Are we any the wiser? Critical Care 3:R25–R28

Webb A R, Moss R F, Tighe D et al 1992 A narrow range, medium molecular weight pentastarch reduces structural organ damage in a hyperdynamic porcine model of sepsis. Intensive Care Medicine 18:348–355

Whitehair K J, Haskins S C, Whitehair J G et al 1995 Clinical applications of quantitative acid–base chemistry. Journal of Veterinary Internal Medicine 9:1–11

Wilkes M M, Navickis R J 2001 Patient survival after human albumin administration. A meta-analysis of randomized, controlled trials. Annals of Internal Medicine 135:149–164

Worthley L I 1986 Hyperosmolar coma treated with intravenous sterile water. A study of three cases. Archives of Internal Medicine 146:945–947

Yatani A, Fujino T, Kinoshita K et al 1981 Excess lactate modulates ionic currents and tension components in frog atrial muscle. Journal of Molecular and Cellular Cardiology 13:147–161

Yu M, Hasaniya N W, Takanishi D M et al 1997 High-volume vs. standard fluid therapy in a septic pig model. Impact on pulmonary function. Archives of Surgery 132:1111–1115

Zadrobilek E, Hackl W, Sporn P et al 1989 Effect of large volume replacement with balanced electrolyte solutions on extravascular lung water in surgical patients with sepsis syndrome. Intensive Care Medicine 15:505–510

Zaloga G P, Sager A, Black K W et al 1992 Low dose calcium administration increases mortality during septic peritonitis in rats. Circulatory Shock 37:226–229

Ziemer E L, Parker H R, Carlson G P et al 1987 Clinical features and treatment of renal tubular acidosis in two horses. Journal of the American Veterinary Medical Association 190:294–296

Zikria B A, King T C, Stanford J et al 1989a A biophysical approach to capillary permeability. Surgery 105:625–631

Zikria B A, Subbarao C, Oz M C et al 1989b Macromolecules reduce abnormal microvascular permeability in rat limb ischemia–reperfusion injury. Critical Care Medicine 17:1306–1309

Drugs and dosages for use in equines

Many drugs have not been approved for use in horses. Products approved for equine use are marked with an asterisk (US) or dagger (Europe). An equine approved product and the label dose should be used whenever possible. It is strongly recommended that the manufacturers' instructions and scientific literature be investigated thoroughly before a drug is used. Drug interactions must be taken into account and adverse reactions can occur.

Drug	Dose	Route
Acepromazine*	0.03–0.10 mg/kg for sedation*† 0.13–0.26 mg/kg for sedation† 0.033–0.055 mg/kg, followed by butorphanol 0.055–0.066 mg/kg 0.04 mg/kg, followed by meperidine 0.6 mg/kg 0.02–0.055 mg/kg, t.i.d. for α receptor blockade 1.5 mg/kg, b.i.d. or t.i.d. for vasodilatation	i.v., i.m., s.c. p.o. i.m., i.v. i.v. i.m.
Acetazolamide	2.2–4.4 mg/kg, b.i.d.	p.o.
Acetic acid	See vinegar	
Acetylcysteine† (10%)	2–5 ml/50 kg, q.i.d.	Aerosol
Acetylcysteine	8 g in 20 g bicarbonate in 200 ml water for meconium impaction	Per rectum
Albendazole	25 mg/kg, b.i.d. for 5 days for *Dictyocaulus arnfieldi* 50 mg/kg, b.i.d. for 2 days for *Strongyloides vulgaris* larvae 4–8 mg/kg, b.i.d. for 1 month for *Echinococcus* spp.	p.o. p.o. p.o.
Albuterol*	0.36–0.9 mg per horse, b.i.d. to t.i.d.	Inhalation
Alfaprostol*	2.7 mg/450 kg for luteolysis; two doses 14 to 18 days apart	i.m.
Allopurinol	5 mg/kg	i.v.
Altrenogest*†	0.044 mg/kg, once daily for 15 days for estrus suppression*† 0.044 mg/kg, once daily for 7 to 10 days for estrus synchronization, followed by a luteolytic dose of prostaglandin $F_{2\alpha}$ 0.44 mg/kg, once daily for pregnancy maintenance 0.44 mg/kg, once daily for 10 days (transitional phase)†	p.o. p.o. p.o. p.o.
Aluminum hydroxide	0.075–0.375 mg/kg	p.o.
Amicarbalide	8.8 mg/kg two doses 24 h apart	i.m.
Amikacin*	2 g in 200 ml sterile saline for 3 days* 6 mg/kg, once daily 20–25 mg/kg, once daily (neonatal foals) 25 mg 125 mg 125 mg diluted for local limb perfusion	Intrauterine i.v., i.m., s.c. i.v., i.m. Subconjunctival Intraarticular i.v. local
Aminocaproic acid	10–20 g, diluted in 1–3 liters saline	Slow i.v.
Aminophylline	2–7 mg/kg, b.i.d. to t.i.d. 5–10 mg/kg, b.i.d.	i.v. p.o.
Aminopropazine fumarate	0.5 mg/kg, b.i.d.	i.m., i.v.
Aminopyrine	2.5–10 mg/450 kg	i.v., i.m.
Ammonium chloride	60–250 mg/kg, once daily (urine acidification)	p.o.
Amoxicillin trihydrate	10 mg/kg, b.i.d.	i.m.

Drug	Dose	Route
Ampicillin sodium or trihydrate*	10–20 mg/kg, t.i.d. to q.i.d. 20 mg/kg (foals) t.i.d. 10 mg	i.v., i.m. p.o. Subconjunctival
Aspirin	10–100 mg/kg, once daily or every other day	p.o.
Atracurium	0.04–0.15 mg/kg	slow i.v.
Atropine[†]	0.03–0.06 mg/kg[†] 1%, every 3–24 h	i.v., i.m., s.c. Ophthalmic
Azithromycin	10 mg/kg	p.o.
Azlocillin	25–75 mg/kg, q.i.d.	i.v.
Bacitracin zinc	10.8 mg/kg, b.i.d. on day 1, once daily day 2	p.o.
Beclometasone	0.5–3.75 mg per horse, b.i.d.	Inhalation
Benzatropine mesylate	8 mg/450 kg	i.v.
Betamethasone*[†]	0.04–0.08 mg/kg[†] 30–60 mg*	i.v., i.m. Intraarticular
Bethanechol	0.02–2.5 mg/kg, b.i.d. to q.i.d. 0.25–0.75 mg/kg, b.i.d. to q.i.d.	s.c. p.o.
Bismuth subsalicylate	0.5–2 ml/kg, every 4–6 h (foals) 2–4 l/450 kg, b.i.d.	p.o. p.o.
Boldenone undecylenate*[†]	1.1 mg/kg, every 3 weeks*	i.m.
Botulinum antitoxin (100–150 IU/ml)	200 ml (foal) 500 ml (adult)	i.v., i.m. i.v., i.m.
Bromocriptine	0.01–0.02 mg/kg, b.i.d.	i.m.
Buparvaquone	4–6 mg/kg, single dose	i.v.
Butorphanol tartrate*[†]	0.05–0.1 mg/kg*[†] (see acepromazine, detomidine and xylazine)	i.v., i.m.
Calcium borogluconate (23%)	0.2–0.4 ml/kg in 1–2 l 5% dextrose	Slow i.v.
Calcium chloride	1–2 g/450 kg	Slow i.v to effect
Cambendazole*	20 mg/kg* for *Strongyloides westeri*	p.o.
Captan	3% solution	Topical
Carbenicillin, indanyl ester	20–30 mg/kg, t.i.d. 100 mg	p.o. Subconjunctival
Carbenicillin sodium	50–80 mg/kg, b.i.d. to t.i.d.	i.v., i.m.
Carbon disulfide	24 mg/450 kg	p.o.
Carprofen[†]	0.7 mg/kg, once or once daily for up to 4 or 9 days (oral)[†]	i.v., p.o.
Casein (iodinated)	5 g, once daily	p.o.

Drug	Dose	Route
Cefaclor	20–40 mg/kg, t.i.d.	p.o.
Cefadroxil	5–40 mg/kg, q.i.d. (neonate) 25 mg/kg, every 4–6 h (foals) 5 mg/kg, q.i.d.	p.o. i.v. i.v.
Cefalexin	10–30 mg/kg, t.i.d. to q.i.d.	p.o.
Cefalotin sodium	20–40 mg/kg, t.i.d. to q.i.d. 100 mg	i.v., i.m. Subconjunctival
Cefamandole	10–30 mg/kg, every 4–8 h	i.v., i.m.
Cefapirin	30 mg/kg, every 4–6 h	i.v., i.m.
Cefataxime sodium	20–30 mg/kg, q.i.d.	i.v.
Cefazolin sodium	15 mg/kg, b.i.d. to t.i.d. 10 mg	i.v., i.m. Subconjunctival
Cefixime	400 mg/kg, t.i.d.	p.o.
Cefonicid	10–15 mg/kg, once daily	i.v., i.m.
Cefoperazone	30–50 mg/kg, b.i.d. to t.i.d.	i.v., i.m.
Ceforanide	5–10 mg/kg, b.i.d.	i.v., i.m.
Cefotaxime	40 mg/kg, q.i.d.	i.v., i.m.
Cefotetan	15–30 mg/kg, b.i.d.	i.v., i.m.
Cefoxitin	30–40 mg/kg, t.i.d. to q.i.d. 20 mg/kg, q.i.d.	i.m. i.v.
Ceftazidine	25–50 mg/kg, b.i.d.	i.v., i.m.
Ceftiofur*[†]	2.0[†]–4.4* mg/kg, once daily	i.v., i.m.*[†]
Ceftizoxime	25–50 mg/kg, b.i.d. to t.i.d.	i.v., i.m.
Ceftriaxone	25–50 mg/kg, b.i.d.	i.v., i.m.
Cefuroxime axetil	25–50 mg/kg, t.i.d. 250–500 mg/kg, b.i.d.	i.v., i.m. p.o.
Charcoal, activated	1–3 g/kg (as 1 g/5 ml water), repeat after 8–12 h if necessary	p.o.
Chloral hydrate*	50 mg/kg for foal restraint 40–100 mg/kg	i.v. p.o.
Chloramphenicol palmitate	4–10 mg/kg, t.i.d. to q.i.d. (foal) 45–60 mg/kg, t.i.d. to q.i.d. (adult)	p.o. i.v., i.m., s.c., p.o.
Chloramphenicol succinate	25 mg/kg, t.i.d. to q.i.d. 50–100 mg	i.v., i.m. Subconjunctival
Chlorhexidine*	1% 1 g	Topical Intrauterine

Drug	Dose	Route
Cimetidine	2.5 mg/kg, t.i.d. to q.i.d., 20 mg/kg b.i.d. (foals) 6.6–10 mg/kg, t.i.d.	p.o. i.v.
Clarithomycin	7.5 mg/kg, b.i.d.	p.o.
Clenbuterol*†	0.8–3.2 μg/kg, b.i.d.*† 0.8 μg/kg, b.i.d.† 200 μg for uterine relaxation	p.o. Slow i.v. Slow i.v., i.m.
Cloprostenol†	125–500 μg†	i.m.
Cloxacillin†	10–30 mg/kg, q.i.d. Single dose†, repeat after 1–3 days if required	i.m. Ophthalmic
Colistin	2500 IU/kg, q.i.d.	Slow i.v.
Corticotropin	1 IU/kg	i.m.
Coumaphos	0.06% wash, 0.1% dust	Topical
Cromoglicate sodium†	80 mg, once daily†	Inhalation
Cyproheptadine	0.25 mg/kg, once or twice daily	p.o.
Dalteparin	50–100 anti–Xa units/kg, once daily	i.v., s.c
Danthon	15–30 ml/kg	p.o.
Dantrolene sodium	10 mg/kg loading dose 2.5 mg/kg, every 2 h maintenance 1.9 mg/kg in saline for acute myopathy 2 mg/kg, once daily to prevent myositis	p.o. p.o. Slow i.v. p.o.
Dembrexine†	0.3 mg/kg, b.i.d.†	p.o.
Demecarium bromide	0.25%, b.i.d.	Ophthalmic
Detomidine*†	0.01–0.08 mg/kg (up to 0.04 mg/kg)*† 0.01–0.02 mg/kg followed by butorphanol 0.025–0.066 mg/kg 0.02–0.04 mg/kg followed by ketamine 2.2 mg/kg	i.v., i.m. i.v. i.v.
Dexamethasone*†	2.5–20.0 mg/horse daily*† 4–6 mg/kg for shock†	i.v., i.m. i.v.
Dexamethasone phosphate	0.1%, every 3–8 h	Ophthalmic
Dextran (6% solution)	8 g/kg, once daily for up to 3 days	i.v.
Diazepam	0.05–2.0 mg/kg in 25–100 mg doses	Slow i.v.
Dichlorvos*	20–41 mg/kg* 0.93% solution	p.o. Topical
Diclazuril	5.5 mg/kg, once daily	p.o.
Dicloxacillin	10 mg/kg, q.i.d.	i.m.
Diethylcarbamazine	1 mg/kg, once daily for 21 days for onchocerciasis 50 mg/kg, once daily for 10 days for verminous myelitis	p.o. p.o.
Diethylstilbestrol	30 mg/450 kg	i.m.

Drug	Dose	Route
Digoxin	0.0022 mg/kg, b.i.d., or as required 0.011 mg/kg, b.i.d.	i.v. p.o.
Dihydrostreptomycin*	11 mg/kg, b.i.d.*	i.m., s.c.
Dimercaprol	2.5–5 mg/kg as 10% solution in oil, every 4 h for 2 days then b.i.d. until recovery	i.m.
Dimethylglycine	1.0–1.6 mg/kg, once daily	p.o.
Dimethyl sulfoxide*	0.5–1.0 mg/kg (10% solution in 5% dextrose–saline) repeat lower doses b.i.d. to q.i.d. 90% solution of gel*	i.v., p.o. Topical
Diminazene	5 mg/kg two doses 24 h apart	s.c.
Dinoprost*†	5† or 10* mg/450 kg	i.m.
Dioctyl sodium sulfosuccinate (DSS) 5% solution	10–20 mg/kg, every 48 h 10 ml in warm water as an enema for retained meconium	p.o. Per rectum
Dioxathion	0.15% wash	Topical
Diphenylhydantoin	See phenytoin	
Diphenyhydramine hydrochloride	0.5–1.0 mg/kg	i.v., i.m.
Dipyrone	5–22 mg/kg	i.v., i.m.
Dobutamine	0.5–15.0 μg/kg/min (250 mg in 500 ml saline infused at 0.45 ml/kg/h)	i.v.
Domperidone	1.1 mg/kg, once daily for fescue toxicosis and milk letdown 1.1 mg/kg, once daily to advance ovulation in transitional mares 0.44 mg/kg, once daily to advance ovulation in transitional mares 0.02 mg/kg, 3, 9 and 15 h postop for ileus	p.o. p.o. s.c. i.v.
Dopamine	1–20 μg/min per kg (200 mg in 500 ml saline infused at 0.45 ml/h per kg)	i.v.
Doxapram*†	0.44 mg/kg*, every 5 min (do not exceed 2 mg/kg in foals) 40–100 mg†	i.v. i.v., i.m., s.c., sublingual
Doxycycline	10 mg/kg, b.i.d.	p.o.
Ecothiophate iodide	0.03%, b.i.d.	Ophthalmic
Enalapril	0.5 mg/kg, once daily	p.o.
Enoxaparin	40–80 anti-Xa units/kg, once daily	i.v., s.c
Enrofloxacin	5–10 mg/kg, once daily	i.v.
Ephedrine sulfate	0.7 mg/kg, b.i.d. 0.03–0.06 mg/kg for hypotension	p.o. i.v.
Epinephrine (adrenaline) 1:1000	0.01–0.02 mg/kg (4–8 ml/450 kg)	i.v., i.m., s.c.
Erythromycin estolate, stearate	25 mg/kg, t.i.d.	p.o.
Erythromycin lactobionate	2.5–5.0 mg/kg, t.i.d. to q.i.d. 20–40 mg	i.v. Subconjunctival

Drug	Dose	Route
Erythromycin phosphate	25 mg/kg, t.i.d. 37.5 mg/kg, b.i.d.	p.o. p.o.
Estradiol-17β	1–10 mg, once daily for management of transitional mares	i.m.
Estradiol benzoate	0.010–0.012 mg/kg (see cypionate)	i.m.
Estradiol cypionate	0.004–0.010 mg/kg, daily for 3 days then every 48 h for urinary incontinence	i.m.
Ethyl alcohol	50%; 5–10 ml/50 kg	Aerosol
Ethylenediamine dihydriodide	0.5–1.5 g/450 kg, once daily	p.o.
Ethylenediamine tetraacetate, calcium disodium	75 mg/kg daily in divided doses for lead poisoning 6.6% solution (1.1 ml/kg), b.i.d. to t.i.d.	Slow i.v. i.v.
Famotidine	4.0 mg/kg, t.i.d.	p.o.
Febantel*	6 mg/kg*	p.o.
Fenbendazole*†	5–10 mg/kg*†, (depending on parasite, p. 65 and 70) 50 mg/kg, once daily for 3 days for verminous arteritis 50 mg/kg for *Strongyloides westeri*	p.o. p.o. p.o.
Fenprostalene	0.5 mg/450 kg	s.c.
Florfenicol	20 mg/kg, every 4–8 h	i.m.
Floxacillin (flucloxacillin)	10 mg/kg, q.i.d.	i.m.
Flumazenil	0.5–2.0 mg	Slow i.v.
Flumetasone*†	1.25–2.5 mg, once daily*	i.v., i.m., intraarticular
Flunixin meglumine*†	1.1 mg/kg*†, once daily for 5 days	i.v., i.m., p.o.
Fluoroprednisolone acetate	5–20 mg/450 kg	i.m.
Fluphenazine	0.05–0.08 mg/kg, every 2 weeks; beware of idiosyncratic reactions	i.m., s.c.
Fluprostenol*	250*–500 μg/450 kg, close to spontaneous delivery; luteolysis*	i.m.
Flurbiprofen sodium	0.03%, t.i.d. to q.i.d.	Ophthalmic
Folic acid	75 mg (foal)	i.m.
Follicle-stimulating hormone*	10–50 mg/450 kg*	i.v., i.m., s.c.
Furazolidone*	4 mg/kg, t.i.d. 4–10%*	p.o. topical
Furosemide (frusemide)*	0.5–4 mg/kg/min 1–3 mg/kg, once or twice daily* 0.5–1 mg/kg	i.v. infusion i.v., i.m. p.o.
Gentamicin*	2–2.5 g, once daily* 2.2 mg/kg, t.i.d. 5–7 mg/kg, once daily 20 mg 250 mg diluted for local limb perfusion	intrauterine i.v., i.m. i.v., i.m., s.c. Subconjunctival i.v. local

Drug	Dose	Route
	5–15 mg/ml every 2–6 h 150 mg 25 mg, ciliary body destruction	Ophthalmic Intraarticular Intraocular
Glucagon	25–50 mg/kg	i.v.
Glycerin	1 g/kg	p.o.
Glycerol	5%; 2–5 ml/50 kg 0.5–2 g/kg (cerebral edema)	Aerosol i.v.
Glycerol guaiacolate	110 mg/kg (convulsions) 0.1–0.2 g/50 kg, q.i.d. (expectorant)	i.v. p.o.
Glycopyrrolate (glycopyrronium)	0.001–0.003 mg/kg	i.v.
Glycosaminoglycan, polysulfated*†	500 mg, every 4 days*†, repeat 6 times 250 mg per joint once weekly*†, repeat 4 times	i.m. intraarticular
Gonadotropin, human chorionic†	1500–3000 U to induce or synchronize ovulation† or for testosterone provocation	i.v., i.m.
Gonadotropin-releasing hormone*†	1 implant (Ovuplant)* 0.05 mg, 2 h and 1 h before breeding for low libido 0.04 mg, 6 h before breeding to induce ovulation†	s.c. s.c. i.v., i.m., s.c.
Griseofulvin*†	2.5 g/450 kg, once daily for not less than 10 days* 10 mg/kg daily	p.o.
Guaifenesin	5–10%; to effect (approximately 110 mg/kg needed for induction) 5% with 4.4 mg/kg thiamylal or 2.5–5.5 mg/kg thiopental 5% with ketamine 1–2 mg/ml and xylazine 0.5 mg/ml	Slow i.v. Rapid i.v. i.v. infusion
Haloperidol decanoate	0.01 mg/kg	i.m.
Heparin	40–150 IU/kg, b.i.d. anticoagulant 40 IU/kg, b.i.d., prevent adhesions 40–100 IU/kg, b.i.d. to q.i.d., acute laminitis	s.c. i.v., then s.c. i.v.
Hetastarch	10–20 ml/h per kg	i.v.
Hyaluronic acid	20–120 mg	Peritendon or intrasynovial
Hyaluronate sodium*†	10–50 mg/joint*† 40 mg†	Intraarticular i.v.
Hydralazine	0.5 mg/kg	i.v.
Hydrochlorothiazide	0.5–0.7 mg/kg	p.o.
Hydrocortisone sodium succinate	1–4 mg/kg	i.v.
Hydroxyzine hydrochloride	0.5–1 mg/kg, b.i.d. to t.i.d.	i.m., p.o.
Hyoscine (scopolamine)	0.14 mg/kg	i.v.
Idoxuridine	0.1% solution every 4–6 h	Ophthalmic
Imidocarb diproprionate*	2 mg/kg, once daily for 2 days for *Babesia caballi** 4 mg/kg, every 3 days for four treatments for *Babesia equi**	i.m. i.m.

Drug	Dose	Route
Imipenem	15 mg/kg, q.i.d. 10 mg/kg, b.i.d.	i.v. in fluids i.m.
Imipramine	2.2 mg/kg to improve ejaculation 0.55 mg/kg, t.i.d. 1.5 mg/kg, t.i.d.	p.o. i.v., i.m. p.o.
Insulin (normal)	0.1–0.4 IU/kg or 0.05 IU/kg/h (starting dose), titrate to maintain blood glucose between 80–110 mg/dl (4.4–6.1 mmol/l)	i.v.
Insulin protamine zinc	0.1–0.4 IU/kg, every 12–24 h	i.m., s.c.
Iodide, sodium	20–40 mg/kg, once daily for several weeks	p.o.
Iodochlorhydroxyquin*	10 g/450 kg, repeat once daily* for 3–4 days, gradually reduce the dose if response obtained	p.o.
Ipratropium bromide	2–4 μg/kg, q.i.d., depends on delivery system	Aerosol
Iron cacodylate	1 g	i.v.
Isoniazid	5–20 mg/kg, once daily	p.o.
Isoproterenol (isoprenaline)	0.05%; 5–10 ml/50 kg, q.i.d.	Aerosol
Isoproterenol (isoprenaline) hydrochloride	0.4 μg/kg by slow infusion (discontinue when heart rate doubles) 0.05–1 μg/min per kg for foal resuscitation	i.v. i.v.
Isoxsuprine hydrochloride[†]	0.6–1.8 mg/kg, b.i.d.[†]	p.o.
Itraconazole	5 mg/kg, once daily for up to 2 months	p.o.
Ivermectin*[†]	0.2 mg/kg*[†] 0.2 mg/kg, twice at 4-day intervals for lice and mange	i.m.*, p.o.*[†] p.o.
Kanamycin	7.5 mg/kg, t.i.d.	i.v., i.m.
Kaolin	1.9–3.7 l/450 kg, b.i.d.	p.o.
Ketamine[†]	2.2 mg/kg[†] (See detomidine and xylazine)	i.v.
Ketoconazole	30 mg/kg, every 12–24 h (dissolve in 0.2 mmol/l HCl)	p.o.
Ketoprofen*[†]	2.2 mg/kg, once daily for up to 5 days*[†]	i.v., i.m.
Lactase	6000 food chemical codex lactase units/foal every 3–6 h	p.o.
Levallorphan tartrate	0.02–0.04 mg/kg	i.v.
Levamisole	8 mg/kg	p.o.
Levothyroxine sodium (thyroxine sodium)	0.01 mg/kg, once daily 10 mg in 70 ml corn syrup, once daily	p.o. p.o.
Lidocaine (lignocaine)	0.25–0.5 mg/kg bolus every 5 min, <2 mg/kg total dose 0.05 mg/min per kg for ileus (see local anaesthetics pp. 297–301)	i.v. i.v. infusion
Lime sulfur	3–5%	Topical
Lindane	3% spray	Topical

Drug	Dose	Route
Loperamide	0.1–0.2 mg/kg, q.i.d.	p.o.
Luprostiol[†]	7.5 mg/horse[†]	i.m.
Magnesium hydroxide (antacid)	200–250 ml, t.i.d.	p.o.
Magnesium sulfate	1–2.5 mg/kg/min (maximum 50 mg/kg) 1–2 mg/kg dissolved in 4 liters warm water, once daily	i.v. p.o.
Malathion	0.5% wash, 5% dust	Topical
Mannitol (20%)	0.25–1.0 g/kg	Slow i.v.
Mebendazole[*][†]	5–10 mg/kg[*][†] 15–20 mg/kg, once daily for 5 days for *Dictyocaulus arnfieldi*[†]	p.o. p.o.
Meclofenamic acid[*][†]	2.2 mg/kg, once daily for 5 to 7 days[*][†]	p.o.
Medetomidine	0.005–0.010 mg/kg	i.v., i.m.
Medroxyprogesterone acetate	250–500 mg/horse	i.m.
Meperidine (pethidine)	0.6–1.0 mg/kg with acepromazine 0.05 mg/kg or xylazine 0.5–1.0 mg/kg	i.v.
Methadone (dolophine hydrochloride)	0.05–0.1 mg/kg 0.2–0.4 mg/kg	i.v. i.m.
Methetharimide	10–20 mg/kg	i.v.
Methicillin	25 mg/kg, every 4–6 h 100 mg	i.m. Subconjunctival
dl-Methionine	20–50 mg/kg	p.o.
Methocarbamol[*]	4.4–55 mg/kg[*] 40–300 mg/kg for convulsions	i.v. p.o.
Methoxychlor	0.5% wash	Topical
Methylcellulose flakes	0.25–0.5 kg/450 kg in 10 l water	p.o.
Methylprednisolone acetate[*][†]	200 mg[*][†] 40–240 mg[*]	i.m. intraarticular
Methylprednisolone sodium succinate	2–4 mg/kg	i.v.
Methylsulfmethoxine	30 g/450 kg, once daily	p.o.
Methylsulfonylmethane	0.5–1.0 g/450 kg, once daily	p.o.
Metoclopramide	0.04 mg/kg/h infusion or 0.25 mg/kg, t.i.d. to q.i.d. 0.6 mg/kg, every 4 h	i.v. in fluids, s.c. p.o.
Metronidazole	15 mg/kg, q.i.d. or 20 mg/kg, b.i.d.	i.v., p.o., per rectum
Mezlocillin	25–75 mg/kg, q.i.d.	i.v.
Miconazole	1%, every 2–4 h	Ophthalmic

Drug	Dose	Route
Midazolam	0.01–0.05 mg/kg	i.v., i.m.
Mineral oil	10 ml/kg, once daily	p.o.
Minocycline	3 mg/kg, b.i.d.	p.o.
Morphine sulfate	0.1–0.4 mg/kg 0.3–0.6 mg/kg with α_2 agonist or phenothiazine	i.m. i.v.
Moxalactam	50 mg/kg, t.i.d.	i.v., i.m.
Moxidectin*†	0.4 mg/kg*†	p.o.
Nafcillin	10 mg/kg, q.i.d.	i.m.
Naloxone	0.01–0.05 mg/kg	i.v.
Naproxen*	5 mg/kg i.v. followed by 10 mg/kg, b.i.d.*	p.o.
Natamycin†	5%, every 2–4 h 0.01% spray, repeat after 4–5 days†	Ophthalmic Topical
Neostigmine*	0.022*–0.050 mg/kg	i.v., s.c.
Netilmicin	2 mg/kg, b.i.d. to t.i.d.	i.v., i.m.
Niclosamide	100 mg/kg	p.o.
Nitrofurantoin	3 mg/kg, b.i.d.	i.m.
Nizatidine	6.6 mg/kg, t.i.d.	p.o.
Norepinephrine (noradrenaline)	0.01–0.75 µg/kg/min	i.v.
Omeprazole*†	0.5 mg/kg, every 12–24 h 4 mg/kg, once daily for treatment of ulcers*† 2 mg/kg, once daily for prevention of recurrence of ulcers*†	i.v. p.o. p.o.
Ouabain	2.5–3 mg/450 kg, every 2 h until heart rate slows or intoxication develops; do not exceed 10 g total dose	i.v.
Oxacillin	25–50 mg/kg, b.i.d. to t.i.d.	i.v., i.m.
Oxfendazole*	10 mg/kg*	p.o.
Oxibendazole*†	10 mg/kg*† 15 mg/kg for *Strongyloides westeri**†	p.o. p.o.
Oxymorphone	0.02–0.03 mg/kg	i.m., i.v.
Oxytetracycline†	2–10 mg/kg† 20 mg/kg, every 72 h (long acting)	i.v., i.m. i.m.
Oxytocin*†	2.5–10 U; 10–40 U† 60–100 U in 1 liter saline 20–100 U*† 1–3 U/450 kg for milk letdown	Slow i.v., i.m. Slow i.v. i.v., i.m., s.c. i.v.
Pancuronium	0.01–0.060 mg/kg	Slow i.v.
Penicillamine D	3–4 mg/kg, q.i.d. for 10 days	p.o.

Drug	Dose	Route
Penicillin G, benzathine and procaine*[†] (benzylpenicillin, benzathine and procaine)	9000*–16 800[†] U/kg, every 48–96 h	i.m.
Penicillin G, procaine*[†] (benzylpenicillin, procaine)	6600*–16 000[†] U/kg, once daily	i.m.
Penicillin G, sodium[†] or potassium (benzylpenicillin, sodium or potassium)	16 0000 U/kg, b.i.d.[†]	i.v.[†], i.m.
Pentazocine*	0.33–1.1 mg/kg*	i.v., i.m.
Pentobarbital*	2–20 mg/kg for convulsions	i.v.
Pentosan polysulfate sodium	250 mg per joint, repeat after 7–10 days	Intraarticular
Pentoxifylline (oxpentifylline)	8 mg/kg, b.i.d.	p.o.
Pentylenetetrazol	6–10 mg/kg	i.v.
Pergolide	1 µg/kg (0.25–3.0 mg per horse)	p.o.
Perphenazine	0.3–0.5 mg/kg, b.i.d	p.o.
Pethidine	see Meperidine	
Phenobarbital	5–25 mg/kg in 30 ml saline for convulsing foals 9 mg/kg, t.i.d. for maintenance 4–12 mg/kg, b.i.d., alter dose according to maintenance of blood levels	i.v. over 30 min i.v. p.o.
Phenothiazine	55 mg/kg 18.3 mg/kg of piperazine – carbon disulfide complex formulation*	p.o. p.o.
Phenoxybenzamine hydrochloride	0.7–1 mg/kg in 500 ml saline, t.i.d. to q.i.d.	i.v.
Phenylbutazone*[†]	2.2–4.4 mg/kg, every 12–24 h*[†]	p.o., i.v.
Phenylephrine	10% 0.1–0.2 µg/kg/min (maximum 0.01 mg/kg)	Ophthalmic i.v.
Phenytoin (diphenylhydantoin)	5–10 mg/kg for convulsing foals and digoxin-induced arrhythmias 1–5 mg/kg, every 4 h for maintenance 10 mg/kg, once daily for digoxin-induced arrhythmias 10 mg/kg, once daily for chronic myositis or intermittent arrhythmias	i.v. i.v., i.m., p.o. p.o. p.o.
Physostigmine	0.1–0.6 mg/kg	i.m., slow i.v.
Pilocarpine hydrochloride	4% gel b.i.d. to q.i.d.	Ophthalmic
Piperazine	88 mg/kg	p.o.
Pipericillin	15–50 mg/kg, b.i.d. to q.i.d.	i.v., i.m.
Ponazuril*	5 mg/kg, once daily*	p.o.
Polymixin B	10 000 IU/kg, q.i.d. 6000 IU/kg, every 6–24 h for endotoxemia	p.o. i.v.
Potassium chloride	40 g in 4–6 liters water b.i.d.	p.o.

Drug	Dose	Route
Potassium iodide	1 g/50 kg, q.i.d.	p.o.
Potassium bromide	10–15 mg/kg, b.i.d.	p.o.
Pralidoxime chloride*	2 g/horse	Slow i.v.
Praziquantel*† with ivermectin or moxidectin	1–2.5 mg/kg*†	p.o.
Prednisolone acetate*	1%, every 3–8 h 50–100 mg*	Ophthalmic Intraarticular
Prednisolone sodium succinate*	0.2*–3 mg/kg, every 12–24 h 2–5 mg/kg for septic shock	p.o., i.m.*, i.v.* i.v.
Prednisone*	100–400 mg/horse*	i.m.
Primidone	1–2 g, b.i.d. to q.i.d. (foal)	p.o.
Procainamide	1 mg/kg/min (total dose 20 mg/kg)	i.v.
Progesterone	150 mg, once daily for 1–10 days to synchronize estrus 300 mg, once daily to maintain pregnancy	i.m.
Promazine*	0.4–1.1 mg/kg* 1–2 mg/kg granules*	i.v., i.m. p.o.
Propantheline bromide	0.014 mg/kg	i.v.
Proparacaine*	0.5%	Ophthalmic*
Propofol	2 mg/kg for induction of anesthesia after premedication	i.v.
Propranolol	0.39–0.78 mg/kg, t.i.d. 0.1–0.3 mg/kg, b.i.d.	p.o. i.v.
Propylene glycol (5%)	3 ml/50 kg	Aerosol
Prostaglandin $F_{2\alpha}$*	10 mg to shorten the estrus cycle	i.m.
Prostalene*	0.005 mg/kg*, two doses 2 weeks apart	s.c.
Psyllium mucilloid	1 g/kg, every 6–24 h	p.o.
Pyrantel pamoate*† (embonate)	6.6 mg/kg* (19 mg/kg†) 13.2(32†) mg/kg for tapeworms	p.o. p.o.
Pyrantel tartrate*	2.6 mg/kg*, as top dressing	p.o.
Pyrilamine maleate*	0.9–1.3 mg/kg*, b.i.d. to q.i.d.	i.v., i.m., s.c.
Pyrimethamine	1 mg/kg, once daily for 30–180 days in combination with a sulfonamide	p.o.
Quinidine gluconate	1.1–2.2 mg/kg, every 10 min, total dose 8–12 mg/kg 0.064% solution, 0.5–2.0 l/h	i.v.
Quinidine sulfate	20 mg/kg, every 2 h for 6 days (maximum 60 g daily)	p.o.
Ranitidine	6.6 mg/kg, t.i.d. 2 mg/kg, t.i.d.	i.v., p.o. i.v., p.o.

Drug	Dose	Route
Rifampin	5–10 mg/kg, once daily 5 mg/kg, b.i.d. with erythromycin, azithomycin or clarithromycin for *Rhodococcus equi*	p.o. p.o.
Romifidine[†]	0.004–0.120 mg/kg followed by 0.02 mg/kg butorphanol[†]	i.v.
Ronnel	2.5% spray	Topical
Saline (hypertonic)	7–7.5%; 4 ml/kg for hypovolemia	i.v. over 20 min
Scopolamine	see Hyoscine	
Selenium (sodium selenite)*	55 mg/450 kg*	i.m.
Sodium bicarbonate	30 g b.i.d.	p.o.
Sodium hypochlorite	0.5%	Topical
Sodium iodide	20–40 mg/kg, once daily	p.o.
Sodium sulfate	1 g/kg dissolved in warm water	p.o.
Sodium thiosulfate (20%)	0.22 ml/kg	Slow i.v.
Spectinomycin	20 mg/kg, t.i.d.	i.m.
Stanozolol*	0.5 mg/kg, every 1 week up to four doses*	i.m.
Stirofos	1% wash	Topical
Streptomycin[†]	10 mg/kg, once daily[†]	i.m.[†], s.c.
Sucralfate	10–20 mg/kg, b.i.d. to q.i.d.	p.o.
Sulfonamides	55–220 mg/kg (check product label for correct dosage)	i.v., i.m., s.c., p.o.
Sulfonamides, potentiated	see Trimethoprim	
Terbutaline	0.02–0.06 mg/kg, b.i.d.	i.v.
Tetanus antitoxin	100 IU/kg, every 3–5 days for therapy	i.m., s.c., i.v.
Tetracycline	6.6–11 mg/kg, every 12–24 h dilute in saline or glucose solution	Slow i.v.
Tetramethin	0.4% solution	Topical
Theophylline	5–15 mg/kg, b.i.d.	p.o.
Thiamine hydrochloride	0.25–1.25 mg/kg, b.i.d.	Slow i.v., i.m.
Thiamylal sodium*	2–4.4 mg/kg*	i.v.
Thiopental[†]	5–10%, 5–10 mg/kg[†]	i.v.
Tiabendazole (thiabendazole)*	44 mg/kg* 88 mg/kg for *Parascaris equorum* 4% solution in saline or 90% dimethyl sulfoxide (DMSO)	p.o. p.o. Topical
Ticarcillin*	40–80 mg/kg, t.i.d. to q.i.d. 6 g per day for 3 days during estrus*	i.v., i.m. i.v.

Drug	Dose	Route
Ticarcillin plus clavulanic acid	50 mg/kg plus 1.67 mg/kg, q.i.d.	i.v.
Timolol maleate	0.5%; b.i.d.	Ophthalmic
Tobramycin	1–1.7 mg/kg, t.i.d. (human dose) 20–40 mg	i.v., i.m. Subconjunctival
Tocopherol acid succinate[†]	0.83–2.48 g/horse, once daily[†]	p.o.
Toltrazuril	5–10 mg/kg, once daily	p.o.
Toxaphene	0.5% wash	Topical
Triamcinolone acetonide[*†]	6–18 mg[*] 0.02–0.04 mg/kg, do not exceed 20 mg[*] 40 mg/ml; 0.25 ml, every 2–4 days 0.01–0.02 mg/kg, b.i.d.	intraarticular i.m., s.c. Subconjunctival p.o.
Trichlorfon	40 mg/kg	p.o.
Trichlormethiazide	200 mg/450 kg	p.o.
Triflupromazine[*]	0.22–0.33 mg/kg[*]	i.v.
Trifluridine	1%, every 2–3 h	Ophthalmic
Trimethoprim–sulfadiazine[*]	15–24[*†] mg/kg, b.i.d. 30 mg/kg, as a single or divided dose[*] 2.5–5 g, once daily	i.v. p.o. i.u.
Trimethoprim–sulfadoxine[†]	15 mg/kg[†]	i.m., slow i.v.
Tripelennamine hydrochloride[*]	1.1 mg/kg[*], b.i.d. to t.i.d.	i.m.
Tromethamine	300 mg/kg	i.v.
Tropicamide	0.5–1%	Ophthalmic
Tylosin	10 mg/kg, b.i.d.	i.m.
Vancomycin	20–40 mg/kg, b.i.d. to q.i.d.	i.v., p.o.
Vedaprofen[†]	2 mg/kg then 1 mg/kg b.i.d. for up to 14 days[†]	i.v., p.o.
Vinegar (acetic acid)	250 ml/450 kg, once daily for enterolith prevention	p.o.
Vitamin E	1500–12 000 IU, once daily	p.o.
Vitamin K_1	0.5–1 mg/kg every 4–6 h for warfarin toxicosis 1–2 mg/kg (divided at several sites) for sweet clover toxicosis 0.5–2 mg/kg (foals)	s.c. s.c. i.m.
Xylazine[*†]	0.6–3.0 mg/kg[*†] 0.33–0.44 mg/kg followed by butorphanol 0.033–0.066 mg/kg 1.1 mg/kg followed by ketamine 1.76–2.2 mg/kg 0.6 mg/kg with acepromazine 0.02 mg/kg 0.66 mg/kg to ejaculate ex copula	i.v., i.m. i.v. i.v. i.v. i.v.
Yohimbine	0.075–0.15 mg/kg for xylazine or detomidine reversal or to restore intestinal motility	Slow i.v.

i.m., intramuscular; i.u., intrauterine; i.v., intravenous; p.o., oral; s.c., subcutaneous.

Index

References to tables and any other non-textual material are in *italics*. Spellings are American. NSAIDs stands for non-steroidal anti-inflammatory drugs.

A

AAEP (American Association of Equine Practitioners) 140, 141, 299
Abaxial sessamoid administration *see* Administration, drugs
Absorption, drugs 2–3
ACE (angiotensin-converting enzyme) inhibitors 212–13
Acepromazine maleate (Phenothiazines)
  esophageal obstruction 96
  opioid analgesics 277, 278, 281
  postpartum problems 187
  reproductive tract/performance 189
  sedatives/tranquillizers 271, 272, 273
  skeletal muscle 138–9
Acetaminophen (paracetamol) 253
Acetate methyl (CH$_3$) group 140
Acetazolamide 165–6
Acetylglucosominadase, β-N-(AGS), urine *see* AGS (β-N-acetylglucosominadase), urine
Acetylation 37
Acetylcholine 87, 141, 269
  Receptors, nicotinic 67
Acetylcysteine 235
Aciclovir 233
Acid-base/electrolyte disturbances *see* Electrolyte/acid-base disturbances
Acidic dissociation constant (pK$_a$) *see* pK$_a$ (acidic dissociation constant)
Acidosis 334, 335, 351–2, 358
Acremonium coenophialum (fungus) 80
ACTH (adrenocorticotropic hormone)
  endocrine system 76, 77, 79, 80
  reproductive system 184, 185
  respiratory system 319, 320
Actinobacillus spp. 26
Active tubular secretion *see* Excretion
Acute inotropes *see* Vasopressors
Acute renal failure (ARF) *see* ARF (acute renal failure)
Adenoma, thyroid gland 81
Adenosine triphosphate (ATP) *see* ATP (Adenosine triphosphate)
ADH (antidiuretic hormone) 164, 168, 169
Administration, drugs 3–4
  abaxial sessamoid route 299, 300
  direct instillation (ophthalmic) 218
  intraarticular route 4, 121–34
  intramuscular route 4, 16, 52, 135–6
  intraocular injections 220

intrauterine administration 25
intravenous route 3
membrane delivery systems (ophthalmic) 219
oral route 4, 16, 52
parenteral administration (ophthalmic) 220–1, 224, 226, 239
patches, topical application 4
perineural infiltration 299
periocular injection 220
pulmonary route 4
regional perfusion 130
retrobulbar injection 220
sub-Tenon's injection 220
subconjunctival injections 219, 220, 223–4, 226
subcutaneous route 4, 16
topical 4
topical instillation (ophthalmic) 218–19
see also Ophthalmic therapeutics
Adnexal disease 218
Adrenaline (epinephrine) *see* Catecholamines
Adrenoceptor agonists/antagonists 95–6, 171
Adrenoceptor agonists
  administration route 270
  anticholinergic agents 205
  bioavailability 270
  duration of effect 270–1
  elimination 271
  horses, major uses in 271
  inhalant bronchodilators 313
  inotropes 207
  mechanism of action 268
  onset of effect 270
  pharmacological effects 268–70
  physicochemical properties 270
  pregnancy therapies (mares) 184
Adrenoceptor antagonists 202–3
Adrenoceptor blockade 208
Adrenocorticotropic hormone (ACTH) *see* ACTH (adrenocorticotropic hormone)
Adrenoreceptors 138
Adverse drug reactions 17
  aminoglycoside antibiotics 30–2
  aminopenicillins 25
  cardiac glyosides 207
  cephalosporins 27
  chloramphenicol/florfenicol 34–5
  extended-spectrum penicillins 25
  fluoroquinolones 42
  lidocaine 201
  macrolides 43–4
  metronidazole 45
  muscle, skeletal 136–7

penicillin G (benzylpenicillin) 23–4
phenytoin 202
procainamide 200
propranolol 203
quinidine 196
rifampin 44–5
sulfonamides, potentiated 37–8
tetracylines 39–40
vasodilators, direct acting 210
Aerosol drug delivery 311, 312, 320, 323
  mask 312, 315, 319, 320, 321
AF (atrial fibrillation)
  cardiac glycosides 206, 207
  procainamide 200
  quinidine 195, 196, 197, 199
Agalactia 89, 186
AGS (β-N-acetylglucosominadase), urine 31
Albumin 341
  electrolyte/acid-base disturbances 356–7
Albuterol sulfate 313, 314, 315, 316, 317
Aldosterone 164
Alfentanil 279–80
Alimentary tract motility 87, 88–91
  aminoguanidine indoles (tegaserod) 90
  benzamides (cisapride, metoclopramide) 88–9
  dopamine antagonists (domperidone, metoclopramide) 89–90
Alkalosis 164, 353
  see also Pentoxifylline; Theophylline
Alpha adrenergic agonists 111–12
Alternaria spp. 229
Altrenogest
  induction during the transitional period 177–8
  estrus synchronization 179
  suppression of estrus in performance mares 180
  early embryonic loss 183
  reduction of aggressive behaviour (stallions) 188
American Association of Equine Practitioners (AAEP) *see* AAEP (American Association of Equine Practitioners)
Amicarbalide 52
Amikacin *see* Antimicrobial agents/therapy
Amiloride 167
Aminoglycoside antibiotics *see* Antimicrobial agents/therapy
Aminoguanidine indoles *see* Tegaserod

Aminopenicillins (amoxicillin/
   ampicillin)
   drug interactions/adverse effects 25
   formulations 25
   indications 24
   pharmacokinetics 24–5
   sustained-release preparations 129
Amiodarone 204
Ammonium chloride 172
Ammonium sulfate 172
Amoxicillin *see* Aminopenicillins
   (amoxicillin/ampicillin)
Amoxicillin-clavulanate 129
Amphoteric drugs 16
Amphotericin B 230
Ampicillin *see* Aminopenicillins
   (amoxicillin/ampicillin)
Anabolic steroids 143–4, 188
Analgesia *see* Opioid analgesics
Anaphylactic reactions, penicillin G
   (benzylpenicillin) 23–4
Anesthetics
   Dissociative (ketamine, tiletamine)
      282–5
   inhalation agents (desflurane,
      halothane, isoflurane,
      sevoflurane, nitrous oxide)
      administration route 295–6
      duration of effect 296–7
      elimination 296–7
      horses, major uses in 297
      MAC values 276, 291, 294
      mechanism of action 290
      onset of effect 295–6
      pharmacological effects 291–5
      physicochemical properties 290–1
   intravenous (ketamine, thiopental,
      propofol) 282–90
   local (bupivacaine; lidocaine
      (lignocaine); mepivacaine)
      297–301
      administration route 298
      duration of effect 298–9
      elimination 298–9
      horse, major uses 299–301
      mechanism of action 297
      morphine 127–8
      onset of effect 298–9
      pharmacological effects 297–8
      physicochemical properties 298
   topical 241
Angiotensin-converting enzyme
   (ACE) inhibitors *see* ACE
   (angiotensin converting
   enzyme) inhibitors
ANP (atrial natriuretic peptides) 159
Antacids 99–100
   aluminum-containing 106
Anthelmintics
   effects 67
   features 65
   pregnancy (mares) 184
   regimens 70
   resistance 70–1

   see also Cambendazole; Fenbendazole;
      Ivermectin; Mebendazole;
      Moxidectin; Oxfendazole;
      Oxibenazole; Piperazine;
      Praziquantel; Pyrantel
Anthroscopy 125
Anti-inflammatory drugs
   central nervous system disorders
      147–9
   corticosteroids/glucocorticoids
      central nervous system disorders
         147–8
      intraarticular medication 121–5
      respiratory disorders 318–22
   dimethyl sulfoxide (DMSO) *see*
      DMSO (Dimethyl sulfoxide)
   hyaluronan 121, 125–6
   intraarticular medication 121–7
   ocular 236–40
      ciclosporin 221, 239–40
      glucocorticoids 236–8
      NSAIDs 238–9
   see also NSAIDs (non-steroidal anti-
      inflammatory drugs)
Antiarrhythmic agents 194–206
   bradyarrhythmias 205
   class I 195
   class Ia 195–200
      procainamide 200
      quinidine 195–200
   class Ib 200–2
      lidocaine 200–1
      phenytoin (diphenylhydantoin)
         201–2
   class Ic 202
   class II 202–3
   class III 203–4
   class IV 204
   magnesium 204–5
Antibiotics *see* Antimicrobial
   agents/therapy
Anticholinergic drugs 110, 205, 269,
   316–17
Antidiuretic hormone (ADH) *see* ADH
   (Antidiuretic hormone)
Antifolate medication
   (diaminopyrimidines) 146
Antimicrobial agents/therapy
   adverse reactions 17
      see also Adverse drug reactions
   amikacin 28, 33, 128, 129, 130
   aminoglycoside antibiotics 28–33
      and chloramphenicol 34
      drug interactions/adverse effects
         30–2
      mechanism 28–9
      pharmacokinetics 29
      resistance mechanisms 29
      respiratory system 323
      urinary tract infections 173
   aminopenicillins 24–5
   appropriate concentrations 16–17
   beta-lactam antibiotics *see* Beta-
      lactam antibiotics

   cephalosporins 25–8
   chloramphenicol/florfenicol 21, 23,
      33–5
   diagnosis 14
   diaminopyrimidines *see*
      Pyrimethamine; Trimethoprim
   distribution volumes 14–15
   dosage regimen design *see* Dosage
      regimen (antimicrobial drugs)
   drug ionization 15–16
   effectiveness of antimicrobial 16
   elimination half-life 17
   extended-spectrum penicillins 25
   gastrointestinal system 115–16
   fluoroquinolones 9, 16, 23, 40–3
   gentamicin *see* Gentamicin
   horses, product approved for 17
   imipenem 28
   infection *see* Infection
   intraarticular medication 128–30
      regional perfusion 130
      sustained-release preparations
         129–30
   intravitreal therapy 226–7
   macrolides 43–4
   metronidazole 21, 45
   neomycin 28, 32
   ophthalmic delivery routes 225–7
      parenteral therapy 220–1, 224,
         226, 239
      subconjunctival therapy 226
      topical therapy 225–6
   organisms 14
      ocular bacteriology 224–5
   pathogens, *in vitro* susceptibility 14
   ophthalmic 227, 230
   penicillin G (benzylpenicillin),
      procaine 22, 24
   penicillin G (benzylpenicillin) 23–4
   protein binding 16
   rational use 13–47
   respiratory system disorders 322–4
   rifampin 21, 44–5
   scope 13
   streptomycin/dihydrostreptomycin
      28, 32
   sulfonamides, potentiated 22, 35–8
   terminology 13
   tetracyclines *see* Tetracyclines
   tobramycin 28, 33
   ulcerative keratitis 227–8
   vancomycin 45–6
Antimuscarinic agents *see*
   Anticholinergic drugs
Antimycotic therapy (ophthalmic
   therapeutics) 228–32
   azoles (clotrimzole, fluconazole,
      itraconazole, ketoconazole,
      miconazole) 230–1
   nucleoside analogs (flucytosine)
      231–2
   ocular mycoses 229
   selection of agents 229–32
Antibiotics *see* Antimicrobial therapy

Antiprotozoal drugs 49–62
  coccidiosis 57–8
  giardiasis 57
  piroplasmosis 49–53
  sarcocystis infections 58–62
  trypanosomiasis 53–7
Antisecretory agents 115
Antiviral therapy (ophthalmic;
     acyclovir, idoxuridine,
     interferon, trifluridine) 233–4
Aplastic anemia 35
Arachidonic acid 247
ARCI (Association of Racing
     Commissioners International)
     299
ARF (acute renal failure)
  NSAIDs 252
  urinary system 155, 157, 158–9, 162,
    166
Arthritis
  carpal 259
  septic 18
Arthropathy 42
Ascarids 66, 67
Aspergillus spp. 229, 230, 231, 232, 234
Aspirin 254–5
Association of Racing Commissioners
     International (ARCI) *see* ARCI
     (Association of Racing
     Commissioners International)
Asthma 315, 319, 321
Ataxia 268, 271
Atenolol 203
Atipamezole 271
ATP (adenosine triphosphate) 87
Atracurium 141–2
Atrial fibrillation (AF) *see* AF (atrial
     fibrillation)
Atrial natriuretic peptides (ANP) 159
Atrioventricular node *see* AV
     (atrioventricular node)
Atropine 110, 205, 240, 316
AUC (frequency distribution) 10
Autonomic nervous system 95
AV (atrioventricular node)
  anticholinergic agents 205
  cardiac rate/rhythm 194
  class IV antiarrhythmic agents 204
Azithromycin 43, 90
Azoles *see* Antimycotic therapy
     (ophthalmic therapeutics)

B

Babesia spp. 49, 50, 72
  B. caballi 49, 50, 51, 52, 53
  B. equi 49, 50, 51, 52, 53
Babesiosis *see* Piroplasmosis
Bacillus cereus 225
Bacteriostatic/bactericidal agents
  19–20
Bacteroides (B.) fragilis 23, 24, 26, 45

Barbiturates
  mechanism of action/
     pharmacological effects 286
  see also Thiopental
Beclometasone dipropionate 319,
    320–1
Benzalkonium chloride 312, 316
Benzamides *see* Cispiride;
    Metoclopramide
Benzathine benzylpenicillin 24
  see also Antimicrobial agents; Beta-
    Lactam antibiotics
Benzeneacetonitriles *see* Diclazuril;
    Ponazuril
Benzimidazoles 64, 66–7, 70, 104
  see also Cambendazole;
     Fenbendazole; Mebendazole;
     Oxfendazole; Oxibenazole
Benzodiazepines 150, 273–5
  administration route 274
  bioavailability 274
  duration of effect 275
  elimination 275
  horses, major uses in 275
  mechanism of action 274
  onset of effect 275
  pharmacological effects 274
  physicochemical properties 274
  see also Diazepam; Midazolam;
     Zolazepam
Benzothiadiazides (thiazide-type
     diuretics) *see* Diuretic agents
Benzylpenicillin *see* Penicillin G
     (benzylpenicillin)
Bertone, Joseph J 1–11, 365–379
Beta adrenoceptor
     agonists/antagonists 112, 243
Beta adrenoceptor antagonists (Beta
     blockers) 203
Beta-endorphin 276
Beta-lactam antibiotics 22–8
  aminoglycoside antibiotics 29
  cephalosporins 26
  combination therapy 21
  mechanism of action 22
  resistance mechanisms 22–3
  respiratory system 323
  see also Aminopenicillins
     (amoxicillin/ampicillin);
     Antimicrobial agents;
     Benzathine benzylpenicillin;
     Cephalosporins; Extended-
     spectrum penicillins; Penicillin
     G (benzylpenicillin); Procaine
     benzylpenicillin
Betamethasone 124–5
Bethanechol
  gastrointestinal system 88, 96, 107,
    109–10
  pharmacokinetics 171
  urine retention 170–1
Bicarbonate 331
Bilirubin 341
Bioavailability

adrenoceptor agonists 270
benzodiazepines 274
dissociative anesthetics 284
ophthalmic therapeutics 217, 221–2,
  223, 224
principles 3, 10
Bismuth subsalicylate (BSS) *see* BSS
     (Bismuth subsalicylate)
Bladder paralysis 169
Blastokinetes 50
Blood
  substitutes 344
  whole 343–4
Blood-aqueous barrier 217
Blood-brain barrier (drug
     distribution) 5
Blood-retinal barrier 217
Boldenone undecylenate 188
Bone, distribution of drugs 5
Bone marrow dyscrasias 257
Bone matrix, demineralized 130
Boophilus microplus see Ticks
Borrelia burgdorferi 225
Bots (*Gasterophilus* spp.) 67
Botulism 137
Bowen, I Mark 193–215
Bradyarrhythmias 195
  antiarrythmic agents 205
Bradycardia 269
Bradykinin 248, 341
Brain 80
Bretylium 203–4
Bromocriptine 79–80
Bronchoconstriction 315–16, 317
Bronchodilator therapy (inhalant)
    313–17
  anticholinergic agents 316–17
  long-acting adrenoceptor agonists
    314–16
  short-acting adrenoceptor agonists
    313–14
Brucella spp., antimicrobial therapy
    29, 34, 41
BSS (bismuth subsalicylate) 94, 115,
    242
Bumetanide 159, 162
Buparvaquone 53
Bupivacaine 300–1
Buprenorphine 281–2
Buspirone 151
Butorphanol 280–1

C

Calcium, electrolyte/acid-base
     disturbances 354–5
Cambendazole 184
cAMP (cyclic adenosine
     monophosphate) 168, 252, 268,
    276
Campylobacter jejunii 43
Candida spp. 229, 230, 231

Captopril *see* ACE (angiotensin converting enzyme) inhibitors
Carbenicillin 25
Carbonic anhydrase inhibitors 165–6, 243
  see also Diuretic agents
'Carboy' fluids 331, 357
Cardiac glycosides 206–7
Cardiovascular system 193–215
  antiarrhythmic agents 194–206
  cardiac rate and rhythm 193–4
  electrocardiograms (ECG) 194, 198, 201, 209
  function 193
  stroke volume 194
    therapy to alter 205–13
Carfentanil 280
Carprofen 253, 254, 260–1
Castor oil 114
Catecholamines epinephrine (adrenaline), norepinephrine (noradrenaline) 87, 209–10, 270, 271, 298
Cathartics 114
Catheters, venous 330, 346–7, 349
Cations 6
CD44 126
Cecal dysfunction/impaction 109
Cefalotin 27
Cefamandole 129
Cefapirin 27
Cefazolin 27, 129
Cefotaxime 27
Cefoxitin 27
Ceftiofur 16, 26, 27, 128–9, 323
Cellulose 87
Centers for Disease Control and Prevention (US) 348
Central compartment, volume (V_c) 9
Central nervous system (CNS)
  anesthetics 283, 284, 286, 288, 289
    local 298
  anti-inflammatory drugs 147–9
  antimicrobial therapy
    penicillin G (benzylpenicillin) 24
    tetracyclines 39
  cardiovascular drugs 201, 205
  distribution of drugs 5
  gastrointestinal drugs 89, 93
  infections, treating 14
  and NSAIDs 250
  opioids 276, 277, 278, 282
  Sarcocystis spp. infections 58, 59, 60
  sedatives/tranquillizers 268, 272, 274, 275
  see also Neurological system
Central venous pressure (CVP) *see* CVP (Central venous pressure)
Cephalosporins 25–8
  drug interactions/adverse effects 27
  formulations 27
  indications 25–7
  pharmacokinetics 27

see also individual agents (Cefalotin, cefamandole, cefapirin, cefazolin, cefotaxime, cefoxitin, ceftiofur)
Cerebrospinal fluid (CSF) *see* CSF (cerebrospinal fluid)
CFC (chlorofluorocarbon) propellant 312, 321
cGMP (cyclic guanosine monophosphate) 211
Chelating agents 235
Chemical cathartics 114
CHF (congestive heart failure)
  angiotensin-converting enzyme (ACE) inhibitors 212
  calcium channel blockers 204
  digoxin 206, 207
  diuretics 210
  hydralazine 211
  quinidine 199
Chlamydia spp.
  antimicrobial therapy 34, 38, 40, 43
  ophthalmic therapeutics 225, 227
Chloramphenicol/florfenicol 33–5
  adverse effects 34–5
  drug interactions 23, 34–5
  formulations 35
  indications 33–4
  infection site 21
  mechanism of action 34
  ophthalmic therapeutics 225
  pharmacokinetics 34
  resistance mechanisms 34
  and sedation 270
  sustained-release preparations 129
Chloride, electrolyte/acid-base disturbances 353
Chlorofluorocarbon (CFC) propellant 312, 321
Chlorpromazine 271, 273
  see also Phenothiazines
Chlortetracycline 39
  ointment 227
Cholinomimetics 88, 109–10
Chondrocytes 122–3, 131
Chondrodestruction (NSAID side effects) 254
Chondroprotection 254
Christley, Robert M 63–74
Chronic obstructive pulmonary disease (COPD) *see* COPD (Chronic obstructive pulmonary disease)
Ciclosporin 221, 239–40
Cilastatin 28
Cimetidine 100, 101, 102, 103, 200
Ciprofloxacin 42, 129, 227
  see also Fluoroquinolones
Circadian pattern 319
Cisapride 89, 107, 111
Clarithromycin 43, 90
Clearance, pharmacokinetics 7
Clenbuterol 96, 184
Clindamycin 43

Clinical signs
  coccidiosis 57
  hypovolemia/dehydration 328–9
  piroplasmosis 50
  sarcocystis infections 58–9, 62
  trypanosomiasis 54
Clostridium spp. 17, 43, 38, 136
  Clostridium botulinum (botulism) 137
  Clostridium difficile 26, 113
  Clostridium perfringens 35, 113, 225
  Clostridium tetani (tetanus) 137
Clotrimazole 231
CNS (central nervous system) *see* Central nervous system (CNS)
Coccidiosis (*Eimeria leukarti*) 57–8, 147
Coliforms 38
Collagen, bovine 340
Colloids 336–42
  albumin 341
  chemical nature 337
  clinical use 342
  crystalloids compared 342
  dextrans 339–40
  gelatins 340–1
  hetastarch 338–9
  hydroxyethyl starches 338–9
  oncotic pressure 337
  plasma 341–2
Combination therapy
  antibiotics 21–2
  respiratory system 317
Congestive heart failure (CHF) *see* CHF (congestive heart failure)
COPD (chronic obstructive pulmonary disease) 76, 316–17
Corley, Kevin T T 327–64
Cornea *see* Ophthalmic therapeutics
Corneal edema 222
Corneal samples, testing 230
Corneal-epithelial barrier 217
Corpus luteum 179–80
Corticosteroids (glucocorticoids)
  adrenosuppressive effects 318
  central nervous system disorders 147–8
  intraaarticular medication 121–5
  ocular therapy 236–8
  pituitary/adrenal glands 75–6
  respiratory disorders 314, 317, 318–22
  thyroid gland 82
  topical 234
see also Beclomethasone, Betamethasone, Cortisone, Dexamethasone, Dexamethasone sodium phosphate, Fluticasone propionate; MPA (methylprednisolone acetate); Methylprednisolone sodium succinate; Prednisolone; Prednisone, Triamcinolone

Corticotrophs 76
Cortisone 122
Corynebacterium spp. 26
Couetil, Laurent 75–83
COX (cyclooxgenase)
  COX1 248–9, 262
  COX2 238, 248, 249, 260
  NSAIDs 247, 249, 250, 251, 253, 255,
    261
  ophthalmic therapeutics 236, 238
Cox, Karina 247–66
Creatinine concentrations 329
Cromoglicate, disodium 322
Cromones (mast cell stabilizers) 322
Cryptococcus 230
Crystalloids
  colloids compared 342
  oral therapy 336
  polyionic solutions 331–6
    dextrose 333–4
    sodium bicarbonate 334–6
    see also Saline solutions
  rehydration phase 350
  requirements 328
CSF (cerebrospinal fluid)
  antimicrobial therapy 16, 34, 36, 42
  and CNS disorders 145, 148
  drug distribution (blood-brain
    barrier) 5
  Sarcocystis spp. infections 58, 59
  sodium concentration 335, 336
Cushing's Disease *see* ECD (Equine
    Cushing's Disease)
CVP (central venous pressure) 329,
    330
Cyathostomes 63, 64, 67, 70
cyclic adenosine monophosphate
    (cAMP) *see* cAMP (cyclic
    adenosine monophosphate)
cyclic guanosine monophosphate
    (cGMP) *see* cGMP (cyclic
    guanosine monophosphate)
Cyclodextrins 222
Cyclooxgenase (COX) *see* COX
    (cyclooxgenase)
Cycloplegics 240–1
Cypermethrin 71
Cyproheptadine 79, 151
Cystic fibrosis 323
Cytochrome P450 enzymes 231, 296
Cytokines 108, 254
Cytosolic carbonic anhydrase 165

D

DDAVP (Desmopressin acetate) 169
D5W (Dextrose, 5%) 334
Dantrolene 142
Dehydration
  clinical signs 328–9
  defined 328
  laboratory signs 329–30

rehydration therapy 350
Dehydronorketamine 285
Deltamethrin 71
Deltoid lateralis muscles 4
Dermacenter spp. *see* Ticks
Desflurane 291, 294
Desfuroylceftiofur 26–7
Deslorelin acetate (GnRH agonist) 179
Desmopressin acetate (DDAVP) *see*
    DDAVP (desmopressin acetate)
Detomidine 95, 107–8, 111, 269, 271,
    282
Dexamethasone
  glaucoma 244
  parenteral 237
  respiratory system 319
  suppression test 76, 77, 79, 80
  urinary system 164
Dexamethasone sodium phosphate
    148
Dextrans 339–40
Dextrose, 5% (D5W) *see* D5W
    (Dextrose, 5%)
DHFR (dihydrofolate reductase) 36,
    60, 146
Diabetes insipidus (DI) 168
Diagnosis
  antimicrobial therapy 14
  coccidiosis 57
  piroplasmosis 51
  sarcocystis infections 62
  trypanosomiasis 54–5
Diamidines, aromatic 51–3, 56–7
Diaminopyrimidines *see*
    Pyrimethamine; Trimethoprim
Diarthroidial joint 131
Diazepam 139, 150, 274, 275
Diclazuril (benzeneacetonitriles) 60,
    145, 147
Dictyocaulus arnfeldi 66
Diffusion, passive 2, 4
Digitilazation 199
Digoxin 199, 206, 207
Dihydropteroate synthetase (DPS) *see*
    DPS (Dihydropteroate
    synthetase)
Dihydrostreptomycin 32
Dihyrofolate reductase (DHFR) *see*
    DHFR (Dihydrofolate
    reductase)
Diltiazem 204
Dimethyl sulfoxide (DMSO) *see*
    DMSO (Dimethyl sulfoxide)
Diminazene aceturate 51
Diminazenes, aromatic 55
Dioctyl sodium sulfosuccinate (DSS)
    114
Diphenylhydantoin 82, 142–4, 150,
    201–2
Dissociative anesthetics 282–5
  administration route 284
  bioavailability 284
  duration of effect 284, 285
  elimination 285

horses, major uses 285
mechanism of action 283
onset of effect 284, 285
pharmacological effects 283–4
physiochemical properties 284
Distribution of drugs 4–5
Distribution volumes, apparent
    (pharmacokinetics) 8–10, 14–15
  terminology 9
  see also V_d (apparent volume of
    distribution)
Diuretic agents 159–68
  benzothiadiazides (thiazide-type
    diuretics) 163–5
  carbonic anhydrase inhibitors
    165–6
  loop (high ceiling) diuretics
    159–63
  osmotic diuretics 166–7
  potassium-sparing 167–8
  stroke volume 210
Divalent metal ion chelating agents 5
DMSO (dimethyl sulfoxide) 121,
    126–7, 148–9, 167
DNA, antiviral therapy 233
DNA-DNA gyrase complex 40, 41
Dobutamine 208–9
Dolophine hydrochloride (methadone)
    279
Domperidone 80, 89–90, 184, 186–7
Dopamine
  antagonists (domperidone,
    metoclopramide) 89–90, 186
  phenothiazines 271
  receptors 1 and 2 88
  renal dysfunction 157–8
  vasopressors 207–8
Dopamine
Dopexamine, vasopressors 208
Dosage regimen (antimicrobial drugs)
    18–22
  administration route 19
  bacteriostatic versus bactericidal
    agents 19–20
  calculation 20–1
  combination antimicrobial therapy
    21–2
  concentration 20
  distribution in body 18–19
  growth rates 19
  host defenses 18
  inhibitory drug dosage 18–19
  prophylactic use 22
  therapeutic index 21
  see also Antimicrobial therapy;
    Infection
Dourine (*Trypanosoma equiperdum*) 53,
    54
Dowling, Patricia M 13–47, 145–54
Doxycycline 38
DPS (dihydropteroate synthetase) 36
Drug administration *see*
    Administration, drugs
Drug interactions *see* Interactions, drug

Drug ionization, antimicrobial therapy 15–16
Drug transfer, physicochemical factors 2
Dry powder inhalants 312, 313
DSS (dioctyl sodium sulfosuccinate) 114
Duodenitis 107, 108–9
  duodenitis/proximal enteritis (DPE) 109, 113
Duodenum 91
Dyspepsia 100

E

E. (Escherichia) coli 92, 180
  anesthetics 297
  antimicrobial therapy
    aminoglycoside antibiotics 32
    beta-lactam antibiotics 26, 28
    chloramphenicol/florfenicol 34
    fluoroquinolones 41
    organisms 14
    sulfonamides 35, 38
    tetracyclines 38
  gastrointestinal drugs 92, 113
  reproductive system 180
ECD (Equine Cushing's disease) 76–80
  dexamethasone suppression test 76, 77, 79, 80
  diagnosis 77
  follow up 80
  and respiratory system 319
  treatment 78–80
ECF (extracellular fluid)
  aminoglycoside antibiotics 29
  crystalloids 330, 331, 332, 333
  infection location 14
  magnesium 355
  principles 8, 10
ECG (electrocardiograms) 194, 198, 201, 209
Echinacea 253
Ectoparasiticides 64, 71–2
ED₅₀ (median effective dose) 21
Edema 222, 330, 337
Edetic acid 312
EDTA (ethylene diamine tetraacetic acid) 77, 235, 312, 316
EEG (electroencephalography) 279, 282
Efluvane 53
Ehrlichia spp. 38, 113
EHV (equine herpes virus) 233
Eicosanoids 247
Eimeria leukarti see Coccidiosis
EIPH (exercise-induced pulmonary hemorrhage) 159, 161, 163
Ejaculation , chemical 189
Ejaculatory dysfunction 188–9
Electrocardiograms (ECG) see ECG (electrocardiograms)

Electroencephalography (EEG) see EEG (electroencephalography)
Electrolyte/acid-base disturbances 351–7
  albumin 356–7
  calcium 354–5
  chloride 353
  lactate 352
  magnesium 355–6
  phosphorus 356
  potassium 353
  sodium 352–3
    isotonic 332
Elimination of drugs see Excretion
ELISAs (enzyme-linked immunoabsorbent assays) 55, 152
Elliott, Jonathan 193–215
Eltenac 262–3
Embonate 67
EMLA cream 298
Enalapril see ACE (angiotensin converting enzyme) inibitors
Endometriosis/endometritis 180–2
Endoparasiticides 63, 64–71
  anthelmintics, features 65
  benzimidazoles 66–7
  clinical disease regimens 69–70
  control programs, internal parasites 67–71, 68
  macrocyclic lactones 64, 66
  piperazine 67
  praziquantel 67
  pyrimidines 67
Endophthalmitis 232
Endophyte-infected fescue toxicosis see Fescue toxicosis
Endoplasmic reticulum 5
Endothelium 131
Endotoxemia 112, 329
  endotoxic shock 147
  endotoxins 341
Enkephalins 93, 115
Enrofloxacin 41, 42, 130, 184
ENS (enteric nervous system) 86, 109
Enteritis 108
Enterobacter spp. 26
Enterobacteriaceae 26
Enterochromaffin cells 98
Enterococci, antimicrobial therapy 26, 30, 38
Enteropathogens 115
Enterotoxigenic bacteria 93
Enzyme-linked immunoabsorbent assays (ELISAs) see ELISAs (Enzyme-linked immunoabsorbent assays)
Epinephrine (adrenaline) see Catecholamines
  reversal 272
EPM (equine protozoal myeloencephalitis) see Sarcocystis infections (EPM)

EPSM (equine polysaccharide storage myopathy) see Muscle, skeletal, disorders
Equine Cushing's Disease (ECD) see ECD (Equine Cushing's Disease)
Equine herpes virus (EHV) see EHV (Equine herpes virus)
Equine metabolic syndrome 81
Equine polysaccharide storage myopathy (EPSM) see Muscle, skeletal, disorders
Equine protozoal myeloencephalitis (EPM) see Sarcocystis infections (EPM)
ERU (equine recurrent uveitis) 221, 237, 238, 239, 243
Erythrolysis 330
Erythromycin
  antimicrobial therapy 21
  macrolides 43, 44
  gastrointestinal system 90, 107
  sustained-release preparations 129
Escherichia coli see E. coli
Esmarch 130
Esmolol 203
Esophagitis, reflux 96–7
Esophagus 95–7
  drugs for relaxation with obstruction 95–6
  reflux esophagitis 96–7
Estradiol 171–2, 179
Estrus suppression (performance mares) 180
Estrus synchronization 179–80
Etacrynic acid 159, 162
Ethylene diamine tetraacetic acid (EDTA) see EDTA (ethylene diamine tetracetic acid)
Excretion (elimination of drugs) 6–7
  gastrointestinal 7
  in milk 6–7
  pulmonary 6
  urinary 6, 27
    tubular secretion, active 6
    tubular reabsorption, passive 6
Exercise-induced pulmonary hemorrhage (EIPH) see EIPH (exercise-induced pulmonary hemorrhage)
Exertional rhabdomyolysis 137, 138
Extended-spectrum penicillins 25
Extracellular fluid (ECF) see ECF (extracellular fluid)

F

Famotidine 100, 101
FARAD (Food Animal Residue Avoidance Databank) 17
FDA (Food and Drug Administration (US)) 211

Fenbendazole 66, 71
Fenger, Clara K 49–62
Fentanyl 279
Fenvalerate 71
Fescue toxicosis 80, 89, 184–5
Fetal membranes, retained 186
Fiber 114–15
Fibrinolytic agents
  intracameral 242
Fipronil 72
5-HT$_3$/HT$_4$ receptor agonist 88, 89, 90
5-hydroxytryptamine (5-HT)
    (serotonin) receptors 88, 138,
    151, 152, 271
5-lipoxygenase 249
15-lipoxygenase 249
Florfenicol see
    Chloramphenicol/florfenicol
Flucloxacillin 129
Fluconazole 231
Flucytosine 231–2
'Fluid bolus' concept, fluid therapy
    348
Fluid therapy 327–64
  blood 343–4
  colloids 336–42
  complications 357–8
  crystalloids see Crystalloids
  delivery 346–51
    disturbances, acid-
      base/electrolyte 351–7
    infusion rates/volumes 348–51
    systems 346–8
  electrolyte/acid-base disturbances
    351–7
  'fluid challenge' 330
  infusion rates/volumes
    maintenance phase 348, 350–1
    rehydration phase 348, 350
    resuscitation phase 348–50
  maintenance 327, 331, 334, 350–1
  parenteral nutrition 344–6
  patients, identifying 328–30
    clinical signs 328–9, 353
    laboratory signs 329–30
  plan
    formulating 327–8
    infusion rates/volumes 348–51
    phases 327, 348–51
  principles
    fluid requirements 330
    formulating plan 327–8
    identifying patients 328–30
  rehydration 327, 348, 350
  requirements 330
  response to 327
    lack of 358
  resuscitation 327, 330, 331, 334,
    348–50
  types of fluid
    colloids 336–42
    crystalloids 330–6
Flumazenil 151, 274, 275
Flunisolide 319, 321–2

Flunixin meglumine, NSAIDs 148,
    250, 254, 258–60, 261
Fluoroquinolones
  and chloramphenicol 34
  distribution volumes 9
  drug interactions/adverse effects 42
  formulations 42–3
  indications 40
  ionization of drugs 16
  mechanism of action 40–1
  ophthalmic therapeutics 225
  and penicillin G (benzylpenicillin) 23
  pharmacokinetics 41–2
  resistance mechanisms 41
Fluphenazine 151–2, 185
Fluprostenol 186
Fluticasone propionate 319, 320, 321
Foals
  'fluid bolus' concept 348
  neonatal
    CVP (central venous pressure)
      measurement 330
    dextrose therapy 333–4
    hypovolemia in 329
    ketoprofen therapy 261
    saline administration 333
  oral replacement therapy 93
  ruptured bladders in 332
  suckling 6–7
  water content 14
Folate supplementation 37
Follicle-stimulating hormone (FSH) see
    FSH (Follicle-stimulating
    hormone)
Food Animal Residue Avoidance
    Databank (FARAD) 17
Food and Drug Administration (FDA)
    see FDA (Food and Drug
    Administration (US)) 211
Frusemide (furosemide) see
    Furosemide (frusemide)
FSH (follicle-stimulating hormone)
  neurological system 151
  reproductive system 179
Fungal infections 229, 230, 231
Furosemide (frusemide) 82, 150,
    155–7, 159–62, 163, 210
Fusarium spp. 229, 230, 231, 232
Fusidic acid 227
Fusobacterium spp. 35, 45

G

GABA (gamma-aminobutyric acid)
  anesthetics 286, 288, 290
  opioids 277
  parasiticides 67
  sedatives/tranquillizers 139, 150,
    274
  seizures 149
  skeletal muscle, drugs affecting
    139, 142

Gametogony 58
Gamma-glutamyltransferase (GGT) see
    GGT (Gamma-glutamyl
    transferase)
Gasterophilus spp. see Bots
Gastric acidity, drugs for 99–106
  antacids 99–100
  H$^+$,K$^+$-ATPase inhibitors
    104–5
  histamine H$_2$ receptor antagonists
    100–3
Gastric emptying 107
Gastric motility, drugs for 107–8
Gastric mucosal protection, drugs for
    106–7
Gastrin 98
Gastroesophageal reflux disease
    (GERD) see GERD
    (Gastroesophageal reflux
    disease)
Gastrointestinal system 85–120
  alimentary tract 87, 88–91
  antimicrobial agents 115–16
  esophagus 95–7
  excretion 7
  gut, electrical rhythm 87
  intestine (small and large) 87,
    108–15
  magnesium 355
  motility 86–8
    alimentary tract 87, 88–91
    gastric 107–8
    intestine (small and large) 108
  neuromuscular stimuli 87
  NSAID side-effects 251–2
  secretion/absorption 91–5
  stomach 97–108
  sympathetic/parasympathetic
    stimuli 87
Gelatins 340–1
Gentamicin
  aminoglycoside antibiotics 28
  combination therapy 21
  formulations 33
  glaucoma 244
  indications 32
  intraarticular agents 128
  NSAIDs 253, 256
  pharmacokinetics 32
  therapeutic drug monitoring 33
GERD (gastroesophageal reflux
    disease) 96–7
Gestation
  late, hastening of fetal maturation
    165
  prolonged 184–5
GFR (glomerular filtration rate) 155,
    157, 158, 159, 166
GGT (gamma-glutamyltransferase),
    urine 31
Giardiasis 57
Glaucoma 243–4
Globulins 337
Glomerular filtration 6, 39

Glomerular filtration rate (GFR) *see* GFR (Glomerular filtration rate)
Glucocorticoids (corticosteroids) *see* Corticosteroids (Glucocorticoids)
Glucuronic acid 270
Glucuronidation 37
Glucuronide 6
Glycerol 166–7
Glyceryl trinitrate 211, 357
Glycopyrrolate 205, 269
Glycoside linkage 28
GM 60001 (ilomastat) 235
GMP (guanosine monophosphate) 211
GnRH (gonadotropin-releasing hormone)
    agonist (deslorelin acetate) *see* Deslorelin acetate (GnRH agonist)
    induction during the transitional period 178
    spermatogenesis 187–8
Gram stains 18, 227
Gram-positive/negative bacteria
    aminoglycoside antibiotics 28, 30, 173
    aminopenicillins 24
    beta-lactam antibiotics 22, 23, 26
    cephalosporins 26
    combination therapy 21
    extended-spectrum penicillins 25
    fluoroquinolones 40, 41
    gentamicin 32
    imipenem 28
    macrolides 43
    metronidazole 45
    nitrothiazoles 61
    ocular bacteriology 224, 227
    organisms 14
    tetracyclines 38
Guaifenesin 140–1, 285, 287, 289, 290
Guanosine monophosphate (GMP) *see* GMP (Guanosine monophosphate)

H

H⁺,K⁺-ATPase inhibitors 97, 98, 104–5
HA (hyaluronan) 121, 125–6
Haemophilus spp., antimicrobial therapy 26, 34, 43, 44
Half-life, pharmacokinetics 7–8
Halothane anesthesia
    and alfentanil 280
    and aminoglycosides 30
    and butorphanol 281
    description 292
    and diazepam 275
    hepatic metabolism 296
    and ketamine 283
    and morphine 278
    and thyroid supplementation 82

Hartmann's solution 331
hCG (human chorionic gonadotropin)
    induction during the transitional period 178
    induction during the breeding season 179
    early embryonic loss 183
    spermatogenesis 188
Headshaking, photic 151
Heart *see* Cardiovascular system
Helicobacter pylori 99
Heme compounds 341
Hemobartonella spp., antimicrobial therapy 34
Hemodynamics 335
Hemoglobin 344
Henderson-Hasselbach equation 2
Heparin 235
Hepatic enzyme systems 6
Hepatotoxins 253
Hetastarch 338–9
HFA (hydrofluoroalkane-134a) 312, 321
High-viscosity carbomer gel 222
Hirsutism 77
Histamine 97
Histamine H₂ receptor antagonists 100–3
Hoffman degradation, spontaneous 141
Homidium bromide 56
Hormonal therapy 151
Host defenses 18
Human chorionic gonadotropin (hCG) *see* hCG (Human Chorionic Gonadotropin)
Hyalomma spp. *see* Ticks
Hyaluronan (HA) *see* HA (Hyaluronan)
Hyaluronidase 298
Hydralazine 210–11
Hydrochloric acid 97, 98, 99
Hydrochlorothiazide 165
Hydrofluoroalkane-134a (HFA) 312, 321
Hydrogen ion activity 99
Hydrolysis 141
Hydroxyethyl starches 338–9
Hydroxylation, aromatic 37
Hydroxymethylaminomethane (THAM) *see* THAM (hydroxymethylaminomethane)
Hydroxypropyl methylcellulose 222
Hyoscine (scopolamine) 110, 205
Hyperchloremia 332, 333
Hypergammaglobulinemia 329
Hyperglycemia 270, 352
Hyperkalemia 141, 332
Hyperkalemic periodic paralysis (HYPP) *see* HYPP (Hyperkalemic periodic paralysis)

Hypernatremia 333, 353
Hyperosmotic agents, topical 242
Hypertension 269
Hyperthermia 280
    malignant 138
Hypertonic sodium chloride solution 222, 330, 332–3
Hypoalbuminemia 341, 342, 356, 357
Hypobiotic cyathostome larvae 66
Hypocalcemia 354, 355
Hypochloremia 353
Hypoinsulinemia 270
Hypokalemia 210, 353, 354
Hypomagnesemia 210, 355
Hyponatremia 165, 352
Hypophosphatemia 356
Hypothyroidism 81, 180
Hypovolemia
    clinical signs 328–9
    defined 328
    hypertonic saline solution 333
    laboratory signs 329–30
    therapy plan 348
        rehydration phase 350
HYPP (hyperkalemic periodic paralysis) 137

I

ICAM-1 (intercellular adhesion molecule-1) 318
ICP (intracranial pressure) 275, 277, 283, 286, 292
Idazoxan 271
Idoxuridine 233
IGF-1 (insulin-like growth factor 1) 124
Ileus, gastrointestinal 108
Ilomastat (GM 60001) 235
Imidocarb dipropionate 52, 72–3
Imipenem 28, 128, 129
Imipramine 172
Incontinence 169–72
Indometacin 92
Induction 185–6
Infection
    environment 19
    location 14
    site of 21
        reaching 14–16
        size of inoculum at 19
Infections
    Borrelia burgdorferi 225
    combination therapy 21
    documenting 17–18
    mixed 19
    Rhodococcus (R.) equi 21, 113, 225
    urinary tract 172–4
    see also Sarcocystis spp. infections (EPM)
Infertility (mares) 180–2

Inhalation therapy (respiratory
    system) 311–25
  anti-inflammatory drugs 318–22
  antimicrobial therapy 322–4
  combination therapy 317
  corticosteroids 314, 317, 318–22
  inhalant bronchodilator therapy
    anticholinergic agents 316–17
    long-acting agonists 314–16
    short-acting agonists 313–14
  mast cell stabilizers 322
Inotropes
  acute 207–10
  novel positive 207
  positive 206–7
  short-acting 207
Insecticides 72
Insulin 82
Insulin-like growth factor 1 (IGF-1)
    124
Interactions, drug
  aminoglycoside antibiotics 30–2
  aminopenicillins 25
  cardiac glycosides 207
  cephalosporins 27
  chloramphenicol/florfenicol 23,
    34–5
  extended-spectrum penicillins 25
  fluoroquinolones 42
  macrolides 43–4
  metronidazole 45
  penicillin G (benzylpenicillin) 23–4
  procainamide 200
  quinidine 200
  rifampin 44–5
  sulfonamides, potentiated 37–8
  tetracyclines 39–40
Intercellular adhesion molecule-1
    (ICAM-1) 318
Interferon 233
Interleukins (IL)
  IL-1 254
  IL-10 318
Interstitial cells of Cajal 86, 87
Intestinal mucosa, drugs acting on
    94–5, 115
Intestinal mucosal cells 86, 106–7
Intestinal secretory disorders,
    pathophysiology 113
Intestine (small and large) 87, 108–15
  agents promoting
    digestion/absorption 115
  antisecretory agents 115
  motility
    clinical conditions 108–9
    drugs acting on 109–13
    pathophysiology 108
  secretion and absorption, drugs
    acting on 113–15
  secretory disorders,
    pathophysiology 113
Intraarticular medication 4, 121–34
  administration 4
  anti-inflammatory drugs 121–7

antimicrobial agents 128–30
local anesthetics 127–8
synovectomy with
    radiopharmaceuticals 130–1
Intracranial pressure (ICP) see ICP
    (intracranial pressure)
Intramuscular drug administration see
    Administration, drugs
Intraocular penetration 221
  injections 220
Intraocular pressure (IOP) see IOP
    (intraocular pressure)
Intrauterine administration see
    Administration, drugs
Intravenous drug administration see
    Administration, drugs
Intravitreal therapy 226–7
Iodine-containing compounds 82
"Ion trapped" 7, 15
Ionized drugs see Drug ionization
Ionized molecules 2
IOP (intraocular pressure) 243
Ipratropium bromide 316–17
Isoflurane 269, 293
Isometamidium chloride 56, 73
Isoproterenol 315
Isothenuria 329
Isotonic sodium chloride solution see
    Saline solutions
Itraconazole 231
Ivermectin 64, 66, 67, 72

J

Jejunum 91
Jet nebulizers see Nebulizers, jet
Jugular vein 347, 349

K

Kanamycin 28
Kava kava 253
KCS (keratoconjunctivitis sicca) 240,
    241
Keratitis 233, 237
  ulcerative 227–8
Keratoconjunctivitis 233
Keratoconjunctivitis sicca (KCS) see
    KCS (Keratoconjunctivitis sicca)
Keratomycosis 229, 230
  treatment protocols 232
Ketamine 282, 283–5
Ketoconazole 231
Ketoprofen 251, 261–2
Ketorolac 262
Kidneys 6
Klebsiella spp.
  aminoglycoside antibiotics 28, 32
  beta-lactam antibiotics 24, 26
  chloramphenicol/florfenicol 34, 35

K. pneumoniae 180
tetracyclines 38
Kollias-Baker, Cynthia 247–66

L

Lactate 329–30, 332, 352
Lactic acidosis 334, 335, 351–2, 358
Lactose-replacement therapy 115
Laminitis 77
Lanreotide 93
Lansoprazole 104
Lasalocid 137
Latanoprost 243–4
Laxatives 113–15
LD$_{50}$ (median lethal dose) 21
LES (lower esophageal sphincter)
  alimentary tract 88, 89
  esophagus 95, 96, 98
Leuconostoc mesenteroides 339
Leukocytes
  intestinal motility disorders 108
  intrarticular medication 122
  NSAIDs 148, 248, 249
  see also PMNs (Polymorphonuclear
    leukocytes)
Leukotrienes (LTs) 247, 249, 250
Levomepromazine
    (methotrimeprazine) 272
Levy, Michael 75–83
LH (luteinizing hormone)
  neurological system 151
  reproductive system 178, 179, 187,
    188
LHRH (luteinizing hormone releasing
    hormone) 178
Lidocaine (lignocaine)
  Class Ib antiarrhythmic agent
    200–1
  and intestinal motility 112–13
  intraarticular medication 127
  local anesthesia 299–300
  and thiopental 287
Lignocaine see Lidocaine (lignocaine)
Lincomycin 43
Lincosamides 43
Lipid solubility 2
Lipocortin production 236
Lipophilicity 315
Lipoxygenase 236
Listeria spp. 26
Liver 16–17
Loading dose 10
Local anesthetics 127–8
Local perfusion, drug administration
    4
Loop of Henle 156, 164, 166
Loop (high ceiling) diuretics
  bumetanide 162
  complications 163
  etacrynic acid 162
  furosemide (frusemide) 159–62

Loperamide 93, 115
Love, Sandy 63–74
Lower esophageal sphincter *see* LES (lower esophageal sphincter)
LTs (leukotrienes) 247, 249, 250
Lubricants 113–14
  ocular 241
Lufenuron 232
Lungworm 67
Luteal inefficiency 182–3
Luteinizing hormone *see* LH (luteinizing hormone)
Luteinizing hormone releasing hormone (LHRH) *see* LHRH (Luteinizing hormone releasing hormone)
Lysosomal enzymes 30

M

MAC (minimum alveolar concentration)
  inhalation agents 276, 291, 293, 294
    halothane 275, 278, 280, 281, 283, 292
  lidocaine 299
  sedatives/tranquillizers 269, 272
MacLeay, Jennifer M 135–44
Macrocyclic lactones 64, 66, 71–2
Macrogametocytes 50
Macrolides 9, 43–4
Magnesium
  antiarrythmic agents 204–5
  electrolyte/acid–base disturbances 355–6
Magnesium sulfate/oxide 114
Maintenance fluids 327, 331, 334, 350–1
Mannitol 158, 166
Mares
  agalactia in 89
  performance 180
  reproduction
    infertility 180–2
    lactation 186–7
    ovulation induction 177–80
    parturition 185–6
    postpartum problems 187
    pregnancy 182–5
Marr, Celia M 193–215
Mason, Diane E 267–309
Mast cell stabilizers 322
Mast cells 86, 98, 315
Mastitis 15
Matrix metalloproteinases (MMPs) *see* MMps (matrix metalloproteinases)
Matthews, Andrew 217–45
Maximum plasma concentration (C_{max}) 10
MBC (minimum bactericidal concentration)

florfenicol 34
fluoroquinolones 42
  inhibitory drug dosage 18
MDI (metered-dose inhalant) devices 312, 319
MDP (methylene diphosphonate) 300
Mean residence time (MRT), pharmacokinetics *see* MRT (mean residence time)
Mebendazole 66
Meclofenamic acid 251, 258
Medetomidine 268, 269, 271
Median effective dose (ED_{50}) 21
Median lethal dose (LD_{50}) 21
Membranes, drug delivery 2, 219
Meperidine (pethidine) 261, 277, 279
Mepivacaine 127, 300
Merogony (asexual reproductive cycle) 57, 58
Merozoites 50, 57
Mesenchymal cells 86
Metabisulfite 312
Metabolic acidosis 334, 351–2
Metabolic syndrome 81
Metabolism, hepatic (biotransformation) 5–6, 296, 299
  metabolites 6
  Presystemic 6
Metered-dose inhalant (MDI) devices *see* MDI (metered-dose inhalant devices)
Methadone (dolophine hydrochloride) 279
Methicillin 128
Methicillin-resistant staphylococci *see* MRSA (methicillin-resistant staphylococci)
Methocarbamol 139–40
Methotrimeprazine (levomepromazine) 272
Methylene diphosphonate (MDP) *see* MDP (methylene diphosphonate)
Methylprednisolone acetate (MPA) *see* MPA (methylprednisolone acetate)
Methylprednisolone sodium succinate 148
Methylprednisone *see* MPA (methylprednisolone acetate)
Metoclopramide
  alimentary tract motility 88–9
  effectiveness 85
  esophagitis 96–7
  fescue toxicosis 80
  gastric motility 107
  intestine 110–11
Metritis 25
Metronidazole 21, 45, 57
Mexiletine 202
MIC (minimum inhibitory concentration)

antimicrobial drug concentration 20
bacteriostatic v bactericidal agent 19, 20
calculation of drug dosage 20, 21
concept 10
fluoroquinolones 41, 42
gentamicin 33
growth of bacteria 19
inhibitory drug dosage 18
intraarticular agents 128, 129
ophthalmic therapeutics 225, 226
respiratory system 323
sulfonamides, potentiated 35, 60
Miconazole 231
Microsomal enzyme system 43
Midazolam 273, 274, 275
Migrating myoelectrical complex (MMC) *see* MMC (migrating myoelectrical complex)
Milk, excretion in 6–7
Milrinone 210
Minimum alveolar concentration (MAC) *see* MAC (minimum alveolar concentration)
Minimum bactericidal concentration (MBC) *see* MBC (minimum bactericidal concentration)
Minimum inhibitory concentration (MIC) *see* MIC (minimum inhibitory concentration)
Minocycline 38
Miotics 241
Misoprostol 94–5, 105, 106, 115
Mitotane (*o,p'*-DDD) 80
MMC (migrating myoelectrical complex) 87, 90, 108, 111
MMPs (matrix metalloproteinases) 123, 228, 234, 235, 236
Monensin 137
Morphine 127–8, 277, 278–9
Motilides 90, 97, 107, 111
Motilin 87
Motility (gastrointestinal system) 86–8
Moxidectin 64, 66, 70, 72
MPA (methylprednisolone acetate) 122–4
  methylprednisone 122
MRSA (methicillin-resistant staphylococci)
  beta-lactam antibiotics 23
  cephalosporins 26
  vancomycin 45–6
MRT (mean residence time), pharmacokinetics 8
Mucor spp. 229
Murray, Michael J 85–120
Murrina *see* Surra
Muscle relaxants 139–42
  centrally acting spasmolytics 139–40
  neuromuscular blockers 140–2

Muscle, skeletal 135–44
  adverse drug reactions 136–7
  agents affecting directly 138–42
    muscle relaxants *see* Muscle
      relaxants
    neuromuscular blockers 140–2
    NSAIDS 138
    tranquillizers 138–9
  agents affecting muscle indirectly
    142–4
  disorders 137–8
    equine polysaccharide storage
      myopathy (EPSM) 137, 138
    polysaccharide storage myopathy
      (PSSM) 137, 138
    recurrent exertional
      rhabdomyolysis (RER) 137,
      138, 141
  intramuscular drug administration
    see Administration, drugs
Mycoplasma spp.
  antimicrobial therapy 34, 38, 40, 41
  ophthalmic therapeutics 225, 227
Mycoses, ocular 229
Mydriatics 240–1
  topical 243
Myoglobin 163
Myotonia 137

N

N-acetylprocainamide (NAPA) *see*
  NAPA (*N*-acetylprocainamide)
Nalidixic acid 40
Naloxone 187, 278, 282
NANC (non-adrenergic, non-
  cholinergic) neurons 87, 88
Nandrolone deconate 188
NAPA (*N*-acetylprocainamide) 200
Naproxen 260
Narcotic agonists/antagonists 90–1
Nasolacrimal epithelium 218
Nasolacrimal lavage system 219
Natamycin (pimaricin) 230
Nebulization, ultrasonic 312, 313,
  316
Nebulizers 312–13, 316
  jet 312–13
Nedocromil sodium 322
Neomycin 28, 32
Neonatal maladjustment syndrome
  (NMS) *see* NMS (neonatal
  maladjustment syndrome)
Neospora hughesi 58
Neostigmine 32, 110
Neotryphodium coenophialum 184
Nephrocalcinosis 163
Nephrolithiasis 163
Nephrotoxicity 30, 31
Netilmicin 129
Neurological system 145–54
  anti-inflammatory therapy 147–9

behavioral disorders 151–2
sarcocystis infections (EPM) *see*
  Sarcocystis infections (EPM)
seizures 149–51
Neuromuscular blockade 31–2
Neuromuscular blockers *see* Muscle
  relaxants, neuromuscular
  blockers
Neuropeptides 276
Neutrophilia 320
Nitazoxanide 61, 147
Nitrates 211
Nitric oxide *see* NO (nitric oxide)
Nitroglycerin (glyceryl trinitrate) 211,
  357
Nitrothiazoles 61, 145, 147
Nitrous oxide 294–5
Nizatidine 100
NMDA (*N*-methyl-D-aspartate)
  receptor 283
NMS (neonatal maladjustment
  syndrome) 147
NO (nitric oxide) 88, 92, 97, 98
  agonists 106–7
Norepinephrine (noradrenaline) *see*
  Catecholamines
Norketamine 285
Normomagnesemia 204
NSAIDs (non-steroidal anti-
  inflammatory drugs) 247–66
  agents 254–63
  aminoglycoside antibiotics 30, 31
  chondroprotection 254
  CNS disorders 148
  eicosanoids 247
  fever 248
  gastrointestinal system 92, 93, 94,
    99, 106, 115
  inflammation, signs of 247
  local anesthetics 127
  mode of action 248–50
  muscle, affecting directly 138
  ocular use 228, 238–9
  pain 248
  pharmacokinetics 250–1
  reproductive system 183, 186, 187
  side effects in horses
    chondrodestruction 254
    coagulation 253–4
    gastrointestinal 251–2
    hepatic 253
    protein binding 253
    renal 252–3
  and thiopental 287
  urinary system 159, 162
  see also Anti-inflammatory drugs
Nucleoside analogs 231–2

O

Octreotide 93
Ocular autonomic drugs 240–1

Ocular bacteriology, antibacterial
  therapy (ophthalmics) 224–5
Ocular drug administration 4
Ocular epithelium 218
Ocular lavage systems, topical drug
  delivery 218–19
Ocular tissue adhesives 242–3
Oedema *see* Edema
Oesophagus *see* Esophagus
Omeprazole 85, 104–6
Onchocerca cervicalis 66
Opioid analgesics 276–82
  agonists (alfentanil, carfentanil,
    fentanyl, meperidine
    (pethidine), methadone
    (dolophine), morphine,
    remifentanil, uses 280–2
  agonists/antagonists
    (buprenorphine, butorphanol,
    pentazocine), uses 280–2
  antagonists (naloxone), uses 151,
    282
  behavioral disorders 151
  mechanism of action 276–7
  pharmacological effects 277–8
Ophthalmic therapeutics 217–45
  antibacterial therapy 224–8
  antimycotic therapy 228–32
  antiviral therapy 233–4
  best practice guidelines 223–4
  bioavailability 217, 221–2, 223, 224
  drug delivery routes 218–21
    antibacterial therapy 225–7
    direct instillation 218
    innovative systems 221
    intraocular injections 220
    membrane delivery systems 219
    obstacles 217
    parenteral administration 220–1,
      224, 226, 239
    periocular injections 220
    retrobulbar injection 220
    sub-Tenon's injection 220
    subconjunctival injections 219,
      220, 223–4, 226
    topical instillation 218–19
  drug preparation 222
  gels 222
  glaucoma 243–4
  injections
    intraocular 220
    periocular 220
    retrobulbar 220
    sub-Tenon's 220
    subconjunctival 219, 220, 223–4,
      226
  intracameral fibrinolytic agents 242
  intraocular penetration 221
    injections 220
  keratomycosis, treatment protocols
    232
  ocular anti-inflammatory therapy
    236–40
  ocular autonomic drugs 240–1

ocular irrigating
    solutions/disinfectants 242
ocular lubricants 241
ocular tissue adhesives 242–3
ointments 222, 227
parenteral administration 220–1,
    224, 226, 239
pharmacokinetics 221–2, 223, 224
pharmacological principles 221–4
    subconjunctival injections 219,
    220, 223–4, 226
solutions 222
suspensions 222
tissue conditions 222
topically applied drugs
    anesthetics 241
    antibacterial therapy 225–6
    antiviral therapy 233
    delivery routes 218–19
    glaucoma 243
    hyperosmotic agents 242
    iodine solution 232
    NSAIDs 238–9
    pharmacological principles 221–3
ulceration therapy 234–6
viscoelastic materials 242
Oral drug administration see
    Administration, drugs
Oral replacement solutions see ORS
Organic anions 6
Organochlorines/organophosphates
    64
ORS (oral replacement solutions) 93–4
Osmotic cathartics 114
Osmotic diuretics 166–7
Ototoxicity 30
Overhydration 357–8
Ovulation, induction 177–80
    breeding season 178–9
    estrus suppression (performance
    mares) 180
    estrus synchronization 179–80
    transitional period 177–8
Oxfendazole 66
Oxibendazole 66
Oxitropium/tiotropium bromides 317
Oxpentifylline see Pentoxifylline
Oxyphenbutazone 256, 257
Oxytetracycline 38, 39, 40, 52, 62
Oxytocin
    esophageal contractility 96
    fetal effects 184
    induction of parturition 185–6
    milk letdown 187
    stimulation of myometrial
    contraction 182

P

pK_a (acidic dissociation constant) 2, 15
P-selectin 108
PABA (para-aminobenzoic acid),

antimicrobial therapy 16, 21, 35, 36
Packed cell volume see PCV
PAE (postantibiotic effect) 20, 29
Pancuronium 141
Pantoprazole 104
Para-aminobenzoic acid (PABA) see
    PABA (para-aminobenzoic acid)
Paracetamol see Acetaminophen
Parasite biology
    coccidiosis 57
    giardiasis 57
    piroplasmosis (antiprotozoal drugs)
    49–50
    sarcocystis infections 61–2
    trypanosomiasis 53
Parasiticides 63–74
    control programs 67–71, 68, 72
    ectoparasiticides 71–2
    endoparasiticides 64–71
    intestinal parasitism 70
Parenteral administration, ophthalmic
    therapeutics see Administration,
    drugs
Parenteral nutrition, fluid therapy
    344–6
Pars intermedia dysfunction see
    Pituitary/adrenal glands 79
Parturition 185–6
Parvaquone 53
Pasteurella spp., antimicrobial therapy
    24, 26, 34, 35, 43
    P. haemolytica pneumonia 323
Patches, topical application see
    Administration, drugs
Pathogenesis
    coccidiosis 57
    prioplasmosis 50
    sarcocystis infections 58, 62
    trypanosomiasis 53–4
Pathogens, antimicrobial susceptibility
    14, 227, 230
PBP (penicillin-binding proteins) 22,
    26
PCV (packed cell volume) 329, 343
PEG (polyethylene glycol) 39, 40
Penicillin G (benzylpenicillin)
    drug interactions/adverse effects
    23–4
    formulations 24
    indications 23
    pharmacokinetics 23
    procaine 22, 24
    sustained-release preparations 129
    see also Aminopenicillins
    (amoxicillin/ampicillin);
    Antimicrobial agents; Beta-
    lactam antibiotics; Extended-
    spectrum penicillins
Penicillin-binding proteins see PBP
Penicillins
    urinary tract infections 173
    see also Aminopenicillins
    (amoxicillin/ampicillin);
    Antimicrobial agents;

Benzathine benzylpenicillin;
    Beta-lactam antibiotics;
    Extended-spectrum penicillins;
    Penicillin G (benzylpenicillin);
    Procaine benzylpenicillin
Penicillium spp. 229
Pentafraction 339
Pentamidine 5–2
Pentapeptides 93
Pentastarch 338, 339
Pentazocine 261, 281
Pentoxifylline 183, 186
    see also Xanthines
Peptic injury 98
Pergolide 78–9
Perineural infiltration see
    Administration, drugs
Periocular injections see
    Administration, drugs
Peristalsis 95
Peritonitis (peritoneal inflammation)
    108, 112
Permethrin 71
Perphenazine 185
Pethidine (meperidine) 261, 277, 279
PGs (prostaglandins) analogs
PGs (prostaglandins)
    alimentary tract protection 94–5
    right dorsal colon ulceration 115
    NSAIDs 247, 248, 250, 251, 252, 253
    PGA_2 248
    PGE_1 248
    PGE_2 248, 262
    PGI_2 248, 252
    $PGF_{2\alpha}$, luteolysis 179, 180, 182
pH measurement, stomach 99, 100–1,
    101, 102, 103
Pharmacodynamics 1, 259
Pharmacokinetics 7–10
    alfentanil 279
    aminoglycoside antibiotics 29
    aminopenicillins 24–5
    angiotensin-converting enzyme
    inhibitors 212
    bethanechol 171
    bromocriptine 79
    cardiac glycosides 206
    cephalosporins 27
    chloramphenicol/florfenicol 34
    clearance 7
    compartmental/non-compartmental
    7
    cyproheptadine 79
    defined 1
    distribution volumes 8–10
    extended-spectrum penicillins 25
    flunixin meglumine 258
    fluoroquinolones 41–2
    gentamicin 32
    half-life 7–8
    horses
    indications for use 250
    side-effects in 251–4
    imipenem 28

Pharmacokinetics (*contd*)
 ketoprofen 261
 lidocaine 201
 macrolides 43
 mean residence time 8
 metronidazole 45
 model-dependent/model-
   independent 7
 nitrates 211
 NSAIDs 250–1
 ophthalmic therapeutics 221–2, 223,
   224
 penicillin G (benzylpenicillin) 23
 phenytoin 202
 procainamide 200
 propranolol 203
 quinidine 196
 ranitidine 101
 rifampin 44
 sulfonamides, potentiated 36–7
 tetracyclines 39
 vasodilators, direct acting 210
Pharmacology, defined 1
Phenamidine isoethionate 51
Phenanthridinium compounds
   (homidium chloride,
   pyrithidium bromide,
   isometamidium chloride) 56
Phenobarbital 82
Phenothiazines 271–3
 and acepromazine 138
 and behavioral disorders 151
 and bromocriptine 80
 duration of effect 273
 elimination 273
 horses, major uses in 273
 mechanism of action 271
 onset of effect 273
 pharmacological effects 271–2
 physiochemical properties 272–3
Phenylbutazone
 aminoglycoside antibiotics 30
 distribution 5
 gastrointestinal system 94, 95, 115
 NSAIDs 250, 253, 254, 255–8, 261
 sulfonamides 37–8
 thyroid gland 82
Phenylephrine 241
 vasopressors 210
Phenytoin (diphenylhydantoin) 82,
   142–4, 150, 201–2
Phosphoinositide system 268
Phospholipase 236, 247
Phospholipids 30, 98, 124
Phosphorus, electrolyte/acid-base
   disturbances 356
Pilocarpine 243
Pimaricin 230
Pimobendan 207
Piperazine 64, 67, 70
Pirbuterol acetate 313, 314
Piretanide 159
Piroplasmosis (Babesiosis)
 clinical signs 50

diagnosis 51
parasite biology 49–50
pathogenesis 50
treatment 51–3, 72
Pituitary/adrenal glands 75–80
 axis, testing 77
 corticosteroids 75–6
 ECD (Equine Cushing's Disease)
   76–80
 pars intermedia dysfunction 76,
   77, 79
PL:CG (poly(*dl*-lactide)-coglycolide)
   130
PLA (polylactic acid) 130
Placental transfer of drugs 5
Placentitis 183
Plasma 329–30, 334, 341–2
Plasma osmolality 353
Plaster of Paris (POP) 130
Platelet aggregation 248, 253–4
PMMA (polymethylmethrylate) 129
PMNs (polymorphonuclear
   leukocytes) 234, 236, 237
POI (postoperative ileus) 85, 89, 109,
   110, 111, 112
Polydipsia 168
Polyenes 230
Polyethylene glycol (PEG) 39, 40
Polylactic acid *see* PLA
Polymethylmethrylate *see* PMMA
Polymorphonuclear leukocytes *see*
   PMNs
Polysaccharide storage myopathy
   (PSSM) *see* Muscle, skeletal,
   disorders of
Polysulfated glycosaminoglycans
   (PSGAGs) 123, 125
 synthetic 235–6
Polyuria 168
Ponazuril 60, 147
Ponies 294, 332, 344
Positive inotropes 206–7
 novel 207
Postantibiotic effect (PAE) 20, 29
Postoperative ileus (POI) 85, 89, 109,
   110, 111, 112
Postpartum problems 187
Potassium, electrolyte/acid-base
   disturbances 353
Potassium bromide 150
Potassium-sparing diuretics 167–8
Potentiated sulfonamides *see*
   Sulfonamides
Praziquantel 64, 67
Prednisolone 76
 sodium succinate 148
Prednisone 122
Pregnancy (mares) 182–5
 embryonic loss, early 183
 gestation
   late, hastening of fetal maturation
     165
   prolonged 184–5
 luteal inefficiency 182–3

placentitis 183
 treatment 183–4
Prekallikrein 341
Presynaptic fibers 87
Proarrhythmias 194, 199, 200
Procainamide 200
Procaine
 Penicillin G (benzylpenicillin) 22,
   24, 38, 272, 299
Progestagen 179, 188
Prokinetic drugs 108, 109
Promazine 271, 273
Prophylaxis 26
Propofol
 duration of effect 289
 elimination 289
 guaifenesin and 290
 horses, major uses in 289–90
 mechanism of action 288
 onset 289
 pharmacological effects 288
 physiochemical properties 289
Propranolol 199, 203
Propylene glycol 40
Prostaglandin analogs *see* PGs
   (prostaglandins)
Prostaglandins (PGs) *see* PGs
   (prostaglandins)
Protein binding
 antimicrobial therapy 16
 NSAID side effects 253
 ocular tissues 222
Proteinase inhibitors 235–6
Proteoglycans 123, 254
Proteus spp.
 antimicrobial therapy
   aminoglycoside antibiotics 28, 32
   beta-lactam antibiotics 24, 26
   chloramphenicol/florfenicol
     34, 35
Proteus mirabilis 27
Pseudomonas spp.
 aminoglycoside antibiotics 30, 32,
   33
 beta-lactam antibiotics 24, 25, 26,
   28
 fluoroquinolones 40, 41
 ophthalmic therapeutics 227, 234,
   241
Pseudomonas aeruginosa 28, 180
 tetracyclines 38
PSGAGs (polysulfated
   glycosaminoglycans) 123,
   125
PSSM (polysaccharide storage
   myopathy) 137, 138
Psyllium administration 114–15
Pulmonary drug administration 4
Pulmonary excretion *see* Excretion
Purkinje cells 194, 202
Purpura hemorrhagica 76
Pyloric stenosis 107
Pyrantel 67, 70, 71
Pyrethroids 71

Pyrimethamine
  antimicrobial therapy 35, 36, 38
  antiprotozoal drugs 59–60, 62
  CNS disorders 145
  pregnancy (mares) 183
Pyrimidines 67
Pyrithidium bromide 56

Q

QRS complex
  Class Ic antiarrhythmic agents 202
  procainamide 200
  quinidine 196, 197
Quinapryamine salts 55, 73
Quinidine 195–200
  adverse reactions 196
  clinical indications 196–7, 199–200
  drug interactions 200
  gluconate 196
  pharmacokinetics 196
  sulfate 196
  therapeutic drug monitoring 196
Quinuronium sulfate 52

R

Racecadotril 93, 115
Radioopaque contrast dyes 82
Ranitidine 100, 101, 102
RBF (renal blood flow) 155, 156, 157–8
Recurrent exertional rhabdomyolysis
    (RER) see Muscle, skeletal,
    disorders
'Refeeding syndrome' 356
Regional perfusion 130
Rehydration 327, 348, 350
Remifentanil 279
Renal blood flow (RBF) see RBF (renal
    blood flow)
Renal dysfunction 155–9
  acute renal failure, effectiveness of
      drug therapy 155, 157, 158–9
  increasing blood flow 157–8
  increasing glomerular filtration rate
      158
  increasing urine output 155–7
  NSAID side effects 252–3
Renal necrosis
  papillary 252
  tubular 39
Renin-angiotensin system 212
Repellents 72
Reperfusion injury 109
Reproductive system 177–91
  mares
    infertility 180–2
    lactation 186–7
    ovulation induction 177–80
    parturition 185–6

postpartum problems 187
pregnancy 182–5
stallions
  ejaculatory dysfunction 188–9
  reproductive tract/performance
      189
  spermatogenesis 187–8
Reproductive tract see Stallions
RER (recurrent exertional
      rhabdomyolysis) see Muscle,
      skeletal, disorders
Reserpine 80, 152
Resistance
  aminoglycoside antibiotics 29
  benzimidazoles 64, 70
  beta-lactam antibiotics 22–3
  chloramphenicol/florfenicol 34
  fluoroquinolones 41
  macrolides 43
  metronidazole 45
  rifampin 44
  sulfonamides, potentiated 36
  tetracyclines 39
Respiratory system, inhalation
      therapy see Inhalation therapy
      (respiratory system)
Resuscitation, fluid therapy 327, 330,
      331, 334, 348–50
Retrobulbar injection 220
Rhabdomyolysis 137, 138, 139, 163
Rhipicephalus bursa see Ticks
Rhodococcus (R.) equi infections 21, 43,
      44, 113, 225
Rickettsia spp., antimicrobial therapy
      34, 38, 40
Rifampin 21, 44–5
Ringer's solution 331, 332
RNA (ribonucleic acid), antimicrobial
      therapy 40, 41, 44
Romifidine 268, 269, 270, 271
Ropivacaine 301
Rush, Bonnie R 311–25

S

Salicylates 94
Saline solutions
  hypertonic sodium chloride 222,
      330, 332–3
  isotonic sodium chloride 330, 331,
      332
Salmeterol 314, 315
Salmonella spp.
  antimicrobial therapy 17, 24, 26, 29,
      34, 35
  gastrointestinal drugs 92, 109, 113
Samarium-153 hydroxyapatite
      microspheres (^{153}Sm) 131
Sarcocystis spp. (Equine protozoal
      myeloencephalitis, EPM) 58–62
  clinical signs 58–9
  parasite biology 61–2

parasiticides 64
pathogenesis 58, 62
pregnancy 183
and thyroid disease 82
Sarcocystis bertrami 61
Sarcocystis equicanis 61
Sarcocystis fayeri 61, 62
Sarcocystis neurona 36, 58, 145, 146, 147
  treatment 36, 37, 38, 59–61, 145–7
SCFA (short-chain fatty acids) 86, 91,
      92
Schizogony (asexual reproductive
      cycle) 57, 58
Schott, Harold C 155–75
Scopolamine see Hyoscine
      (scopolamine)
Secretion (gastrointestinal), drugs
      affecting 92–3
Sedatives/tranquillizers 267–75
  adrenoceptor agonists (detomidine,
      romifidine, xylazine) 268–71
  benzodiazepines (diazepam,
      midazolam, zolazepam) 273–5
  phenothiazines (acepromazine)
      271–3
  skeletal muscle, affecting 138–9
  stallions 189
Seizures 149–51
Seldinger technique 346, 347
Selenium sulfide 72
Sensitivity testing see Pathogens,
      antimicrobial susceptibility
Septic shock 343
Serotonin 88, 138, 151, 152
Serratia spp. 26
Sevoflurane 293–4
Sexually transmitted infections 180
Shigella spp. 35
'Shock dose' concept, fluid therapy
      348
Short-chain fatty acids (SCFA) 86, 91,
      92
Side effects see Adverse drug
      reactions; Interactions, drug
Sinus rhythm 197
Skeletal muscle see Muscle, skeletal
Sodium, electrolyte/acid-base
      disturbances 332, 352–3
Sodium cromoglicate see Cromoglicate
Sodium hyaluronate see HA
      (Hyaluronan)
Sojka, Janice E 75–83
Somatostatin analogs 93
Spasmolytics, centrally acting 139–40
Spermatogenesis see Stallions
Spironolactone 167–8
Sporozoites 50
Stabling 72
Stallions
  reproductive system 187–9
    ejaculatory dysfunction 188–9
    reproductive tract/performance
        189
    spermatogenesis 187–8

Stanozolol 188
Staphylococci
  aminoglycoside antibiotics 32
  beta-lactam antibiotics 25, 26
  chloramphenicol/florfenicol 34
  macrolides 43
  sulfonamides 35
  tetracyclines 40
Staphylococcus aureus
  antimicrobial therapy 24, 27, 34, 41, 44
  betamethasone 124
Starling's law of the heart 194, 327
Steroids *see* Anabolic steroids;
      Corticosteroids
Stomach, drugs for 97–108
  gastric acidity 99–106
  gastric motility 107–8
  gastric mucosal protection 106–7
  pH measurement 99, 100–1, *101*, *102*, *103*
Streptococcus spp.
  antimicrobial therapy 14, 26, 30, 34, 35, 43
  and skeletal muscle 136
  Strep. equi 180
    subsp. *zooepidemicus* 187, 225
Streptomycin 28, 32
Stroke volume 205–13
  acute inotropes/vasopressors 207–10
  contractility 194
  diastolic load 194
  diuretics 210
  positive inotropes 206–7
    novel 207
  preload 194
  vasodilators 210–13
Strongyles 67
Strongyloides westeri 66
Strongylus vulgaris 63, 67, 70
Sub-Tenon's injection *see*
      Administration, drugs
Subconjunctival injections *see*
      Administration, drugs
Subcutaneous *see* Administration, drugs
Subpalpebral lavage system 219
Succinylcholine chloride *see*
      Suxamethonium
Sucralfate 106
Sulfadiazine 59–60, 145, 146, 173
Sulfadimidine 57
Sulfamethazine 57
Sulfamethoxazole 173
Sulfamethoxine 57
Sulfonamides
  combination therapy 22
  drug interactions/adverse effects 37–8
  folate supplementation 37
  formulations 38
  indications 35–6
  mechanism of action 36

NSAIDs 256
  parasiticides 72
  pharmacokinetics 36–7
  potentiated 35–8, 145, 146–7, 173
  pregnancy (mares) 183
  resistance mechanisms 36
  sarcocystis infections 36, 37, 59, 145, 146–7
  thyroid disease 82
  urinary tract infections 173
  see also Sulfadiazine, Sulfadimidine,
      Sulfamethazine,
      Sulfamethoxazole,
      Sulfamethoxine
Sulpiride 185
Suramin 55–6, 73
Surfactants 114
Surra (or murrina) 54
Sustained-release preparations 129–30
Suxamethonium 140–1
Suxibuzone 258
Sympatholytics 112
Sympathomimetics 111–12
Synovectomy, with
      radiopharmaceuticals 130–1
Synthetic polysulfated
      glycosaminoglycans *see*
      PSGAGs
Systemic inhibitors *see* Ulceration
      therapy

T

T$_3$ (triiodothyronine) 81, 82
T$_4$ (blood thyroxine) 81, 82
  Racing thoroughbreds, thyroid
      hormone concentrations 82
Tabanus spp. 49, 54
Tachyarrhythmias 202, 206
Tachycardias 203, 204, 280, 329, 358
Tapeworms 67
Taylorella equigenitalis (contagious
      equine metritis) 180
Tegaserod 90
Tenon's capsule 220
Tetanus 137
Tetracyclines 38–43
  antiprotozoal therapy 52–3
  bone, accumulation in 5
  buparvaquone 53
  combination therapy 22
  drug interactions/adverse effects 23, 39–40
  efulvane 53
  formulations 40
  indications 38
  infection site 21
  ionization of drugs 16
  mechanism of action 39
  pharmacokinetics 39
  resistance mechanisms 39
Trypan blue (red) 53

ulceration therapy (ophthalmic) 235
  urinary tract infections 173
THAM
      (hydroxymethylaminomethane)
      336
Theileria equi 50
Theophylline 168
Therapeutic drug monitoring
  cardiac glycosides 206–7
  gentamicin 33
  quinidine 196, 197
Therapeutic index 261, 320
Thiazide-type diuretics 163–5
Thiopental
  administration route 287
  bioavailability 287
  duration of effect 287
  elimination 287
  horses, major uses 287–8
  onset of effect 287
  physicochemical properties
      286–7
3-hydroxymepivacaine 300, 301
Thrombophlebitis 357
Thromboxanes (TXs) *see* TXs
      (thromboxanes)
Thyroid gland disease 80–2
  baseline hormone measurements
      81–2
  diagnosis 81–2
  metabolic syndrome 81
  treatment 82
  see also
Thyroid hormone responsive
      syndrome 81
Thyroid-releasing hormone (TRH) *see*
      TRH
Thyroid-stimulating hormone (TSH)
      see TSH
Thyroxine, blood (T$_4$) *see* T4
Tiamulin 43
Ticarcillin 25, 30
Ticarcillin-clavulanic acid 128
Ticks 49, 50
  Boophilus microplus 50
  Dermacenter marginatus and
      reticulatus 49
  Dermacenter nitens 49
  Hyalomma spp. 49
  Rhipicephalus bursa 49
Tiletamine 273, 282, 284, 285
Tilmicosin 43
TIMPs (tissue inhibitors) 234
Tiotropium bromide 317
Tissue plasminogen activator (tPA)
      220, 242
TIVA (total i.v. anesthetic) techniques
      283, 284, 289
TNF (tumor necrosis factor) 183
Tobramycin 28, 33, 129
Tocainide 202
Tolazoline 271
Toltrazuril 60–1, 72, 147
Tolypocladium inflatum 239

Topically applied drugs *see* Administration, drugs
Torasemide 159
Torsades de pointes 204–5
Torulopsis spp. 229
Total i.v. anesthetic (TIVA) techniques *see* TIVA techniques
Total parenteral nutrition (TPN) *see* TPN
Toxicity
  antimicrobial therapy 17
    see also Adverse drug reactions; Interactions, drug
  and enterotoxigenic bacteria 93
  and nephrotoxicity 30, 31
  and ototoxicity 30, 31
  see also Fescue toxicosis
Toxicology, defined 1
TPA (tissue plasminogen activator) 220, 242
TPN (total parenteral nutrition) 334, 345, 346
Tranquillizers *see* Sedatives/tranquillizers
Transcellular compartments 5
TRH (thyroid-releasing hormone) 76, 80
Triamcinolone 124, 319
Triamterene 167
Triazinones, symmetrical (ponazuril, toltrazuril) 60–1, 145, 147
Trichlormethiazide
  and dexamethasone 165
Trichomonas vaginalis 61
Trifluridine 233
Triiodothyronine (T$_3$) *see* T3
Trimethoprim
  antimicrobial therapy 35, 36, 37
  antiprotozoal drugs 59, 60
  CNS disorders 146
Trimethoprim–sulfamethoxazole 129, 183
  see also Sulfonamides, potentiated
Tromethamine 336
Tropicamide 240
Tricyclic antidepressants 151, 189
Trypan blue (red) 53
Trypanocidal drugs 73
Trypanosomes (Trypanosoma spp.) 53
  T. brucei 51, 53, 55, 56, 73
  T. congolense 51, 54, 55, 56, 57, 73
  T. equiperdum 53, 54, 55, 57
  T. evansi 52, 54, 55, 57, 73
  T. vivax 51, 54, 55, 56, 57, 73
Trypanosomiasis 53–7
  clinical signs 53–4
  diagnosis 54–5
  parasite biology 53
  pathogenesis 53–4
  prophylaxis recommendations 56–7
  treatment 55–7
Tsetse flies 53

TSH (thyroid-stimulating hormone) 76, 81
Tuberoinfundibular system 79
TXs (thromboxanes) 247, 248, 254
  TXA$_2$ 248
Tylosin 43

U

Ulcerative keratitis *see* Keratitis
Ulcer
  gastric 102, 105
  therapy (ophthalmic) 234–6
    heparin 235
    ilomastat (GM 60001) 235
    polysulfated glycosaminoglycans (PSGAGs), synthetic 235–6
    proteinase inhibitors 235–6
    systemic inhibitors 235
Ultrasonic nebulization *see* Nebulization, ultrasonic
Urea compounds, complex (amicarbalide, imidocarb dipropronate, quinuronium sulfate), piroplasmosis treatment 52
Urinary excretion *see* Excretion (elimination of drugs)
Urinary system 155–75
  antidiuretic agents 168–9
  diuretic agents 159–68
  renal dysfunction 155–9
  urine retention/incontinence 169–72
  UTIs (urinary tract infections) 172–4
Urinary tract infections (UTIs) *see* Urinary system
Urine
  acidifying agents 172
  retention 169–72
  specific gravity 329
Urolithiasis 172
UTIs (urinary tract infections) *see* Urinary system
Uveitis, acute interior 237

V

Vancomycin 45–6, 129
  resistant enterococci (VRE) *see* VRE
Vasodilators 210–13
  direct acting 210–11
  indirectly acting 212
Vasopressors 207–10
  dobutamine 208–9
  dopamine 207–8

dopexamine 208
milrinone 210
norepinephrine (noradrenaline) 209–10
phenylephrine 210
V$_c$ (volume of central compartment) 9
V$_d$ (apparent volume of distribution)
  calculation of drug dosage 20
  drug ionization 16
  principles 8, 9
V$_{dss}$, apparent volume of distribution at steady state 9
Vecuronium 141
Vedaprofen 262
Ventricular fibrillation 203, 204
Venturi effect 312
Verapamil 204
Viscoelastic materials (ophthalmic) 242
Vitamin K antagonism 27
Vivrette, Sally 177–91
Volume of distribution *see* Vd and Distribution volumes (pharmacokinetics)
VRE (vancomycin-resistant enterococci) 45

W

Warfarin 5, 256

X

Xanthines (alkylxanthines) 43, 168
  see also Pentoxifylline; Theophylline
Xylazine
  dissociative anesthetics 285
  esophageal obstruction 95
  gastric motility 107–8
  intestinal motility 111
  opioid analgesics 278, 281
  sedative/tranquillizers 269, 270, 271

Y

Yarbrough, Tom 121–34
Yohimbine 112, 271

Z

Zolazepam 273, 282, 284, 285

Printed in the United States
By Bookmasters